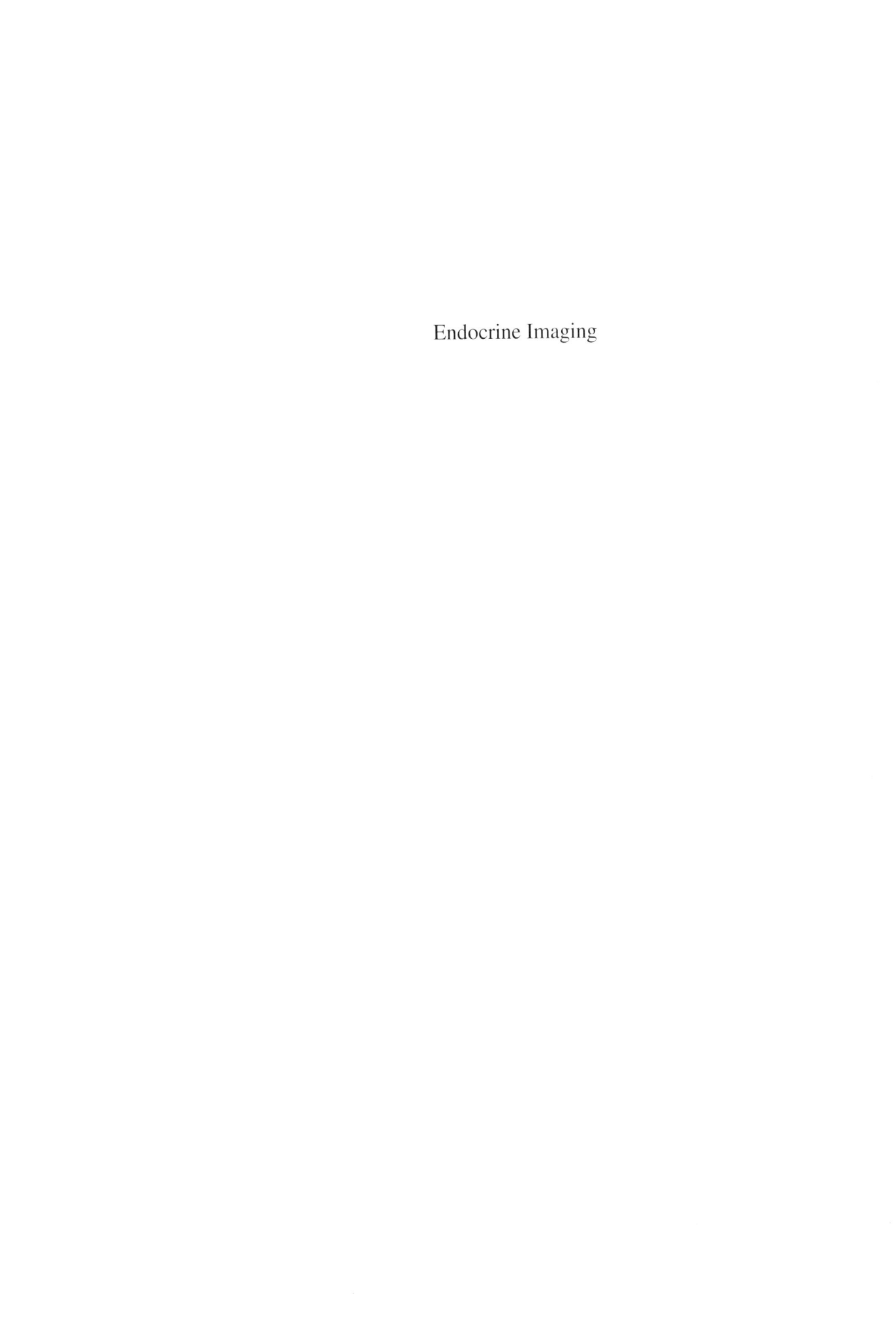

Endocrine Imaging

Endocrine Imaging

Textbook and Atlas

Edited by C. B. Higgins and W. Auffermann

with contributions by:

L. Abet	K.-J. Gräf	S. Majumdar	W. Schörner
A. M. Aisen	S. Grampp	H. P. Molsen	P. Schubeus
G. Albertini Petroni	S. Gust	L. Moltz	R. Sörensen
W. Auffermann	R. A. Halvorsen	C. Muhr	J. Spiteri-Grech
G. Barzen	C. B. Higgins	R. Nagel	D. D. Stark
H. E. Bechtel	N. Hosten	G. Natali	J. Staudt
M. Bezzi	H. Hricak	F. Neumann	P. Steiger
L. Broglia	M. Jergas	K. Öberg	T. Steinmüller
G. P. Cardone	Y. S. Kang	F. Orsi	S. K. Stevens
C. Catalano	A. Kern	R. Passariello	E. Sugimoto
K. J. Cho	U. Keske	P. Pavone	P. Vassallo
O. H. Clark	B. P. Kreft	M. J. Popovich	C. Zwicker
M. Di Girolamo	P. Lang	P. Ricci	
I. R. Francis	M. Langer	H.-D. Röher	
R. Friedrichs	R. Langer	K. Rosenkranz	
H. K. Genant	W. R. Lanksch	M. Rossi	
C. Glüer	L.-E. Lörelius	P. Rossi	
G. A. W. Gooding	A. Lunderquist	F. M. Salvatori	

Forewords by A. R. Margulis and H.-K. Beyer

619 illustrations

1994
Georg Thieme Verlag
Stuttgart · New York

Thieme Medical Publishers, Inc.
New York

Library of Congress Cataloging-in-Publication Data

Endocrine imaging : textbook and atlas / edited by
  C. B. Higgins and W. Auffermann ; with contributions by
  L. Abet . . . [et al.] ; forewords by A. R. Margulis and
  H.-K. Beyer.
    p.   cm.
  Includes bibliographical references and index.
  ISBN 3-13-116001-2. -- ISBN 0-86577-512-5
  1. Endocrine glands -- Imaging. 2. Endocrine glands –
  Imaging-Atlases. I. Higgins. Charles B. II.
  Auffermann, W. (Wolfgang)
  [DNLM: 1. Endocrine Diseases – diagnosis.
  2. Endocrine Glands-pathology. 3. Diagnostic Imaging.
  WK 100 E51288 1993]
RC649.E5163 1993
616.4'0754–dc20
DNLM/DLC
for Library of Congress   93-38768
                                                      CIP

Cover drawing by Renate Stockinger

Important Note: Medicine is an ever-changing science undergoing continual development. Research and clinical experience are continually expanding our knowledge, in particular our knowledge of proper treatment and drug therapy. Insofar as this book mentions any dosage or application, readers may rest assured that the authors, editors and publishers have made every effort to ensure that such references are in accordance with the state of knowledge at the time of production of the book.

Nevertheless this does not involve, imply, or express any guarantee or responsibility on the part of the publishers in respect of any dosage instructions and forms of application stated in the book. Every user is requested to examine carefully the manufacturers' leaflets accompanying each drug and to check, if necessary in consultation with a physician or specialist, whether the dosage schedules mentioned therein or the contraindications stated by the manufacturers differ from the statements made in the present book. Such examination is particularly important with drugs that are either rarely used or have been newly released on the market. Every dosage schedule or every form of application used is entirely at the user's own risk and responsibility. The authors and publishers request every user to report to the publishers any discrepancies or inaccuracies noticed.

Some of the product names, patents and registered designs referred to in this book are in fact registered trademarks or proprietary names even though specific reference to this fact is not always made in the text. Therefore, the appearance of a name without designation as proprietary is not to be construed as a representation by the publisher that it is in the public domain.
This book, including all parts thereof, is legally protected by copyright. Any use, exploitation or commercialization outside the narrow limits set by copyright legislation, without the publisher's consent, is illegal and liable to prosecution. This applies in particular to photostat reproduction, copying, mimeographing or duplication of any kind, translating, preparation of microfilms, and electronic data processing and storage.

© 1994 Georg Thieme Verlag,
Rüdigerstraße 14, D-70469 Stuttgart, Germany
Thieme Medical Publishers, Inc., 381 Park Avenue South,
New York, NY 10016

Typesetting by Druckhaus Götz GmbH,
D-71636 Ludwigsburg
System CCS Textline (Linotronic 630)

Printed in Germany by K. Grammlich GmbH

ISBN 3-13-116001-2 (GTV, Stuttgart)
ISBN 0-86577-512-5 (TMP, New York)   1 2 3 4 5 6

Forewords

Rarely has a book dedicated to the imaging of an organ system achieved in its first edition the high quality of this multi-authored text. The rigorous attention to detail and the encyclopedic breadth covering the anatomy, endocrinology, and imaging techniques are given further depth by adding the overview from the standpoint of the radiologist and, whenever indicated, by the surgeon. In addition to the imaging of the normal and diseased endocrine organs, namely the pituitary, thyroid, parathyroids, adrenals, endocrine pancreas, testes, and ovaries, the editors have concisely yet clearly described the basic modern imaging techniques employed. The idea of including the tumors of the enterochromaffin cells, carcinoid, which are similar to apudomas, is an example of broad vision and contributes to the completeness of this book. The imaginative expansion to the quantification of osteoporosis, which is a clinically most important consequence of menopause, and Positron Emmission Tomography (PET), which is assuming increasing value in imaging receptors and metabolic mapping, significantly adds to the value of this book.

The high quality of this text, the wealth of important, relevant, and up-to-date references, the clarity of appropriate drawings, and the excellence of illustrations reflect the choice of contributors who are leaders in their field. The many authors from Germany, Italy, Sweden, the United States, and Japan, as well as the editors who selected them and conceived and organized this work, can be proud of their achievement.

Alexander R. Margulis, M.D.
Vice-Chancellor
Medical School
University of California, San Francisco

The manifold diseases of the endocrine organs feature prominently in general medical diagnostics. Credit goes to the authors for having tackled the often complicated and highly differentiated pattern of diagnostic problems. This book meets a need for a comprehensive presentation, which has so far been lacking in available textbooks. The authors have succeeded admirably in presenting the various current diagnostic imaging methods for the multifarious endocrine diseases with valuable pointers as to ranking and reliability.

The target group aimed at by the authors is surely a mixed one. The book appeals both to radiologists and to endocrinologists as well as to gynecologists and surgeons—all of whom are supplied with an efficient guide to a complex discipline. The requirements of and relations to medical practice are always preeminent.

The dramatic upswing in imaging, which has resulted in a multitude of diagnostic possibilities, makes it imperative to be discriminating in selecting the most rational diagnostic procedures. Here, too, the authors give valuable advice.

Another attractive feature of the book is the impressive array of competent and renowned authors. The editors deserve to be congratulated for having succeeded in enlisting their help.

Professor Dr. med. H.-K. Beyer
Chairman
Department of Radiology
University of Bochum
Germany

Preface

Endocrine Imaging aims to be a comprehensive textbook that covers the clinical features and imaging characteristics of diseases of the endocrine organs with contributions from the most advanced and experienced authors in this field from Europe and the United States. The book comprises a wide variety of techniques, from the conventional X-ray to X-ray angiography, venous sampling, computed tomography, nuclear medicine, positron emission tomography, ultrasound, and magnetic resonance imaging. Interventional procedures are also mentioned where they are appropriate.

The diagnosis of endocrine disease requires a complex morphologic, functional, and metabolic approach, which cannot be covered either by a single technique or by an individual specialist. Imaging is an ever-growing component in this field because the development of a more targeted, integrated pharmacologic and surgical approach requires exact demonstration of small morphologic structures related to specific functional issues. Moreover, the arsenal of current imaging techniques offers an ever increasing opportunity not only to give a morphologic diagnosis, but to obtain comprehensive anatomic, physiologic, and biochemical information.

For most radiologists, an encounter with a diagnostic problem related to endocrine disease is relatively infrequent. An enigma in selecting or advising the optimal imaging study may arise because of the ever-changing capabilities of the various imaging modalities. With this in mind, the current volume describes the application of the appropriate techniques by radiologists with considerable experience. In addition an overview of the topic is provided by a clinician or surgeon in order to distill the relative clinical value and practical effectiveness of the proposed diagnostic approaches.

Endocrine Imaging is directed to a wide variety of physicians in many disciplines as well as to medical students. Practicing radiologists may find it useful as a reference guide for the diagnostic evaluation of endocrine disease. The book is also intended to serve as a guide to clinicians seeking the optimal imaging approach for their patients with suspected endocrine abnormalities. Experienced clinicians from internal medicine, surgery, and urology have contributed their practical views on the clinical impact of imaging on their disciplines.

We gratefully acknowledge all the authors from Ann Arbor, Berlin, Bonn, Boston, Düsseldorf, Hamburg, Lund, New York, Rome, San Francisco, and Uppsala for contributing their expertise in the preparation of this book. We have been fortunate to work with Achim Menge, Harlich Kübler, Monique Scheer, and Helmut Schäfer at Thieme Verlag and thank them for their invaluable advice, constructive criticism, and contributions in the field of publishing arts.

Autumn 1993

Charles B. Higgins, San Francisco
Wolfgang Auffermann, Hamburg

Addresses

PD Dr. med. L. Abet
Radiologische Abteilung
Ev.-Freikirchliches Krankenhaus Rüdersdorf
Waldstraße
15562 Rüdersdorf
Germany

A. M. Aisen, M. D.
Associate Professor of Radiology
Co-Director of Magnetic Resonance Imaging
Department of Radiology, Box 30
University of Michigan Hospitals
University of Michigan School of Medicine
1500 E. Medical Center Drive
Ann Arbor, MI 48109-0030
USA

G. Albertini Petroni, M. D.
Department of Radiology
University of Rome "La Sapienza"
Policlinico Umberto I
Viale Regina Elena 325
00161 Rome
Italy

Dr. med. W. Auffermann
Praxisklinik Bergedorf
Radiologie und Nuklearmedizin
Alte Holstenstraße 16
21031 Hamburg
Germany

Dr. med. G. Barzen
Grafenberger Allee 84
40237 Düsseldorf
Germany

Dr. med. H. E. Bechtel
Medizinische Klinik
Universitätsklinikum Rudolf Virchow
Spandauer Damm 130
14050 Berlin
Germany

M. Bezzi, M. D.
Department of Radiology
University of Rome "La Sapienza"
Policlinico Umberto I
Viale Regina Elena 325
00161 Rome
Italy

L. Broglia, M. D.
Department of Radiology
University of Rome "La Sapienza"
00161 Rome
Italy

G. P. Cardone, M. D.
Department of Radiology
Ospedale Riuniti of Livorno
Livorno
Italy

C. Catalano, M. D.
Department of Radiology
University of Rome "La Sapienza"
Policlinico Umberto I
Viale Regina Elena 325
00161 Rome
Italy

K. J. Cho, M. D.
Professor of Radiology and
Director of Division of Cardiovascular and
Interventional Radiology
Department of Radiology
University of Michigan Hospitals
1500 E. Medical Center Drive
Ann Arbor, MI 48109
USA

O. H. Clark, M. D.
Professor and Chief of Surgery
University of California San Francisco
Mount Zion Hospital
1600 Divisadero Street
San Francisco, CA 94115
USA

M. Di Girolamo, M. D.
Department of Radiology
University of Rome "La Sapienza"
Policlinico Umberto I
Viale Regina Elena 325
00161 Rome
Italy

I. R. Francis, M. D.
Professor of Radiology
Department of Radiology
University of Michigan Hospitals
University of Michigan School of Medicine
1500 E. Medical Center Drive
Ann Arbor, MI 48109-0030
USA

Dr. med. R. Friedrichs
Urologische Klinik der Freien Universität Berlin
Universitätsklinikum Rudolf Virchow
Augustenburger Platz 1
13344 Berlin
Germany

H. K. Genant, M. D.
Professor of Radiology, Medicine,
and Orthopedic Surgery
Chief, Skeletal Section
Department of Radiology
Director, Osteoporosis Research Group
University of California San Francisco
Parnassus Avenue
San Francisco, CA 94143
USA

C. Glüer, Ph. D.
Adjunct Assistant Professor of Radiology
Department of Radiology
Associate Director, Osteoporosis Research Group
University of California San Francisco
Parnassus Avenue
San Francisco, CA 94143
USA

G. A. W. Gooding, M. D.
Professor and Vice Chairman
Department of Radiology
University of California San Francisco
Veterans Administration Medical Center
4150 Clement Street
San Francisco, CA 94121
USA

PD Dr. med. K.-J. Gräf
Abteilung Innere Medizin und Poliklinik
Freie Universität Berlin
Universitätsklinikum Rudolf Virchow
Spandauer Damm 130
14050 Berlin
Germany

S. Grampp, M. D.
Research Associate
Department of Radiology
University of California San Francisco
Parnassus Avenue
San Francisco, CA 94143
USA

Dr. med. S. Gust
Radiologie und Nuklearmedizin
Praxisklinik Bergedorf
21031 Hamburg
Germany

R. A. Halvorsen, Jr., M. D.
Professor of Radiology
University of California, San Francisco
Chief, Department of Radiology
San Francisco General Hospital
1001 Potrero Avenue
San Francisco, CA 94110
USA

C. B. Higgins, M. D.
Professor of Radiology and Chief of Magnetic
Resonance
Department of Radiology
University of California San Francisco
Parnassus Avenue
San Francisco, CA 94143
USA

Dr. med. N. Hosten
Strahlenklinik und Poliklinik (Radiology)
Universitätsklinikum Rudolf Virchow
Augustenburger Platz 1
13353 Berlin
Germany

H. Hricak, M. D., Ph. D.
Professor of Radiology, Urology,
and Radiation Oncology
Department of Radiology
University of California San Francisco
Parnassus Avenue
San Francisco, CA 94143
USA

M. Jergas, M. D.
Research Associate
Department of Radiology
University of California San Francisco
Parnassus Avenue
San Francisco, CA 94143
USA

Y. S. Kang, M. D.
Department of Radiology
University of California, San Francisco
Parnassus Avenue
San Francisco, CA 94143
USA

Dr. med. A. Kern
Strahlenklinik und Poliklinik (Radiology)
Universitätsklinikum Rudolf Virchow
Spandauer Damm 130
14050 Berlin
Germany

Dr. med. U. Keske
Strahlenklinik (Radiology)
Universitätsklinikum Rudolf Virchow
Augustenburger Platz 1
13353 Berlin
Germany

Dr. med. B. P. Kreft
Department of Radiology
Universität Bonn
Sigmund-Freud-Straße 25
53127 Bonn
Germany

Dr. med. P. Lang
Department of Radiology
University of California San Francisco
Parnassus Avenue
San Francisco, CA 94143
USA

Prof. Dr. med. M. Langer
Head, Division of Radiologic Diagnostics
Radiologische Klinik
Hugstetterstr. 55
79106 Freiburg
Germany

Prof. Dr. med. R. Langer
Strahlenklinik (Radiology)
Universitätsklinikum Rudolf Virchow
Augustenburger Platz 1
13353 Berlin
Germany

Prof. Dr. med. W. R. Lanksch
Chairman
Abteilung für Neurochirurgie (Neurosurgery)
Universitätsklinikum Rudolf Virchow
Augustenburger Platz 1
13344 Berlin
Germany

L.-E. Lörelius, M. D., Ph. D.
Department of Diagnostic Radiology
University Hospital, Uppsala
Akademiska Sjukhoset
75185 Uppsala
Sweden

A. Lunderquist, M. D.
Professor of Radiology
Svenska vägen 48
22639 Lund
Sweden

S. Majumdar, Ph. D.
Assistant Professor of Radiology
Department of Radiology
University of California San Francisco
Parnassus Avenue
San Francisco, CA 94143
USA

PD Dr. med. H. P. Molsen
Strahlenklinik (Radiology)
Universitätsklinikum Rudolf Virchow
Augustenburger Platz 1
13353 Berlin
Germany

Prof. Dr. med. L. Moltz
Institut für Gynäkologische Endokrinologie,
Fertilität und Familienplanung
Knesebeckstraße 35
10623 Berlin
Germany

C. Muhr, M. D.
Professor of Neurology
Department of Neurology
Uppsala University
Akademiska Sjukhuset
75185 Uppsala
Sweden

Prof. Dr. med. R. Nagel
Direktor
Urologische Klinik und Poliklinik
Universitätsklinikum Rudolf Virchow
Augustenburger Platz 1
13353 Berlin
Germany

G. Natali, M. D.
Department of Radiology
University of Rome "La Sapienza"
00161 Rome
Italy

Prof. Dr. med. F. Neumann
Schering AG
Müllerstraße 178
13342 Berlin
Germany

K. Öberg, M. D., Ph. D.
Associate Professor
Head, Endocrine Unit
Department of Internal Medicine
Akademiska Sjukhuset
75185 Uppsala
Sweden

F. Orsi, M. D.
Department of Radiology
University of Rome "La Sapienza"
00161 Rome
Italy

R. Passariello, M. D.
Professor of Radiology & Director
Department of Radiology
University of Rome "La Sapienza"
Policlinico Umberto I
Viale Regina Elena 325
00161 Rome
Italy

P. Pavone, M. D.
Department of Radiology
University of Rome "La Sapienza"
Policlinico Umberto I
Viale Regina Elena 325
00161 Rome
Italy

M. J. Popovich, M. D.
Department of Radiology
University of California San Francisco
Parnassus Avenue
San Francisco, CA 94143
USA

P. Ricci, M. D.
Department of Radiology
University of Rome "La Sapienza"
00161 Rome
Italy

Prof. Dr. med. H.-D. Röher
Direktor
Chirurgische Klinik und Poliklinik (Surgery)
Heinrich-Heine-Universität Düsseldorf
Moorenstraße 5
40225 Düsseldorf
Germany

Dr. med. K. Rosenkranz
Strahlenklinik und Poliklinik (Radiology)
Universitätsklinikum Rudolf Virchow
Augustenburger Platz 1
13353 Berlin
Germany

M. Rossi, M. D.
Department of Radiology
University of Rome "La Sapienza"
Policlinico Umberto I
00161 Rome
Italy

P. Rossi, M. D.
Professor of Radiology & Director
Department of Radiology
Quarta Cattedra
University of Rome "La Sapienza"
Policlinico Umberto I
00161 Rome
Italy

F. M. Salvatori, M. D.
Department of Radiology
University of Rome "La Sapienza"
00161 Rome
Italy

Prof. Dr. med. W. Schörner
Radiologische Klinik
Klinikum Braunschweig
38126 Braunschweig
Germany

Dr. med. P. Schubeus
Strahlenklinik und Poliklinik (Radiology)
Universitätsklinikum Rudolf Virchow
Augustenburger Platz 1
13353 Berlin
Germany

PD Dr. med. R. Sörensen
Strahlenklinik und Poliklinik (Radiology)
Universitätsklinikum Rudolf Virchow
Augustenburger Platz 1
13353 Berlin
Germany

J. Spiteri-Grech M. D., Ph. D.
The Population Council and Rockefeller University
1230 York Avenue
New York NY 10021
USA

D. D. Stark, M. D.
Professor of Radiology
Department of Radiology
Massachusetts General Hospital
Harvard Medical School
32 Fruit Street
Boston, MA 02114
USA

Prof. Dr. med. J. Staudt
Direktor
Institut für Anatomie
Universitätsklinikum Charité
Medizinische Fakultät der Humboldt-Universität
zu Berlin
Schumannstraße 20/21
10098 Berlin
Germany

P. Steiger, Ph. D.
Adjunct Assistant Professor of Radiology
Senior Scientist, Hologic Inc., Waltham, MA
Department of Radiology
University of California San Francisco
Parnassus Avenue
San Francisco, CA 94143
USA

Dr. med. T. Steinmüller
Chirurgische Klinik (Surgery)
Universitätsklinikum Rudolf Virchow
Augustenburger Platz 1
13353 Berlin
Germany

S. K. Stevens, M. D.
Department of Radiology
University of California San Francisco
Parnassus Avenue
San Francisco, CA 94143
USA

E. Sugimoto, M. D.
Department of Radiology
Saitama Medical School
38-Morogongo
Moroyama, Iruma-gun
Saitama 350-04
Japan

P. Vassallo, M. D., Ph. D.
Department of Radiology
Memorial Sloan-Kettering Cancer Center
1275 York Avenue
New York NY 10021
USA

PD Dr. med. C. Zwicker
Virchowstraße 12
78224 Singen
Germany

Contents

1 Technique ... 1

Computed Tomography ... 1
C. Zwicker

MR Imaging ... 1
W. Auffermann

Digital Subtraction Angiography ... 3
R. Langer, and M. Langer

Nuclear Imaging ... 4
U. Keske

Imaging Devices ... 4
Imaging Methods ... 5
Radioisotopes ... 5
Radiopharmaceuticals ... 5
References ... 5

2 Pituitary ... 7

Anatomy ... 7
J. Staudt

Endocrinology ... 9
K.-J. Gräf

Physiology ... 9
Endocrine Disorders ... 10
    Pituitary Insufficiency ... 10
    Pituitary Adenomas ... 11
    Diseases of the Posterior Pituitary ... 16
References ... 16

Radiography ... 16
W. Auffermann, and S. Gust

Technique ... 16
Normal Sella ... 16
Pathological Findings ... 17
References ... 18

Computed Tomography ... 18
A. Kern, and U. Keske

Normal Findings ... 20
    Transverse Plane ... 20
    Coronal Plane ... 22
Pathology ... 22
Outlook ... 26
References ... 27

MR Imaging ... 27
P. Schubeus, and W. Schörner

Technique ... 27
Normal Anatomy ... 28
Pituitary Adenomas ... 30
Differential Diagnosis ... 33
    Empty Sella ... 33
    Cysts ... 33
    Craniopharyngeomas ... 33
    Meningiomas ... 35
    Gliomas of the Optic Nerve ... 35
    Aneurysms ... 35
    Rare Causes of Pituitary Disturbance ... 35
References ... 35

Angiography ... 35
H. P. Molsen

Technique ... 35
Normal Findings ... 36
Pathological Findings ... 36
References ... 39

A Radiologist's View ... 40
W. Auffermann

Adenoma ... 40
Meningioma ... 41
Craniopharyngeoma ... 41

Aneurysm	41
Other Lesions	41
References	41

A Surgeon's View	41
W. R. Lanksch	

3 Thyroid Gland 43

Anatomy 43
J. Staudt

Endocrinology 46
K.-J. Gräf

Physiology	46
Examination Methods	46
Diseases of the Thyroid	46
Goiter	46
Inflammations of the Thyroid	47
Hyperthyroidism	47
Hypothyroidism	49

Ultrasound 50
K. Rosenkranz

Method	50
Normal Findings	51
Pathological Findings	51
Diffuse Thyroid Diseases	51
Nodular Thyroid Diseases	51
References	54

Computed Tomography 55
C. Zwicker

Technique	55
Normal Anatomy	55
Pathological Changes	55
Summary	56
References	56

MR Imaging 57
W. Auffermann, and C. B. Higgins

Technique	57
Normal Thyroid	58
Pathological Findings	59
Goiter	59
Graves Disease	60
Thyroiditis	61
Adenoma	61

Cysts or Cystic Degeneration	63
Carcinoma	63
References	68

Nuclear Medicine 69
U. Keske

Method	69
Radiopharmaceuticals	69
Thyroid Scintigraphy	69
Thyroid Uptake	69
Special Tests	70
Scintigraphic Findings	70
Normal Findings	70
Goiter	70
Thyroid Nodules	71
Graves Disease	73
Thyroiditis	73
Ectopic Thyroid	74
Whole Body Scintigraphy in Thyroid Carcinoma	74
Method	74
Scintigraphic Findings	75
Medullary Carcinoma	75
References	76

Diagnostic Imaging in Graves Ophthalmopathy 76
N. Hosten

Clinical Presentation and Pathophysiology	76
Examination Technique and Diagnostic Criteria	77
Differential Diagnosis	78
References	81

A Surgeon's View 81
T. Steinmüller

Multinodular Goiter	81
Hyperthyroidism	81
Malignancies	82
References	83

4 Parathyroid Gland 85

Anatomy 85
J. Staudt

Endocrinology 85
K.-J. Gräf

Physiology	85
Hypoparathyroidism	85
Hyperparathyroidism	85

Ultrasound 86
G. A. W. Gooding

Ultrasound Imaging Technique 86
Normal Findings 87
Pathologic Findings 87
   Parathyroid Cysts 89
   Pitfalls 89
   Clinical Setting 90
   Variants 91
   Secondary Hyperparathyroidism 91
   Familial Hyperparathyroidism 91
   Multiple Endocrine Neoplasia (MEN) 91
   Risk Factors 92
   Parathyroid Biopsy 92
   Parathyroid Variants 93
   Parathyroid Hyperplasia 94
   Parathyroid Cancer 94
   Treatment 95
   Future Considerations 96
Perspectives in Imaging 96
References 97

Computed Tomography 98
B. P. Kreft, and D. D. Stark

Technique 99
Normal Anatomy 100
Pathology 100
   Parathyroid Hyperplasia 100
   Parathyroid Adenoma 101
   Ectopic Parathyroid Adenomas 101
   Persistent or Recurrent
   Hyperparathyroidism 102
   Parathyroid Carcinoma 103
Summary 103
References 103

MR Imaging 104
C. B. Higgins, and W. Auffermann

Technique 104
Anatomy 104
Hyperparathyroidism 105
   Preoperative Localization of Abnormal
   Parathyroid Glands 106

Imaging Characteristics of Parathyroid
   Disorders 106
Pitfalls in the Detection of Abnormal
   Parathyroid Glands by MRI 109
MR Contrast Media: Effect on Signal
   Intensity of Abnormal Parathyroid Glands .. 111
Results Using MRI for Preoperative
   Localization in Recurrent or Persistent
   Hyperparathyroidism 111
Comparison of Diagnostic Techniques in
   Hyperparathyroidism 112
References 112

Angiography and Venous Sampling 113
R. Sörensen

Parathyroid Veins 113
Autotransplanted Parathyroid Tissue 117
Venous Sampling Technique 117
Road-mapping of Sampling 118
Sampling Results 119
Parathyroid Arteries 120
Intra-arterial Digital Subtraction Angiography .. 121
Complications 121
Treatment 122
References 122

Nuclear Medicine 123
U. Keske

Imaging Technique 123
Scintigraphic Findings 124
References 125

A Radiologist's View 125
W. Auffermann

Recurrent or Persistent Hyperparathyroidism 125
Ectopic Adenomas 125
References 126

A Surgeon's View 127
O. H. Clark

References 128

5 Adrenal Gland 129

Anatomy 129
J. Staudt

Endocrinology 131
K.-J. Gräf

Physiology 131
Hyperaldosteronism 131
Hypoaldosteronism 132

Hypercortisolism (Cushing Syndrome) 132
Hypocortisolism 132
Congenital Adrenal Hyperplasia (CAH) 133
Adrenocortical Tumors 134
Hypertrichosis and Hirsutism 134
Adrenal Medulla 134
   Pheochromocytoma 134

Ultrasound 135
L. Abet

Investigative Technique 135
Normal Findings 135
Pathology 135
Summary 142

Computed Tomography 142
C. Zwicker

Technique 142
Anatomy 142
Pathology 142
   Tumors of the Adrenal Cortex 142
   Carcinoma 143
   Adrenal Hyperplasia 143
   Tumors of the Adrenal Medulla 143
   Other Tumors 144
Summary 145
References 146

MR Imaging 146
I. R. Francis, and A. M. Aisen

Techniques 146
Normal Glands 147
   Anatomy 147
   MR Appearance 147
Nonfunctioning Tumors 147
   Adrenal Cysts 147
   Adrenal Myelolipomas 147
   Hematomas 147
Hyperfunctioning Adrenal Tumors 148
   Adrenal Cortical Hyperfunction 148
Adrenal Cortical Carcinoma 149
   Adrenal Medullary Hyperfunction 150
   Adenomas or Metastasis 153
Conclusion 156
References 158

Angiography 159
K. J. Cho

Vascular Anatomy 159
Technique 159
Hypercorticoidism 161

Primary aldosteronism 162
Adrenal Cortical Carcinoma 163
Pheochromocytomas 164
Conclusion 168
References 168

Nuclear Medicine 169
G. Barzen

Principles of Scintigraphic Imaging of the
Adrenal Cortex 169
   Technique 169
   Normal Distribution 170
   Pathological Findings 170
Principles of Scintigraphic Imaging of the
Adrenal Medulla 171
   Technique 172
   Normal Distribution 173
   Pathological Findings 174
   Typical Findings 175
Principles of Receptor Imaging of the Adrenal
Gland 175
   Technique 176
   Normal Distribution 176
   Pathological Findings 177
References 177

A Radiologist's View 177
W. Auffermann

   Hyperplastic Glands 177
   Adenoma 177
   Hemorrhage 177
   Calcification 178
   Myelolipoma 178
   Cyst 178
   Carcinoma 178
   Metastasis 178
   Pheochromocytoma 178
References 178

A Surgeon's View 178
H.-D. Röher

Localization and Diagnosis of Adrenal Tumors . 178
References 179

6 Pancreas 180

Anatomy 180
J. Staudt

Endocrinology 180
R. A. Halvorsen Jr.

Computed Tomography 182
*M. Bezzi, F. Orsi, P. Ricci, F. M. Salvatori,
L. Broglia, P. Rossi*

Technique 182
Normal Findings 183
Pathological Findings 184
Diagnostic Accuracy 188
   Insulinoma 188
   Gastrinoma 188
Interpreting the International Literature on the
Localization of Endocrine Pancreatic Tumors .. 188
References 189

MR Imaging 190
P. Pavone, M. Di Girolamo, G. Cardone, C. Catalano,
G. Albertini Petroni, and R. Passariello

MRI of the Pancreas: Method of Study 190
Normal Findings 191
Pathological Findings 191
Conclusions 194
References 194

Angiography 194
M. Bezzi, F. M. Salvatori, F. Orsi, M. Rossi,
G. Natali, and P. Rossi

Technique 194
Normal and Pathological Findings 195
   Diagnostic Accuracy 201
Transhepatic Portal Venous Sampling (PVS) ... 202
Intra-arterial Stimulation Test (IAS) 202
References 205

A Radiologist's View 206
R. A. Halvorsen Jr.

Imaging Techniques 206
   Sonography 206
   Computed Tomography 206
   Magnetic Resonance Imaging 206
   Arteriography 206
   Transhepatic Percutaneous Portal Venous
   Sampling 206
   Intraoperative Ultrasound 207
Insulinoma 207
Gastrinoma 207
Summary 208
References 208

A Surgeon's View 209
H.-D. Röher

References 210

7 Carcinoid 211

Anatomy 211
J. Staudt

Endocrinology 211
H. E. Bechtel

Carcinoid Tumors 211
   Carcinoid Syndrome 212
   Diagnosis 212
References 213

Computed Tomography 214
L.-E. Lörelius and E. Sugimoto

References 221

Angiography and Interventional Radiology .. 221
L.-E. Lörelius

Normal Vascular Anatomy 221
Carcinoid Tumors 221

   Carcinoid Anatomy 222
   Angiographic Findings 222
   Differential Diagnoses 224
   Liver Metastases 225
Interventional Radiology 227
   Contraindications 229
   Preparation of the Patient 229
   Embolization Technique 231
   Adverse Reactions 231
References 232

Nuclear Medicine 232
U. Keske

Imaging Technique 232
Scintigraphic Findings 232
References 233

A Radiologist's View 233
A. Lunderquist

References 234

8 Multiple Endocrine Neoplasia 235

Endocrinology 235
K. Öberg

Multiple Endocrine Neoplasia Type I (MEN I) . 235
   Clinical Features 235
   Biochemical Diagnosis 238
Multiple Endocrine Neoplasia Type II
(MEN II) 238
   MEN II b (MEN III) 239

   Biochemical Screening Program 239
Summary 239
References 240

Imaging 240
L.-E. Lörelius

References 245

9 Testis 246

Anatomy 246
J. Staudt

Endocrinology 247
F. Neumann, and K.-J. Gräf

Physiology 247
Clinics 248
    Puberty and Pubertal Disorders 248
Fertility Disorders 250
    Congenital Anorchism, Mono-orchism 251
    Cryptorchidism 251
    Varicocele 251
    The Most Common Endocrine Syndromes
    Associated inter alia with Infertility .. 251
    Rare Symptoms Associated with
    Hypogonadism 252
Testicular Tumors 252
Prostatic Carcinoma 252
Benign Prostatic Hyperplasia (BHH) 253
Tumors of the Seminal Vesicles, Epididymides,
Vas Deferens and Testicular Capsule 253
Tumors of the Penis 253
References 253

Ultrasound 253
P. Vassallo, and J. Spiteri-Grech

Indications and Diagnostic Value of Testicular
Ultrasonography 253
Harware and Examination Technique 254
Normal Ultrasonic Appearance of the Scrotal
Contents 255
Congenital Anomalies of the Scrotum 255
    Abnormal Migration 255
    Arrested Descent 255
    Polyorchia 256
    Macro-orchia 256
    Aplasia of the Epididymis, Epididymo-
    Testicular Dissociation and Absence
    or Atresia of the Vas Deferens 257

Acute Scrotal Disease 257
    Primary Orchitis 258
    Secondary Orchitis 259
    Idiopathic or Primary Testicular Infarction ... 259
Testicular Tumors 260
Other Structural Abnormalities of the Testes 262
    Hydroceles 262
    Varicoceles 263
    Testicular Atrophy 263
    Testicular Cysts 263
    Fibrosis and Calcification of the Tunica
    Albuginea 264
    Testicular Calcifications 264
Conclusion 265
References 265

MR Imaging 267
Y. S. Kang, M. J. Popovich, and H. Hricak

Major Clinical Indications 267
Safety 267
Technique 267
Anatomy 268
Pathology 269
    Congenital Anomalies 269
    Inflammatory Processes 269
    Torsion 270
    Neoplasm 271
    Miscellaneous 274
    Fluid Collections and Benign Scrotal
    Masses 276
References 278

A Surgeon's View 279
R. Friedrichs, and R. Nagel

Testicular Tumors 279
Acute Scrotum 280
Conclusion 280
References 280

10 Ovary 282

Anatomy 282
J. Staudt

Endocrinology 283
F. Neumann, and K.-J. Gräf

Physiology 283
Clinics 283
    Puberty and Disorders of Puberty 283
    Ovarian Agenesis and Dysgenesis 283
    Amenorrhea 286

Polycystic Ovary Syndrome (PCO) 286
Idiopathic Hirsutism 287
Ovarian Hyperthecosis 287
Adrenogenital Syndrome (AGS) 287
Cushing Syndrome 287
Hyperprolactinemia (Galactorrhea-
Amenorrhea Syndrome) 287
Ullrich-Turner Syndrome 287
Swyer Syndrome 287
Rokitanski-Küster-Hauser Syndrome 288

Kallmann Syndrome in Women 288
Endometriosis 288
    Glandular Cystic Endometrial Hyperplasia ... 288
    Ovarian Carcinoma 288
    Endometrial Carcinoma 289
    Cervical Carcinoma 289
Vaginal Carcinoma, Vulvar Carcinoma 289
References 289

MR Imaging 289
S. K. Stevens

Major Clinical Indications 289
    Imaging Techniques 290
    MRI Appearance of Normal Ovaries 291
Ovarian Pathology 292
    Disorders of Sexual Differentiation 292
    Endometriosis 295
    Nonneoplastic Cysts 297
    Ovarian Tumors 298
References 312

Hyperandrogenism 314
R. Sörensen, and L. Moltz

Anatomy 314
Endocrinology 315
    Clinical History 318
    Physical Examination 319
    Laboratory Tests 319
    Stress 319
    Normal Women 319
    Nontumorous Hyperandrogenism 320
    Polycystic Ovary Syndrome 320
    Ovarian Hyperthecosis 321
    Androgen-secreting Ovarian Neoplasm 321
Catheterization Techniques 321
    Side Effects 322
    Radiation Exposure 322
Conclusion 322
References 322

11 Quantification of Osteoporosis 324
P. Lang, S. Grampp, M. Jergas, P. Steiger, S. Majumdar, C. Glüer, and H. K. Genant

Single Photon Absorptiometry 325
Dual Photon Absorptiometry 326
Dual X-ray Absorptiometry 326
Quantitative Computed Tomography 331
    Technical Aspects of Vertebral QCT 331
Finite Element Analysis 336
Ultrasound 336
Magnetic Resonance Imaging 338
Clinical Use of Bone Densitometry 339

Evaluation of Patients with Metabolic
Disease Affecting the Skeleton 339
Evaluation of Perimenopausal Women for
Initiation of Estrogen Therapy 339
Detection of Osteoporosis and Assessment
of its Severity 339
Monitoring of Treatment, Evaluation of
Disease Course 340
References 340

12 Positron Emission Tomography in Endocrine Disease 344
C. Muhr

Metabolic Mapping 344
Receptor Studies 345
Evaluation of Medical Treatment 346
Hyperprolactinemia – Prolactin-secreting
Pituitary Adenoma 346
Differential Diagnosis of Hormonally Inactive
Pituitary Adenomas versus Suprasellar
Meningiomas 347

Pharmacokinetics and Pharmaceutical
Distribution 348
Parathyroid Adenomas 349
References 349

Index 351

Abbreviations

ACTH	Adrenocorticotropic hormone	HPT	Hyperparathyroidism
ADH	Antidiuretic hormone	5-HT	5-hydroxytriptamine
AFP	Alpha-fetoprotein	5-HTP	5-hydroxytryptophan
AGS	Adrenogenital system	IGF	Insulin-like growth factor
AP	Anteroposterior (projection)	IIH	Insulin-induced hypoglycemia
APUD	Amine precursor uptake and decarboxylation (cells)	i. m.	Intramuscular
		IU	International Unit
AVM	Arteriovenous malformation	KeV	Kiloelectron volt
BMC	Bone mineral content	kV	Kilovolt
BMD	Bone mineral density	kV(p)	Kilovolt (peak)
BPH	Benign prostatic hyperplasia	LH	Luteinizing hormone
BVA	Broadband ultrasound attenuation	MAR	Mixed antiglobulin reduction (test)
CAH	Congenital adrenal hyperplasia	mEq	Milliequivalent
cAMP	Cyclic adenosine triphosphate	MRI	Magnetic resonance imaging
CBG	Corticosteroid-binding globulin	MSH	Melanocyte-stimulating hormone
CEA	Carcinoembyonic antigen	NPY	Neuropeptide Y
CGRP	Calcitonin gene-related peptide	OHP	17α-hydroxyprogesterone
CNS	Central nervous system	o,p'DDD	Mitotane
CRH	Corticotropin-releasing hormone	P	Proton density
CSF	Cerebrospinal fluid	PAP	Prostatic acid phosphatase
CT	Computed tomography	PCO	Polycystic ovary (disease)
DDAVP	Desmopressin acetate	PDGF	Platelet-derived growth factor
DHEA-S	Dehydroepiandrosterone	PP	Pancreatic polypeptide
DHT	5a-dihydrotestosterone	PRL	Prolactin
DMSA	Succimer (meso-2,3)-Dimercapto-succinic acid	PSA	Prostate-specific antigen
		PTH	Parathyroid hormone
DPA	Dual-photon absorptiometry	pTNM	Pathological tumor node metastasis (staging)
DPD	Diphenamid		
DSA	Digital subtraction angiography	PTP	Percutaneous transhepatic portography
DXA	Dual–X-ray absorptiometry	PVS	Portal venous sampling
DZX	Diazoxide	RF	Radiofrequency
ECG	Electrocardiogram	RFLP	Restriction fragment lengths polymorphis (analysis)
18FDG	18-fluorodesoxyglucose		
FEA	Finite element analysis	ROI	Region of interest
FIGO	Féderation Internationale de Gynécologie et d'Obstétrique	ROPE	Respiratory-ordered phase encoding
		SHBG	Sex hormone-binding globulin
FOV	Field of view	SIADH	Syndrome of inappropriate ADH secretion
FSH	Follicle-stimulating hormone		
GDA	Gastroduodenal artery	SMA	Superior mesenteric artery
Gd-DTPA	Gadolinium diethylene-triamine penta-acetic	SMC	^{75}Se-6β-selenomethyl-19-nor-cholesterol
GEP	Gastroenteropancreatic system	SOS	Speed of sound
GH-RH	Growth hormone–releasing hormone	SPA	Single photon absorptiometry
GnRH	Gonadotropin-releasing hormone	SPECT	Single photon emission computed tomography
HAE	Hepatic artery embolization		
5-HIAA	5-hydroxyindoleacetic acid	SPGR	Spoiled gradient-recalled imaging

SRIF	Somatostatin	T_4	Thyroxine
SXA	X-ray tube	TBG	Thyroxine-binding hormone
T	Tesla, Testosterone	TG	Thyroglobulin
T_1	Spin-lattice relaxation, transverse relaxation time constant	TRIAC	Tiratricol
		TRH	Thyrotropin-releasing hormone
T_2	Spin-spin relaxation, longitudinal relaxation time constant	TSH	Thyroid-stimulating hormone
		U	Unit
T_{2*}	Decay constant	VIP	Vasoactive intestinal polypeptide
T_3	Triiodothyroxine	VmA	Vanilylmandelic acid

1 Technique

Computed Tomography

C. Zwicker

Computed tomography (CT) was developed by Ambrose and Hounsfield in 1973 (2). CT allows computer-based, high-resolution image reconstruction of transverse slices from absorption measurements in defined slices (2). The emitted X-ray beam is registered by a detector (crystal coupled to a photo diode or inert gas) after transmission through the patient. Each tomographic slice requires a complete rotation of the transmitter–detector system. Each image point (pixel) represents an absorption value which is proportional to the linear absorption coefficient of the transmitted substance. This relative absorption coefficient (CT value) is called the Hounsfield unit (HU). The CT value of water is defined as zero. Air has a CT value of -1000 HU, and cortical bone has a CT value of more than $+1000$ HU. The density values of adipose tissue are on the order of -100 HU, whereas the density of unenhanced soft tissue is in the range of 20 to 80 HU.

Image reconstruction is based on the transformation of the measured absorption value profile by an analog–digital converter into computer readable, digital raw data. The final image is the result of bending and back projection. The density values of the pixels are displayed as gray values. Because the human eye is not able to differentiate 2000 gray levels, window techniques are used for visual image analysis. The window technique makes it possible to display important diagnostic image information extracted from the entire data set by varying the window level and width (3, 4, 5).

Whereas early CT scanners required up to 6 minutes measuring time per slice and where therefore suitable for cranial applications only, modern devices need less than 1 second per slice due to the continuous rotation of the X-ray tube and the detector (6). Moving artifacts can be thereby minimized. Depending on the size of the target organ, slice thickness can be varied from 1 mm to 100 mm in soft tissue diagnostic imaging. Moreover, contrast media distribution curves can be acquired in a dynamic series by rapid, repetitive scanning of a single slice as a function of time (1, 6).

Optimal delineation of vascular and soft tissue structures requires contrast-enhanced dynamic CT with continuous table movement. Automatic intravenous bolus injection with a total dose of 100–200 mL at a flow of 1–2 mL per slice is superior to continuous infusion (6). Quantitative analysis of contrast media enhancement with dynamic CT requires constant table movement and the injection of a definite contrast bolus of 1 mL per kg body weight and an injection speed of 4–8 mL/sec.

References

1 Claussen CD, Lochner B. Dynamische Computertomographie. Berlin: Springer; 1983.
2 Hounsfield GN. Computerized transverse axial scanning (tomography). Part 1. Description of system. Br J Radiol. 1973;46:1016–1022.
3 Lee JKT, Sagel SS, Stanley RJ. Computed body tomography with MRI correlation. New York: Raven Press; 1989.
4 Linke G, Pfeiler M. Grundlagen und Verfahren in der Röntgen-Computertomogaphie. In: Schinz HR. Radiologische Diagnostik, Hrsg v. Frommhold W, Dihlmann W, Stender HS, Thurn P. Band I/1. Stuttgart: Thieme; 1987:139–189.
5 Wegener OH. Ganzkörpercomputertomographie. Basel, München, Paris: S. Karger; 1981.
6 Zwicker C, Langer M, Astinet F, Langer R, Ulrich V, Felix R. Differenzierung maligner Lebertumoren mit schneller dynamischer CT. ROFO. 1990;152:293–302.

MR Imaging

W. Auffermann

In ^{1}H-magnetic resonance (MR) imaging, radio-frequency (RF) pulses interact with hydrogen nuclei (protons) within the human body in the presence of a strong homogeneous magnetic field. After termination of the RF pulse, the protons return to their equilibrium state, thereby generating a signal. The frequency distribution of this signal depends on the location, the proton density, and the internal structure of the investigated tissue or body region and can be received by an RF coil. MR signal contrast within an image reflects the relative rates at which those protons return to their equilibrium state. The resulting MR image is a three-dimensional map of signal intensities along the transverse, sagittal, and coronal planes of the body. The signal intensities are composed of multiple, temporarily overlapping parameters, which include proton density (ρ), spin-lattice relaxation (T1), spin-spin relaxation (T2), blood flow, chemical shift, and magnetic susceptibility. T1 represents the transverse relaxation time constant, whereas T2 represents the longitudinal component.

Application of these basic principles to generate MR images of the human body began about 20 years ago. Since then, significant progress has been made in the engineering of homogeneous magnets and RF coils, in the development of new pulse sequences including fat suppression, fast MRI, three-dimensional imaging, angiography sequences, artifact suppression techniques, and in the synthesis of a variety of new MR contrast agents (1–8).

Spin-echo imaging remains the mainstay for clinical evaluation of the body, offering a wide scale of contrast between various tissues of the human body. Whereas T1 relaxation time constants vary between 150 ms (fat) and 2000 ms (water), T2 constants vary from about 40 ms (liver, pancreas) to approximately 250 ms (water). In a given clinical MR system, the efficacy of spin-lattice energy transfer (T1 relaxation) is related to the inherent molecular mobility of the tissue. Water molecules are small and have a high molecular mobility causing an inefficient relaxation with long T1 and T2. Thus, tissues with higher water content have longer relaxation times than tissues with lower water content. Large molecules, however, such as triglycerides and proteins, show a low molecular mobility due to their state of inertia and intermolecular friction, which cause relatively short T1 and T2 time constants. Adipose tissue normally exhibits very short intrinsic T2 constants because of its high compartmentalization within membranes restricting molecular motion. The transverse spin-spin relaxation process is influenced by the loss of magnetization from the inhomogeneity of the magnet. The time constant T2* characterizes the rate of magnetization loss. If the magnetic field were totally homogeneous, the decay constant T2* would be equal to T2, the transverse relaxation time constant. Multiecho sequences allow the calculation of T1 and T2 relaxation time constants.

In order to assure optimal image quality and to obtain the required morphologic and functional information, a specific imaging protocol has to be designed for the target organ. The design of an imaging sequence protocol includes the patient's position, the choice of a coil, pulse sequences, imaging plane, administration of contrast media, and perhaps the application of saturation pulses, ECG gating, and other motion artifact reduction techniques. An important consideration for the design of a protocol is the total time required for the investigation of a patient.

The required hardware can be considered as a set of separate components integrated into the MR system. The heart of the system is the magnet, which can be a permanent, resistive, or superconducting magnet. The central bore has to be large enough to accomodate the patient. Optimal field strength for clinical imaging is currently between 0.5 and 1.5 T. The higher the magnetic field strength, the higher is the signal-to-noise ratio allowing better spatial resolution. However, with increasing field strength, artifacts from motion and eddy currents may become more apparent. Furthermore, MR systems require shimming coils, gradient coils, and radiofrequency antennas. Normally, three computers are required, one for the control of pulse sequences, another for data acquisition and processing, and a third for parallel image processing and review. When considering the large number of RF coils available, the optimal coil has to be chosen for each imaging protocol in order to obtain satisfactory image quality for a specific diagnostic purpose. In general, the smaller the coil, the better the signal-to-noise ratio and also the ROI that can be visualized.

In spin-echo imaging, a 90° pulse is followed by a 180° pulse. After termination of the pulse, protons start to return to their initial positions. The possibility of ECG gating makes MR suitable for mediastinal imaging. T2 characteristics of tissue can be studied by multiecho sequences. Gradient-echo imaging can reduce the imaging time from the order of minutes per series to the order of seconds per series by using low flip angles. This enables three-dimensional as well as dynamic imaging studies. With the recent development of turbo gradient-echo and echo planar imaging, acquisition times can even be reduced down to the order of milliseconds. Using various modifications, these sequences can be tailored individually for certain applications. Chien and Edelman give a detailed review of recent fast imaging sequences (3).

If native tissue contrast does not allow sufficient discrimination, it may be enhanced by increasing or decreasing signal intensity of one tissue versus another. Contrast enhancement can be positive or negative. The ideal contrast agent improves tissue discrimination by selectively enhancing the target tissue. The concentration of paramagnetic agents is critical to the degree of observed relaxation enhancement. Paramagnetic contrast media currently in clinical use are gadopentetate dimeglumine (Gd-DTPA) as well as gadodiamide (Gd-DTPA-BMA). The key biologic factors determining the usefulness of MR contrast media are biodistribution and toxicity. Paramagnetic contrast media may also be applied in patients who are allergic to iodinated contrast media or are in hyperthyroid states. The optimal imaging protocol including hardware and software requirements will be discussed in the specific organ chapters.

References

1 Atlas SW. Magnetic resonance imaging of the brain and spine. New York: Raven; 1991.
2 Bellon EM, Haake EM, Coleman PE, Sacco DC, Steiger DA, Gangarosa RE. MR artifacts. A review. AJR 1986;147:1271–1281.

3 Chien D, Edelman RR. Fast magnetic resonance imaging. In: Higgins CB, Helms CA, Hricak H, eds. Magnetic Resonance Imaging of the Body. New York: Raven, 2nd ed., 1992, pp. 175–198.
4 Crooks LE: Instrumentation and techniques. In: Higgins CB, Helms CA, Hricak H (eds.): Magnetic Resonance Imaging of the Body. 2nd ed. New York: Raven; 1992:137–150.
5 Kneeland JB. Specialized radiofrequency coils. In: Higgins CB, Helms CA, Hricak H, eds. Magnetic Resonance Imaging of the Body. 2nd ed. New York: Raven; 1992:151–156.
6 Kucharczyk J, Chew WM. Basic principles. In: Higgins CB, Helms CA, Hricak H, eds. Magnetic Resonance Imaging of the Body. 2nd ed. New York: Raven; 1992:127–136.
7 Moseley ME. Imaging Techniques. Pulse sequences from spin-echo to diffusion. In: Higgins CB, Helms CA, Hricak H, eds. Magnetic Resonance Imaging of the Body. 2nd ed. New York: Raven; 1992:157–174.
8 Ruggieri PM, Laub GA, Masaryk TJ, Modic MT. Intracranial circulation. Pulse sequence considerations in three-dimensional (volume) MR angiography. Radiology. 1989;171:785–791.
9 Watson AD, Rocklage SM. Theory and mechanisms of contrast-enhancing agents. In: Higgins CB, Helms CA, Hricak H, eds. Magnetic Resonance Imaging of the Body. 2nd ed. New York: Raven; 1992:1257–1287.
10 Wehrli FW. Principles of magnetic resonance. In: Stark DD, Bradley WG, eds. Magnetic resonance imaging. St. Louis: Mosby; 1988:3–23.

Digital Subtraction Angiography

R. Langer and M. Langer

Digital subtraction angiography (DSA) is based on the principles of cut film subtraction technique. A radiogram without opacification of the arteries is subtracted from an identical image with contrast enhancement. The result of this procedure is a radiogram that shows only the vascular system without interference from superimposed structures such as bones.

Since the introduction of DSA in clinical radiology in the late 1970s and early 1980s, a considerable change in technology and clinical application can be registered.

DSA was first designed to evaluate the arterial system by injecting contrast medium into a peripheral vein. This technique did not fulfill all clinical requirements and today, DSA is essentially used with intra-arterial contrast medium application. Nevertheless, because digital images allow different postprocessing procedures, the contrast medium volume as well as the catheter size and the injection speed could be reduced for DSA in comparison to plain film angiography. These developments made intra-arterial DSA a suitable angiographic technique for inpatient and outpatient studies.

When DSA is performed in fluoroscopic or continuous mode, a plain image is built up in an image intensifier television chain by a continuous X-ray beam. When DSA is done in the pulsed mode, pulsed, or intermittent X-ray beam is emitted by the X-ray tube. The frequency of the impulses can be regulated up to a maximum of 25 to 30 per second. This mode is the established state-of-the-art DSA technique.

The images are immediately digitized and filed in an intermediate memory as digital image information. The image is not stored in an analog form. A digital signal value is assigned to each picture element (pixel) and can be retrieved at any time from the appropriate image store. The number of pixels available depends on the size of the matrix of the image grid. Today, a matrix size of 1024 by 1024 pixels is standard for high-resolution DSA. For intravenous studies a matrix size of 512 by 512 pixels is sufficient.

Today the most widely distributed method of image subtraction is the so-called real-time subtraction technique or the time-dependent subtraction technique. A mask, the equivalent of the plain television picture, is created at the start of the examination before contrast enhancement of the vascular system. By choosing an appropriate integration factor for the mask, this frame can be obtained from a few images in the case of objects with slow intrinsic movements or from a long series of images in the case of objects with rapid intrinsic movements in order to produce a blurred, poorly defined mask. A second sequence of images analog to the mask is determined by a second integration of a previous number of single images, the minimum is one image at the time of maximum contrast medium density in the vessel. Electronic subtraction of these two frames from each other results in the subtraction image that is visible on the monitor.

One of the major advantages of this technique is the good subtraction of high contrast structure, which is immediately available during the examination. A disadvantage of this procedure is its high sensitivity to motion artifacts, because every difference in the image information between the mask and the contrast scan is electronically amplified before reproduction.

The further development of computer software has made it possible to perform not only digital subtraction angiograms but also digital angiography without subtractions (with visible bone structure), in clinical routine. These nonsubtracted studies or subtracted studies with underlying anatomic background give excellent contrast resolution on one hand and sufficient topographic anatomic information on the other hand.

Awareness of potential artifacts sources is essential for the evaluation of digital subtraction angiograms because the former can mimic pathological findings in the vascular system.

A distinction must therefore be made between equipment-related factors and patient-related factors. The equipment-related factors include image noise, overexposure artifacts, underexposure artifacts, and insufficient spatial resolution due to a matrix that is too small. Patient-related factors include all kinds of voluntary and involuntary patient movement. Secondarily, especially for intravenous studies, a prolonged transit time of the contrast medium bolus injected into a central vein or the right atrium and a reduced cardiac output have to be considered as potential factors that reduce the image quality.

All angiographic examinations including all DSA studies should begin with a detailed explanation of the procedure to the patient by the radiologist. During the procedure of obtaining an informed consent, the patient must be asked whether he or she is hypersensitive to contrast media or suffers from any thyroid or kidney function disorders.

The physician should also be familiar with any pertinent history of heart, lung, or kidney disease, so that the examination can be tailored to these pathological conditions.

With a defined signal-to-noise ratio and other fixed examination parameters, the quality of a digital subtraction angiogram is essentially determined by the concentration and duration of the contrast medium bolus. The magnitude of the intravascular iodine concentration is the decisive factor in DSA. Increasing the contrast medium concentration in the artery to be examined results in a greater difference in X-ray attenuation between the vessel and adjacent tissues and provides better delineation of the vessel.

Today it is proven that nonionic contrast media have a significantly lower side effect rate. The incidence of pain following arterial injection of low osmolal nonionic contrast agents is generally low. Anesthesia is no longer required. Selective intra-arterial contrast medium injection gives excellent angiographic results when an iodine concentration of about 150 to 250 mg iodine per ml is injected. An intra-arterial iodine concentration between 50 and 200 mg iodine per ml blood in the arteries of the target region gives the best results.

The detailed angiographic examination techniques and special problems of angiographic examinations of endocrine organs are discussed and illustrated in the specific chapters.

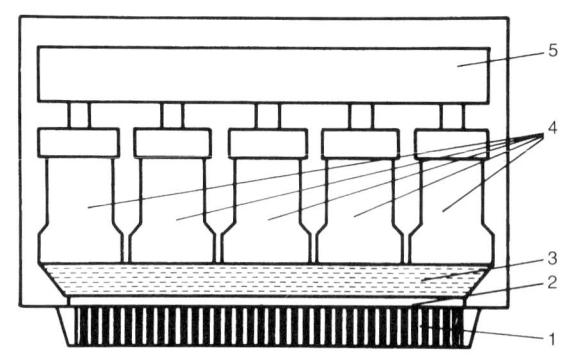

Fig. 1.**1** Gamma camera head. The collimator 1. focuses the gamma rays emitted by the radiopharmaceutical and reduces scattered radiation. The crystal 2. converts the gamma rays into visible photons, which are passed on by a light pipe 3. The photons are localized by photomultipliers 4., which transfer them into electrons and amplify them. The electrons are then passed on to the summing network 5., an electronic preamplifier (adapted from 5)

Nuclear Imaging
U. Keske, Berlin

Introduction

In nuclear imaging, a radionuclide is incorporated into the body, where its activity distribution is measured. In order to study the function of an organ, the radionuclide may be bound to a pharmaceutical. The resulting substance is called a radiopharmaceutical. It is taken up by the organ and, depending on the function of the organ, metabolized. Nuclear imaging is always functional imaging, because it is based on a functioning organ.

Radioactive tracers were first used in 1923 to study biologic systems. In the 1930s, radioactive iodine was introduced for thyroid studies. Technetium was first used for medical purposes in 1961.

Imaging devices

The **gamma camera,** developed by Anger in 1959 (1), has become the most common imaging device in nuclear medicine (8). Static and dynamic investigations are possible and imaging data can be postprocessed in a computer system. The gamma camera consists of two major components: the detector head (Fig. 1.**1**) and the console. The detector head consists of a sodiumiodine **crystal** with a diameter of 20–42 cm and a thickness of 0.62–1.25 cm. Due to the photoeffect, this crystal transforms gamma rays into visible light (photons). The efficacy of the crystal to convert gamma rays depends on the gamma energy. Below 200 keV, the efficacy is relatively hight at 80%, but above 300 keV it drops to 25% (5, 6, 7). The photons are then located by **photomultipliers,** which convey the energy of the light photons to electrons. A positional network transfers the impulses into a two-dimensional image. In modern imaging devices, the images are digitized and inhomogenities are corrected.

A lead **collimator** is placed in front of the sodium iodine crystal to reduce scattered radiation. It consists of a lead sheet, about 2.5 cm thick, with many holes (up to 15 000). Gamma rays that travel in directions not parallel to the collimator holes are absorbed by the collimator septa (the material between the holes). The design of the collimator determines the spatial resolution and sensitivity of the gamma camera. If the diameter of the holes is increased, sensitivity increases, and spatial resolution decreases (7, 9). By varying the diameter, it is possible to construct high-resolution and low-resolution collimators (3). The most commonly used collimators are parallel-hole collimators. They have replaced converging collimators that reduce the image. For thyroid studies, a special single-hole ("pinhole") collimator that magnifies the image may be used (7).

Imaging Methods

In **static scintigraphy**, a two-dimensional image of the activity distribution of the body is acquired. The camera is positioned in one place over the body, and impulses are collected and added up to form a single image. When multiple images are made with the gamma camera fixed in the same position, dynamic changes of the activity distribution can be seen **(sequential scintigraphy)**. For regions of interest, global and regional time-activity curves for certain organs may be calculated **(dynamic study)**.

For **whole body scintigraphy**, the total body image is recorded. This is achieved by a constantly moving the gamma camera crystal over the body. Alternatively, multiple images of the whole body may be obtained with gamma camera that has a large field of view.

With "Single Photon Emission Computed Tomography" **(SPECT)**, tomographic images of the body can be acquired. This is achieved by a rotating gamma camera. The patient is positioned on a table, and the gamma camera rotates over an angle of 360° (in some cases 180°) around the patient. Usually, an image is acquired every 6° with a matrix of 64×64 pixels. Acquisition time varies between 10 minutes and 30 or more minutes. By filtered back projection, several contiguous tomographic sections are reconstructed. For SPECT, special dual camera systems with two opposed rotating camera heads have been designed (2).

Radioisotopes

The ideal radioisotope is a pure gamma radiation emitter that provides optimal emission for the imaging device, and a very high photon density, yet delivers minimal radiation to the patient (10). **Iodine-131** (^{131}I) is a nuclear by-product with a relatively long half-life of 8.1 days. It emits gamma radiation with a relatively high energy of 364 keV and beta radiation. Due to the high gamma energy, the collimator septa have to be relatively thick. Thus, only medium and high energy collimators, which offer a relatively low spatial resolution are used (6).

Iodine-123 (^{123}I) has a much shorter half life (13.3 hours) and a relatively low gamma energy of 159 keV; it emits no beta radiation. Detection efficacy in the crystal of the Anger camera is about 90%, which is three times higher than that of ^{131}I (364 keV). I-131 is a cyclotron product, and the cost of its production and its radiopharmaceuticals is fairly high (10).

Thallium-201 (^{201}Tl) has a relatively long half-life of 73.5 hours. It principally emits X-rays (93%) of 69 keV and 80 keV and gamma rays of 135 keV and 168 keV and is usually furnished as thallium chloride.

Technetium-99m (^{99m}Tc) has become the most commonly used radioisotope in clinical nuclear medicine. Its half-life is relatively low (6 hours). The major gamma radiation is found at 140 keV (98.6%); there is no beta radiation. It is easily available in every nuclear medicine department, because it is supplied by generators, which are commercially available. These generators contain Molybdenum-99. The daughter, ^{99m}Tc, is eluted with sterile physiological saline as sodium pertechnetate (Na^{99m}TcO$_4$). About 95% of the photons are absorbed by about 1 mm of lead. Usually, the septa of the collimator are only 0.25 mm thick. Three different types of collimators are in use: high-resolution, all-purpose and high-sensitivity (6). For almost all studies, short-life radionuclides like ^{99m}Tc are advantageous because they permit the employment of larger doses resulting in higher photon fluxes and a reduced radiation dose.

Selenium-75 (^{75}SE) has a long half-life (120 days) and decays by electron capture; there are ten gamma rays ranging in energy from 25 keV to 460 keV. For imaging, the gamma rays at 264 keV and 279 keV or a wide band of 200–400 keV is used (4, 5, 10). Due to its long physical half-life, it delivers a relatively high radiation dose to the body, and the amount injected has to be kept very low (4). Nowadays it is rarely used for adrenal imaging.

Radiopharmaceuticals

For imaging, radionuclides are bound to a pharmaceutical. The resulting radiopharmaceutical is incorporated into the body and then taken up by the organ and possibly metabolized. The ideal radiopharmaceutical is a substance that is specific for a particular function or provides excellent organ localization (10).

For **thyroid imaging**, sodium iodine with the isotopes ^{131}I, ^{123}I, or pertechnetate is used. For medullary thyroid carcinoma, thallium chloride, pentavalent Succimer (DMSA), or antibodies against carcinoembryonic antigen (CEA) may be used.

The **parathyroids** are examined with ^{201}Tl in combination with a thyroid scan performed with pertechnetate. For the **adrenal cortex**, cholesterol derivatives are used. They may be labeled with ^{131}I or with ^{75}Se. For **adrenal medullary** and **carcinoids**, a guanidine derivative labeled with ^{131}I or ^{123}I is used.

References

1. Anger HO, Rosenthall DJ. Scintillation camera and positron camera. In: Medical Radioisotope Scanning. Vienna: International Atomic Energy Agency; 1959:59.
2. Budiger TF. Single Photon Emission Computed Tomography. In: Gottschalk A, Hoffer PB, Potchen EH, eds. Diagnostic Nuclear Medicine. Baltimore: Williams & Wilkins; 1988:108–127.
3. de Bruin M. Radioactivity: Measurements and Instrumentation. In: van Rijk PP, ed. Nuclear Techniques in Diagnostic Medicine. Dordrecht: Martinus Nijhoff; 1986:1–66.
4. Eckelman WC. Radiopharmaceuticals. In: Gottschalk A, Hoffer PB, Potchen EH, eds. Diagnostic Nuclear Medicine; vol. 1. 2nd ed. Baltimore Hong Kong London Sydney: Williams & Wilkins; 1988:150–163.

5 Feine U, zum Winkel K. Radiopharmakologie und Radiopharmazeutik. In: Feine U, zum Winkel K, eds. Nuklearmedizin-Szintigraphische Diagnostik. 2. Auflage. Stuttgart: Thieme; 1980:85–111.
6 Heller SL, Goodwin PN. Nuclear imaging. In: van Rijk PP, ed. Nuclear Technique in Diagnostic Medicine. Dordrecht-Boston-Lancaster: Martinus Nijhoff; 1986:67–98.
7 Jahns E, Lange D. Physikalische Grundlagen und Technik. In: Feine U, zum Winkel K: Nuklearmedizin-Szintigraphische Diagnostik. 2. Auflage. Stuttgart: Thieme; 1980:1–70.
8 Muehllehner G. The Anger Scintillation Camera. In: Gottschalk A, Hoffer PB, Potchen EH, eds. Diagnostic Nuclear Medicine; vol. 1. 2nd ed. Baltimore Hong Kong London Sydney: Williams & Wilkins; 1988:71–81.
9 Tsui BMW, Gunther DL, Beck RN. Physics of Collimator Design. In: Gottschalk A, Hoffer PB, Potchen EH, eds. Diagnostic Nuclear Medicine; vol. 1. 2nd ed. Baltimore Hong Kong London Sydney: Williams & Wilkins; 1988:42–54.
10 Tubis, M. Radiopharmaceuticals. In: van Rijk PP, ed. Nuclear Techniques in Diagnostic Medicine. Dordrecht-Boston-Lancaster: Martinus Nijhoff; 1986:99–134.

2 Pituitary

Anatomy

J. Staudt

The pituitary gland is approximately the size of a hazelnut and weighs about 600 mg. It is surrounded by a rigid connective tissue capsule fixed to the base of the diencephalon. On the other side, it is immovably fixed within its bony cavity, the sella turcica. It is only connected to the cerebral base through a median hole in the sellar diaphragm, which is penetrated by the hypophyseal stalk (i. e., infundibulum) (Fig. 2.**1**). The sellar floor varies in appearance depending largely on the degree of aeration of the underlying sphenoid sinus.

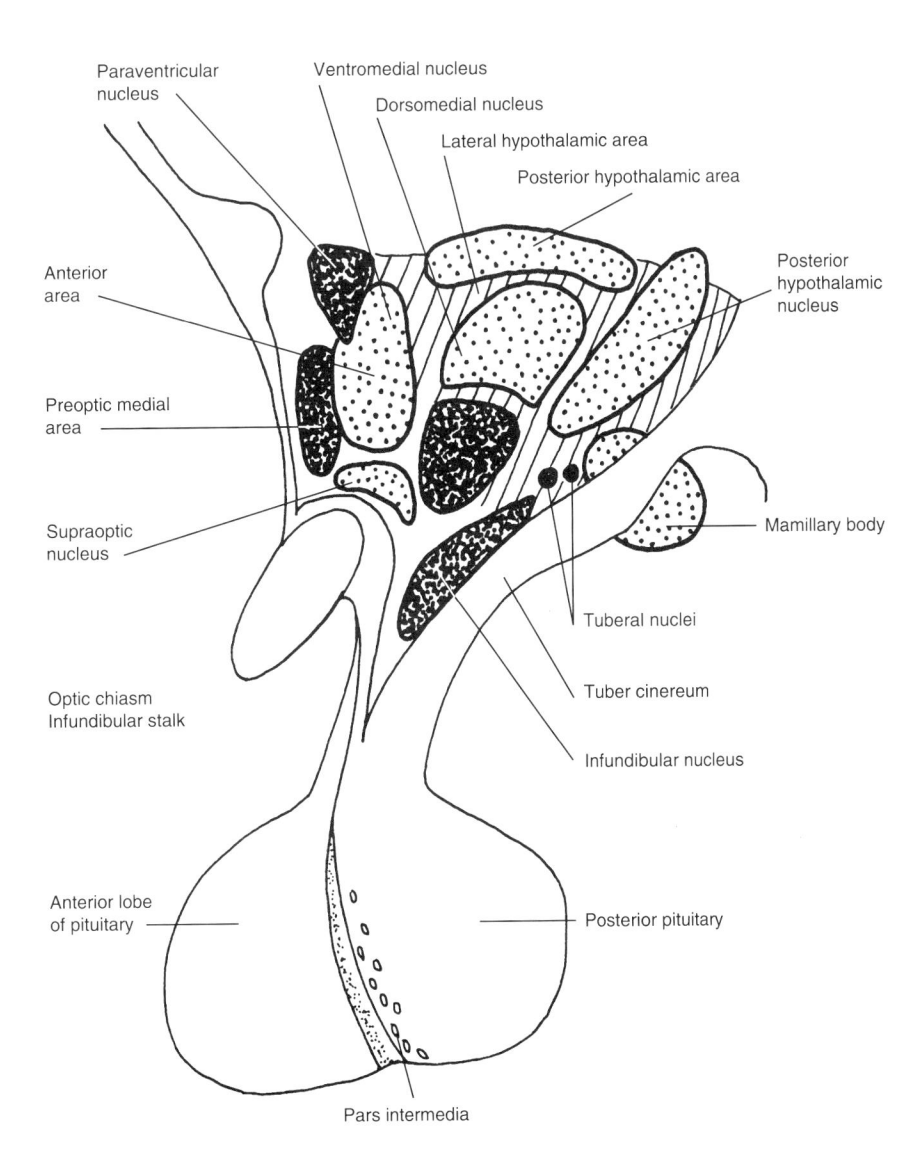

Fig. 2.**1** Hypothalamic–hypophysis system

8   2 Pituitary

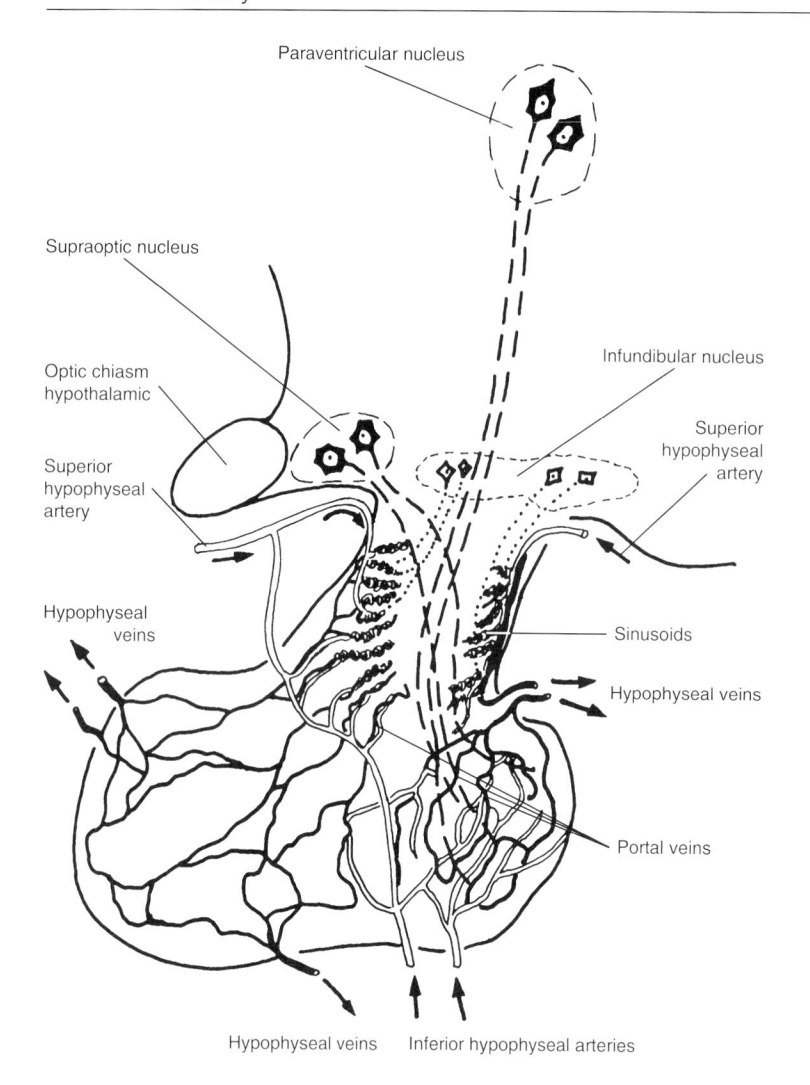

Fig. 2.2 Blood vessels and hypothalamic–pituitary axis

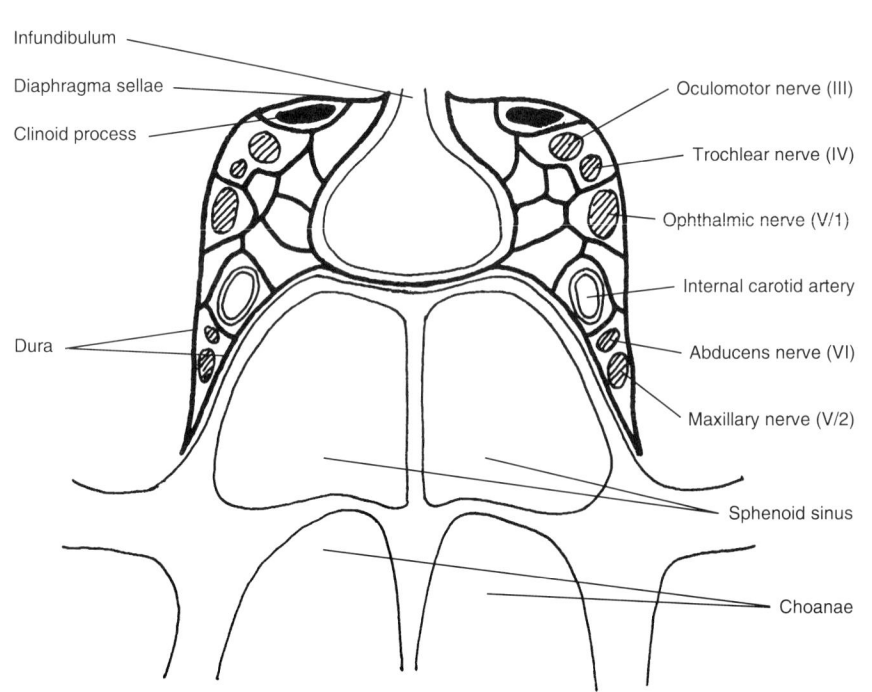

Fig. 2.3 The cavernous sinus and the hypophysis

Embryologically, physiologically, and anatomically, the gland can be divided into the adenohypophysis, which forms the anterior lobe, and the neurohypophysis, which forms the posterior lobe. The adenohypophysis originates from the ectodermal roof of the oral invagination (Rathke's pouch) by segmentation, which ventrally approaches the later infundibulum. The anterior lobe represents about three-fourths of the organ weight with its distal part, the tuberal part at the pituitary stalk, and the intermediary part.

Its function as a senior endocrine gland for the production of glandotropic hormones is reflected in the vascular architecture (Fig. 2.2). Two separate pairs of arteries, the superior pituitary arteries from the internal carotid artery and the inferior pituitary arteries from the circulus arteriosus form two capillary networks in the outer zone of the pituitary stalk. The blood then flows into the portal vessels of the adenohypophysis with its anastomosing vascular sinuses. These sinuses surround the cells and represent another capillary network connected in series ahead of the actual venous drainage.

The venous system has numerous connections to the cavernous sinus (Fig. 2.3). The cavernous sinus represents a dural venous groove, in which the third cranial nerve and the ophthalmic (V1) and maxillary (V2) devisions of the fifth cranial nerve are identified in cranio–caudal order as hypointense structures within the lateral wall.

Endocrinology

K.-J. Gräf

Physiology

The hypothalamic–pituitary axis is the central control system for the function of various endocrine target organs (Fig. 2.4). This is where numerous external, and internal signals such as emotion, light, temperature, and rhythm are registered and modulated. The hypothalamus coordinates all the important information—from the central nervous system (CNS) as well as from the periphery (via feedback control mechanisms)—in order to ensure a humoral equilibrium of hormonal secretion. The complex activity of the hypothalamus results in the release of specific hypophysiotropic peptide hormones (releasing and in-

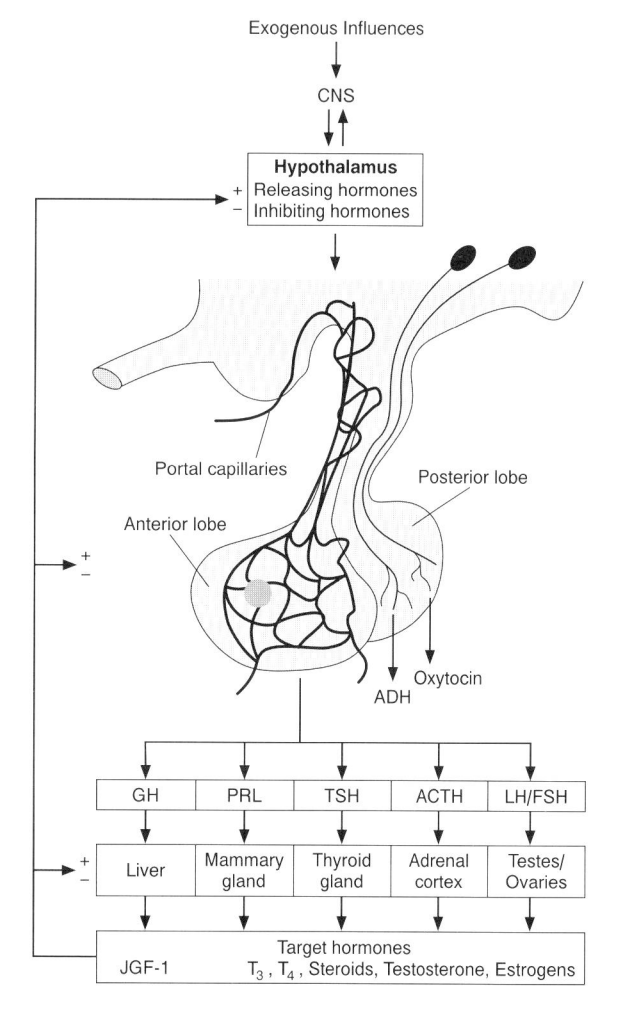

Fig. 2.4 The hypothalamo-pituitary regulatory system and its feedback control mechanisms

hibiting hormones), modulatory neuropeptides, and neurotransmitter substances into the hypothalamic hypophyseal portal capillaries, which connect the median eminence and the anterior pituitary lobe (adenohypophysis). In contrast, the endocrine function of the posterior lobe (neurohypophysis) is independent of control by the peptides and neurotransmitters released into the portal vein system (see p. 7f. and Fig. 2.**4**). The hormones oxytocin and vasopressin (antidiuretic hormone) are synthesized in nerves originating in the supraoptic and paraventricular nuclei, transported in axons down to the nerve endings at the neurohypophysis, and released into the peripheral blood. Whereas vasopressin secretion depends mainly on plasma osmolality, blood pressure, and blood volume, oxytocin secretion increases because of vaginal (vaginal distension during parturition) and nipple stimulation.

The main physiological actions of the pituitary hormones are summarized in Table 2.**2**.

Endocrine Disorders

Pituitary Insufficiency

Pituitary insufficiency means a total or partial loss of endocrine function of the pituitary (mostly of the anterior lobe, seldom of the posterior lobe). The various causes of hypopituitarism are summarized in Table 2.**3**. The clinical features depend on the degree of decrease in hormone secretion and whether the deficiency occurs before puberty or in adolescence.

Prepubertal TSH deficiency leads to growth retardation and cretinism. In adults, the typical clinical symptoms of hypothyroidism are obvious (see Chapter 3).

Untreated GH deficiency causes short stature in children, whereas its clinical importance in adults is under discussion. LH and FSH deficiency results in hypogonadism with oligo(menorrhea or amenorrhea in women and reduction or loss of libido and spermiogenesis in men (see Chapters 9 and 10).

Reduction or loss of ACTH secretion is followed by adrenal insufficiency and loss of pigmentation due to concomitantly reduced MSH secretion.

Isolated prolactin deficiency is very rare. Its potential clinical importance in women is lactation failure, whereas its consequence in men is still unknown.

Antidiuretic hormone (ADH) insufficiency results in diabetes insipidus, and the clinical importance of lowered oxytocin secretion is unclear.

Table 2.**1** Hypothalamic hypophysiotropic hormones

Releasing hormone	Function
Thyrotropin-releasing hormone (TRH; thyroliberin)	Stimulates thyroid-stimulating hormone (TSH) and prolactin (PRL) secretion
Gonadotropin-releasing hormone (Gn-RH; gonadoliberin)	Stimulates luteinizing hormone (LH) and follicle-stimulating hormone (FSH) secretion
Growth hormone–releasing hormone (GH-RH; somatoliberin)	Stimulates growth hormone (GH) secretion
Corticotropin-releasing hormone (CRH; corticoliberin)	Stimulates adrenocorticotropic hormone (ACTH) secretion
Inhibiting hormones/factors	
Somatostatin	Inhibits GH and TSH secretion
Dopamine	Inhibits PRL and TSH secretion

Table 2.**2** Major physiological actions of pituitary hormones

Hormone	Main mode of action
TSH	Synthesis and release of thyroid hormones
LH	In women, maturation of ovulation and steroidogenesis; in men, stimulation of steroidogenesis in Leydig's cells
FSH	Maturation and function of granulosa cells of the ovary and sertoli cells of the testes (initiation of spermatogenesis)
Prolactin	Initiation and maintenance of lactation, impairment of gonadal function (during physiological post-partum lactation)
GH	IGF-1 synthesis in the liver, skeletal maturation, organ growth (anabolic, lipolytic activity and others)

Pituitary Adenomas

Pathophysiology and General Management

Pituitary tumors are usually benign adenomas, carcinomas being rare exceptions. They account for about 10% of all intracranial tumors. Currently, pituitary adenomas are classified by their endocrine activity as nonfunctioning (endocrine inactive) and functioning (endocrine active) adenomas (see Table 2.**4**). The old classification in acidophilic, basophilic, and chromophobic adenomas has been abandoned in favor of immunohistological staining techniques detecting the hormone production in the tumor cell itself. Furthermore, a distinction should be made between microadenomas (diameter less than 10 mm) and macroadenomas (diameter greater than 10 mm). Nonfunctioning pituitary adenomas are clinically evident only because of complications in patients with macroadenomas, e.g., chiasma syndrome, headaches, and symptoms due to pituitary insufficiency, especially hypothyroidism, adrenal insufficiency, hypogonadotropic hypogonadism with cycle disturbances, infertility, loss of libido, or both. The clinical features of functioning adenomas are characterized by the hormone or hormones secreted in excess, and in the case of macroadenomas, also by symptoms due to tumor mass expansion, as in nonfunctioning adenomas.

The diagnostic workup for pituitary adenomas includes CT, and even better, MR imaging studies with enhancement. In the case of macroadenomas, ophthalmological assessment of visual field defects and reduction of vision is also necessary. The endocrinological studies include measurement of all the hormones of the adenohypophysis (basal levels of ACTH, TSH, LH, FSH, PRL, and GH) together with the target hormones cortisol, testosterone (in men), estradiol (in women), and the thyroid hormones triiodothyronine and thyroxine. Dynamic tests are required for functioning tumors secreting GH (acromegaly) and ACTH (Cushing disease).

Nonfunctioning Adenomas

About a third of all pituitary adenomas are classified as nonfunctioning adenomas with no detectable hormone excess of clinical relevance. The clinical feature depends on tumor size and hormone insufficiency in macroadenomas, while nonfunctioning microadenomas are generally asymptomatic. The growth rate may be very slow and clinically silent for years before these tumors are diagnosed incidentally or due to neurological complications (e.g., headaches) or ophthalmological symptoms (e.g., visual field defects). Therapy of choice is neurosurgical adenectomy via the transsphenoidal or transcranial approach. Irradia-

Table 2.**3**   Causes of hypopituitarism

Primary hypopituitarism

Pituitary adenomas

Tumors other than pituitary adenomas
  meningioma, lymphoma, craniopharyngioma, metastatic carcinomas, dermoid and epidermoid cysts, carotid artery aneurysm, pinealoma, chordoma, optic nerve glioma, plasmacytoma, osteosarcoma

Pituitary infarction
  postpartum (Sheehan syndrome)
  others (shock, diabetes mellitus, vasculitis, trauma, cavernosus sinus thrombosis, sickle cell disease, infections)

Infiltrations
  hemochromatosis, sarcoidosis, histiocytosis, infections (tuberculosis, syphilis, mycosis, autoimmune disease, hypophysitis)

Empty sella syndrome

Iatrogenic
  surgical, radiological, steroid treatment (withdrawal syndrome)

Secondary hypopituitarism

Pituitary stalk injury
  trauma, surgical, aneurysms, suprasellar arachnoid cysts, suprasellar tumours (besides pituitary adenomas e.g. teratoma, harmartoma, ganglioneuroma, astrocytoma, glioblastoma, fibroma, fibrosarcoma)

Hypothalamic/pituitary stalk infitration
  lymphoma, leukamia

Idiopathic
  hypoplasia, aplasia (familial: Kallmann syndrome)

Acromegaly

Acromegaly is caused by an excessive secretion of GH. In most cases, GH excess is due to an adenoma of the adenohypophysis, which accounts for about 10–20% of all pituitary adenomas. In about 20–30% of all cases, these adenomas cosecrete prolactin in addition to GH. In some very rare cases, GH excess is due to an ectopic (paraneoplastic) secretion of GH-RH (bronchial and gastrointestinal carcinoid, pancreas tumors). The clinical symptoms of acromegaly are listed in Table 2.4 (see also Fig. 2.5). Acromegaly is a chronic disease with silent clinical manifestations. In most cases, the tumor can be visualized by CT or MR imaging. However, some microadenomas are not detectable with any of the available radiological techniques. Thus, the diagnosis of acromegaly always requires the endocrinological detection of GH excess. Because of fluctuations, the measurement of basal GH levels is useless. The determination of IGF-1 levels and the use of several function tests are much more reliable for diagnostic purposes. The most suitable dynamic test is based on the measurement of GH under an overload of glucose (oral glucose test), which suppresses GH secretion to levels below 1 ng/ml in healthy subjects.

Acromegaly may be cured by neurosurgery. Irradiation is only indicated when a neurosurgical approach is not possible or refused, and in patients with invasive tumor growth postoperatively. For medical treatment, somatostatin has been shown to be very effective in the suppression of GH secretion and in tumor size reduction as well. However, the need for

Table 2.4 Classification of pituitary adenomas

Endocrine active tumors	75%
Prolactinomas	35%
GH-producing adenomas (Acromegaly)	20%
Cosecretion of GH and prolactin	6%
ACTH-producing adenomas (Cushing disease)	12%
Glycoprotein hormone–producing adenomas	2%
– TSH	
– Mixed, (TSH, Prolactin, GH, LH)	
– FSH	
– LH	
– Cosecretion of FSH and LH	
– Mixed (FSH, LH, GH, prolactin)	
– α-Subunit	
– Mixed (α-Subunit; GH, prolactin, ACTH)	
Endocrine inactive tumors	25%

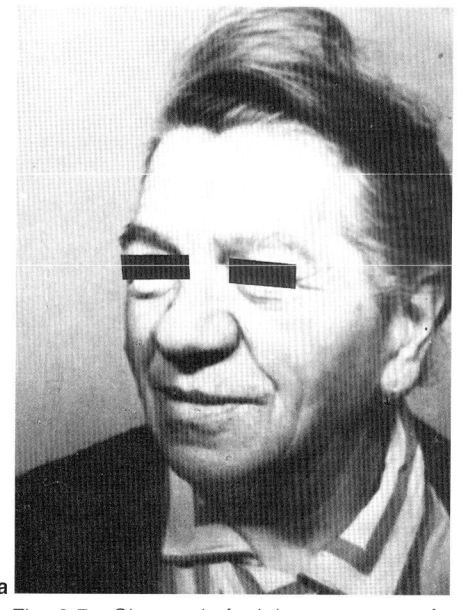

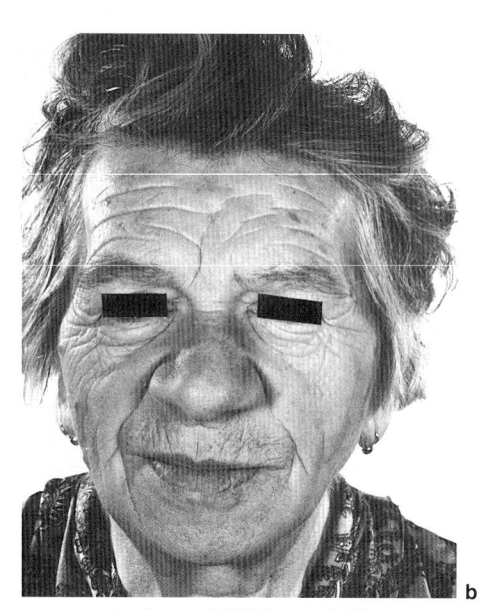

Fig. 2.5 Change in facial appearance of a patient with acromegaly **a)** aged 50 **b)** aged 77

long-term subcutaneous therapy with its side effects (abdominal pain, diarrhea, gallstones and others) is a limiting factor.

Table 2.**5** Typical clinical findings in acromegalic patients

Acral growth, visceromegaly, soft tissue thickening
Menstrual disorders, amenorrhea
Decreased libido and impotence
Weight gain
Headaches
Hypertension
Paresthesias (carpal tunnel syndrome)
Arthralgias
Impaired glucose tolerance, diabetes mellitus
Weakness
Hypertrichosis

Prolactinoma

Prolactinomas—the most common hormone secreting pituitary adenomas—account for about one-third of all pituitary adenomas. No special endocrinological tests are necessary. The diagnosis depends on the magnitude of a single basal prolactin level in serum. Concentrations higher than 100 ng/ml are most likely due to a prolactinoma. In cases with only slightly elevated prolactin levels (20–100 ng/ml), it should be remembered that several drugs are known to enhance prolactin secretion (Table 2.**6**). Increased prolactin levels may also be caused by nipple stimulation, pituitary stalk injury, stress, primary hypothyroidism, chronic renal failure, and other factors. In patients with prolactin levels higher than 100 ng/mL, MRI or CT imaging is necessary to exclude a hypothalamic or hypophyseal cause.

The main clinical features are secondary amenorrhea and menstrual disorders in women and decreased libido in men. In macroprolactinomas, signs of pitu-

Table 2.**6** Physiological, pathophysiological, and pharmacological, effects on prolactin secretion

Physiological hyperprolactinemia
Stress
Sleep
Cohabitation
Postpartal lactation
Pregnancy
Suckling stimulus; nipple stimulation

Pathological (endogenous) hyperprolactinemia
Prolactinoma
Suprasellar masses; inflammation
Ectopic prolactin production (hypernephroma, lung cancer, and others)
Thorax trauma
Prostate carcinoma/hyperplasia
Chronic renal failure
Primary hypothyroidism

Hyperprolactinemia caused by pharmaceuticals

Estrogens	H_2-receptor antagonists (e. g., cimetidine)
Oral contraceptives	Antihypertensives (e. g., Reserpine, Methldopa)
Antiandrogens	Neuroleptics
Prostaglandins	Phenothiazine and related agents (e.g., Chlorpromazine)
Endorphins	Butyrophenone and related agents (e.g., Haloperidol)
Morphine	Others (e.g., Sulpiride, Thioxanthine)
TRH	Antidepressants (e.g., benzazopine derivatives, Imipramine)
3-iodine-L-thyroxine	Antiemetics and related agents (e.g., Metoclopramide, Domperidone)
GABA	
5-hydroxytryptophan	Antihistamines and related agents
L-tryptophan	
Histamine	

Hypoprolactinemia caused by pharmaceuticals
L-Dopa
Dopamine
Dopamine agonists
Fenclonine (DL-p-Chlorphenylalanine)

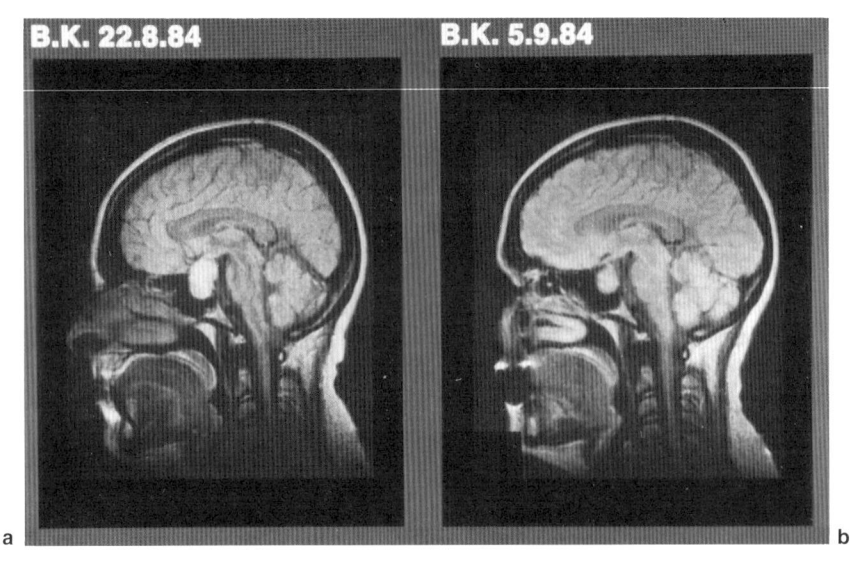

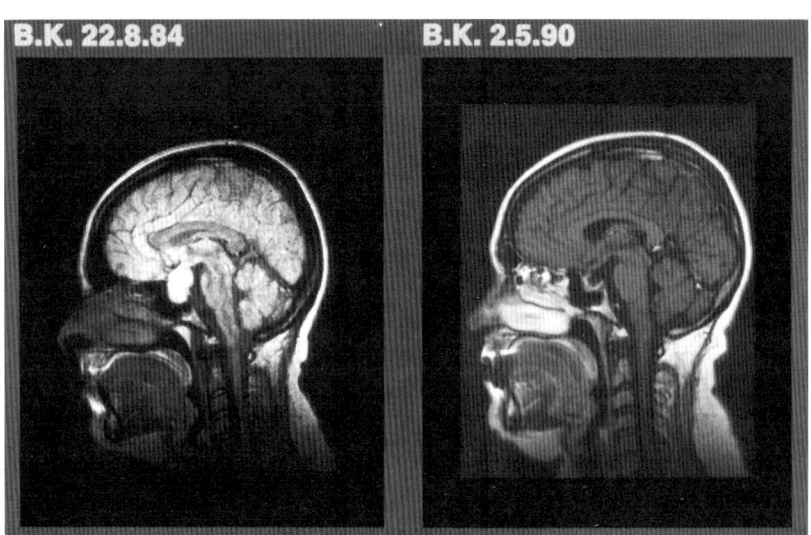

Fig. 2.6 MRI scans of a woman with a macroprolactinoma (sagittal sections). (**a**) and (**c**) before treatment; (**b**) after 2 weeks of treatment with the partial dopamine agonist terguride; (**c**) after 5 years of treatment with terguride

itary insufficiency may occur as well as symptoms due to tumor mass expansion. The therapy of choice is treatment with dopamine agonists (bromocriptine, lisuride, and others). In most patients, these drugs effectively suppress prolactin secretion and also lead to reduction of tumor size (Fig. 2.**6**). Nowadays, transphenoidal neurosurgical adenectomy is only required in a few patients with the chiasm syndrome or in patients with intolerance or resistance to dopamine agonists.

Cushing Disease

In about 90% of all cases, Cushing disease is due to an ACTH-secreting adenoma of the adenohypophysis (for Cushing syndrome see Chapter Adrenal Gland). These tumors—which account for about 5–10% of all pituitary adenomas—are mostly very small, which makes their radiological elevation rather difficult.

The best results are obtained with contrast-enhanced MR imaging or high-resolution CT studies. Ectopic CRH secretion as a cause of orthotopic ACTH excess is a very rare disease. Nelson syndrome is the ACTH-producing pituitary adenoma following bilateral adrenalectomy due to the loss of inhibitory feedback control by corticosteroids. The clinical characteristics of Cushing disease are mainly related to the excess of glucocortico- and androgenic steroids secreted by the adrenal cortex (Table 2.**7** and Fig. 2. **7**).

For screening purposes the dexamethasone test (1 or 2 mg given orally at 11 p. m. and measurement of serum hydrocortisone level at 8 a. m. the next day) as well as the standard dexamethasone test (0.5 mg given every 6 hours for 1 or 2 days) are well established. In addition, and probably as one of the best parameters, it is suggested to measure the total free hydrocorti-

Endocrinology 15

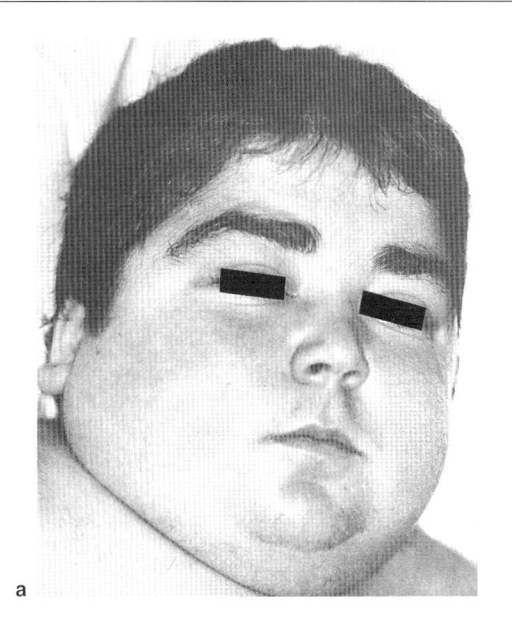

Table 2.7 Typical clinical findings in Cushing disease

Moon face, plethora
Hypertension
Weight gain, abdominal fat, buffalo hump
Hirsutism, hypertrichosis
Diabetes mellitus
Amenorrhea
Osteoporosis
Thin skin (arms and legs)
Striae
Enhanced bruisability (ecchymosis)
Muscular weakness
Poor wound healing

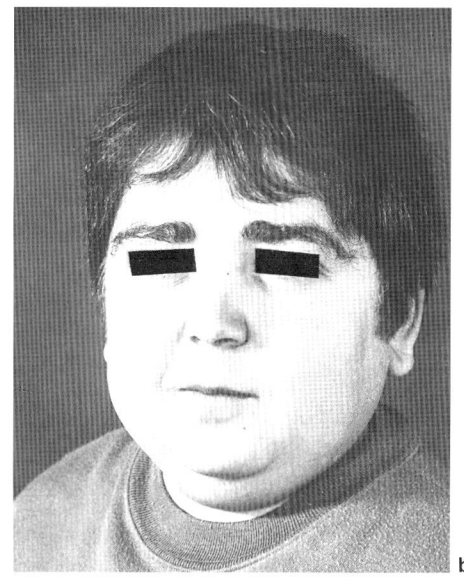

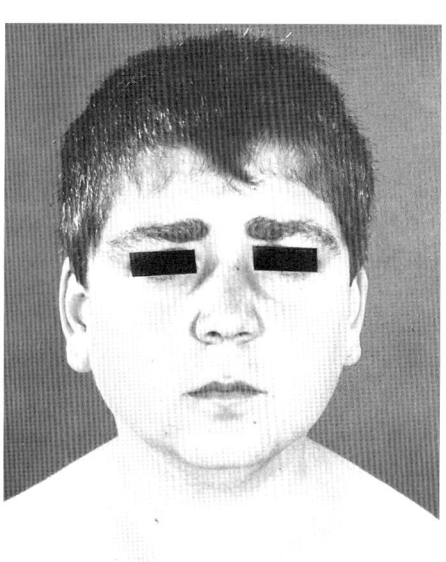

Fig. 2.7 Clinical features of Cushing disease: (a) before treatment; note the typical "moon face" (b) 3 months after start of treatment with mitotane; (c) 6 months after start of treatment with mitotane

sone and corticoid metabolite concentrations in a 24-hour urine collection before and after dexamethasone suppression. Furthermore, basal ACTH measurement as well as the ACTH and hydrocortisone increase due to CRH stimulation may be helpful in distinguishing between Cushing syndrome (pituitary independent excess of glucocorticoid secretion) and Cushing disease. In Cushing disease the therapy of choice is selective transsphenoidal adenectomy. The cure rate in specialized neurosurgery centers is between 70% and 90%. However, long-term follow-up studies indicate that the relapse rate is unexpected high. Alternatives, which are inferior to neurosurgery, are external radiotherapy and medical treatment to inhibit steroid synthesis by the adrenal cortex using e. g., ketoconazole, metyrapone, aminoglutethemide, or mitotane (o, p'-DDD).

Thyrotropin-producing Adenoma

The TSH-secreting adenoma is rare, accounting for less than 1% of all pituitary adenomas. This disease is characterized by the clinical symptoms of goiter and thyrotoxicosis with the endocrinological constellation of elevated thyroid hormones and increased or not suppressed TSH levels. Interestingly, most of these patients secrete TSH together with its α-subunit. The treatment of choice is the neurosurgical approach. TSH suppression may also be achieved with triacetic acid (Triac), dopamine agonists and somatostatin. However, both medical treatment and radiotherapy are only second-line regimens.

The inappropriate TSH secretion syndrome (Refetoff syndrome) is characterized by elevated thyroid hormone secretion together with "inappropriately" high TSH levels but normal TSH α-subunit levels. In these patients, a relative resistance to the action of thyroid hormones (with reduced inhibitory feedback control), and not a TSH secreting tumor causes the TSH excess.

Gonadotropin-secreting Adenoma

The FSH- and/or LH-secreting pituitary adenoma with or without α-subunit cosecretion is, like the TSH-secreting adenoma, relatively rare.

The main clinical characteristics are menstrual disorders in women and hypogonadism (lowered or subnormal testosterone levels) with decreased libido in men. In patients with macroadenomas, symptoms related to tumor size expansion are also possible. Neurosurgery is the treatment of choice; only little experience has been made using radiotherapy and medical treatment with dopamine agonists, somatostatin, and LH-RH agonists and antagonists.

Diseases of the Posterior Pituitary

Diabetes insipidus

Diabetes insipidus is due to an absolute or relative reduction of ADH secretion. It can be familial, due to head injury (trauma or postsurgery), tumor infiltration, infections, or vascular lesions. However, the cause remains unclear in many cases. The typical laboratory findings are a specific gravity of the urine below 1005 and urinary osmolality below 300 mosm/kg. The ADH serum levels may be lowered, undetectable, or even normal. In most cases it is necessary to perform the water deprivation test. The main clinical symptoms are polyuria and polydipsia. The treatment of choice for diabetes insipidus is administration of the vasopressin analog, desmopressin acetate (DDAVP).

Syndrome of Inappropriate ADH Secretion Schwartz–Bartter Syndrome (SIADH)

SIADH is a clinical disorder with hyponatremia, excessive renal sodium excretion, and inappropriate retention of body water due to an "inadequate" excess of ADH secretion. SIADH may be caused by various tumors (e.g., small-cell carcinoma of the lung and other malignancies, especially brain tumors), respiratory disorders (e.g., tuberculosis, aspergillosis, pneumonia of various origin, bronchial asthma, and positive pressure ventilation), infections of the CNS (meningitis and encephalitis), head injury, cerebral hemorrhage, thrombosis or porphyria, as well as by several other severe diseases. Furthermore, many drugs such as vincristine, vinblastine, cisplatin, cyclophosphamide, chlorpropamide, carbamazepine, amitryptyline, phenothiazine, thiacides, chlofibrate, morphine, histamine, and others have been potentially implicated in the induction of this syndrome. Therapy should be initially aimed at removing the underlying cause. If this is not possible, fluid restriction and slow substitution of sodium is necessary. In addition, medical treatment with lithium, phenytoin, demeclocycline or oxilorphan may be used to inhibit ADH release or ADH activity.

References

1. Grossmann A, ed Clinical Endocrinology, 1st ed. Oxford: Blackwell Scientific Publications, 1992.
2. Wilson JD, Foster DW, eds. Williams Textbook of Endocrinology, 8th ed. Philadelphia: Saunders, 1992.
3. Yen, SSC, Jaffe RB, eds. Reproductive Endocrinology, 3rd ed. Philadelphia: Saunders, 1991.
4. Klibanski A, Zervas NT, Diagnosis and management of hormone-secreting pituitary adenomas. N Engl J Med 1991;324:822–31.

Radiography

W. Auffermann and S. Gust

Technique

Radiographic documentation of the sella turcica should be obtained in frontal and lateral projections. In order to avoid misinterpretation, exact positioning of the patient is a prerequisite for diagnostic evaluation. The measurement of the sella can be important when the intracranial pressure is increased, in case of direct pressure erosion or with intrasellar expanding processes. The size of the sella can be estimated from the following:

1. The craniocaudal and the anteroposterior diameters (1)
2. The area on the lateral projection (4)
3. Volumetric measurements (2) (Fig. 2.**8**)

Whereas method 1 is most easily performed, method 3 is the most exact and should be applied in suspicious cases (3).

Normal Sella

The diagnostic value of conventional radiography for the diagnostic evaluation of endocrine disorders of the pituitary gland is limited, because the variability of the normal size and shape of the sella turcica is wide (volume ranges from 240 mm^3 to 1092 mm^3 with a mean value of 594 mm^3, and the gland itself is not visible. Only indirect signs of pituitary enlargement may be visible when the bony structures of the sella turcica are affected. Nevertheless, in many centers, the radiograph is still part of the basic diagnostic schedule for the pituitary gland, because it is easy, cheap, and fast (Fig. 2.**9**).

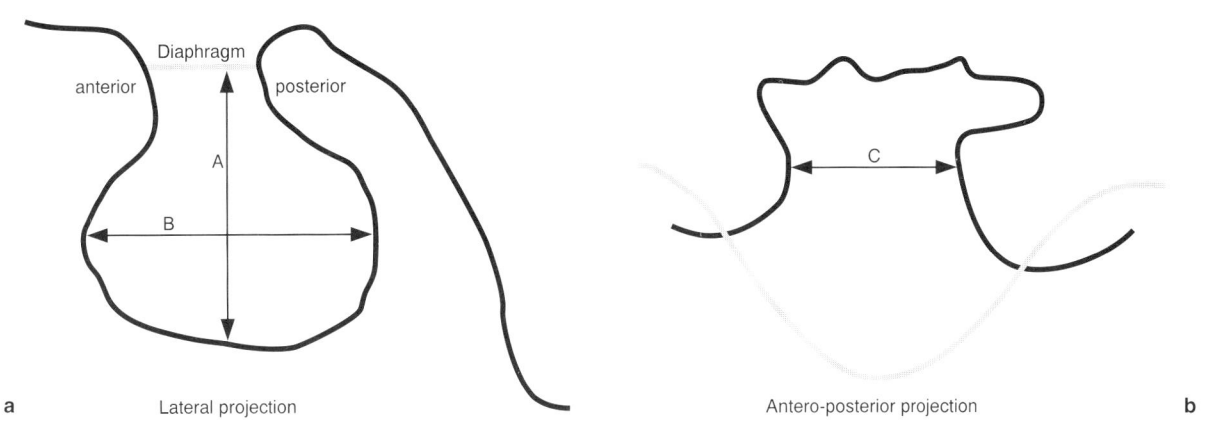

Fig. 2.8 Measurement of (**a**) craniocaudal (A) and anteroposterior (B) as well as (**b**) lateral (C) diameters of the sella turcica for volumetric estimation (1, 2)

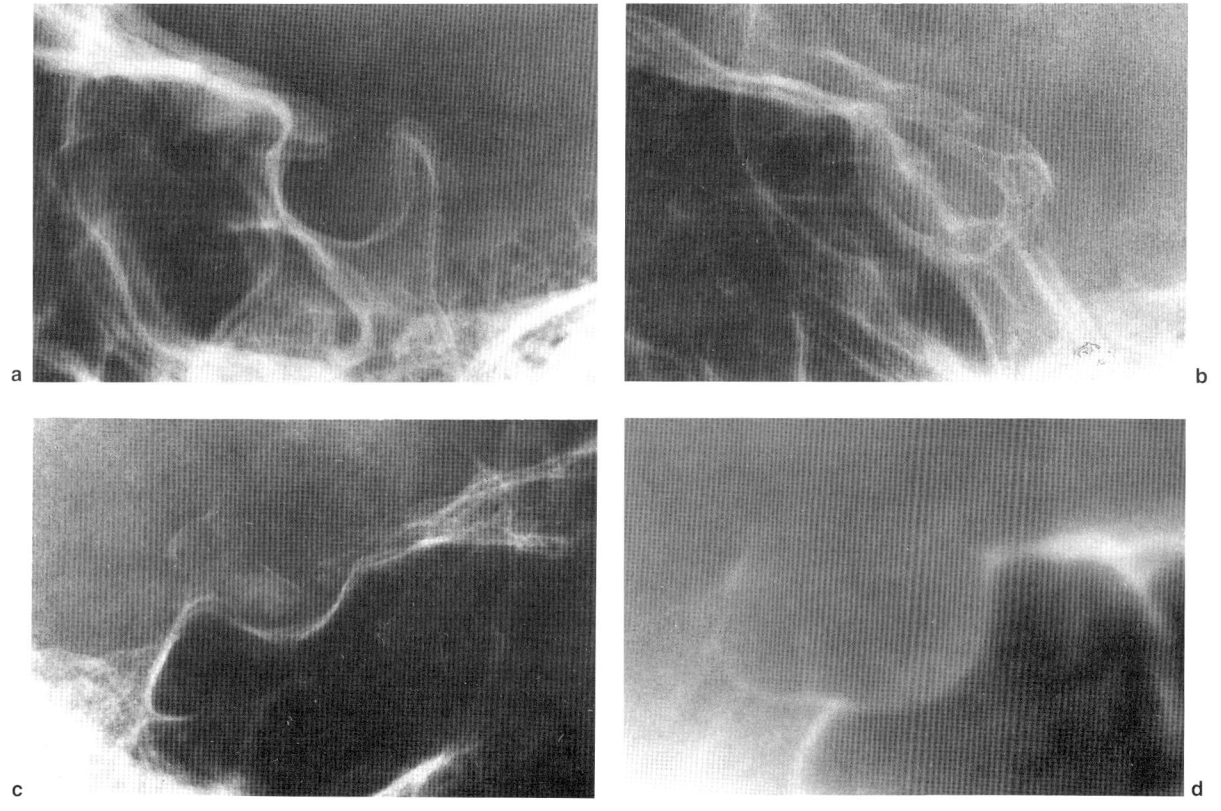

Fig. 2.9 Radiography of the sella turcica: (**a**) normal sella; (**b**) pontine sella as a normal variant; (**c**) excavation of the sella with erosion of posterior clinoid processes by increased intracranial pressure from an extrasellar lesion; (**d**) enlargement of the sella and bulging of the sellar contour by a pituitary macroadenoma

Pathological Findings

Intrasellar tumors originating from the pituitary gland can cause thinning, excavation, and a double contour of the sellar floor. The dorsum sellae can be thinned, elongated, and displaced posteriorly. All parts except the remaining clinoid processes can be eroded or destroyed. If erosion is asymmetric, conventional tomography offers supplementary information on the regional extension of intrasellar processes. Erosion of the sella turcica may be caused by pituitary adenomas as well as by craniopharyngeomas. Extrasellar processes which cause a rise in intracranial pressure can also cause excavation of the sella, but do not erode the floor or the clinoid processes of the sella. Small pituitary adenomas and particularly microadenomas may not cause a significant excavation or erosion of the sella and are not visible on radiographs. Therefore, the contribution of conventional radiography to the diagnosis of endocrine disorders of the pituitary gland remains limited.

References

1 Camp JD. Normal and pathologic anatomy of the sella turcica as revealed at necropsy. Radiology. 1923;1:65–73.
2 DiChiro G, Nelson KB. The volume of the sella turcica. Am J Roentgenol. 1962;87:989–1008.
3 Meschan I. Analysis of Roentgen Signs. Philadelphia: Saunders; 1973.
4 Silverman F. Roentgen standards for size of the pituitary fossa from infancy through adolescence. Am J Roentgenol. 1957;78:451–460.

Computed Tomography

A. Kern and U. Keske

The CT diagnosis of pituitary lesions is hampered by the complex anatomy, the close topographic connections, and the small size of the organ, which has a height of about 4 mm and a transverse extension of 5 mm × 6 mm. Extensive tumors within the pituitary grove associated with excavation and bony destruction of the sella turcica are easily recognized on the conventional radiograph, but smaller intrasellar or merely suprasellar lesions escape radiographic detection (1, 2).

The most common tumors of the sellar region are pituitary adenomas, followed by meningeomas, craniopharyngeomas, and pilocytic astrocytomas (5). Metastases, cysts, chordomas, ectopic pinealomas, malignant lymphomas, epipharyngeal tumors, and histiocytosis are found less frequently (5, 6, 8).

The evolution of CT has accelerated significantly since its introduction in 1973 and has improved the diagnostic competence of noninvasive radiologic imaging. High-resolution CT, which was introduced into the diagnostic evaluation of sellar disorders in the early 1980s, has contributed to an improvement in spatial resolution and thereby, to increased detectability of tumors. However, artifacts from beam hardening and aliasing by surrounding bony structures deteriorate image quality and hamper the evaluation of CT studies (3, 6, 8). Therefore, spatial resolution within the sella, even with modern systems, is not beyond 1.5–2.0 mm². Scanning parameters and artifact reduction techniques have to be optimized for the delineation of the sellar region.

The transverse plane is the standard CT plane for the pituitary region. According to Bonneville (2), the plane should be angled 10° anteriorly from the orbitomeatal line in order to minimize beam hardening and streak artifacts from the petrous bone. Figure 2.**10** shows the position of the standard transverse plane for the investigation of the pituitary gland compared to the orbitomeatal line.

Additional information is gained from the primary coronal plane and from secondary coronal and sagittal reconstructions. In 1986, Bonneville recommended the coronal plane as the standard view for the pituitary gland.

Since then, CT technique has advanced and improved significantly. The quality difference between primary coronal scans and secondary coronal reconstructions has diminished. Moreover, one should consider that primary coronal scans are often poorly tolerated, particularly by elderly patients, because of the required prone position or reclination of the head in the supine position, respectively. Motion and respiration artifacts may additionally deteriorate the quality of primary coronal CT scans. Dental prostheses may also result in significant beam hardening and aliasing artifacts in the coronal plane (3, 6).

Most questions can be answered sufficiently by a high-resolution thin sliced multiaxial reconstruction technique applied before and after contrast injection. Primary coronal scanning should be reserved for special indications.

For exact delineation of the anatomic structures of the sellar region, thin slices between 0.5 mm and 1.5 mm are required in the transverse as well as in the coronal plane. The reconstruction matrix should contain either 512 × 512 pixels or 1024 × 1024 pixels.

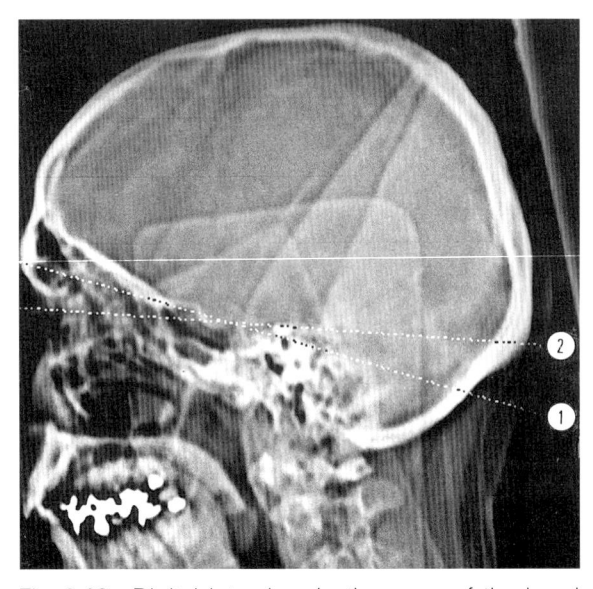

Fig. 2.**10** Digital lateral projection scan of the head with tracing of the orbitomeatal line (1) and of the standard transverse plane for the pituitary gland (2). The latter is angulated 10° anteriorly from the orbitomeatal line

Computed Tomography 19

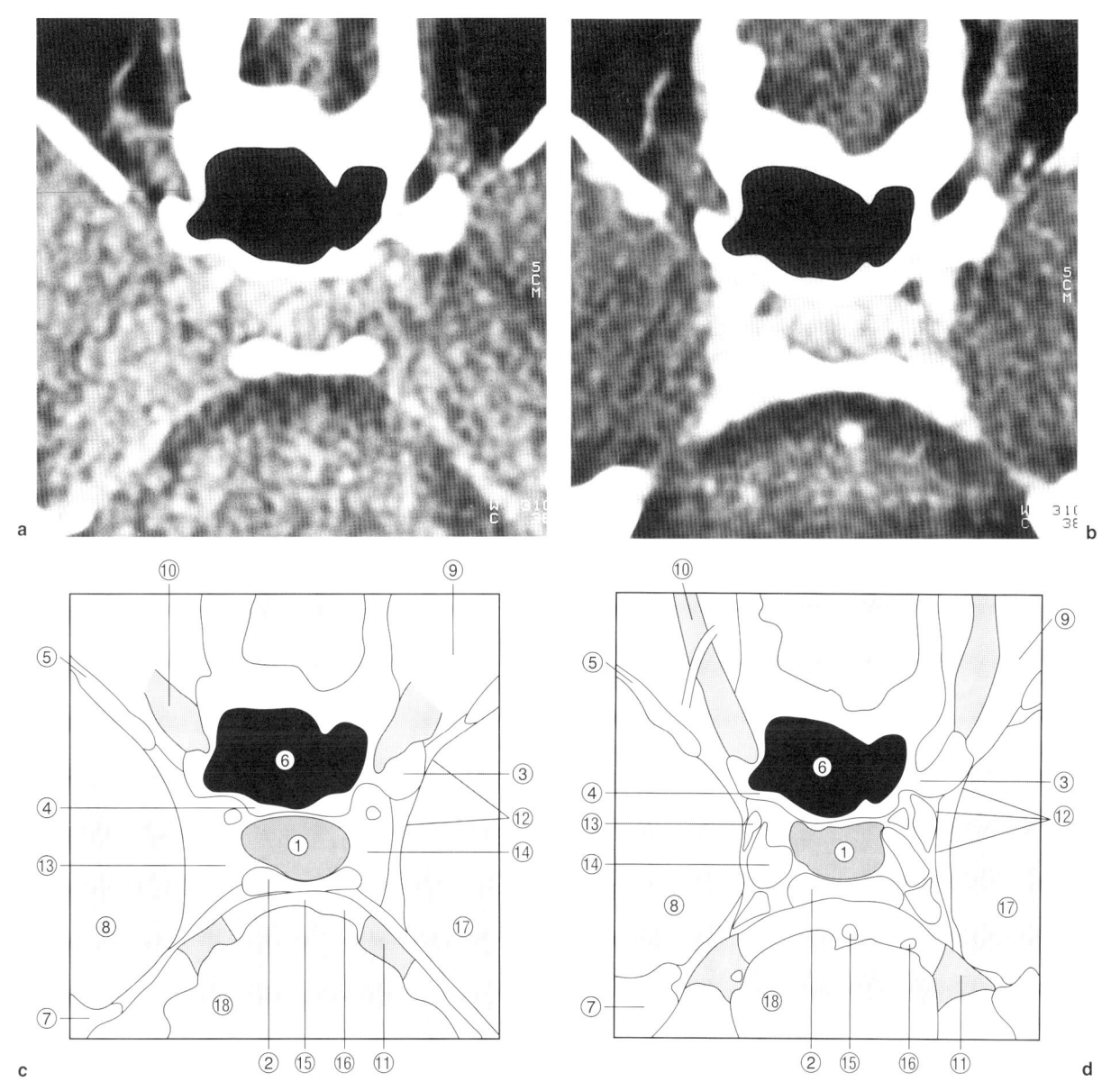

Fig. 2.**11 a** Anatomy of the sellar region in the transverse plane with 1 mm slice thickness on a precontrast scan

b Anatomy of the sellar region in the transverse plane with 1 mm slice thickness on a postcontrast scan

c Schematic drawing corresponding to (**a**) (precontrast scan). 1. Pituitary gland 2. dorsum sellae 3. anterior clinoid process 4. sphenoid limb 5. sphenoid wing 6. sphenoid sinus 7. apex of the petrous bone 8. medial cranial fossa 9. orbital funnel 10. optic nerve 11. trigeminal nerve 12. dura mater 13. cavernous sinus 14. internal carotid artery 15. basilar artery 16. pontine branches of the basilar artery 17. medial temporal lobe 18. pons

d Schematic drawing corresponding to (**b**) (postcontrast scan). For legend see (**c**)

While maintaining this matrix, the field of view (FOV) should be limited to the sellar region and the adjacent anatomic structures (Fig. 2. **11**). The zoom factor should be about 7 to 9. High-kV technique at 110–130 kV and a photon flux of 300–700 mA is recommended. This technique offers good soft tissue contrast. Scanning times are on the order of 0.7 to 5.0 seconds per slice. Spiral CT with 1 mm table feed per second may result in an additional improvement of spatial resolution.

Each study of the pituitary gland starts with a precontrast scan. Sixteen to 20 contiguous slices, 1 mm thick, are normally sufficient to cover the entire organ from the sellar floor to the hypothalamus. The study is repeated after contrast media injection (Fig. 2.**11b**). A nonionic iodine-containing agent should be given intravenously with a flow of 0.7 to 3 mL per second. Because of better bolus geometry, automatic injection is preferable to manual bolus injection. Infusion alone does not guarantee sufficient enhancement of the pituitary gland and the adjacent vascular structures. A total amount of 80–120 mL is required. If the available CT system has dynamic scanning properties, an initial bolus of 50 mL is followed by an additional 50–70 mL infusion throughout the study.

Normal Findings

Transverse Plane

Figure 2.**11** shows the anatomy of the sellar region on transverse slices of 1 mm thickness. The zoom factor is 7; the matrix has 512 × 512 pixels. A soft tissue window with a width of 310 Hounsfield units (H) and a center of 38 H is used. Figure 2.**12a** shows a precontrast scan; figure 2.**11b** a postcontrast scan.

The pituitary fossa consists of a groove in the posterior part of the sphenoid bone, which is separated anteriorly from the sphenoid sinus (6) by a thin bony lamina, the sphenoid limb (4). This bony lamina has a transverse crest: the tuberculum sellae. At their chiasmal passage, the optic nerves (10) run along the optic groove, which is located above the tuberculum sellae. The sphenoid limb, which forms the anterior border of the sella turcica, is located between the optic groove and the sphenoid plane. The anterior clinoid processes (3) and the lesser sphenoid (5) wings form the anterolateral, natural border to the medial cranial fossa (8), the medial temporal lobes (17), and the orbital tunnels (9). The sellar floor is bilaterally framed by the cavernous sinus (13), which is embedded into a duplicature of the dura mater (12) and embraces the carotid arteries (14) like a cushion. The pituitary gland is also embraced by dural structures, which coat the lateral walls of the sella turcica, the sella floor, and the upper sellar aperture. The upper sellar aperture is covered by the sellar diaphragm, which consists of a

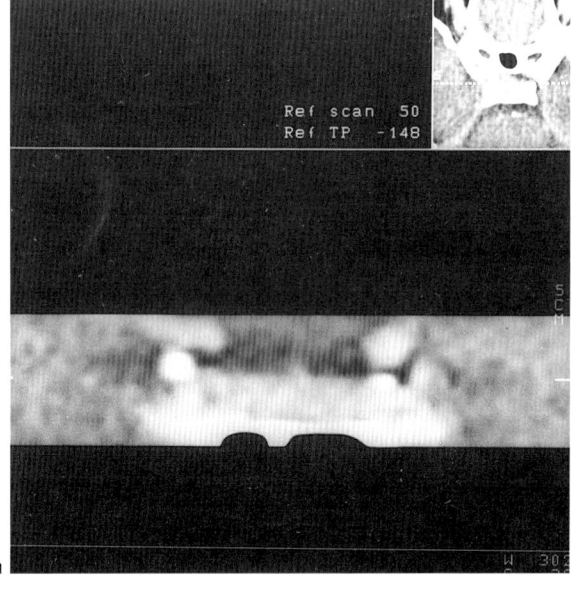

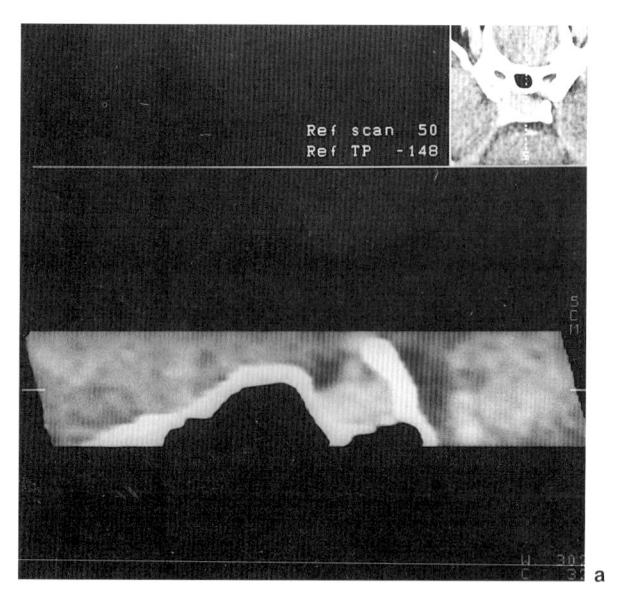

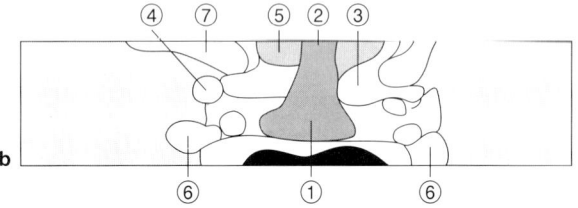

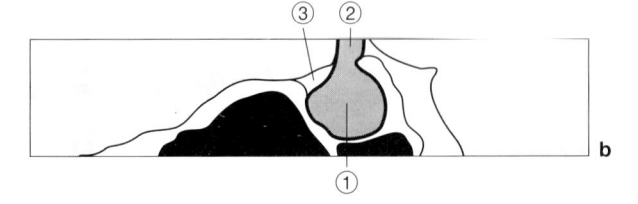

Fig. 2.**12 a** Anatomy of the sellar region, coronal reconstruction through the center of the sella from a postcontrast transverse series
b Schematic drawing corresponding to (**a**) 1. pituitary gland 2. hypophyseal stalk 3. suprasellar cistern 4. anterior clinoid process 5. optical tract 6. internal carotid artery 7. medial cerebral artery

Fig. 2.**13 a** Anatomy of the sellar region, sagittal reconstruction from a postcontrast transverse series
b Schematic drawing corresponding to Fig. (**a**). For legend see Fig. 2.**12b**

sellar duplicature. The sellar diaphragm is less than 1 mm thick and usually not visible on CT. Posteriorly, the dorsum sellae (2) separates the sellar region from the brain stem with the pons (18) and the brain stem cisterns (19). The basilar artery (15), with its pontine branches (16), runs ventrally to the pons. Ventrolaterally, the trigeminal nerve exits the brain stem and forms, below the given slice level, the semilunar ganglion (gasserian ganglion) at the medial border of the medial cranial fossa (8).

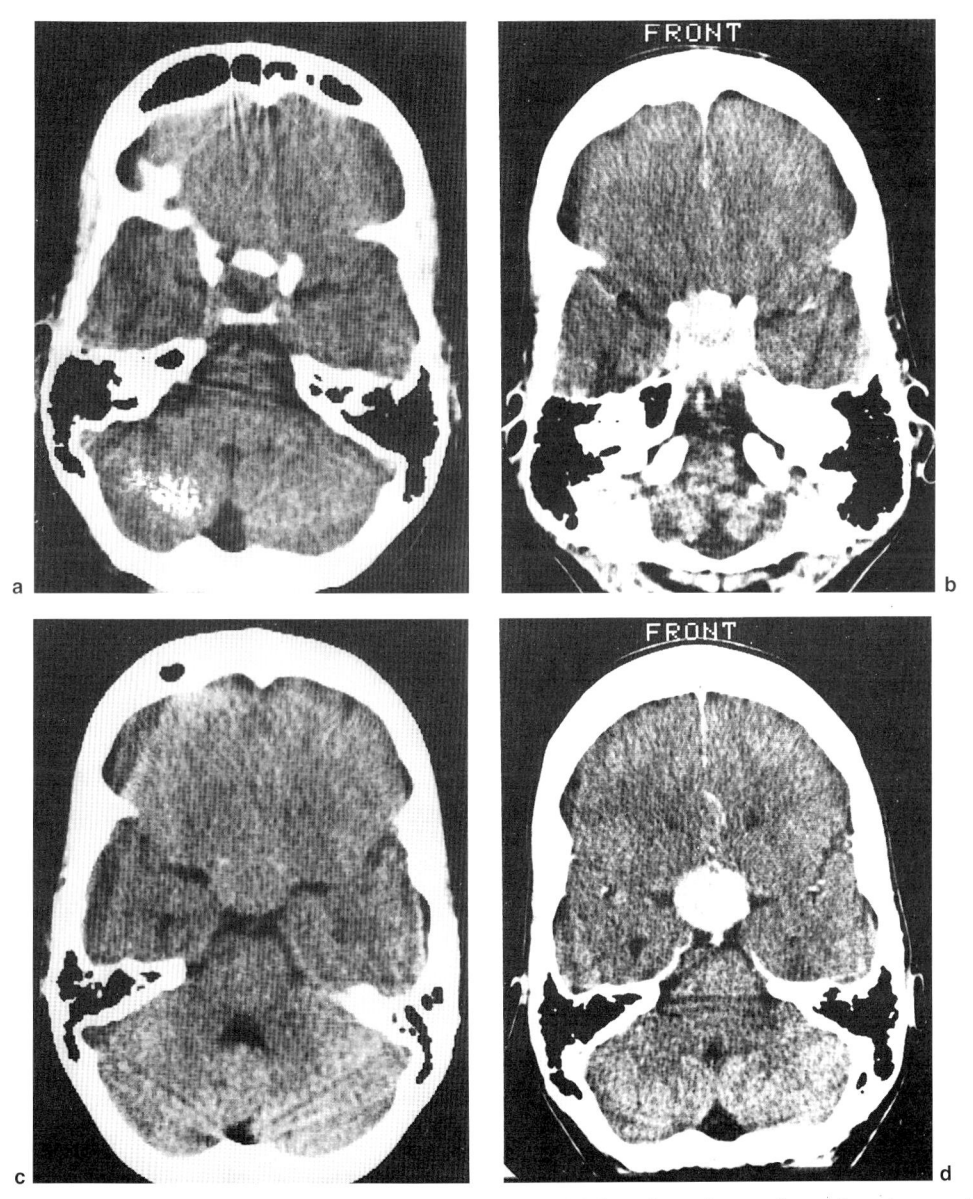

Fig. 2.**14** Solid pituitary adenoma (Prolactinoma) The 21-year-old, female patient suffered from increasing headache and visual loss for about 6 months at the time of the CT study. Clinical neurological examination discovered a chiasmatic syndrome with bitemporal hemianopsia. Serum levels of prolactin were markedly increased to 1798 ng/mL. The CT study revealed an excavation of the bony structures of the sella turcica by a round expansile mass with a density of 38–45 H (**a**). The tumor had invaded the opticochiasmatic cistern and displaced the optic chiasm (**c**). Tumor tissue was slightly hyperdense compared to the remaining brain tissue.
Following infusion of contrast media, tumor tissue enhanced intensely to a density of 88 ± 7 H (**b, d**). The basilar artery could be clearly demarcated at the posterior face of the tumor due to its intense contrast enhancement. Case # 1 demonstrates the typical solid pituitary adenoma (prolactinoma) with suprasellar growth, characterized by the bony atrophy of the sella and its isodense or slightly hyperdense structure compared to the remainder of brain tissue as well as by its strong contrast enhancement

Coronal Plane

Figures 2.**12** and 2.**13** show coronal and sagittal reconstructions from 1 mm transverse slices of the same patient as in Figure 2.**10**. The reconstruction volume has a depth of one voxel. Images are presented in a soft-tissue window centered at 32 H with a width of 302 H.

Pathology

Pituitary adenomas are classified according to size. Up to 10 mm in size, they are called microadenomas. Above 10 mm, they are called macroadenomas. According to Bonneville (3), the pituitary gland is considered pathologically enlarged if its height exceeds 8 mm. Some of the adenomas are already visible on radiographs and on conventional tomographs due to either a double contour, signs of bony erosion, or an asymmetric excavation of the sellar floor.

Depending on the tumor's extension, one should strictly separate entirely intrasellar adenomas from adenomas with suprasellar extension. The diaphragm is normally only lifted above a tumor size of 8 mm, causing invasion of the opticochiasmatic cistern. There-

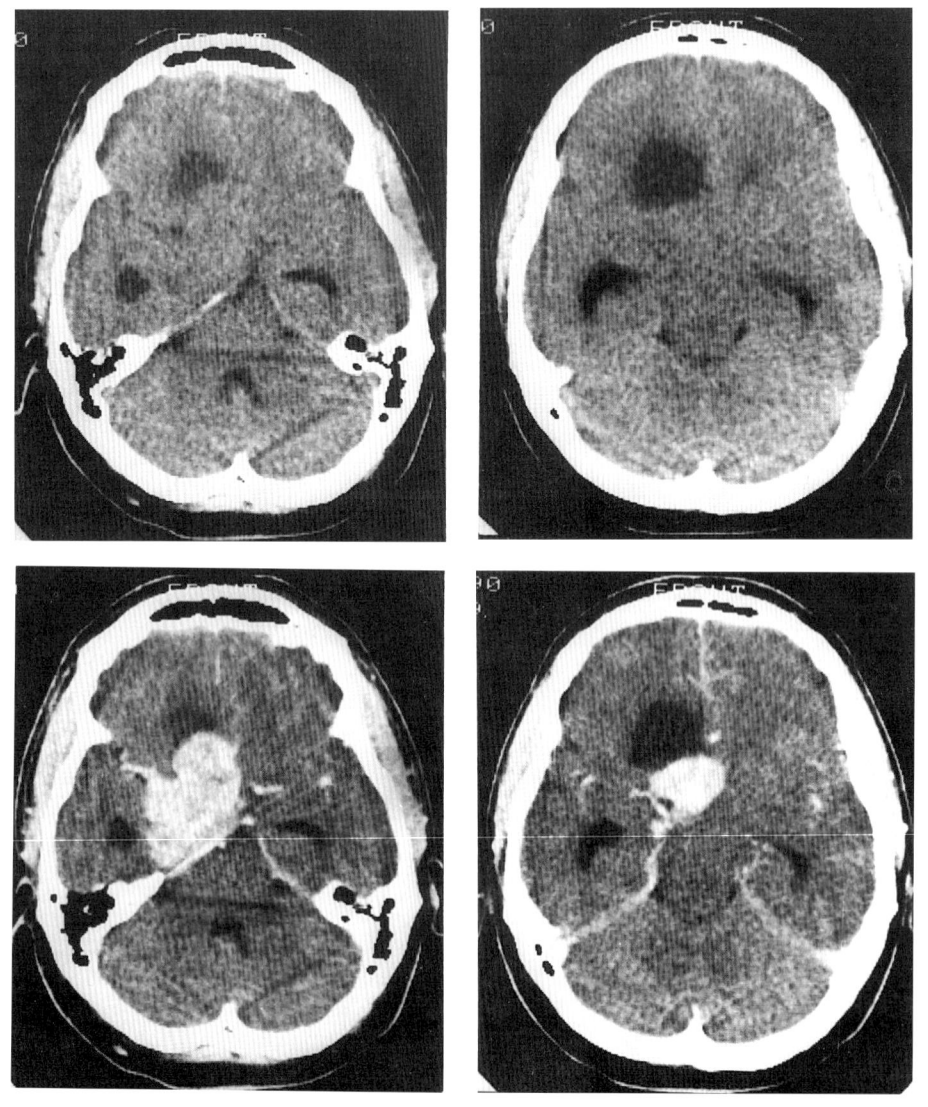

Fig. 2.**15** Solid pituitary adenoma (Prolactinoma) This 27-year-old, male patient suffered from heavy, paroxysmally increasing headache. He demonstrated a left-accentuated bitemporal hemianopsia and a distinct right-sided temporal theta-delta focus in the electrophysiologic examination. Computed tomography (**d**) demonstrated an extensive, expansile mass with intense contrast enhancement, which originates from the sella turcica, invades the opticochiasmatic cistern, and expands far into the medial cranial fossa. The tumor has embedded the right-sided cavernous sinus, the right medial cerebral artery, and the right posterior cerebral artery. Prolactin levels were excessively elevated to more than 2000 ng/mL

fore, microadenomas are strictly intrasellar, whereas macroadenomas may extend into the intra- and suprasellar region or both.

Classification of pituitary adenomas according to their histologic staining pattern into eosinophilic, basophilic, chromophobe, and mixed adenomas has been stopped recently. Since then, classification according to endocrinologic criteria is preferred; i.e., hormonally active tumors are separated from inactive tumors. For this differentiation, immunohistochemical and cell culture techniques are required (5). Prolactin, growth hormone, thyroxine-stimulating hormone, and mixed adenomas are separated. These groups of secreting pituitary adenomas are segregated from the nonsecreting ones. Nonsecreting tumors cannot be differentiated from secreting ones by CT.

CT criteria for the classification of pituitary masses are:

1. Hounsfield density
2. Contrast enhancement
3. Morphology of the lesion
4. Tumor extension and relation to surrounding structures

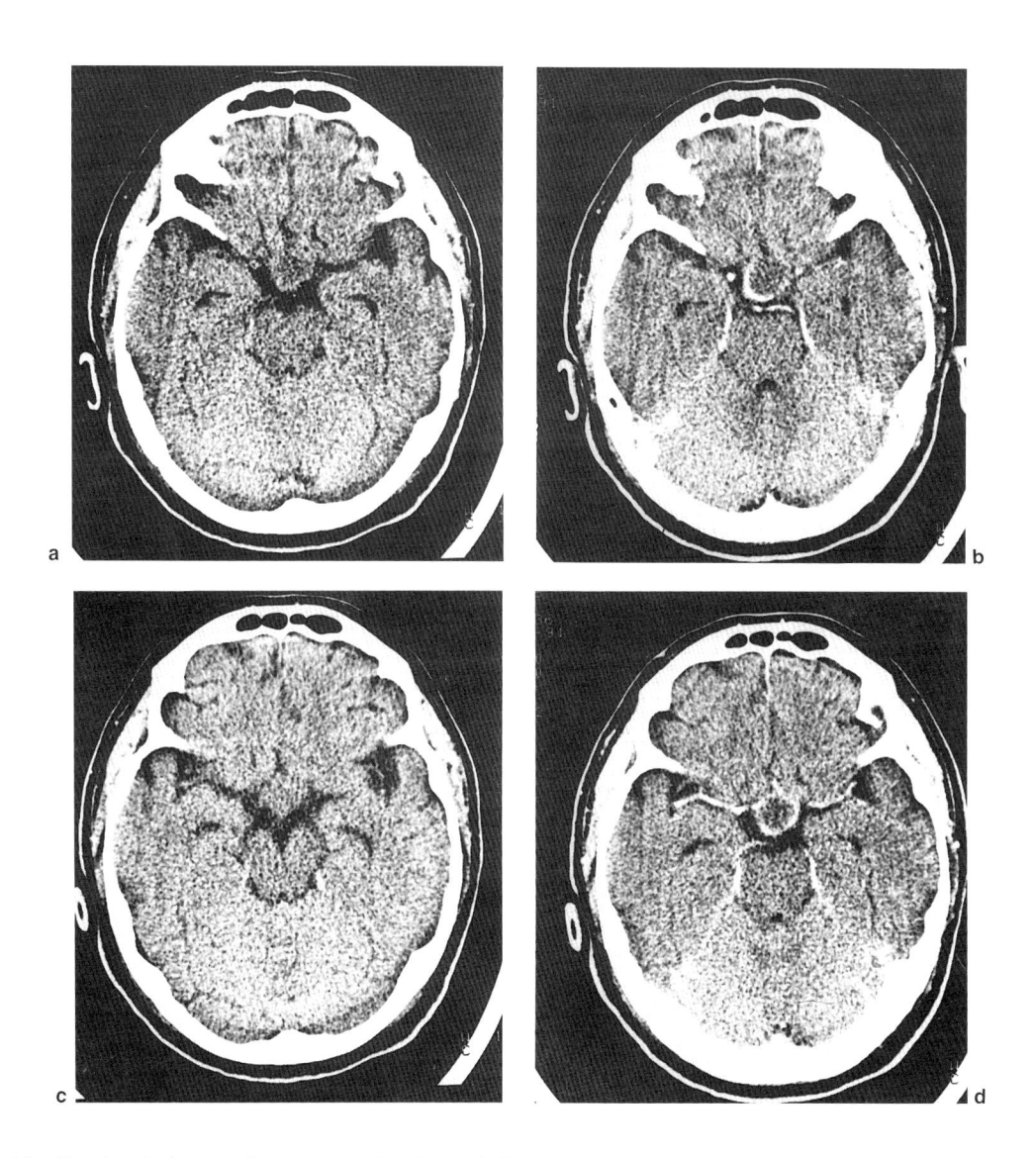

Fig. 2.**16** Cystic pituitary adenoma (prolactinoma) The 40-year-old, male patient suffered from headache, fatigue, and exhaustion. The CT shows a hypodense, expansile, centrally cystic lesion with a slightly iso- to hypodense margin. Within the suprasellar cistern, the surrounding border shows intense contrast enhancement. The tumor does not reach the medial cerebral artery. Despite displacement of the optic chiasm, no chiasmatic syndrom was present on neurologic examination

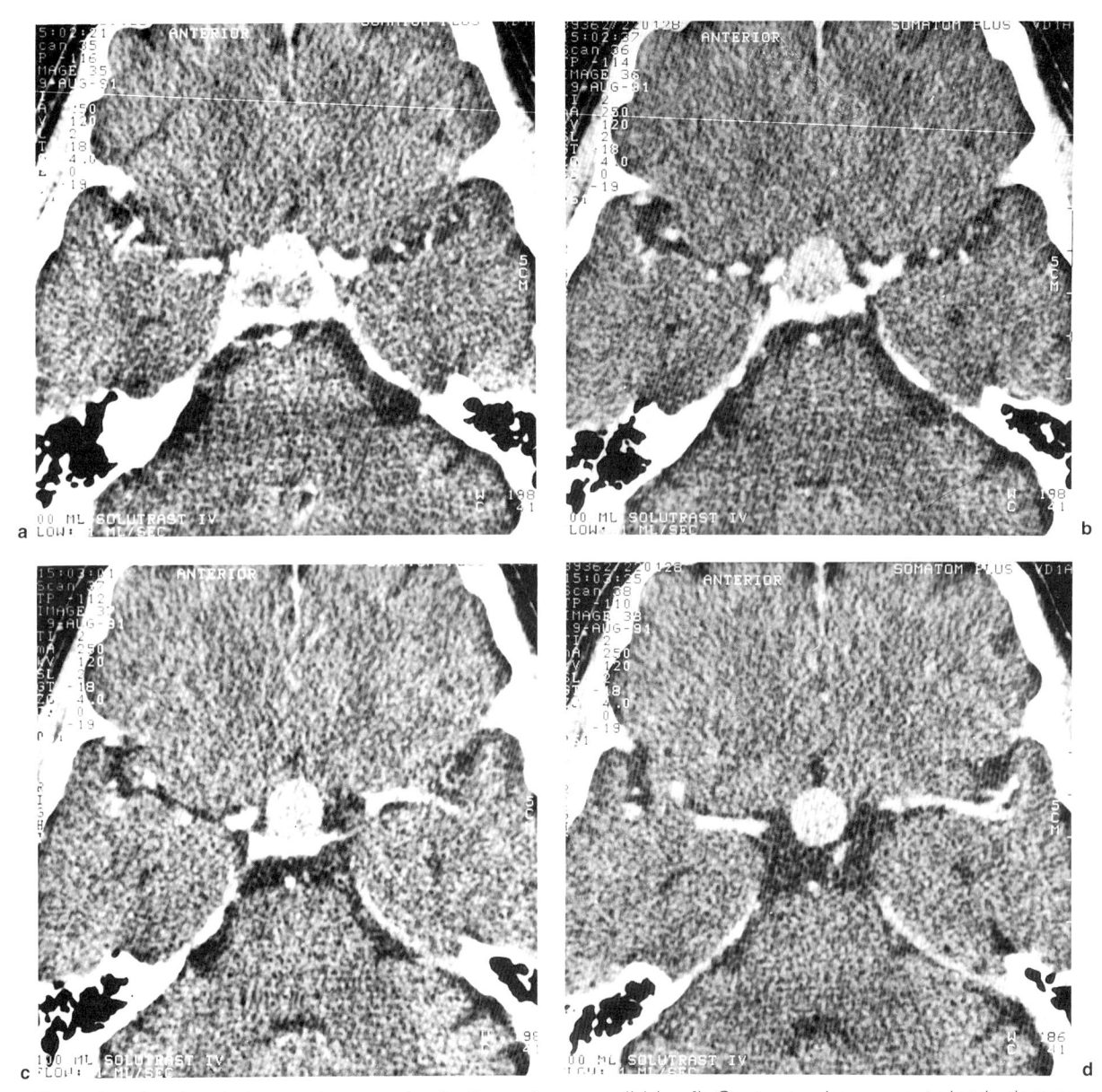

Fig. 2.**17** Cystic pituitary adenoma (prolactinoma) This 38-year-old, male patient suffered from a chiasmatic syndrom. CT revealed a partially cystic pituitary tumor at the level of the sella turcica (**a**, **b**). Those parts of the tumor lying within the opticochiasmatic cistern are solid (**c**, **d**). Contrast enhancement clearly demarcates cystic from solid tumor parts. Extensively elevated serum levels of prolactin supported the diagnosis of prolactinoma

Computed Tomography 25

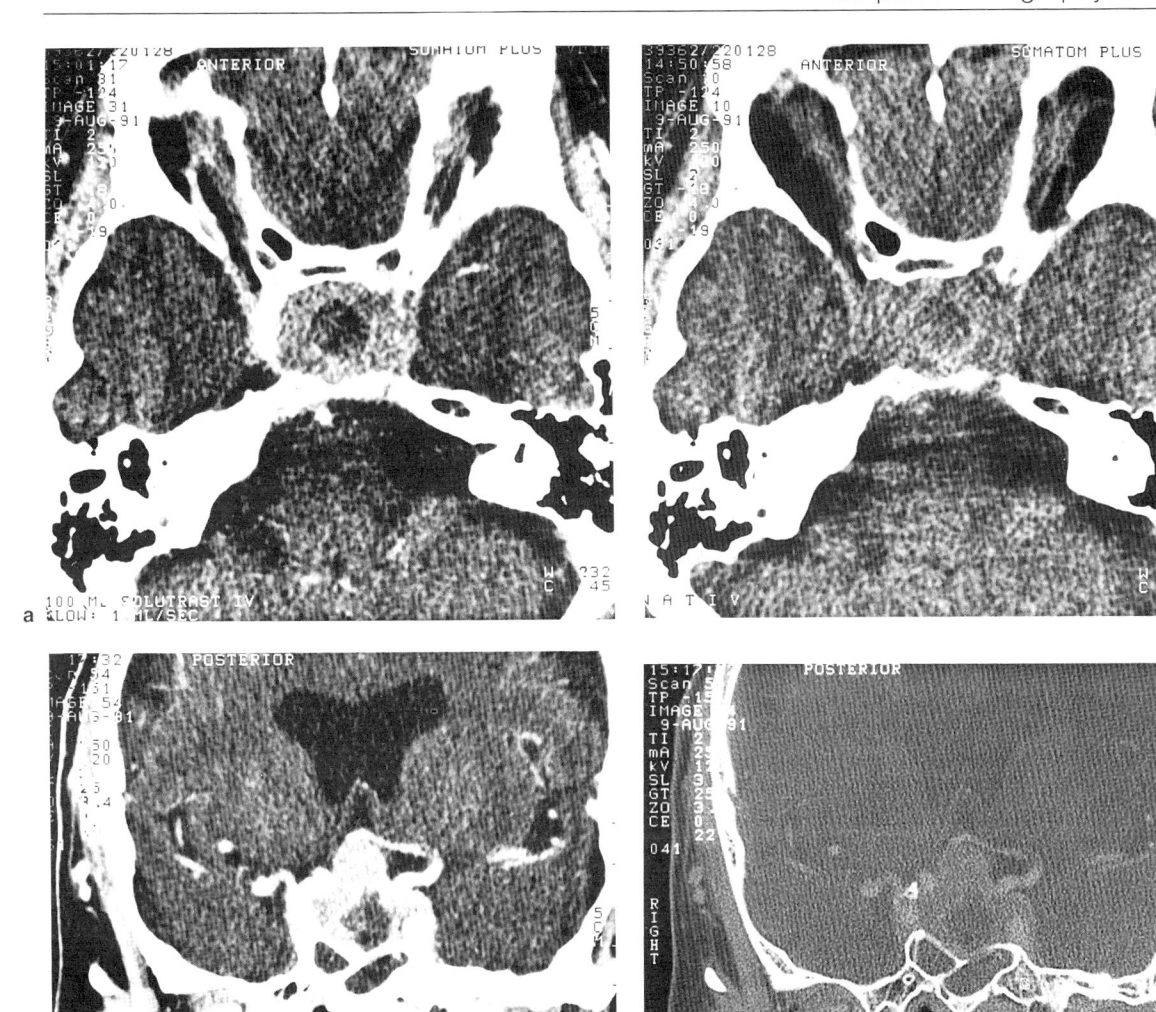

Fig. 2.**18** Cystic pituitary adenoma (prolactinoma) In this 29-year-old, male patient with a chiasmatic syndrom, CT showed a cystic as well as a solid pituitary adenoma (**a**, **b**). The contrast enhanced coronal view clearly demonstrates that the tumor has embedded the carotid arteries bilaterally, has displaced the medial cerebral arteries and has elevated the leftsided anterior cerebral artery. Bony erosion of the sellar floor towards the left sphenoid sinus is clearly demonstrated in the bone window view (**b**)

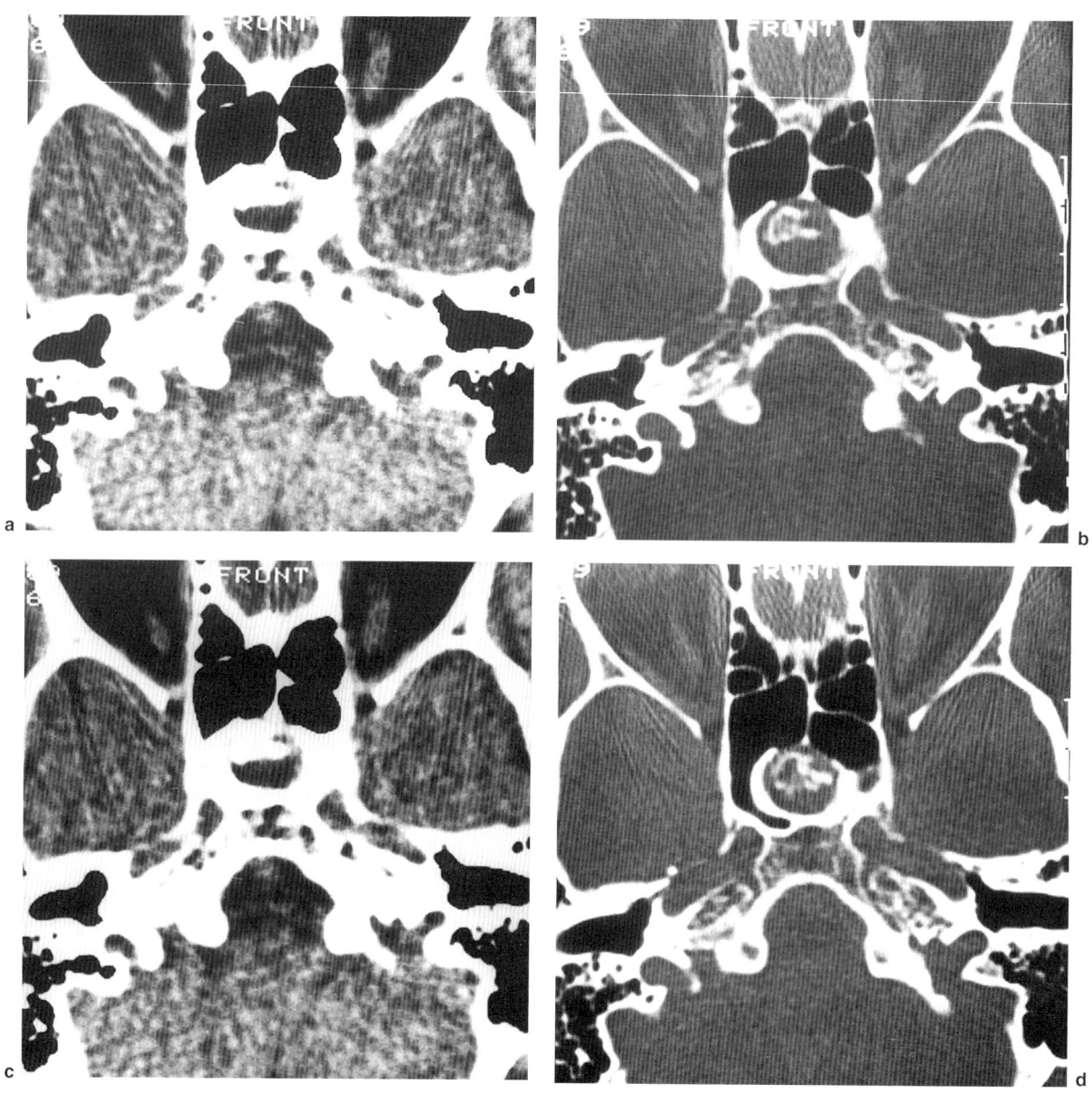

Fig. 2.**19** Calcified pituitary adenoma In this 45-year-old male patient with extensive Marie disease, CT shows a solid pituitary adenoma with plaque-shaped intrasellar calcifications (**a**, **b**). In the bone window, calcified areas can be clearly demarcated from solid tumorous portions (**b**, **d**). Those calcified areas probably represent secondary calcifications after microinfarctions of the pituitary gland

Outlook

Multiaxial high-resolution CT of the sellar and parasellar region has significantly improved diagnostic capabilities for diseases of the pituitary in recent years. A three dimensional reconstruction of the sellar region and frontal cranial base is given in Figure 2.**21**. The anatomic relation of the clinoid processes, the sphenoid limbs, and the dorsum sellae is clearly visible. This technique, however, is not suitable for three-dimensional representation of soft tissue structures. Because data input at a distinct threshold level is required, data loss may result. Figure 2.**21** gives an example of a thin bony lamella of the lamina cribrosa, which is lost after three-dimensional reconstruction, so that one can look through the floor of the anterior cranial fossa directly into the nasal cavity. The development of software techniques and the advancement of computer technology may help to eliminate current problems in three-dimensional reconstruction and should lead to a better two-dimensional resolution and improved diagnostic capability of CT for diseases of the pituitary gland.

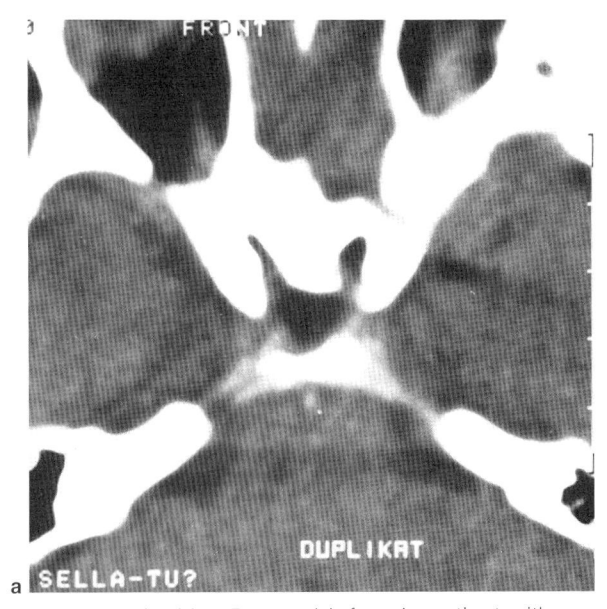

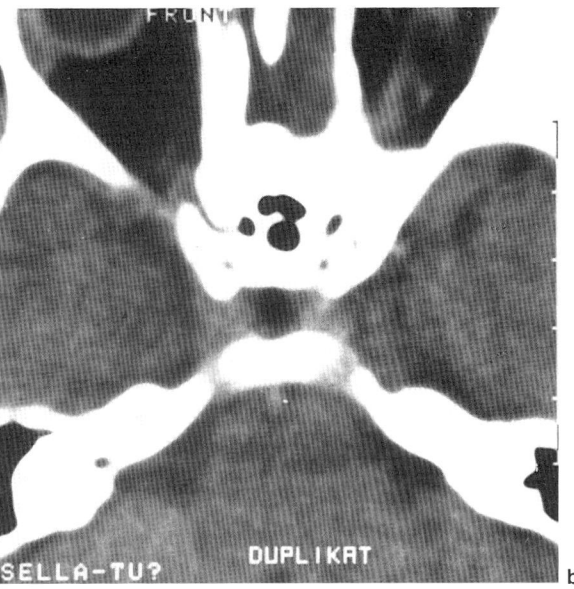

Fig. 2.**20** In this 15-year-old, female patient with unspecific headache, CT revealed a liquor-dense cystic lesion within the sella turcica, confirming the diagnosis of a primarilly empty sella (**a** , **b**)

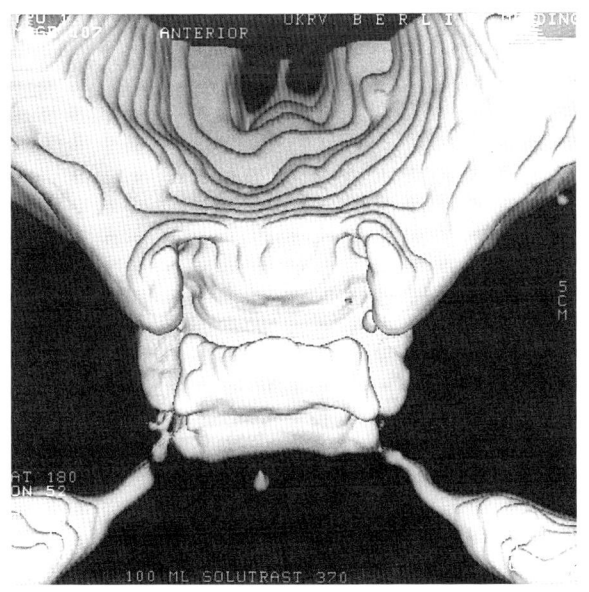

Fig. 2.**21** 3-dimensional surface reconstruction of the sella turcica from a high-resolution CT dataset of 2 mm transverse slices

References

1 Azar Kia B, Palacios E, Churchill RJ. Diagnosis of sellar and parasellar leasons by CT and other diagnostic modalities. CT. 1977;1:249–256.
2 Bonneville JF, Poulignot D, Cosch G, Portha C, Cuttin F, Bacha M. Radiological techniques in the diagnosis of microprolactinoma. In: Molinatti GM, ed. A clinical problem: Microprolactinoma. Diagnosis and treatment. Amsterdam, Oxford, Princeton: Excerpta Medica; 1982:57.
3 Bonneville JF, Cuttin F, Dietemann JL (1986). Computed tomography of the pituitary gland. Berlin.
4 Dietemann JL, Bonneville JF. Radiological diagnosis of pituitary diseases. In: Imura H, ed. Pituitary gland. New York: Raven Press; 1974:341–361.
5 Kazner E, Wende S, Grumme T, Stochdorph O, Felix R, Claussen C. Computer- und Kernspintomographie intracranieller Tumoren aus klinischer Sicht. Berlin, 1988.
6 Lange S, Grumme T, Kluge W, Ringel K, Meese W. Cerebrale und spinale Computertomographie. Berlin, 1988.
7 Rilliet B, Mohr G, Robert F, Hardy J. Calcifications in pituitary adenomas. Surg Neurol 1981;15:249–255.
8 Taylor S. High resolution computed tomography of the sella. Radiologic clinics of North America. 1982;20:183–192.
9 Vannier MW, Marsh JL, Warren JO. Three dimensional CAD for cranial facial surgery. Electronic imaging 1983;2:48–54.

MR Imaging

P. Schubeus and W. Schörner

Technique

Exact positioning of the patient is necessary to obtain a symmetrical image of the pituitary region. It is recommended to use the head coil, as surface coils provide no signal gain because of the central position of the pituitary. Slice thickness should be reduced to 3 mm or 5 mm at 1.5 T or 0.5 T, respectively. The interslice gap should not exceed 1 mm; the field of view should be reduced to 20 cm. Using a 256 × 256 matrix, a nominal anatomic resolution of 0.8 × 0.8 mm is obtained. To obtain a sufficient signal-to-noise ratio, the

Table 2.8 Applied sequences

	T1-WI	T2-WI
TR (ms)	400–500	2500
TE (ms)	15–30	70–90
NEX	3–4	1
Slice thickness (mm)	3–5	3–5
Acquisition time	5–8.5	10.5

TR repetition time
TE echo time
NEX number of excitations

number of excitations has to be increased compared to the standard protocol. Because this results in increasing acquisition time and motion artifacts, a compromise has to be found. Three to four excitations are recommended for T1-weighted imaging of the pituitary.

Contrary to MRI examinations of other brain regions, axial imaging is not the most useful imaging plane to visualize the pituitary gland. Coronal and sagittal images are preferred in pituitary imaging. Coronal images are well suited to visualize displacement of the infundibulum, asymmetric expansion of the gland, and the relationship of the carotid artery and the cavernous sinus to the tumor. The infra- or suprasellar extension of a tumor is best demonstrated on sagittal images. Furthermore, these images allow a simple correlation with conventional X-rays of the sellar region. MR examinations start with a fast sagittal "localizer" followed by coronal and sagittal imaging.

In the sellar region, spin-echo sequences should be preferred to gradient-echo imaging. Gradient-echo sequences allow for shorter acquisition times. But susceptibility, differences of brain tissue, CSF, and air-containing sinuses cause artifacts with diffuse signal enhancement or signal void, which may degrade the diagnostic value of gradient-echo images. With three-dimensional gradient-echo sequences, three-dimensionally reconstructable thin slices can be generated. Since these sequences are sensitive to susceptibility and motion artifacts as well, results are still inferior to spin-echo images.

In cerebral MRI, T2 weighting is used as a screening procedure for most pathologies. For imaging of the pituitary region, however, T1-weighted imaging is recommended as a screening technique. T2-weighted imaging of the pituitary is compromised by limited anatomical resolution and artifacts caused by CSF pulsation. Furthermore, contrast between pathologic, normal, and pituitary tissues on T1-weighted images is equal to that on T2-weighted images. Therefore, the use of T2-weighted sequences in the sellar region is restricted to cases, in which the remainder of the brain to be examined, or the consistency of pituitary tumors has to be evaluated. Cystic parts of a tumor are displayed with higher signals intensity than solid areas on T2-weighted images.

It is well known that demonstration of brain tumors in MRI can be improved by administration of Gd-DTPA, if the tumor's blood–brain barrier is impaired. After contrast administration, tumors are displayed with higher signal intensity compared to normal brain tissue, which has an intact blood–brain barrier. For the pituitary gland this is only partly true: the normal gland shows contrast enhancement, whereas different enhancement behaviors are described for pituitary tumors. As a result, demarcation of a pituitary tumor from the normal gland is not improved by contrast administration in all cases, while demarcation of the tumor tissue from the remaining brain tissue is generally improved. Contrast enhancement is therefore useful in macroadenomas, whereas the diagnostic benefit in microadenomas may be small. Contrast administration should be performed if definition of the tumor on the plain scan is poor. Contrast enhancement is not necessary in cases that are clearly defined on unenhanced images.

Normal Anatomy

The sella turcica is a saddle-shaped excavation of the sphenoid bone. It is bordered anteriorly, inferiorly and posteriorly by the sphenoid, laterally by the cavernous sinuses, and superiorly by the diaphragma sellae. The sella contains the adenohypophysis and the neurohypophysis as well as the infundibulum. The superior part of the infundibulum, the optic nerves and the optic chiasm are located in the suprasellar cistern. The cavernous sinus contains the carotid artery and the cranial nerves III, IV, V, and VI.

Bony structures are displayed without signal in MRI because of the absence of resonating protons. Therefore, the sellar floor can not be delineated from the hypointense air-containing sphenoid sinus, unless it contains swollen mucosa, which is displayed hyperintense compared to cortical bone. The dorsum sella contains hyperintense fat and is easily delineated with MRI.

The adenohypophysis exhibits intermediate signal intensity on T1- and T2-weighted images similar to normal brain tissue (Fig. 2.22). It can be visualized at the floor of the sella with a height of 3–8 mm and a flat or concave superior surface. In young or pregnant women, the superior surface can be convex and the height can be up to 10 mm. An asymmetric bulge of the superior surface, however, is always suggestive of a pituitary tumor.

The neurohypophysis is located posteriorly to the adenohypophysis and represents the smaller part of the gland. As a rule it is displayed with high signal in all sequences, which is due to a high amount of intracellular fat. In some cases, however, neurohypophysis and adenohypophysis may be difficult to differentiate from each other with MRI.

MR Imaging 29

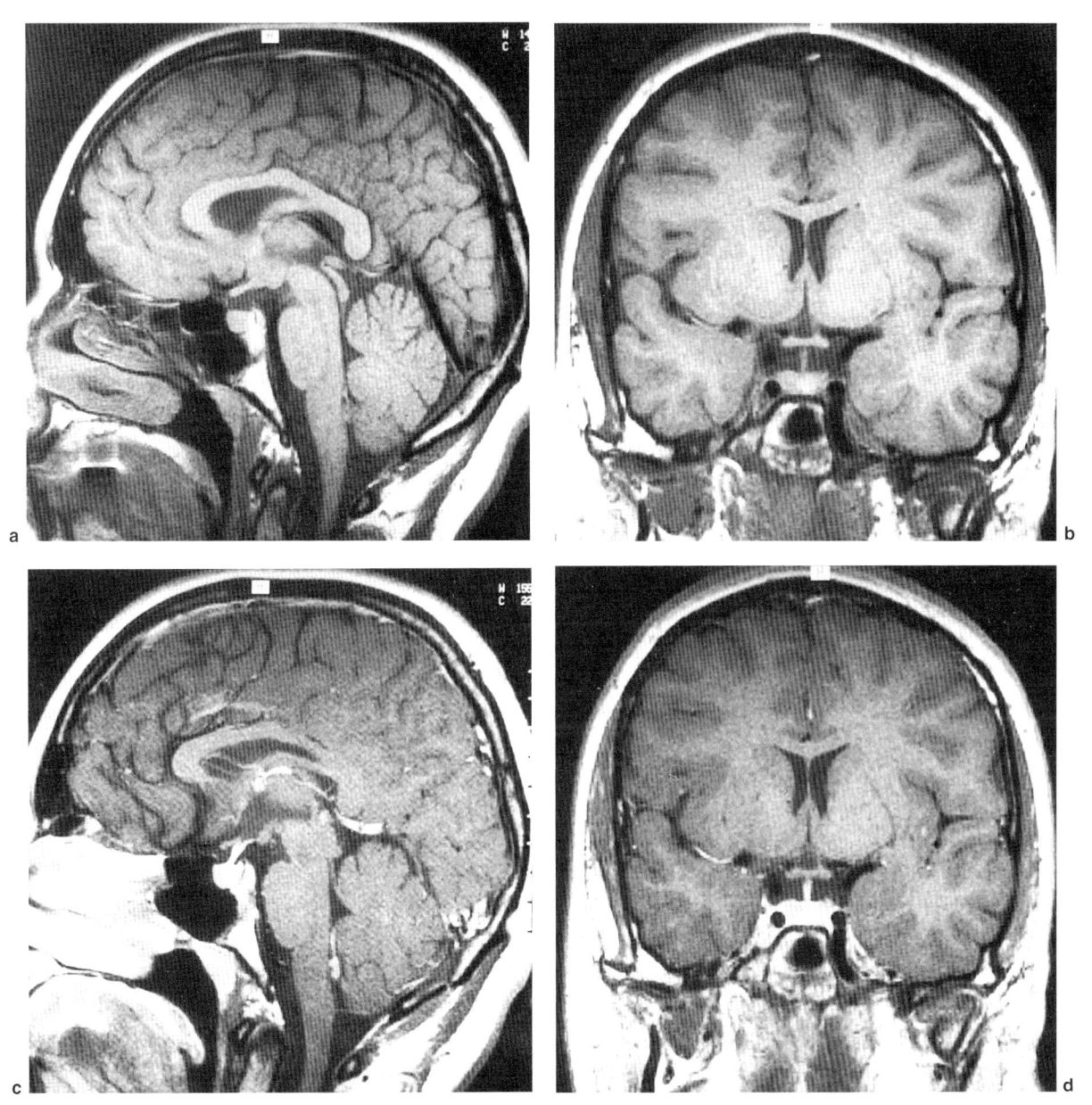

Fig. 2.**22** Normal anatomy of the pituitary gland (14-year-old girl)
a T1-weighted image, sagittal, precontrast. The sagittal image shows a flat, nonconvex superior surface of the gland and a normal suprasellar cistern
b T1-weighted image, coronal, precontrast. There is no enlargement of the gland and no displacement of the infundibulum

c T1-weighted image, sagittal, postcontrast. After contrast administration, the gland shows a homogeneous enhancement
d T1-weighted image, coronal, postcontrast. Homogeneous contrast enhancement of the gland without focal hypointense areas is also demonstrated on the coronal view

The infundibulum originates from the hypothalamus and extends from the optic chiasm to the pituitary gland. It is 1 mm to 1.5 mm thick and isointense to the adenohypophysis. Thickening and signal changes may indicate a tumor of the infundibulum. Displacement often reveals a displacement of the pituitary gland and is a sensitive, indirect sign of a pituitary tumor.

The sellar diaphragm is a horizontal structure that separates the suprasellar cistern from the sella. It is a fibrous dural fold, which is not directly visualized with MRI. With high anatomical resolution, however, it can be visible on T2-weighted images because of its high contrast to the surrounding hyperintense CSF. A displacement of the diaphragm has to be regarded as abnormal.

The suprasellar cistern contains the optic nerves, which extend from the optic foramina to a medial position and form the optic chiasm anteriorly to the infundibulum. From there, the optic tracts extent posterolaterally. The nerves are displayed with intermediate signal intensity and can easily be differentiated from the CSF. The chiasm and the optic nerves have to be evaluated for displacement or encasement by suprasellar extending tumors.

The cavernous sinuses border the sella laterally. On plain images, the sinuses exhibit intermediate signal intensity. After application of Gd-DTPA, the sinus shows marked contrast enhancement. The carotid artery is easily recognized by its signal void on spin echo images, whereas it can be displayed with high signal on gradient echo images. The cranial nerves III, IV, V, and VI can be identified after contrast enhancement at high anatomical resolution as small hypointense structures within the sinus. Other hypointense areas after enhancement may indicate tumor invasion into the sinus.

Pituitary Adenomas

Pituitary adenomas represent about 8% to 15% of all intracranial neoplasms. Most of them are benign tumors, arising from the adenohypophysis. The tumors are most common from 30 to 60 years of age. Clinical symptoms are caused by hormone overproduction or pituitary insufficiency with compression of the normal gland. Furthermore, large tumors can cause symptoms by impairing surrounding structures. Suprasellar extension with compression of the optic nerves or the optic chiasm causes scotoma, e.g., bitemporal hemianopsia or atrophy of the optic nerve. Progressive suprasellar extension may lead to obstructive hydrocephalus with compression of the third ventricle. Parasellar invasion may cause an impairment of the cranial nerves.

Secreting and nonsecreting adenomas can be differentiated by endocrinological methods. About 30% of pituitary adenomas are nonsecreting. Secreting adenomas are classified according to the secreted hormones. Prolactinomas are often diagnosed as small tumors because of their characteristic symptoms, e.g., galactorrhea or amenorrhea in women and loss of libido in men. ACTH-producing adenomas causing Cushing disease are also diagnosed early. HGH-producing adenomas lead to gigantism in children and acromegaly in adults. TSH-, FSH- and LH-producing tumors are rare.

The different forms of secreting and nonsecreting tumors can not be differentiated by MRI. Nonsecreting tumors, however, are often larger than secreting tumors, because nonsecreting adenomas only cause symptoms by suprasellar or parasellar extension. Cystic degeneration exhibits low signal on T1-weighted images and high signal on T2-weighted images and occurs frequently in prolactinomas and nonsecreting adenomas. Subacute hemorrhage exhibits high signal intensity in all sequences and is often found in prolactinomas and HGH-producing adenomas. Hemorrhage results in acute severe headache, visual loss or pituitary insufficiency. In rare cases, prolactinomas show calcifications. Calcifications may be difficult to detect with MRI because of their high signal loss.

In addition to the detection of a pituitary neoplasm, demonstration of the tumor's extent is important in planning the surgical strategy. Because of its high contrast resolution and multiplanar capabilities, MRI is the ideal preoperative imaging modality. Adenomas less than 10 mm are classified as microadenomas, those larger than 10 mm as macroadenomas. As a rule, microadenomas can be resected transsphenoidally, whereas in macroadenomas, depending on the tumor's extent, a transsphenoidal or a transcranial approach may be chosen.

Microadenomas often are only a few millimeters in size and require an optimal imaging technique. For the detection of microadenomas, direct and indirect signs are used (Fig. 2.**23**). The tumor tissue is displayed hypointense on T1-weighted and hyperintense on T2-weighted images compared to normal pituitary tissue in most cases. After contrast administration, the tumor initially remains hypointense, but may become hyperintense on delayed images. Therefore, contrast-enhanced images have to be acquired in the initial phase after contrast administration to detect microadenomas. The tumor can be located laterally from the gland or in the center of the gland. In cases of Cushing disease, the gland is often diffusely enlarged. A convex-shaped superior surface of the gland suggests an adenoma, especially if the bulge is asymmetric. Furthermore, an asymmetric inferior surface of the gland and a displaced infundibulum are indicative of a microadenoma. Microadenomas may invade the sphenoid sinus and the cavernous sinus. Regressive changes such as cysts and hemorrhage are identified by their characteristic signal intensity patterns.

Macroadenomas may have large suprasellar, parasellar and retrosellar extension and impair adjacent structures (Figs. 2.**24** and 2.**25**). Preoperatively, it has to be evaluated, whether the tumor is resectable transsphenoidally or a craniotomy has to be performed. Small tumors with sharp margins can often be resected transsphenoidally, whereas encasement of the optic chiasm, the optic nerves or the carotid artery (Fig. 2.**26**), requires transsphenoidal surgery.

Like microadenomas, macroadenomas appear hypointense on T1-weighted and hyperintense on T2-weighted images compared to normal brain tissue. After application of Gd-DTPA, macroadenomas are

MR Imaging 31

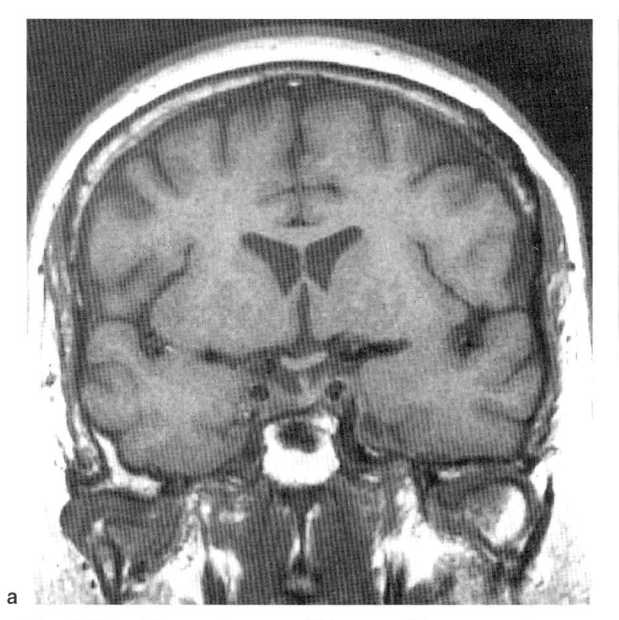

Fig. 2.**23** Microadenoma (64-year-old woman, hyperprolactinemia)

a T1-weighted image, coronal, precontrast. Displacement of the infundibulum to the left side and right-sided downward bulging of the intrasellar soft tissue indicate a microadenoma on the plain image

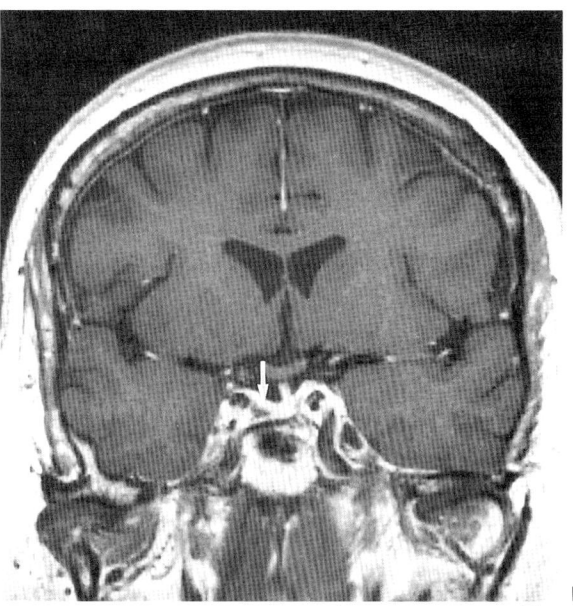

b T1-weighted image, coronal, postcontrast. After contrast administration, demarcation of the hypointense microadenoma (arrow) from the enhancing gland is improved

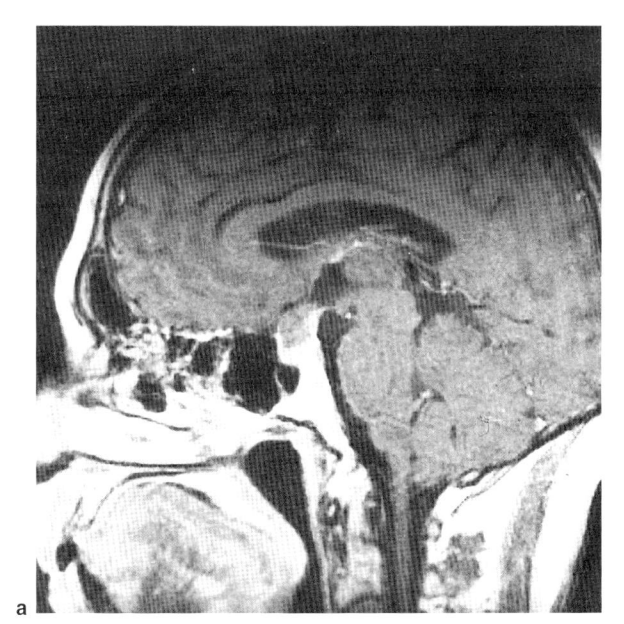

Fig. 2.**24** Macroadenoma with suprasellar extension (59-year-old woman, bitemporal hemianopsia)

a T1-weighted image, sagittal, postcontrast. An intrasellar mass with suprasellar extension is demonstrated

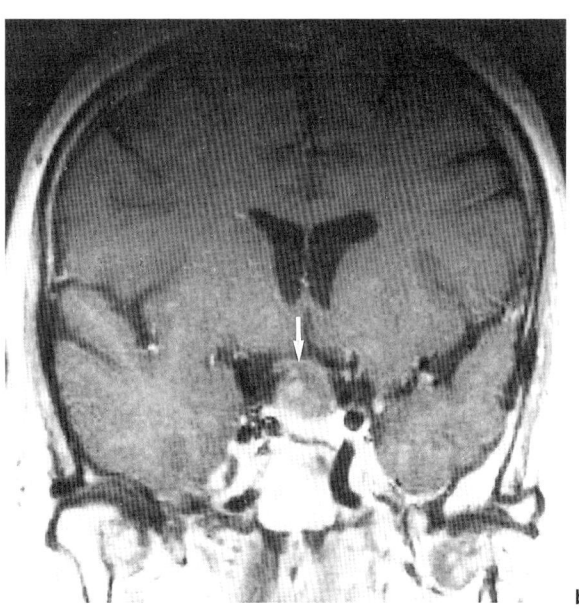

b T1-weighted image, coronal, postcontrast. The coronal view reveals impairment of the optic chiasm (arrow). There is no evidence of a parasellar extension

32   2 Pituitary

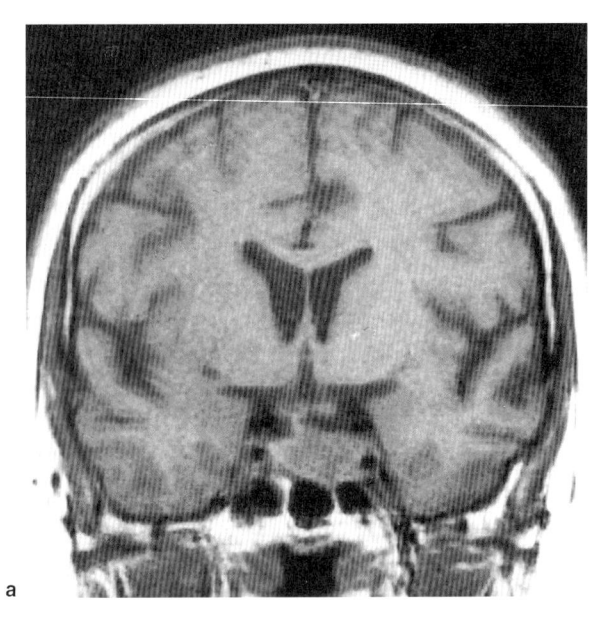

Fig. 2.**25** Macroadenoma with parasellar extension (62-year-old woman, nonsecreting adenoma)
a T1-weighted image, coronal, precontrast. On the plain image an intrasellar mass is demonstrated on the left side. There no suprasellar extension, the parasellar extension cannot be determined

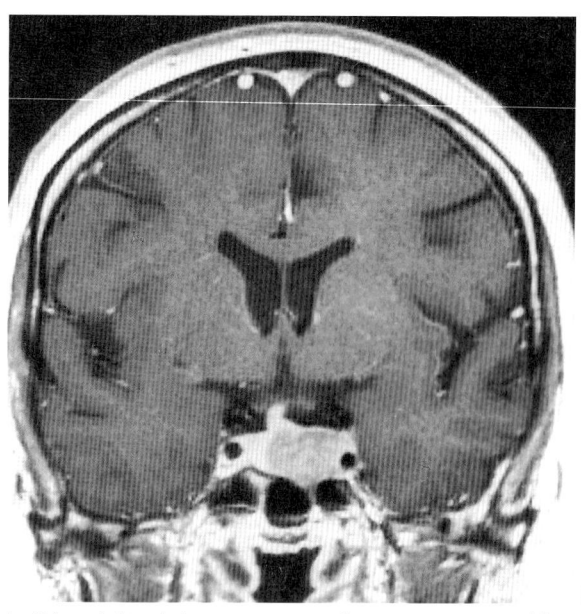

b T1-weighted image, coronal, postcontrast. After contrast administration, the tumor appears hypointense compared to the cavernous sinus. The tumor infiltrates the left cavernous sinus

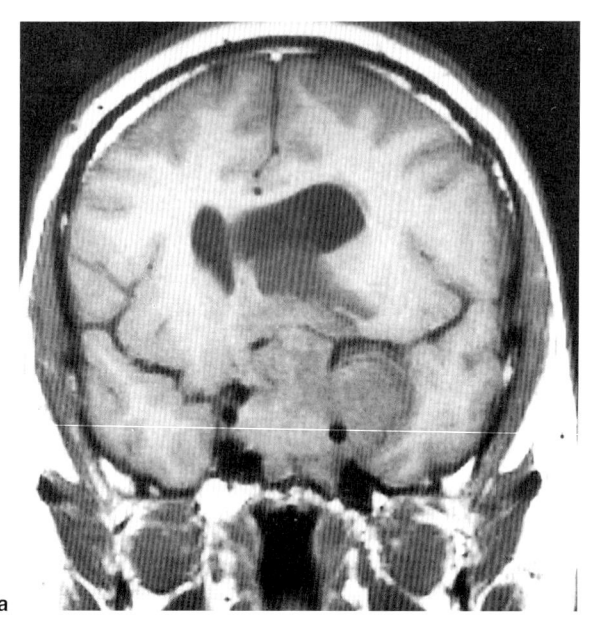

Fig. 2.**26** Macroadenoma with encasement of the carotid arteries (48-year-old patient, hyperprolactinemia)
a T1-weighted image, coronal, precontrast. On the precontrast image an intra-, para- and suprasellar mass is demonstrated, but demarcation from the surrounding brain tissue is not sufficient

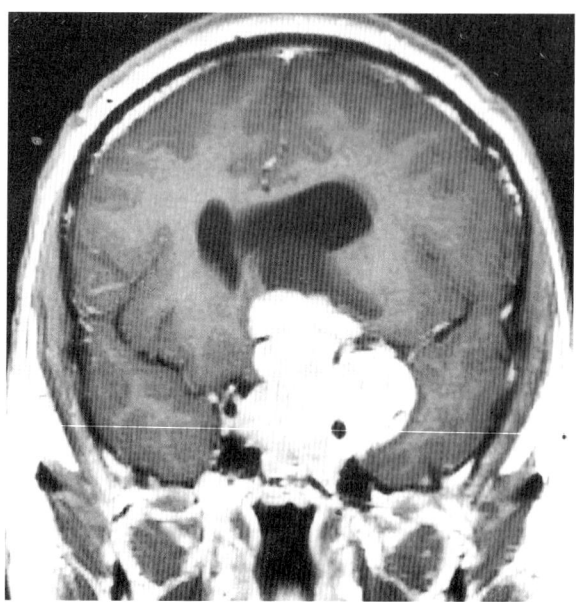

b T1-weighted image, sagittal, precontrast. After contrast administration, the tumor tissue shows intensive enhancement. Both carotid arteries are encased by the huge prolactinoma. Furthermore, there is no demarcation of the optic chiasm

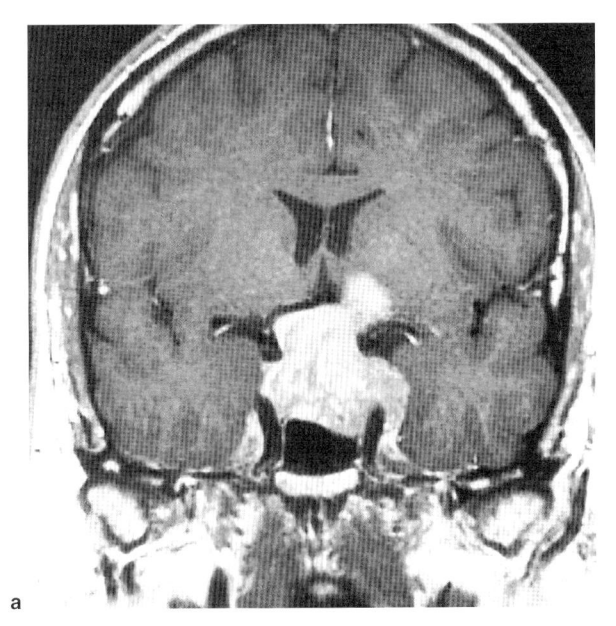

Fig. 2.**27** Postoperative follow-up (53-year-old man, right-sided visual loss)
a Preoperative T1-weighted image, coronal, postcontrast. A macroadenoma with supra- and parasellar extension is demonstrated. No definition of the optic chiasm

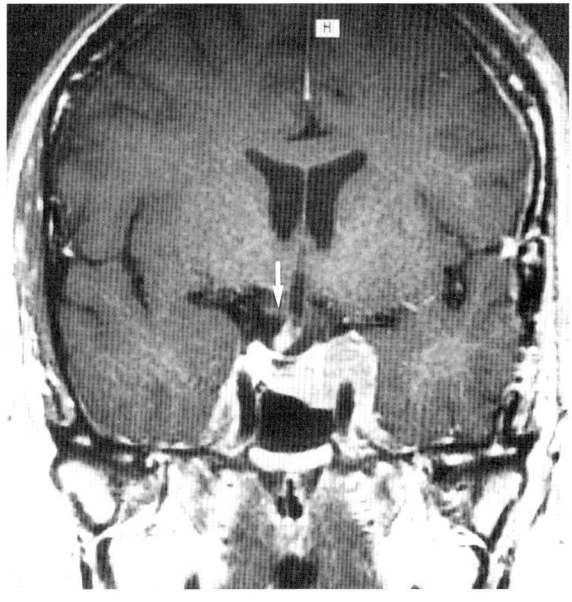

b Postoperative T1-weighted image, coronal, postcontrast. After the suprasellar portion of the tumors has been resected, the chiasm can be clearly defined (arrow). However, there is evidence of residual intra- and parasellar tumor

displayed with higher signal intensity than brain tissue. In large tumors, the normal gland is often not detectable. Regressive changes like hemorrhage or cysts in macroadenomas are more frequent than in small tumors. Large cysts may even show a fluid–fluid level.

In addition to its preoperative value, MRI is useful in posttherapeutic evaluation (Fig. 2.**27**). Except prolactinomas, which can be treated conservatively, patients with pituitary adenomas have to be referred to surgery. If no MR examination has been performed immediately after surgery, tumor recurrence may be difficult to detect. Asymmetry of the gland or the infundibulum as well as soft tissue in the sphenoid sinus may reflect postoperative changes. Extrasellar masses, however, indicate residual or recurrent tumor tissue. If a baseline postoperative examination is available, any progressive mass effect is suggestive of a recurrent tumor, whereas postoperative scar tissue generally retracts.

Differential Diagnosis

Pituitary adenomas have to be differentiated from other sellar pathologies. The lesions may affect the sella either primarily or secondarily.

Empty Sella

The "empty sella" represents a herniation of the suprasellar cistern into the sella, caused by a natural or acquired defect of the sellar diaphragm. A flattening of the pituitary gland results, which may be accompanied by hormonal disturbance. With MRI a crescent-shaped gland is found at the floor of an "empty" sella (Fig. 2.**28**). The infundibulum is located close to the dorsum sella, but does not show any midline shifting.

Cysts

Intrasellar cysts are arachnoid cysts or they arise from the Rathke cleft. Clinical symptoms may be caused by displacement of the gland, the infundibulum, or the chiasm. In MRI, the signal intensity of arachnoid cysts is similar to that of CSF. Differentiating these cysts from cystic tumors may be difficult. Rathke cleft cysts arise from the pars intermedia and most of them remain small. Because of their mucoid content, these cysts often exhibit high signal intensity in all sequences.

Craniopharyngeomas

Most craniopharyngeomas are suprasellar tumors with secondary extention into the sella, but primary intrasellar tumors occur as well. Craniopharyngeomas

34   2 Pituitary

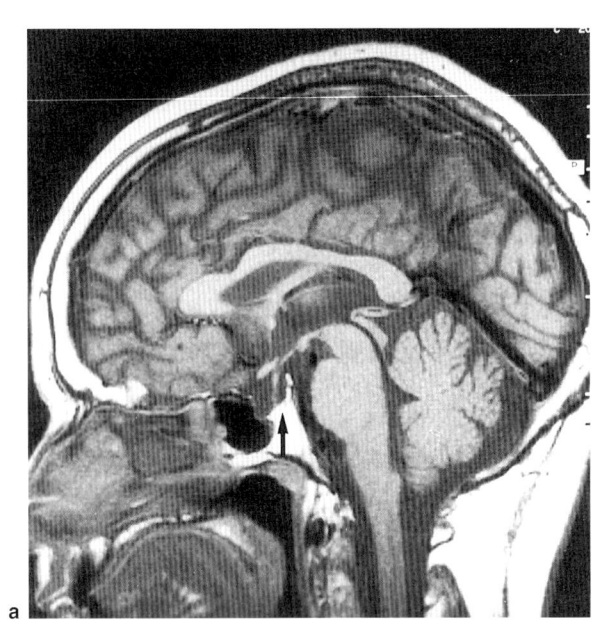

Fig. 2.**28** Empty sella (48-year-old man, pituitary insufficiency)
a T1-weighted image, sagittal, precontrast. The gland is demonstrated at the floor of the sella and is crescent shaped (arrow). The sella seems to be "empty"

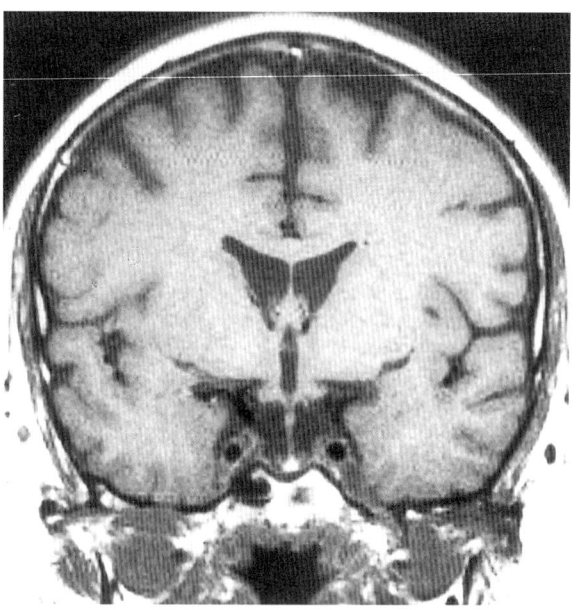

b T1-weighted image, coronal, precontrast. The infundibulum is oriented vertically without any midline shifting

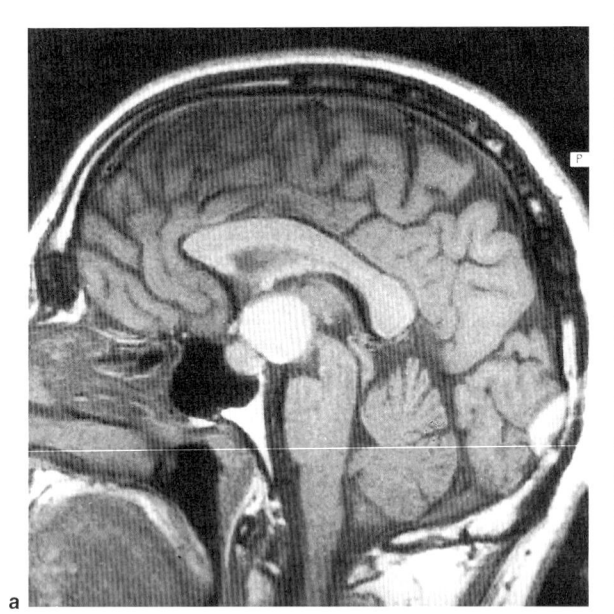

Fig. 2.**29** Craniopharyngeoma (36-year-old patient, visual disturbance)
a T1-weighted image, sagittal, precontrast. A cystic intra- and suprasellar mass is demonstrated. The content of the cyst is hyperintense compared to normal brain tissue

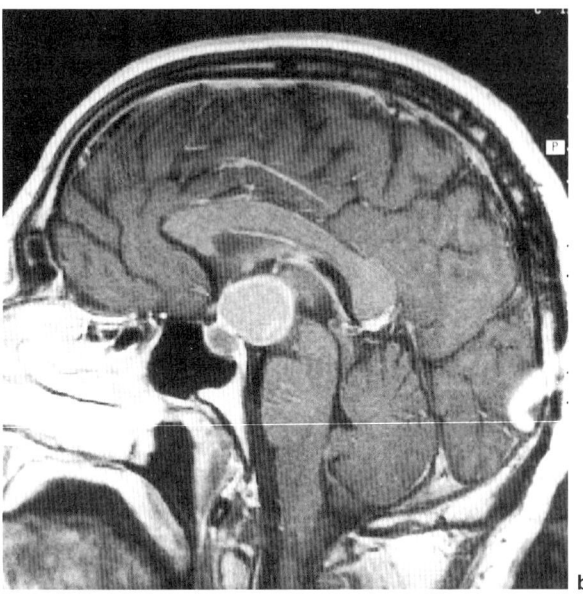

b T1-weighted image, sagittal, postcontrast. The cyst shows a rim-shaped enhancement. There is no evidence of solid tumor parts

are relatively rare and comprise about 1% of all intercranial tumors. Contrary to pituitary adenomas, these tumors are more common at an early age. Craniopharyngeomas may cause pituitary insufficiency, visual impairment, hydrocephalus and hypothalamic disturbance. With MRI, they can be differentiated from pituitary adenomas by their consitency and location. As a rule, large cysts are visible, and can be signal intense because of hemorrhage or high cholesterol levels (Fig. 2.**29**). Typical calcifications are demonstrated as areas of signal loss. Solid parts of the tumor show intensive contrast enhancement.

Meningeomas

Most meningeomas are benign tumors, which occur frequently in elderly women. Suprasellar meningeomas may expand into the sella, but primary intrasellar tumors occur as well. They can cause symptoms by impairing the cavernous sinus and the chiasm. In MRI, meningeomas show close contact to meningeal structures and an intense contrast enhancement. Furthermore, these tumors are accompanied by osteoplastic changes with no enlargement of the sella.

Gliomas of the Optic Nerve

Gliomas of the optic nerve mainly occur at an early age and are frequent in patients with Recklinghausen disease. They rarely expand into the sella. In MRI, the tumors are hypointense on T1-weighted images and hyperintense on T2-weighted images compared to normal brain tissue. Their extension along the optic nerves and their low contrast enhancement are characteristic, whereas, contrary to craniopharyngeomas, cysts and calcifications are not present in gliomas of the optic nerve.

Aneurysms

Aneurysms of the intracranial arteries may be located within the sella. Prior to pituitary surgery the presence of an aneurysm has to be ruled out. MRI has proven accurate in this question, so that preoperative angiography can be omitted in most cases. Perfused parts of the aneurysm are signal-free on spin-echo images, whereas thrombotic areas are hyperintense.

Rare Causes of Pituitary Disturbance

Chordomas and gliomas of the hypothalamus may invade the sella. These tumors can be identified with MRI according to their location. Furthermore, the pituitary gland can be affected by malignant lymphomas or metastases. These tumors are diagnosed analogically to other brain regions, considering MR findings and clinical history. Rarely, primary or postoperative inflammatory pituitary lesions may cause endocrinologic disturbance. In these cases, the correct diagnosis can only be made considering the clinical course of the patient.

References

1 Brant-Zawadski M, Norman D. Magnetic resonance imaging of the central nervous system. New York: Raven; 1987.
2 Huk WJ, Gademann G, Friedmann G. Magnetic resonance imaging of central nervous system disease. Berlin/Heidelberg: Springer; 1990.
3 Kazner E, Wende S, Grumme T, Stochdorph O, Felix R, Claussen C. Computed tomography and magnetic resonance tomography of intracranial tumors. Berlin/Heidelberg: Springer; 1989.
4 Lange S, Grumme T, Kluge W, Ringel K, Meese W. Cerebral and spinal computerized tomography. Berlin: Schering; 1989.
5 Pomeranz SJ. Craniospinal magnetic resonance imaging. Philadelphia: WB Saunders; 1989.
6 Wehrli FW, Shaw D, Kneeland JB. Biomedical magnetic resonance imaging. New York: VCH; 1988.

Angiography

H.P. Molsen

Technique

Transarterial catheterization of the internal carotid artery is the usual approach in the angiographic visualization of the sella region. If the transfemoral approach is selected, the carotid artery can be visualized bilaterally as opposed to direct puncture in the neck area, which used to be the standard procedure. More recently, an approach via the brachial artery has gained importance. Thanks to greater technical sophistication, thin catheters can be used and the angiographic investigation can be carried out on an outpatient basis, obviating the bedrest required after puncture of the femoral artery.

Although the arterial as well as the venous phase can be assessed in transarterial angiography, contrast enhancement of the cavernous sinus, which encompasses the pituitary gland, is usually not sufficient. If the indication requires this, visualization with a venous approach may be necessary, along with the approaches used for intervention in this area, e. g., arteriovenous fistulas in the cavernous sinus. Possible access modes may be provided by a frontal vein, the angular vein, and in particular, the transfemoral–transjugular approach via the inferior petrosal sinus to the cavernous sinus.

From a radiological point of view, DSA sets the quality standard for angiographic investigations. Because the pituitary region poses some problems in angiographic delineation due to the bony superimposition of the base of the skull, photographic subtraction technique was implemented a number of years ago. However, this procedure could only be realized after the intervention had already taken place (Fig. 2.**31**). DSA makes an immediate evaluation during the investigation possible and thus, a targeted delineation of pathological findings. If optimal equipment is available, such as a high-resolution 1024 × 1024 matrix, finely delineating conventional angiography, including magnification angiography, is abundant.

An intravenous survey of the whole skull with overlapping and unfocussed simultaneous demonstration of all intracranial arteries is insufficient for the sellar region. Intraarterial selective angiography, however provides considerably more information. It is still too early to determine the extent to which MR angiography will be able to replace catheter angiography, one prerequisite for this is the development of more sophisticated technology.

It is in part due to the high-resolution and strong contrast enhancement of the DSA technique that the sophistication of catheter material for selective and possibly superselective angiography has reached a point at which 4-5 French catheters can be used. This has the advantage that only small amounts of contrast medium have to be administered. The usual tip configuration of the catheters used for cerebral angiography is used. In special situations, for example, arteriovenous fistulae, aneurysms, or tumors in the sellar region, superselective angiography via microcatheters may be required, especially if embolization is being considered (4, 6).

The isotonic contrast media that are currently used are also employed for selective and superselective (Fig. 2.**33**) angiography of the sellar region. The amounts of contrast medium and the concentrations vary from vessel to vessel and depend on the local flow. If there is an allergic disposition or a previous contrast medium reaction, the risk must be carefully weighed or an appropriate prophylaxis implemented.

Normal Findings

The angiographic evaluation of the pituitary region usually requires imaging of both carotid arteries. In individual cases, unilateral catheterization with compression of the contralateral carotid artery for visualisation of the contralateral side may be sufficient. The need for angiography of the vertebral artery is limited to few indications with carotid occlusion or pronounced carotid fistulae.

The lateral view of the carotid artery at the level of the cavernous sinus resembles a siphon (Fig. 2.**30**) with many variations in shape. It is important to distinguish them from signs of parasellar growth of an intrasellar mass, which can usually be identified by a V-shaped change of the siphon.

In the lateral view, the anterior part of the circulus arteriosus with the pars circularis of the anterior cerebral artery (A1 segment) is relevant. It's location and shape as well as its communication with the other side have to be visualized. Usually the A1 segment is slightly bow-shaped, turns horizontally at its medial part and has approximately the same diameter on both sides. Since variations of the circulus arteriosus are not uncommon, there may be clear differences between the two sides of A1, with hypoplasia or aplasia on one side and a corresponding twofold supply of the anterior cerebral arteries from the other side (Fig. 2.**30 a, b**). This situation may gain special relevance for the surgical approach to the sella if both anterior cerebral arteries are supplied from one side only and a large suprasellar mass impedes the substitute circulation from the contralateral side.

The blood supply of the pituitary can rarely be demonstrated because of the small diameter of the vessel. It is not until pathological conditions have led to vascular hypertrophy that angiographic visualization becomes possible (Fig. 2.**31 a**). This is particularly true for the meningohypophysial trunk and the lower pituitary branches from the cavernous sinus section of the carotid artery (7, 10). The upper pituitary branches rarely lend themselves to angiographic visualization.

Visualization of the cavernous sinus is usually most sucessful with a venous approach. Orbital phlebography, for example, shows orbital drainage into the cavernous sinus and the characteristic bilateral filling of the parasellar spaces.

Pathological Findings

Sellar or perisellar masses are usually the indication for the angiographic visualization of the pituitary area. These questions tend to concern pituitary adenomas but may also involve craniopharyngiomas, meningiomas, or larger carotid aneurysms simulating a tumor.

The basal extension of a pituitary tumor can already be seen in the plain skull film by the corresponding erosion of the base (usually a so-called double base contour with unequal emphasis on each side) with infiltration into the sphenoid sinus. If information on the suprasellar or parasellar extent of the tumor is needed, angiography is, however, more helpful (8). Growth in a cephalad and ventral direction results in the typical elevation and stretching of the circular part of the anterior cerebral artery (A1 segment, according to Fischer), it usually involves the same vessel on the other side and can then be especially well visualized in the anteroposterior projection with compression of the contralateral carotid artery (1). This elevation of the A1 segment could also be a normal variation; however, taking the course of the vessel into consideration, as well as other findings such as the widening of the sellar entrance or clinical signs of a suprasellar mass such as a bitemporal hemianopsia, differentiation is usually possible. The significance of other anomalies of the circulus arteriosus, such as unilateral hypoplasia of the A1 segment for

Angiography 37

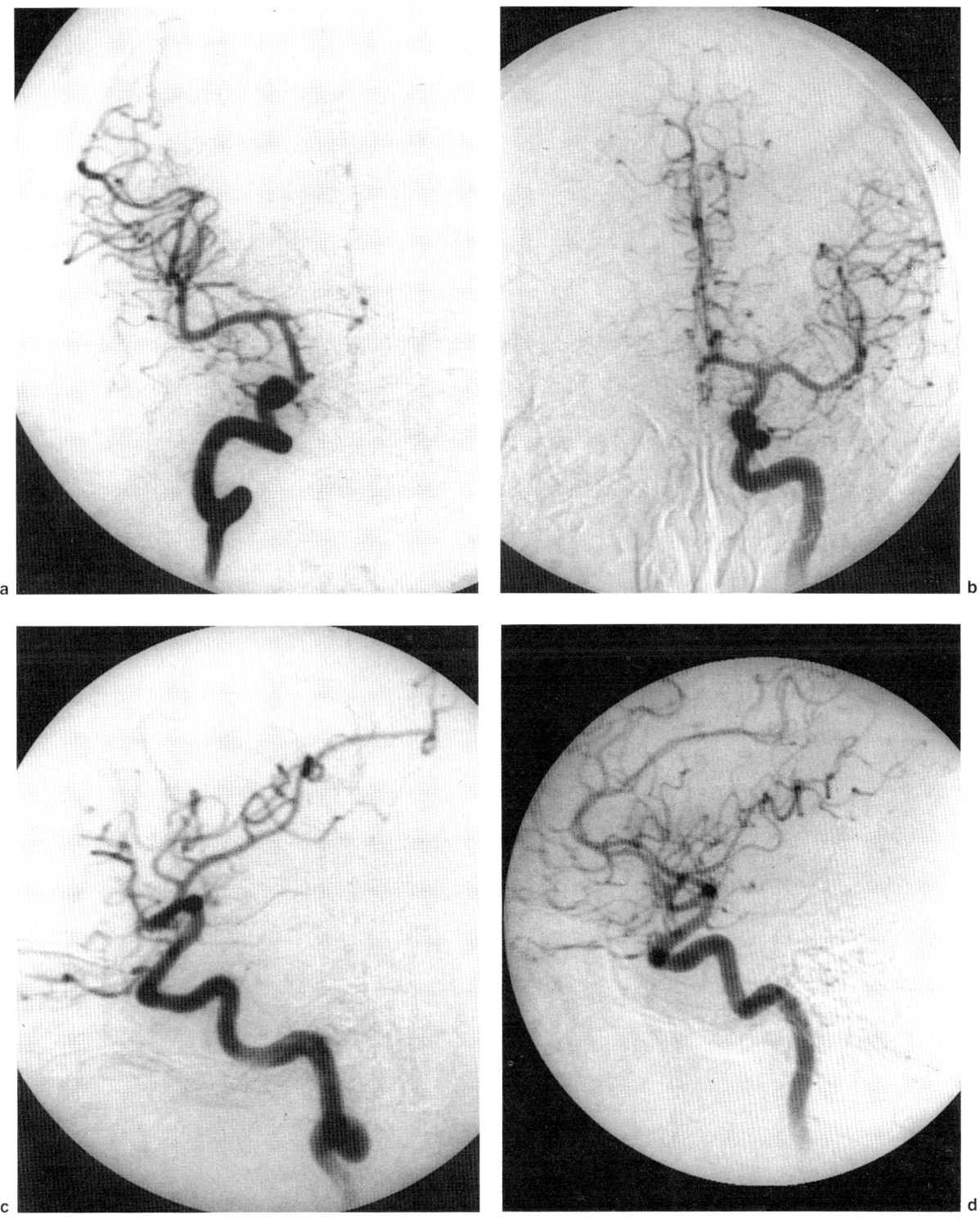

Fig. 2.**30** Chromophobic hypophyseal adenoma with hypoplasia of A1 as variant (**a**) with enhanced contrast of A1 to the left with suprasellar tumor extension (**b**); dual feeding of the cerebral anterior arteries from the left (**b**); *V*-shaped carotid siphon signifying lateral growth of the tumor to the right (**c**) contrary to normal carotid image lateral to the left (**d**)

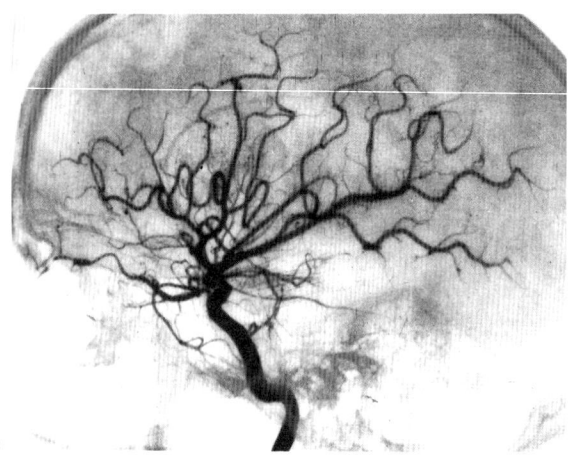

Fig. 2.**31** Prominent intrasellar and parasellar tumor with hypertrophy of the lower hypophyseal arteries with siphon bent upward (**a**); stenosis of the carotid artery due to lateralization and compression at the anterior clinoid process, as well as hypoplasia (or extension?) of A1 to the left (**b**)

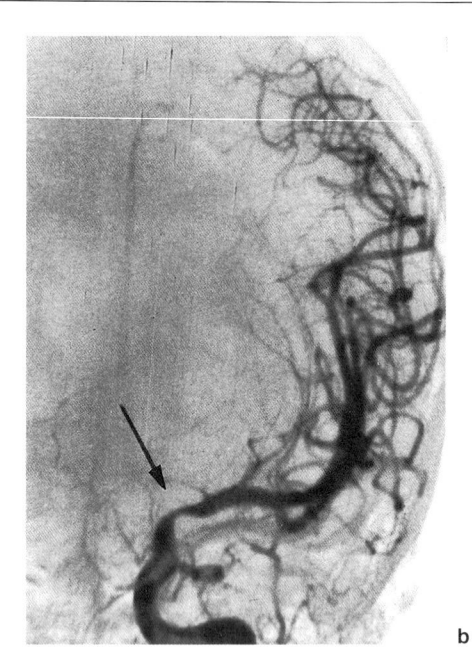

the frontobasal surgical approach, have already been mentioned.

If the suprasellar tumor grows in a more dorsal direction, the elevation of the A1 segment may be missing. Visualization of the growth direction used to be facilitated by pneumoencephalography; currently sagittal MR scans are the best option. More pronounced suprasellar masses in connection with blockage of the third ventricle may lead to hydrocephalic changes with an elevation of the anterior venous angle and a large bowed course of the anterior cerebral arteries.

The parasellar extension of a pituitary adenoma is demonstrated in the lateral arteriogram by an increasing opening of the usual carotid siphon (Fig. 2.**30 d**) to a V shape (Fig. 2.**30 c**) or an almost complete stretched out position (Fig. 2.**31 a**). In the anteroposterior projection, a lateralization of the carotid artery is shown. In very pronounced cases, the additional hydrocephalus may even lead to a stenosis of the carotid artery (5) (Fig. 2.**31 b**). Likewise, the posterior communicating artery as well as the beginning of the anterior choroidal artery may appear lateralized in a ap-projection (2). If the pituitary adenoma extends even more laterally ("breaking-out type") the angiographic appearance of a temporal mass with elevation of the middle cerebral artery may result. This leads to a compression of the cavernous sinus, which can no longer be demonstrated in arteriography or phlebography. Tumors with less lateral growth show partial buging into the cavernous sinus (2).

The lower pituitary branches from the meningohypophyseal trunk, which emerge from the bow-shaped (arched) transition of the carotid artery from the petrous segment to the lower siphon branches, usually supply the posterior pituitary lobe (3). These arteries hypertrophize if a tumor develops in the sella enabling angiographic visualization in 50% of the cases (2). One third of all pituitary adenomas show homogeneous tumor staining (Fig. 2.**32**). In a series in which magnification angiography and substraction were used, virtually all pituitary tumors showed pathological vessels (1).

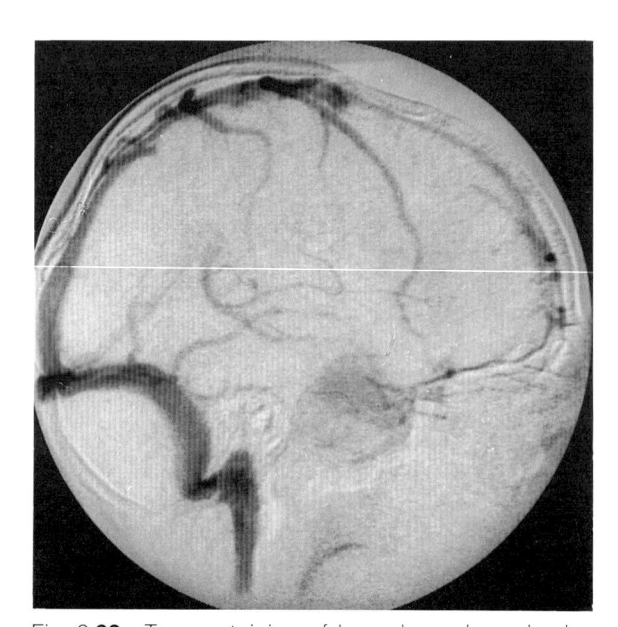

Fig. 2.**32** Tumor staining of large hypophyseal adenoma with suprasellar extension in the late phlebogram; image of the anterior venous angle not yet enhanced; no imaging of the cavernous sinus

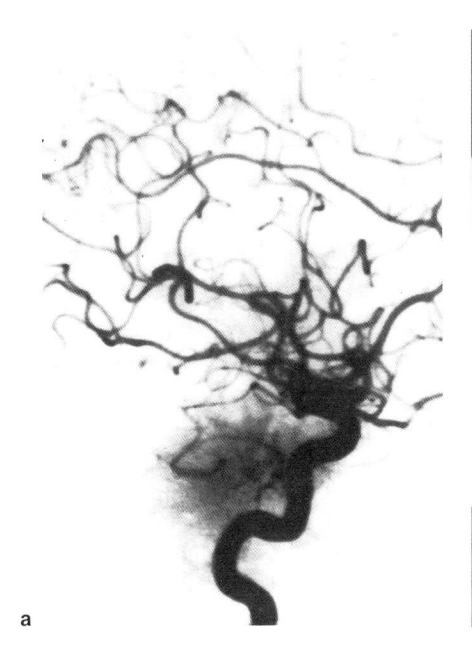

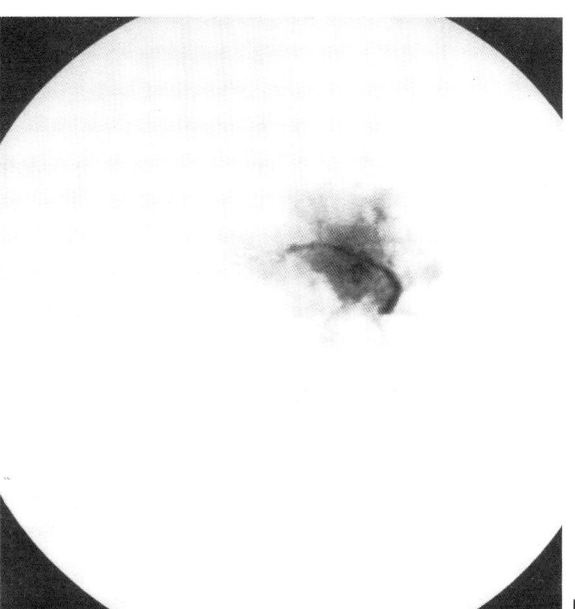

Of the other tumors of the sella region, meningeomas are most likely to simulate the angiographic image of tumor vessels from the meningohypophysial trunk and their staining pattern (Fig. 2.**33**). Craniopharyngiomas, optical gliomas or tumors growing upward from the base of the skull or from the sphenoid sinus are usually not difficult to distinguish from pituitary adenomas.

Ruling out an aneurysm as the cause of a sellar alteration is a very important indication for angiography in intrasellar masses. This may also involve the exclusion of an aneurysm as a second finding besides a pituitary adenoma, which could in the course of surgical management, lead to disastrous bleeding. This is of special significance if the transsphenoidal approach is used. Although the area between the two carotids can be controlled by an image intensifier in the anteroposterior projection, rupture of an unsuspected aneurysm may occur (Fig. 2.**34**). Furthermore, clipping is not really possible under these circumstances. Invasive angiographic imaging should remain the investigation of choice until MR is able to prove or exclude an aneurysm with a comparable degree of reliability.

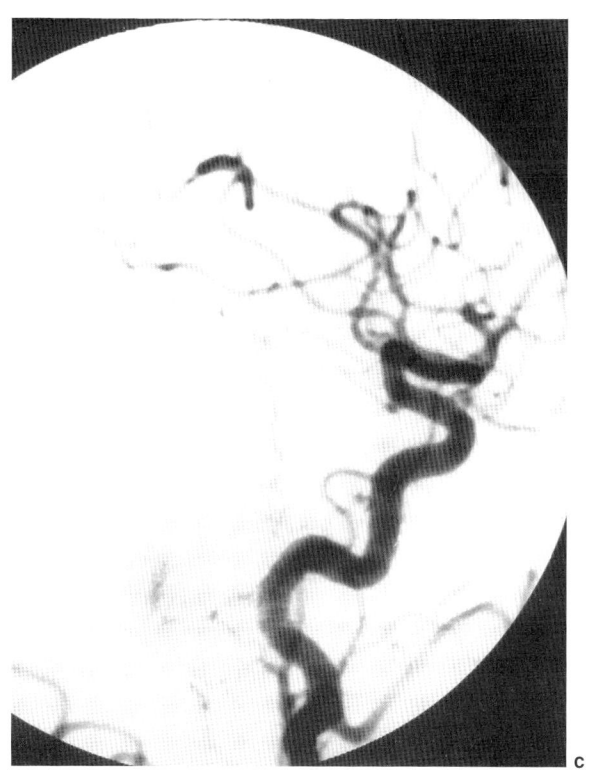

Fig. 2.**33** Tumor staining of a meningioma via hypertrophied meningohypophyseal branches (**a**); superselective angiography of the meningohypophyseal trunk (**b**); condition after preoperative embolization of tumor (**c**)

References

1 Baker H. The angiographic delineation of sellar and parasellar masses. Radiology. 1972;104:67.
2 Bentson JR. Relative merits of pneumographic and angiographic procedures in the management of pituitary tumors. In: Kohler PO and Ross GT, eds. Diagnosis and treatment of pituitary tumors Amsterdam: Excerpta Medica, 1973:86–99.
3 Lehrer HZ. Angiographic visualization of the posterior pituitary and clinical stress. Radiology. 1970;94:7.
4 Manelfe C, Berenstein A. Treatment of carotid-cavernous fistulas by venous apporach. J Neuroradiol. 1980;7:13–21.
5 Molsen HP. Seltene Form einer tumorbedingten Stenose der A. carotis interna. Radiol Diagn. 1980;21:479–481.

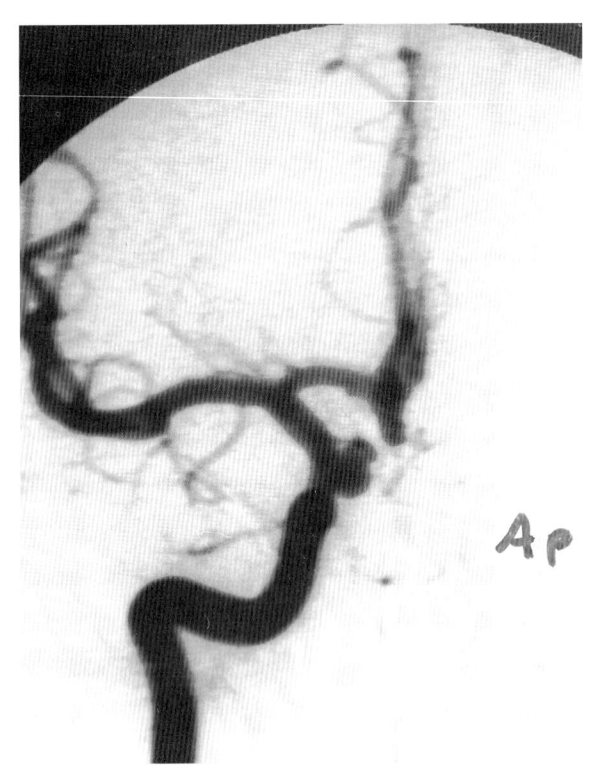

Fig. 2.**34** Aneurysm of the carotid artery, right supraclinoidal, with medial extension (potential risk in hypophyseal tumor surgery)

6 Molsen HP, Friedrich U, Kintzel D, Nisch G, Siedschlag WD, Winkelmann H. Interventionsradiologie in der Neurochirurgie – zum Einsatz der endovaskulären Ballonokklusion. Zent bl Neurochir. 1988;49:263–269.
7 Parkinson D. Collateral circulation of cavernous carotid artery: anatomy. Canad J Surg. 1964;7:251–268.
8 Powell DF, Baker HL, Laws ER. The primary angiographic findings in pituitary adenomas. Radiology. 1974;110:589–595.
9 Shiu P, Hanafee W, Wilson G, Rand R. Cavernous sinus venography. Am J Roentgenol. 1968;104:57.
10 Wallace S, Goldberg HI, Leeds NE. The cavernous branches of the internal carotid artery. Am J Roentgenol. 1967;101:34.

A Radiologist's View

W. Auffermann

Patients are generally referred for pituitary imaging because of pituitary axis dysfunction, which includes a wide variety of endocrine disorders, or for partial or complete visual loss. On the premises of availability, MRI has supplanted other imaging techniques (CT, angiography, radiography) as the modality of choice for primary evaluation of the sellar and parasellar region. Imaging of the complex anatomy of this region is promoted by the inherent capabilities of MRI, which offers a multiplanar approach with superior tissue contrast differentiation. Most common sellar and parasellar abnormalities are in the order of incidence: macroadenoma, microadenoma, meningioma, craniopharyngioma, glioma, and aneurysm comprise around three-fourths of all sellar lesions. The precise radiographic differential diagnosis of sellar and parasellar lesions is facilitated by dividing them by location into intrasellar, suprasellar, and parasellar lesions and combinations thereof.

If a sellar or parasellar lesion is suspected, the imaging approach is guided by the clinical symptoms. If an isolated endocrine abnormality indicating a sellar mass is the leading symptom, an unenhanced T_1-weighted coronal MR scan should be the primary approach. After additional, optional T_1-weighted axial scanning and T_2-weighted images, the study should be completed with a contrast-enhanced scan. If there is an indication of pituitary hyperplasia in a child, contrast media injection might be waived in favor of a repeat study after endocrine replacement therapy.

If cranial nerve symptoms predominate or clinical symptoms point to hypothalamic dysfunction, a parasellar lesion is to be expected. In this case, a multi-planar MR imaging approach, including contrast enhancement, should be chosen. If involvement of the skull base is expected, an initial radiograph should be followed by high-resolution CT in coronal and transverse planes to assess the extent of bone erosion. If MR images suggest a parasellar aneurysm, additional flow-sensitive MR sequences may complete the study, but should be followed by either conventional angiography or, if available, MR angiography for definitive diagnosis.

Adenoma

Adenomas are by far the most common intrasellar lesions. They are classified by size. Microadenomas are less than 10 mm in size; macroadenomas measure 10 mm or more. Contrast-enhanced MR imaging is the only modality that offers sufficiently high sensitivity for the detection of microadenomas, which, because of their hypovascularity, appear hypointense compared to the remainder of the gland after contrast enhancement. Dynamic gradient-echo sequences offer the highest accuracy for the detection of microadenomas because they avoid the effect of isoenhancement relative to the remaining pituitary tissue. Infundibular deviation or upward convexity of the pituitary gland, however, constitute less confident signs.

In macroadenomas, the mass effect usually dominates the symptoms of hormonal excess. Macroadenomas may already be detected on unenhanced MR images. In most cases, CT offers similar sensitivity for this disorder. However, the relation of pituitary adenomas to surrounding structures is significantly better visualized using MRI. Unilateral carotid artery encasement and cavernous sinus invasion are best assessed by MR imaging because of its superior soft tissue contrast.

There are three major reasons for an angiographic evaluation of the pituitary region. One is the exclusion of an aneurysm at the cause of an intrasellar mass. In the absence of MR, angiography is an important adjunct to CT for the evaluation of the relation of the tumor to the carotid arteries and to the cavernous sinus. The third indication for angiography is related to the preparation for a possible interventional radiologic procedure. However, with the advancement of MR imaging, the demand for angiography will probably recede.

Meningeoma

Meningeomas are most comprehensively evaluated with MR imaging. Arising from either a supra- or parasellar location, meningeomas may cause visual loss by compression of the optic chiasm. Due to their highly vascular nature, contrast enhancement is usually equally rapid and intense on either MR or CT. Intratumoral calcification and accompanying hyperostosis are best shown on unenhanced CT scans. The dural tail is best visualized on enhanced T_1 weighted MR images. Angiography does not play a major role in the diagnostic evaluation of meningeomas.

Craniopharyngeoma

Craniopharyngeomas are associated with a wide variety of neurologic symptoms such as chronic headache, visual defects, disturbance of liquor circulation and hypothalamic–hypophyseal axis dysfunction. MR imaging contributes to the evaluation of lesion extension in preoperative planning and in the detection of tumor recurrence. CT is an important adjunct, as it provides superior delineation of tumor calcification and, thus, may allow more specific histogenetic classification of the tumor mass.

Aneurysm

If MRI is not available or the patient has contraindications to MR imaging, CT may replace MR in the second row. If an enhancing intrasellar mass is seen on CT, the patient should proceed to cerebral angiography, in order to confirm the presence of a parasellar aneurysm. Use of MRI may obviate the need for CT and, in particular, for diagnostic angiography, because flow-sensitive sequences as well as MR angiography offer promising alternatives for the detection and characterization of intracranial aneurysms.

Other Lesions

Lesions from another histogenesis only form one-fourth of sellar and parasellar lesions and should undergo MRI first. MR is superior to CT except in the demonstration of bone changes and tumor calcification (2). In case of bone erosions, conventional radiography (including tomography) and high-resolution CT constitute an important adjunct. CT is useful as a supplementary modality when detailed information on bone anatomy is required, particularly if a transsphenoidal surgical approach is considered.

References

1 Kucharczyk W, Montanera WJ. The sellar and parasellar region. In: Atlas SW ed. Magnetic Resonance Imaging of the Brain and Spine. New York: Raven; 1991:625–667.
2 Lundin P, Bergström K, Thomas KA, Lundberg PO, Muhr C. Comparison of MR imaging and CT in pituitary macroadenomas. Acta Radiol. 1991;32:189–196.
3 Sartor K. Tumours of the sellar region and base of skull. In: Sartor K, ed. MR Imaging of the Skull and Brain. Berlin: Springer; 1992:379–452.

A Surgeon's View

W. R. Lanksch

Cranial CT has significantly improved diagnostic capabilities in intrasellar masses with and without suprasellar, parasellar, and retrosellar as well as subfrontal extension. The separation from normal structures, such as the sellar floor, the cavernous sinus, the opticochiasmatic cistern, the optic chiasm, the internal carotid artery, the anterior cerebral arteries, and the third ventricle is more precise with CT. CT has enabled diagnosis of millimeter-sized pituitary microadenomas. However, conventional tomography of the sellar floor has usually been added for the proof of local bony excavation. Confirmation of preoperative differential diagnosis between pituitary adenoma, aneurysm, metastasis, suprasellar meningeoma, ectopic pinealoma, craniopharyngeoma, and chordoma could often be achieved when considering plain CT, contrast-enhanced CT, clinical symptoms, and serum hormone analysis.

Before designing the surgical intervention by either the transsphenoidal or the transcranial approach, CT evaluation usually had to be completed using bilateral carotid angiography. From the angiograms, surgically important information on the displacement of the carotid, vertebral, and anterior cerebral arteries was provided. Irregularities of the vascular wall indirectly suggested tumor encasement with infiltration of the vascular wall. With the guidance of CT and angiography, surgical strategy could be designed using the transsphenoidal approach for all medially located intrasellar and purely suprasellar processes, which therefore lie within the field of vision of the operation microscope; the transcranial approach was used for more extensive intra-, supra-, para-, and retrosellar masses.

CT allows the definite proof of postoperative space-occupying hemorrhages in the surgical region. The diagnosis of residual tumor tissue, however, can only be achieved after fading of postoperative tissue alteration (hemorrhages, etc.). Using contrast-enhanced CT, the diagnosis of recurrent tumors is possible with equally high accuracy as that of the primary tumor.

For the design of the surgical approach and the intraoperative strategy of sellar and parasellar masses, MRI has the following advantages over CT:

1. Significantly improved recognition of normal anatomic structures and pathological processes
2. Visualization of the investigated object in three spatial planes
3. Improved tissue characterization and simultaneous visualization of vascular structures
4. Visualization of blood vessels using MR angiography

Pituitary microadenomas (less than 10 mm) are characterized by their reduced contrast enhancement compared to the normal pituitary gland on T_1-weighted MR images. An additional criterion for the presence of a microadenoma is the displacement of the hypophysial stalk, which is directed toward the tumor side in tumors close to the sellar floor, but directed toward the contralateral side in more cranially located masses. In microadenomas located close to the sellar floor, there may be an additional excavation of the sellar floor which, like the clivus, appears hyperintense on T_1-weighted images due to its high lipid content. The exact delineation of a mass on MR images facilitates the transsphenoidal approach, it makes a targeted search for the microadenoma possible.

Intrasellar pituitary adenomas enhance less after contrast administration than the normal pituitary on T_1-weighted images. With MRI, the localization of the compressed hypophysial gland is possible in at least two imaging planes, enabling precise surgical approach in order to preserve the remainder of the gland. Unilateral or bilateral parasellar invasion of pituitary adenomas into the cavernous sinus is decidedly demonstrated on MR images, and thereby enables the surgeon to avoid the dreadful complication of iatrogenic carotid artery injury.

In suprasellar and parasellar extending adenomas, the normal or altered topography of the suprasellar basal arteries shows whether the tumor displaced the basal vessels superficially or if it has embedded them. In the latter case, the surgeon has to be aware of encountering vessels within the tumor, which should not be injured under any circumstances. The larger the pituitary mass, the more inhomogeneous the contrast enhancement usually is (due to necrosis and cysts). This aggravates differentiation from the compressed and displaced remainder of the hypophysis.

The demonstration of large suprasellar and retrosellar space-occupying lesions in the sagittal plane points the surgeon clearly to the transcranial approach: fronto-lateral, bifrontal, transventricular, or transcallosal. Due to this subtle surgical design, the surgeon succeeds more and more in totally resecting para-, supra-, and retrosellar adenomas, craniopharyngeomas, and chordomas, in preserving functionally important structures, and thereby in minimizing the patient's risk.

It remains to be seen, how far the newest generation of CT devices (including spiral CT) with the possibility of three-dimensional reconstruction, will further improve preoperative diagnosis and advance operative design and surgical performance.

3 Thyroid Gland

Anatomy

J. Staudt

The thyroid gland is a soft, brownish organ surrounded by a strong fibrous capsule (outer capsule), which separates the gland into different lobules (inner capsule). Macroscopically, a finger-wide single medial part (isthmus) can be separated from both lateral parts (right and left lobule). In the adult, the isthmus crosses ventrally over the second and third tracheal cartilage. The thyroid isthmus is firmly connected to the trachea and follows the movement of the larynx during swallowing (Fig. 3.1). The shape of the thyroid resembles the letter H. The lobules are parallel to the long axis of the body and are covered by the sternocleidomastoid muscle. One lobule is about 6 cm long, 4 cm wide and 2–2.5 cm deep, and its weight ranges

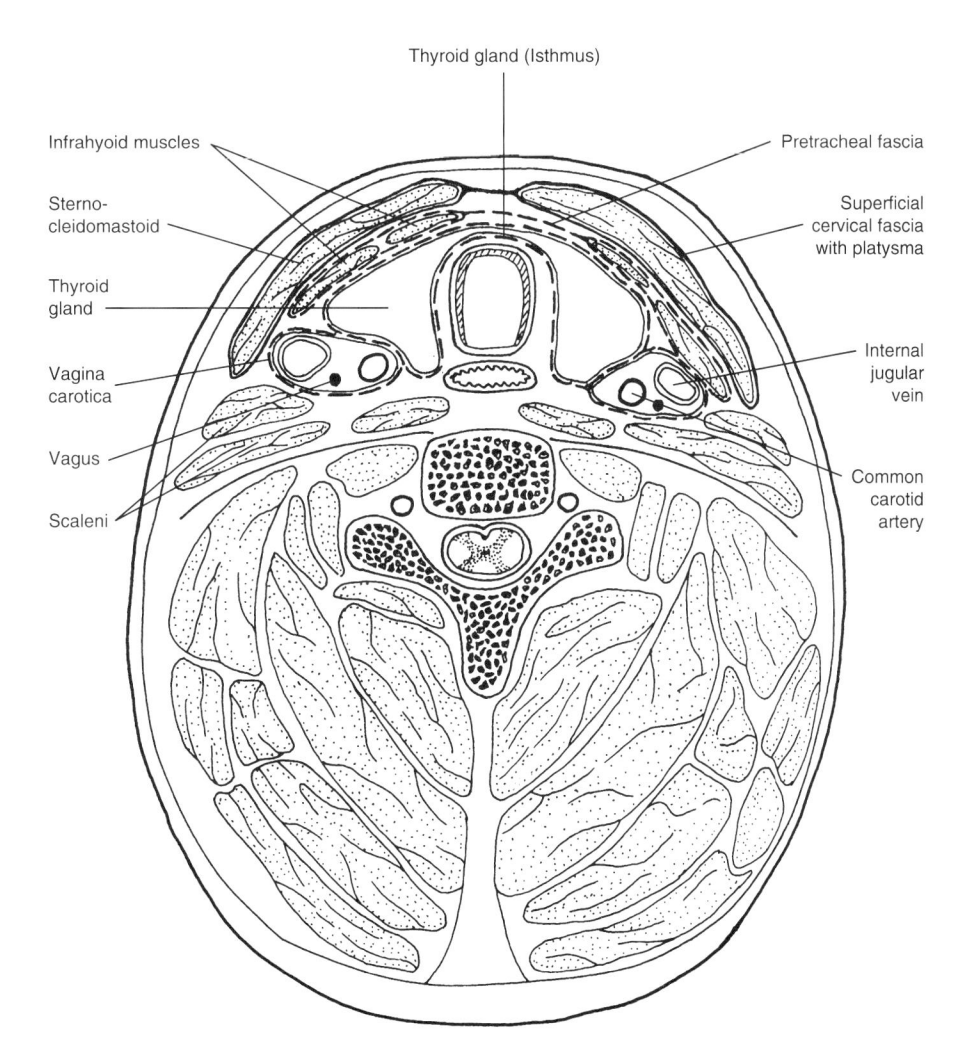

Fig. 3.1 Thyroid gland with pyramidal lobe

from 25 g to 50 g. Normally, the inferior margin does not cross the border of the upper thoracic aperture (Fig. 3.2). About half of the human population has a pyramidal lobe in the area of the thyroid isthmus, which may reach up to the cricoid cartilage. The pyramidal lobe is a remnant of the thyroglossal duct. The development of the thyroid starts at the pharyngeal arch and reaches its final position by descent. Median cervical cysts and fistulas are also derived from remnants of the thyroglossal duct and accessory thyroid glands may have a similar origin. Ten percent of humans do not have a thyroid isthmus.

Histologically, the gland is composed of two tissue compartments, the supporting scaffold of stroma containing blood vessels and nerves and the glandular tissue or parenchyma which forms the thyroid follicles. The follicles consist of cavities with a diameter of .05–.5 mm, which are mostly coated by mono-

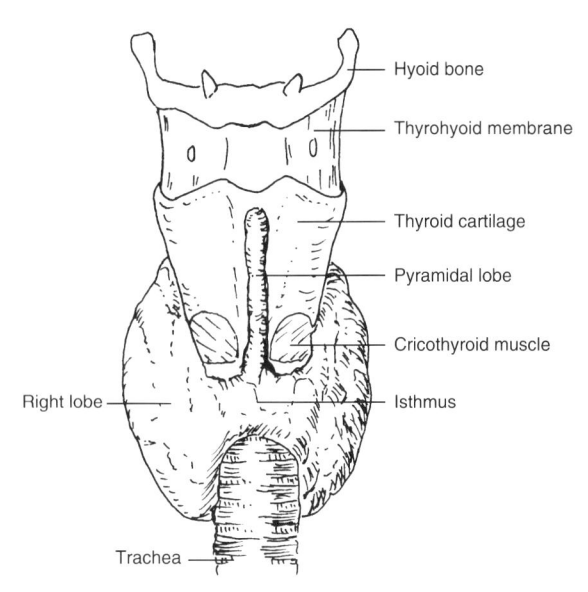

Fig. 3.2 Relation of the thyroid gland

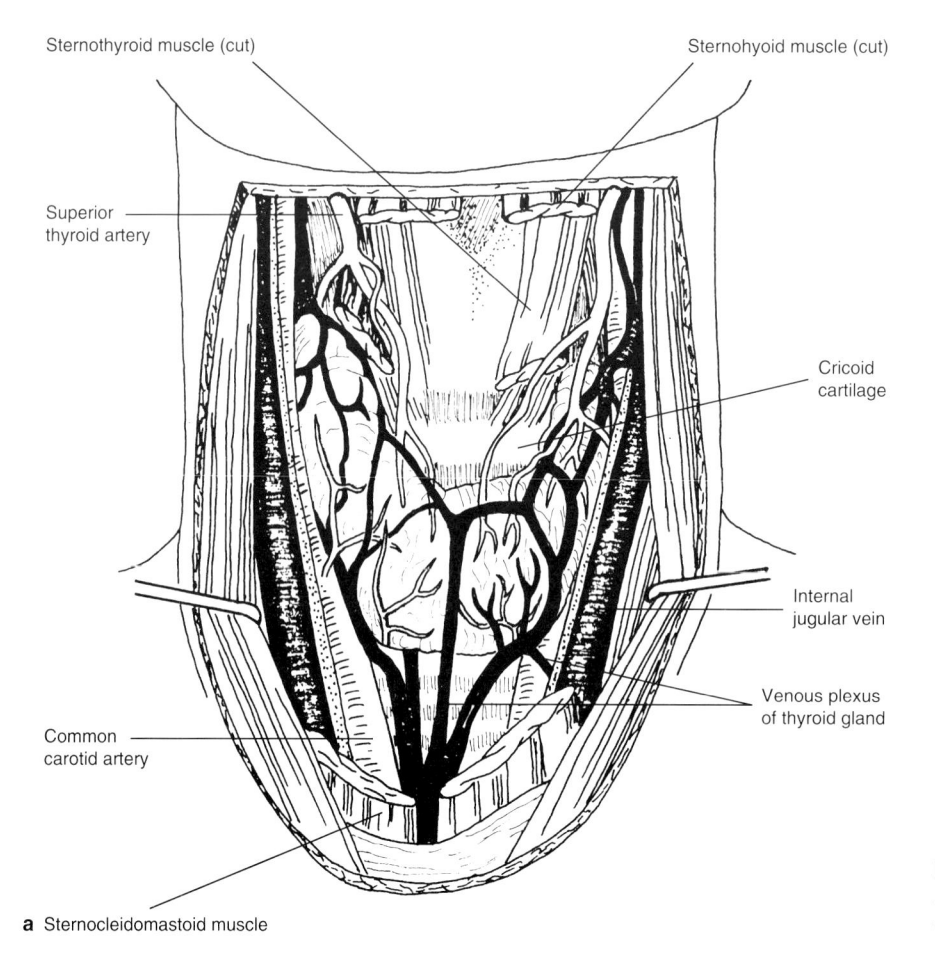

Fig. 3.3 Anterior (3.3a) and Posterior (3.3b) view of the thyroid gland

stratal, cubic epithelium. Within these follicles, follicular cells exceed the other glandular cells that secrete iodine-containing hormones. The follicles are small and the cells are high in case of increased hormonal demand. Moreover, there are numerous resorption vacuoles. Resting follicles consist of flat cells with large follicles. Parafollicular cells, i.e., C cells, originate from the neural crest and produce calcitonin. The C cells belong to the amine precursor uptake and decarboxylation (APUD) system.

Blood supply to the gland comes largely from the superior thyroidal artery, derived from the external carotid artery, and from the inferior thyroidal artery, derived from the thyrocervical trunk from the subclavian artery (Fig. 3.**3**). The inferior thyroidal artery supplies the inferior pole and the posterior part of the thyroid. These arteries dispose of considerable reserve length, which is required for the movement of the gland during swallowing. All four thyroidal arteries are connected with each other like a network on the surface and in the substance of the gland, which prevents circulatory disturbance in case of the occlusion of a single artery. The neighboring organs also have numerous branches. A solitary lowest thyroid artery, originating from the brachiocephalic trunk or from the aortic arch, is present in about 6% of humans. The right lobe of the thyroid is frequently more densely vascularized and slightly larger than the left. It also tends to enlarge more in disorders associated with a diffuse increase in glandular size. A wide capillary network surrounds each follicle. Veins accompany the arteries and drain the blood from the gland on three different levels via the superior and medial thyroidal veins which flow into the internal jugular veins, and via the inferior jugular veins (i.e., plexus thyroideus impar), which flow into the left bra-

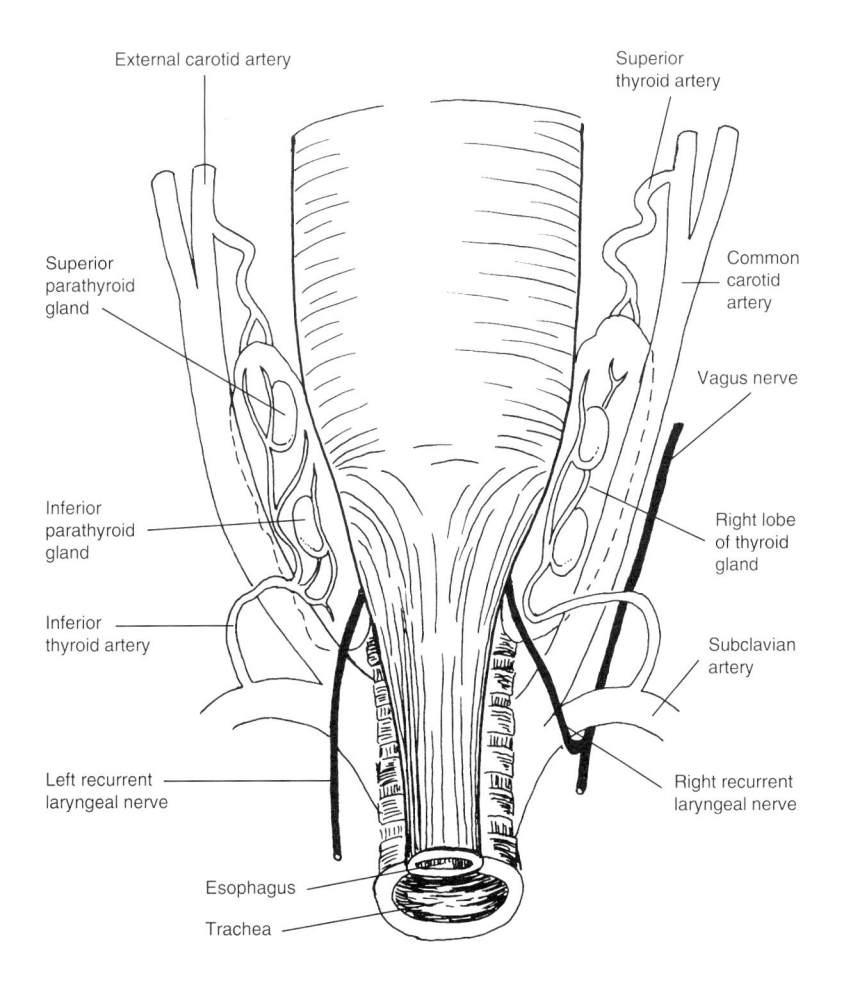

Fig. 3.**3b**

chiocephalic vein. The thyroid is richly supplied with lymphatics, which drain into the lower cervical and mediastinal lymph nodes.

Topographically important is relation of the thyroid to the recurrent nerve and the sympathic trunk, since the recurrent nerve follows the inferior thyroidal artery and directly attaches the posterior face of the thyroid (Fig. 3.**3**). The cervical lymphatic trunk runs laterally and separated from the thyroid gland along the posterior sheat of the prevertebral fascia and often forms a slope around the subclavian artery.

Endocrinology

K.-J. Gräf

Physiology

The endocrine function, of the thyroid like that other target organs, is governed by the familiar hypothalamo-pituitary feedback mechanisms (see Fig. 2.**4**). The thyroid produces and secretes two hormones: triiodothyronine (T_3) and thyroxine (T_4). Within the gland itself, the thyroid hormones are bound overwhelmingly to thyroglobulin (TG, intracellular type of storage). The major part of the serum T_3 concentration—which is about two to three times more potent than T_4—comes from deiodination of thyroxine in the periphery. In blood, the thyroid hormones are bound to an extent of more than 99% to proteins (about 60% to TBG = thyroxine-binding globulin, about 30% to albumin, and about 10% to prealbumin). Only the hormones not bound to protein — less than 0.5% — are biologically active.

Examination Methods

Every case of thyroid disease demands a careful exploration of the patient's history followed by a thorough physical examination, which should emphasize the thyroid, the cervical lymph nodes, the eyes, cardiac auscultation, and measurement of the pulse and blood pressure. The size of the thyroid is graded in three stages as classified by the World Health Organization:

I. Thyroid enlargement palpable (per thyroid lobe, transverse diameter greater than the end phalanx of the patient's thumb).
II. Thyroid enlargement clearly visible on close inspection.
III. Thyroid enlargement visible from a distance of several meters.

Important supplementary examination methods are sonography, thyroid scintigraphy, computered tomography, and X-ray examination of the thoracic organs, if applicable, with spot films of the trachea. Fine-needle biopsy is an important diagnostic procedure, but it should always be preceded by sonography and thyroid scintigraphy.

Thyroid function can be adequately assessed by in vitro diagnosis only. The parameters to be determined are the concentrations of T_4 and T_3, with particular preference being given to the free, i.e., not protein bound, hormones in the case of methodologically reliable assays. The determination of TSH with the most sensitive assays is also essential, if necessary in addition to the TRH test. It may also be advisable to determine the following antibodies: microsomal antibodies (comparable to the antibodies to thyroid peroxidase), thyroglobulin antibodies, and thyrotropin-receptor antibodies.

Determination of the thyroglobulin concentration is of clinical relevance only in tumor aftercare; it is superfluous as a tumor indicator in the screening program. Of importance is the determination of the calcitonin concentration is suspected C cell carcinoma. Furthermore, the pentagastrin test is of great diagnostic value for family screening of multiple endocrine neoplasia (MEN) patients.

Diseases of the Thyroid

Goiter

Thyroid enlargement, or goiter, is the most common disease of the thyroid gland. The enlargement may diffuse or nodular and can be accompanied by thyroid inflammation, normal thyroid function (euthyroidism), underfunction (hypothyroidism) or overfunction (hyperthyroidism). The definition of thyroid enlargement is a gland volume of greater than 18 mL in women and greater than 25 mL in men. The pathogeneses of goiter is not fully known. An iodine deficit apparently plays an important role. The daily dose of iodine required to avoid goiter should not be less than 150 µg. Other causes are the development of autonomy and the growth of adenomas and carcinomas. The influence of growth-stimulating immunoglobulins has also been discussed recently. The volume of the thyroid can increase in acromegaly and during pregnancy and lactation. It is also known that numerous drugs can lead to the development of goiter, e.g., all thyrostatics (some members of the cabbage family also contain thyrostatics), lithium, aminoglutethimide, sulphonamides and sulphonyl ureas.

The clinical symptoms of euthyroid goiter depend almost entirely on the local complications. Goiter can be very painful if the thyroid is inflamed. In general, however, thyroid enlargement causes significant complaints only if it displaces other organs. Subjectively, the patients often report a feeling of a lump or tightness in the region of the neck. Large goiters can lead to difficulty in swallowing and respiratory distress with stridor (on tracheal constriction of more than 70–80%). Large intrathoracic goiters in particular may also lead to an upper influx blockade and, possibly, to irritation of the laryngeal nerve and, hence, to trachyphonia (suggestion of malignancy!). The diagnostic work up of goiter must always include thyroid sonography and functional diagnosis (determination of the thyroid hormones, T_3, T_4, TSH, and, if applicable, the TRH test). Thyroid scintigraphy and fine-needle puncture should also be performed in the case of nodular goiter. X-ray examinations of the trachea and the thoracic organs, and possibly CT may also be indicated, particularly in the case of large retrosternal and intrathoracic goiters.

The therapeutic management of goiter is guided essentially by the local finding, the functional status, the scintigraphic results, and the clinical symptoms. In general, diffuse thyroid enlargement without nodes in patients with a euthyroid metabolic status can be treated antigoitrogenously with a gradually increasing dosage of l-thyroxine, and possibly with iodide alone or in combination with l-thyroxine. The presence of thyroid autonomy must be ruled out before this therapy is instituted, which means that a thyroid scintigram and TSH determination—and possibly a TRH test—are advisable in such cases before the start of therapy. Nodular goiter always raises the question of malignancy. Surgical exploration is essential in the case of solitary nodes, in particular in scintigraphically nonstoring nodes ("cold nodes"), in the case of rapid nodular growth, and in cases with cervical lymph node enlargement. Because of the increased surgical risks (paresis of the laryngeal nerve, etc.), the pros and cons of an operation must be weighed very carefully in the case of recurrent goiter. Radioiodine therapy is an option only in diffusely storing goiter or in patients with thyroid autonomy.

Inflammations of the Thyroid

Thyroid inflammation is relatively rare. Table 3.1 shows a breakdown of the different types of thyroiditis. Acute bacterial thyroiditis is usually highly sensitive to touch. The patients also display fever, and clinical chemistry reveals all the typical signs of inflammation. The therapy of choice is, of course, antibiotic treatment aimed at the particular or suspected pathogen.

Subacute thyroiditis is likewise a very painful disease with typical clinical and chemical signs of inflammation; it can occur with or without fever. No thyroid antibodies are demonstrable. The thyroid scintigram is usually marked by distinctly reduced or even a total absence of nuclide uptake. Similarly, thyroid sonography shows an inhomogeneous, reduced echostructure.

The Hashimoto type of chronic lymphocytic thyroiditis is clinically silent, without any signs of inflammation. The diagnosis is often made by chance.

Typical antibody constellations are normal with this disease, e.g., an increase in thyroglobulin antibodies and, above all, of microsomal antibodies (however, only very high titers are pathognomonic); aspiration cytology may be necessary to confirm the diagnosis.

Chronic fibrous thyroiditis (Riedel disease) is an extremely rare disease characterized mainly by the local finding of usually unilateral iron-hard goiter. There are no typical clinical or chemical constellations in this disease. The diagnosis is confirmed only by aspiration cytology or histology.

Hyperthyroidism

Hyperthyroidism is defined as an increased secretion of thyroid hormones—usually an increase in the concentration of both T_4 and T_3, but sometimes of an in-

Table 3.1 Classification of thyroid inflammations

Nature of inflammation	Causes	Clinical finding	Laboratory finding
Acute thyroiditis	Bacterial infection	Inflammation, painful palpation, usually fever	Nonspecific signs of inflammation, leucocytosis, (left shift)
Radiation thyroiditis	Radioiodine	No abnormal discovery	None
Subacute thyroiditis (de Quervain thyroiditis)	Virus infection, manifestation latency 2–12 weeks p.i.	Signs of inflammation; very painful palpation finding	Nonspecific signs of inflammation, leucopenia lymphocytosis
Chronic thyroiditis (Hashimoto lymphocytic thyroiditis)	Autoimmune	Nonspecific, hypothyroidism as late symptom	Thyroid peroxidase, MAK and TAK positive
Fibrous thyroiditis Riedel disease	Unknown	Uncharacteristic; firm thyroid palpation finding and hypothyroidism in late stage	Nonspecific

Table 3.2 Clinical symptoms of hyperthyroidism

Mild excitability, inner restlessness, nervousness
Tachycardia, arrhythmias, palpitations
Hyperkinesia, tremor of the fingers
Dyspnea on exertion, tiredness on exertion, dyspnea and tiredness on exertion
Diarrhea
Endocrine orbitopathy (only in Graves disease)

crease of T_3, and, in very rare cases, of T_4 alone. The different causes of hyperthyroidism are discussed below; the main clinical symptoms are listed in Table 3.2.

Graves Disease, Graves Type Hyperthyroidism, Endocrine Orbitopathy

Graves disease consists of the symptom complex of hyperthyroidism, goiter and ocular symptoms, e.g., exophthalmos, lid elevation or retraction, ophthalmoplegia, inflammation of the conjunctives, periorbital swelling (Merseburg triad). It is considered to be an autoimmune disease; immunogenic hyperthyroidism caused by stimulatory autoantibodies to thyrocytes. The immunological connection with endocrine orbitopathy is still unclear. Women are affected 4–5 times more often than men. The diagnosis of Graves disease is usually made clinically. Clinical chemistry reveals not only increased concentrations of thyroid hormones with simultaneous TSH suppression, but also distinctly increased microsomal antibodies and thyroid-stimulating antibodies. Of importance to the clinician is that endocrine orbitopathy need not simultaneously occur with hyperthyroidism. It is quite possible for ocular symptoms to develop before or after the occurrence of thyroid dysfunction. The clinical and chemical demonstration of the typical antibody constellations of increased microsomal and thyroid-stimulating antibodies in existing hyperthyroidism without ocular symptoms is therefore classified as the Graves type of hyperthyroidism.

The treatment of choice for the initial management of hyperthyroidism is always thyrostatic therapy, usually with thiamazole or propylthiouracil, alternatively with perchlorate. Treatment with thyrostatics must be carefully supervized because of the possible side effects (particularly the risk of bone marrow suppression, rush, etc.) and also because of the problems of overdosage, which could cause hypothyroidism. Our standard regimen is thiamazol 10 mg for the initial treatment, which should be reduced further in the course of therapy—L-T_4 has to be added alternatively—depending on the clinical symptoms and the thyroid hormone levels. The importance of the L-thyroxine supplementation in addition to thyrostatics for the relapse problem is still under discussion. Because of the high recurrence rate of Graves disease (about 60–70%), a definitive indication for treatment by surgery or radioiodide therapy is generally advisable after a euthyroid metabolic status has been achieved.

While the hyperthyroid symptoms respond well to thyrostatics within a few weeks, the treatment of endocrine orbitopathy is by no means as satisfactory. It must be stressed here that the development of endocrine orbitopathy may occur completely independently of the development of hyperthyroid metabolism status. None of the therapeutic approaches currently available for endocrine orbitopathy is satisfactory. An attempt at therapy with glucocorticoids should always be tried as soon as symptoms become clinically relevant (e.g., double images, ophthalmoplegia, etc.). Alternative therapeutic approaches with cyclosporin or recently, with octreotide or immunglobulins do not appear to be coming up to expectations. Retrobulbar irradiation is also by no means always successful. Surgical correction is required as a last resort if the results of the various attempts at conservative management are unsatisfactory.

Thyroid Autonomy

Thyroid autonomy (TSH-independent thyroid hormone production) occurs as solitary "autonomic adenoma", or diffusely as "disseminated", or "multifocal autonomy". It can develop with (decompensated autonomy) or without (compensated autonomy) hyperthyroidism. The condition of autonomy is demonstrated definitively in the suppression scintigram in only. Hyperthyroidism is demonstrated by the finding of elevated thyroid hormones; the secretion of TSH is suppressed. As in immune hyperthyroidism, thyrostatics are always employed for the initial treatment of hyperthyroidism in autonomy. Radioiodine therapy is particularly important as definitive treatment, especially in decompensated autonomous adenoma. Surgery is preferred to radioiodine therapy in very large goiters with diffuse or multifocal autonomy. The therapy of compensated autonomy is optional and, in general, prophylactic. Initial thyrostatic treatment is not necessary here. Otherwise, the same therapeutic principles apply as for decompensated autonomy with hyperthyroidism. If a decision is made not to treat compensated autonomy, the patient must avoid any exposure to iodine (iodine salt, iodine-containing drugs or disinfectants, iodinated contrast media).

Thyroid Storm

Thyroid storm is the term given to a severe, life-threatening form of hyperthyroidism. The clinical symptoms are characterized by tachycardiac arrhythmias, hyperthermia, hyperkinesia, dehydration, and disturbances of consciousness such as disorientation, stupor, somnolence, and coma. The causes of the thyrotoxic crisis are unclear. It is, however, known that the administration of iodine in particular is important as a trigger factor. Any thyrotoxic crisis demands besides high dosage of thyrostatics multifactorial, intensive medical care.

Hypothyroidism

Underfunction of the thyroid can have completely different causes (Table 3.3). The symptoms of hypothyroidism are, in general, typical (Table 3.4) but are frequently missed because of the insidious course. In adulthood, hypothyroidism occurs more frequently between the ages of 40 and 70, usually as a result of Hashimoto's thyroiditis (ratio of women to men is 5:1). Hypothyroidism is treated by oral replacement with l-thyroxine; the maintenance dose is generally between 100 and 200 µg/day. Normalization of endogenous baseline TSH secretion can be regarded as the yardstick for the correct dosage. Replacement should be performed slowly—in step-up dosage—in elderly patients and in patients with long-standing hypothyroidism. After thyroidectomy and, where necessary, radioiodine therapy, thyroid carcinoma patients require the highest possible replacement dose of l-thyroxine with the aim of complete TSH suppression.

Table 3.3 Causes of hypothyroidism

Connatal hypothyroidism

Acquired hypothyroidism
- Primary hypothyroidism
  - Inflammatory
  - Neoplastic
  - Extreme iodine deficiency
  - Iatrogenic (postoperative, postirradiation, medicinal)
- Secondary hypothyroidism
  - Anterior pituitary lobe insufficiency
  - Thyroid hormone resistance

Table 3.4 Clinical symptoms of hypothyroidism

Tiredness, lack of drive, slowing down
Weight increase
Sensitivity to cold
Depression
Arthralgia, myalgia
Dry scaling skin, brittle nails
Lumpy speech, croaky, deep voice
Oedema (face, lids but also generalized)
Bradycardia
Constipation
Menstrual disorders, decrease of libido and potency

Primary Hypothyroidism

Hormone dysgenesis (poor utilization of iodine) and thyroid aplasia and dysplasia predominate in neonates (connatal hypothyroidism). In adults, (acquired hypothyroidism), thyroid inflammations, neoplasias, and drugs can lead to hypothyroidism. It can also result from external irradiation after radioiodine therapy or postoperatively (when replacement is not performed). The diagnosis of primary hypothyroidism is confirmed by the demonstration of reduced serum-serum T_3 and T_4 concentrations with simultaneously elevated baseline or TRH-stimulated TSH secretion. Latent hypothyroidism is defined as a constellation of still normal thyroid hormone concentrations in peripheral blood, but an exaggerated response of TSH secretion to TRH stimulation (TRH test).

Secondary Hypothyroidism

Secondary hypothyroidism is characterized by a reduction of thyroid hormones in peripheral blood secondary to reduced TSH secretion. Possible causes here are, above all, pituitary and hypothalamic processes (see Chapter 2). Secondary hypothyroidism can develop due to a macroadenoma of the pituitary postoperatively after neurosurgery in the pituitary/hypothalamus region, or after irradiation of this region (notice the considerable latency period for the development of hypothyroidism). It is important to remember in these cases that the feedback control mechanisms no longer function, which means that TSH secretion cannot be used as a parameter for assessing underfunction of the thyroid.

Malignant Thyroid Tumors

Carcinoma of the thyroid is rare and accounts for less than 1% of the total number of all carcinomas. The mean incidence in central Europe is 3 per 100 000 inhabitants. It is increased in patients with nodular goiter and particularly in those with solitary nodes. The clinical symptomatology of thyroid carcinoma is extremely variable and usually uncharacteristic. The fresh occurrence of nodes which are fastgrowing, firm, hardly movable (if at all), scintigraphically cold, and a low-echo sonographic texture is suggestive. Sonography, thyroid scintigraphy, and possibly puncture cytology should always be performed in nodular goiter.

In medullary thyroid carcinoma, and particularly in the MEN type IIa and III, calcitonin is of crucial diagnostic importance as a tumor indicator. The determination of TG is of no importance whatsoever as a screening examination in the diagnosis of thyroid carcinoma.

Malignant thyroid tumors are generally categorized using the 1988 WHO classification (Table 3.5). The Tumor-node-metastasis (TNM) and pTMN classification of these tumors is shown in Table 3.6.

Table 3.5 WHO classification of malignant thyroid tumors

I. Ephitelial tumors	II. Nonepithelial tumors
A. Benign	III. Malignant lymphomas
1. Follicular adenoma	IV. Various tumors
2. Others	
B. Malignant	
1. Follicular carcinoma	V. Secondary tumors (metastases)
2. Papillary carcinoma	
3. Medullary carcinoma (C cell carcinoma)	VI. Unclassifiable tumors
4. Undifferentiated (anaplastic) carcinoma	VII. Tumor-like lesions
5. Others	

The histopathological classification is extremely important as regards the prognosis and, consequently, also plays an important role in therapy planning. Differentiated thyroid carcinomas have a good prognosis with a 10-year survival probability of 60% for follicular, of 70–80% for papillary, of 55% for medullary, and only about 3% for anaplastic carcinoma.

Primary squamous cell carcinoma, mucoepidermoid carcinoma, thyroid sarcomas and hemangioendotheliomas are very rare malignant tumors of the thyroid. Malignant lymphoma of the thyroid is, overall, a rare finding, accounting for about 2% of all lymphomas and for less than 5% of all malignant tumors of the thyroid. In general, intrathyroid metastatic disease is also unusual; in the order of probability, the following malignant tumors may metastasize: Hypernephroma, bronchial carcinoma, mammary carcinoma, melanoma.

The therapy of choice for thyroid carcinoma is, in general, thyroidectomy, if applicable with simultaneous resection of lymph node metastases. Because of the highly favorable prognosis in papillary thyroid carcinoma, lobectomy may be sufficient in patients with favorable prognostic criteria (e. g., patients less than 40 years of age and local tumor limitation to stages T1, T2, and N0).

After surgery and radioiodine therapy, all thyroid carcinoma patients should undergo therapy with the highest possible dose of l-thyroxine in order to completely suppress TSH secretion.

The measurement of TG is important as regards tumor aftercare. It has largely replaced routine nuclear-medical diagnosis (whole-body scintigraphy), which is now required only when the clinical finding or an increase of the TG concentration raises the suggestion of recurrent malignancy.

Ultrasound

K. Rosenkranz

Ultrasound of the thyroid gland is a simple, noninvasive method, which provides morphological information and thus complements the results of scintigraphy and laboratory tests. In addition to primary diagnosis and follow-up of pathological findings, sonography of the thyroid gland enables fine needle biopsy of focal lesions.

Method

Real-time sonography of the thyroid gland is performed using linear scanners with high-frequency

Table 3.6 Classification of malignant thyroid tumors

Stage TNM		pTNM
T0	No evidence for primary tumor	pT0 No evidence for primary tumor
T1	Unilateral solitary node	pT1 Solitary node up to 1 cm, without capsular rupture
T2	Unilateral multiple nodes	pT2 Solitary node >1 cm but <4 cm, without capsular rupture
T3	Bilateral tumor or isthmus tumor	pT3 Tumor >4 cm, multiple nodes, unilateral and/or isthmus nodes, all without capsular rupture
T4	Tumor breaks out of the thyroid	pT4 Tumor breaks out of the thyroid capsule
N0	No involvement of regional lymph nodes	No involvement of regional lymph nodes
N1	Movable, homolateral lymphomas	Movable homolateral lymphomas
N2	Contralateral, bilateral or medial lymph nodes	Contralateral, bilateral or medial lymph nodes
N3	Fixed lymphomas	Fixed lymphomas

Each T category can be further subdivided into a) solitary tumor b) multifocal tumor pTNM-pathological TNM

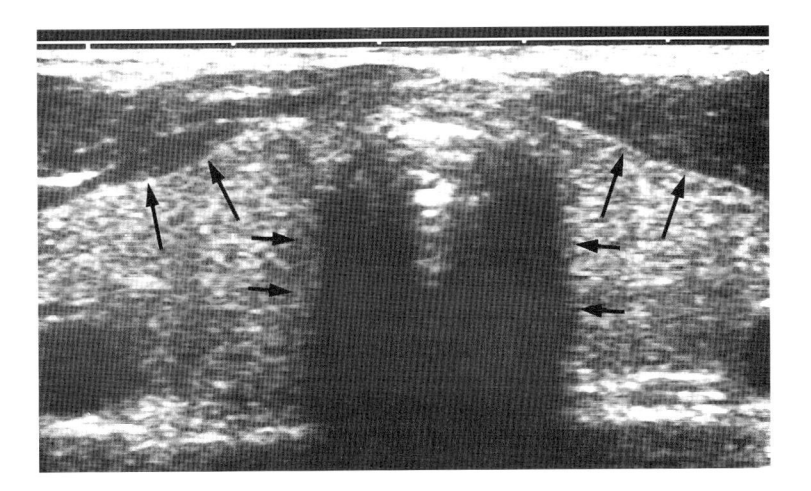

Fig. 3.**4** Sonogram of both thyroid lobes: transverse section. The hyperechoic thyroid parenchyma can be easily differentiated from the hypoechoic anterior neck muscles (big arrows). The trachea is marked by the small arrows

transducers (5 to 7.5 MHz) and—if necessary—a water path. In cases with goiter and retrosternal parts, 3,5 MHz sector scanners should be used in order to assess thyroid volume. This is determined according to Brunn (3): $V_L = L \times W \times T \times C$ (V_L = thyroid volume, L = length, W = width, T = thickness, C = correction factor). The empirically optimized correction factor (C = 0.479) (3) is replaced by the factor 0.5 (8). The echogenicity and echographic pattern of thyroid parenchyma are also analyzed.

Color-coded duplex sonography is actually performed in order to assess different vascularization (10, 11). Blood flow velocity and direction are color coded.

Normal Findings

Due to its uniform echogenicity, the normal gland can be easily differentiated from surrounding tissue by sonography (Fig. 3.**4**). The thyroid gland is hyperechoic in comparison with the muscles of the anterior neck. Normal thyroid volume should be up to 12 mL for each lobe.

Color-coded duplex sonography shows no or only few Doppler signals within thyroid parenchyma. Capsular vessels and major supplying vessels can be detected.

Pathological Findings

Diffuse Thyroid Diseases
Diffuse goiter

Diffuse nontoxic goiter results in a general enlargement of the gland with a normal echostructure and echogenicity at the beginning. In long-term disease, degenerative processes result in a coarsened, inhomogeneous pattern. Disseminated thyroid autonomy in diffuse goiter cannot be excluded by sonography. Therefore, radionuclide evaluation by scintigraphy and laboratory tests are necessary in order to rule out functional disorders of the thyroid gland.

Graves Disease

In Graves disease, the echogenicity of the thyroid parenchyma is homogeneously reduced (Fig. 3.**5**, 5, 6). The gland shows a normal size or an enlargement, particularly in the sagittal plane. These signs can also occur in other autoimmune thyroid disorders, e. g., Hashimoto disease. On the other hand, a normal echo pattern does not enclude Graves disease (5). Sonographic follow-up studies during therapy often show normalization of echostructure due to remission (6).

Color-coded duplex sonography often shows increased Doppler signals in patients with Graves disease due to hypervascularization (11). Therapy results in a decrease or normalization of color-coded duplex findings.

Autoimmune Thyroiditis (Hashimoto Disease)

In autoimmune thyroiditis, thyroid parenchyma shows diffuse inhomogeneous reduction of echogenicity (Fig. 3.**6**, 5.**6**). Concerning differential diagnosis, Graves disease, subacute thyroiditis (de Quervain), and the extremely rare acute thyroitis must be considered. Subacute thyroiditis is usually easily differentiated by pathognomonic laboratory tests and physical findings. In some cases, needle biopsy for differentiation of chronic autoimmune thyroiditis and thyroid malignoma is required.

Nodular Thyroid Diseases
Benign Nodular Goiter

Thyroid nodules represent the main indication for sonography. The functional activity of such nodules cannot be assessed by this method, and most of them require further radionuclide evaluation. Four types

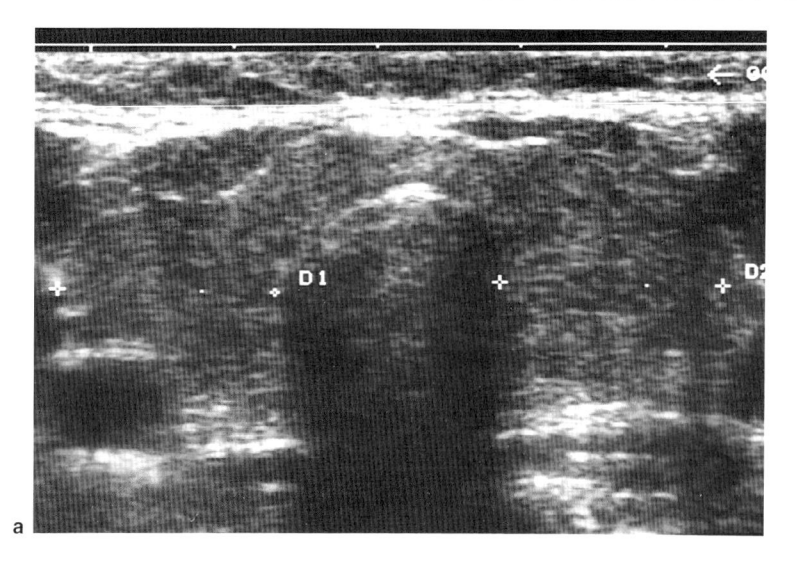

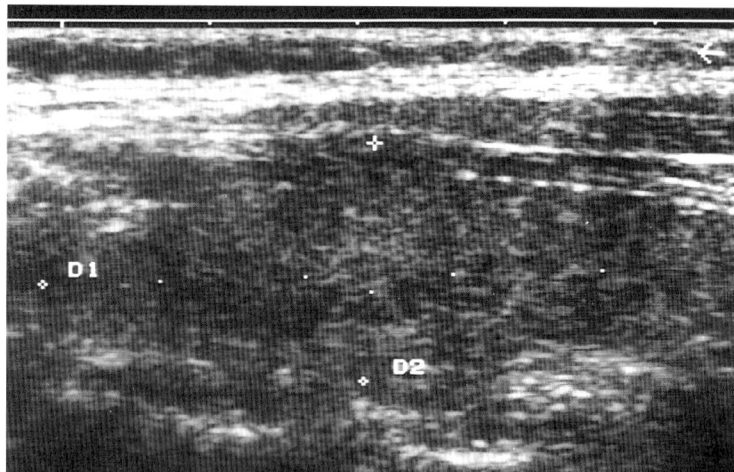

Fig. 3.5 Transverse section of both thyroid lobes (**a**) and longitudinal section of the right lobe (**b**) in Graves disease. It is difficult to differentiate the thyroid gland from surrounding tissues due to reduced echogenicity. In this case, the echostructure is discretely inhomogeneous

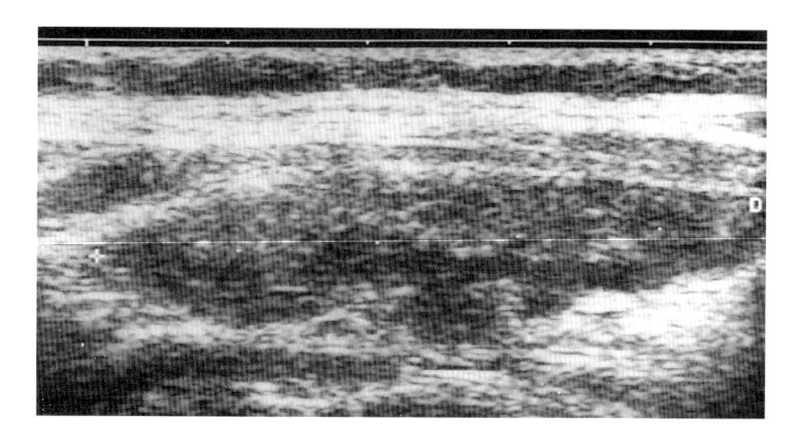

Fig. 3.6 Longitudinal section of the right thyroid lobe in autoimmune thyroiditis (Hashimoto disease). The parenchyma shows multiple hypoechoic areals

can be differentiated according to their sonographic feature.

Hyperechoic and Isoechoic Nodules (Fig. 3.7)

Hyperechoic and isoechoic nodules displacing and compressing normal thyroid tissue often lead to the formation of a rim of decreased echogenicity, or a "halo" around the nodule (Fig. 3.7). Most of them are benign macrofollicular adenomas. The "halo," although mostly found in benign lesions, does not exclude malignancy. Several examples of malignant tumors with a "halo" have been reported (9).

Fig. 3.**7** Longitudinal (left) and transverse section (right) of a hyperechoic nodule in the right thyroid lobe. The perifocal rim of decreased echogenicity is marked by the arrows ("halo"). The histological correlate is a benign macrofollicular adenoma

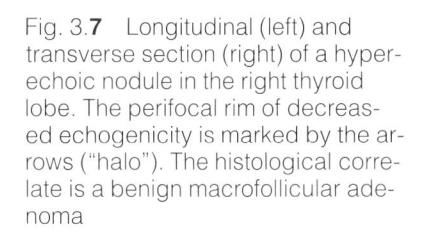

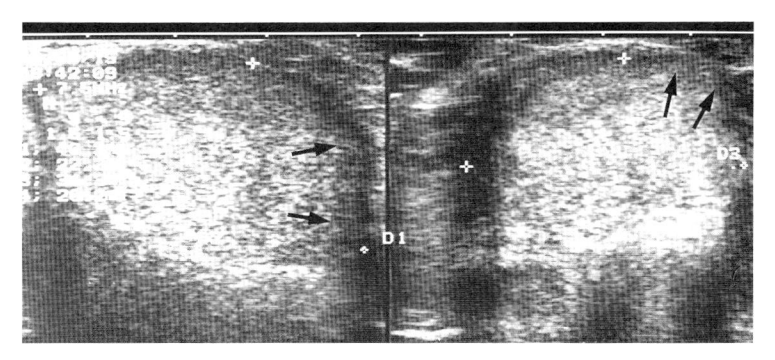

Hypoechoic Nodules (Fig. 3.**8**)

The presence of a hypoechoic nodule requires further radionuclide evaluation, because 50–75% of microfollicular autonomous adenomas are reported to be hypoechoic (1, 7). In addition, thyroid carcinoma should be excluded. A large number of microfollicular, scintigraphically "cold" adenomas are also hypoechoic (6).

Echofree Nodules (Fig. 3.**9**)

An echofree area with enhanced distal echogenicity is the typical sonographic finding for cysts. Some of them show central hyperechoic or hypoechoic structures due to internal hemorrhage (Fig. 3.**9**) or septae. In these cases, further diagnostic evaluation (scintigraphy, needle biopsy) is required to exclude cystic malignancy. Cysts can develop in benign and malignant nodules.

Mixed Echoic Nodules (Fig. 3.**10**)

In most cases, mixed echoic nodules are benign macrofollicular adenomas with regressive degeneration. They often show central cystic lesions, calcifications as hyperechoic structures with decreased distal echogenicity (Fig. 3.**10**), or both. If a sonographically mixed echoic nodule is shown to be "cold" in scintigraphy, needle biopsy should be performed because malignant lesions can sometimes show this pattern (2, 9).

Autonomous Adenoma (Fig. 3.**8**)

As mentioned above, most cases of microfollicular autonomous adenoma appear hypoechoic in sonography with sharp margins. However, because of regressive degeneration, autonomous adenoma can also show hyperechoic, isoechoic, or mixed echoic patterns (1, 7, 8). Color-coded duplex sonography shows increased Doppler signals within the nodules due to hypervascularization (10, 11).

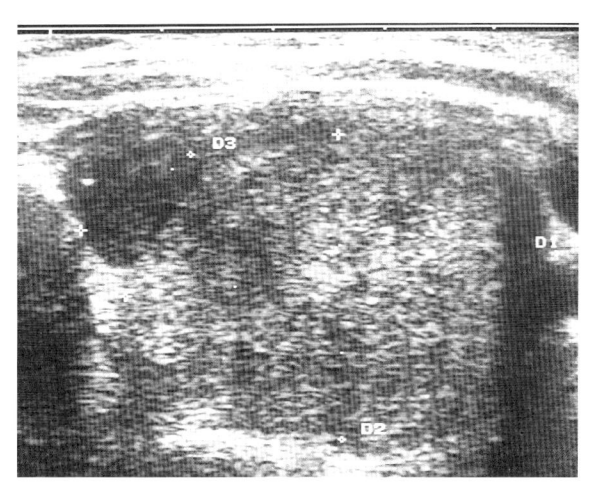

Fig. 3.**8** Transverse section of the left thyroid lobe with a small autonomous adenoma (scintigraphically "cold") in the ventromedial region. Laterally, a hyperechoic nodule (scintigraphically "cold") is shown

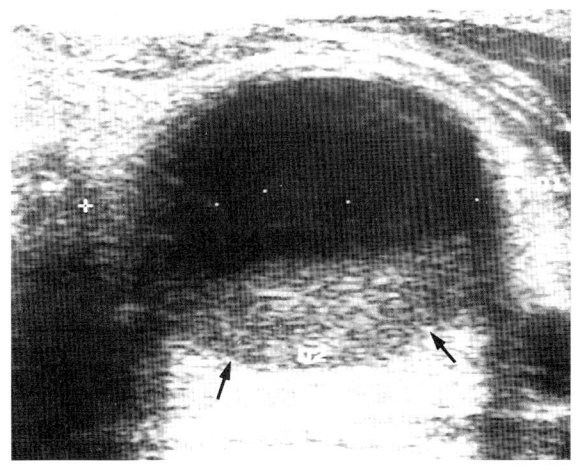

Fig. 3.**9** Transverse section of the left thyroid lobe that shows a large cyst. The latter is echofree with enhanced distal echogenicity. Hyperechoic material on the bottom marked by the arrows is the sonographical correlate of internal hemorrhage

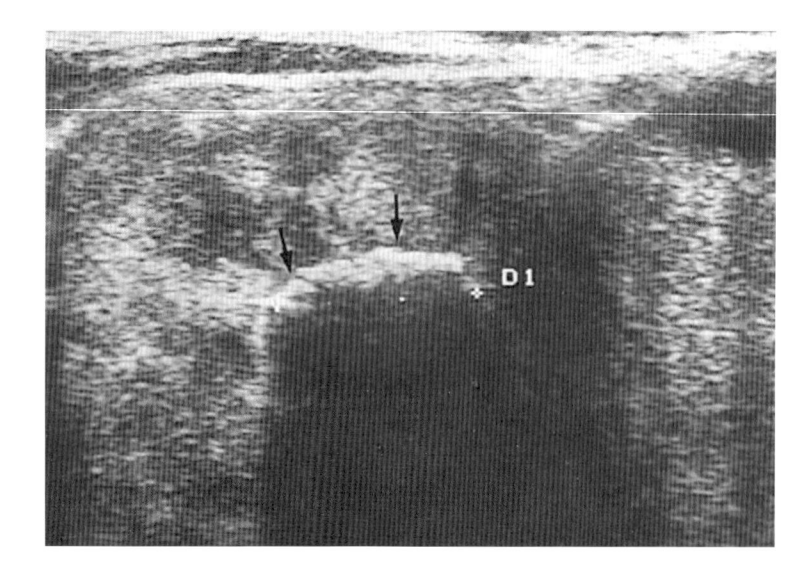

Fig. 3.10 Transverse section of the right thyroid lobe in benign nodular goiter. A large mixed echoic nodule with central calcification as hyperechoic structure with distal ultrasound absorption (arrows)

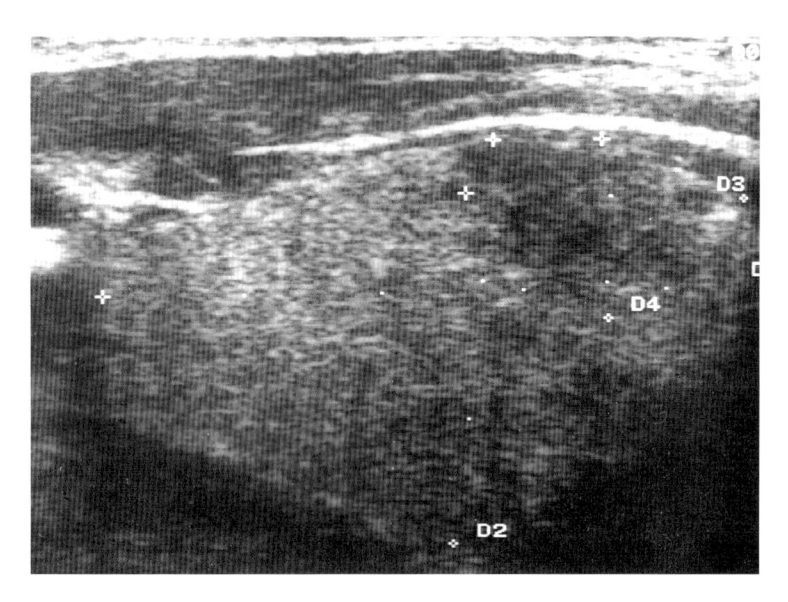

Fig. 3.11 Longitudinal section of the right thyroid lobe with a hypoechoic nodule in the caudo-ventral region. It is difficult to differentiate this focal (scintigraphically "cold") lesion from the surrounding parenchyma. Needle biopsy showed a papillary carcinoma

Thyroid Malignoma (Fig. 3.11)

Particular sonographic signs that permit exclusion or prove malignancy do not exist. Most malignant thyroid tumors (papillary, follicular, anaplastic, etc.) are found in hypoechoic nodules (2, 4, 9). Some cases show an isoechoic pattern or mixed echoic nodules because of central cystic or hyperechoic areas. Calcifications are rare. Hypoechoic, scintigraphically "cold" nodules require further evaluation by needle biopsy. In contrast, the incidence of malignancy in hyperechoic and echofree nodules is extremely low (2, 9).

References

1 Becker W, Börner W, Gruber G. Szintigraphie und Sonographie bei der Diagnostik der Schilddrüsenautonomie. Dtsch Med Wschr. 1986;111:1630–1635.
2 Börner W, Becker W. Stellenwert von Szintigraphie, Sonographie und Zytologie in der Diagnostik von Schilddrüsenkrankheiten. Krankenhausarzt 1985;58:277–294.
3 Brunn J, Block U, Ruf G, et al. Volumetrie der Schilddrüsenlappen mittels Real-time-Sonographie. Dtsch Med Wschr 1981;106:1338–1340.
4 Hirsch H. Diskussionsbemerkung zu den Vorträgen „Sonographische Befunde bei Knotenstrumen". Akt Endokrinol Stoffw 1983;4:127.
5 Leisner B. Ultrasound Evaluation of thyroid diseases. Horm Res 1987;26:33–41.
6 Pfannenstiel P. Heutiger Stellenwert und Indikationen der Sonographie der Schilddrüse. Akt Endokrinol Stoffw 1983; 4:142–150.
7 Reiners C, Wiedemann W. Kombination von Sonographie und Szintigraphie – Bestimmung des Impuls-Dickenquotienten. Akt Endokrinol Stoffw 1983;4:130–135.
8 Rosenkranz K, Langer R, Cordes M. Eine vergleichende Studie sonographischer und szintigraphischer Befunde bei nodösen und diffusen Strumen. Röntgenpraxis 1990;43:81–87.
9 Solbiati L, Volterrani L, Rizzatto G, et al. The thyroid gland with low uptake lesions: evaluation by ultrasound. Radiology 1985;155:187–191.

10 Thomas C, Bautz W, Müller-Schauenburg W, Feine U. Angiodynographie bei umschriebenen Schilddrüsenveränderungen. Fortschr Röntgenstr 1989;150:72–75.
11 Treisch J, Schneider F, Langer R, Felix R. Farbkodierte Duplex-Sonographie der Schilddrüse vor und nach Radiojodtherapie. Ultraschall Klin Prax 1990;5:170.

Computed Tomography

C. Zwicker

Though contrast-enhanced CT is helpful in the evaluation of larynx and pharynx tumors and in lymph node staging of the neck, the possible interaction of decoupled iodine with thyroid metabolites limits its use in the evaluation of the thyroid.

Technique

Investigation of the thyroid should be performed with a slice thickness of 4–5 mm. Artifacts caused by swallowing and movement can be avoided by short scanning periods of 1–2 seconds and breathing instructions (commands). On plain CT, the delineation of the thyroid against blood vessels and lymph nodes is often difficult, thus necessitating i. v. contrast administration. This should take place by way of a slow injection of contrast bolus (e. g., 100 mL contrast medium, 1 mL/s speed of injection). The body's own deiodinases always lead to an increase of the free iodine pool (1). This means that the thyroid is blocked for scintigraphy and radioiodine therapy for at least 8 weeks. In addition, patients with Graves disease, thyroiditis and nodular goiter risk an exacerbation of their symptoms. In cases in which contrast medium administration cannot be avoided, iodine transport into the thyroid should be inhibited with perchlorate. Sixty drops per os and continuation of medication over a period of 8 days after the investigation is advisable (3 × 30 drops) (4).

Normal Anatomy

The two lobes of the thyroid gland are on either side of the trachea and the isthmus is immediately ventral to it. The laterodorsal border is formed by the common carotid arteries; the lateroventral border by the internal jugular veins, which may differ greatly in caliber (Fig. 3.12). The outer contour of the gland is smooth, and because of its high iodine content (0.65 mg I/g), its noncontrast-medium enhanced density is considerably higher than that of musculature. The thyroid gland's good vascularization leads to an intense increase in density after i. v. contrast administration (7). The ventral borders are formed by the sternothyroid and sternohyoid muscles. The cervical longissimus muscle lies on the dorsal side of the thyroid.

Pathological Changes

In addition to nodular thyroid enlargement, multinodular goiter is characterized by an inhomogeneous absorption pattern with regressive calcifications and cystic changes. The extent of retrosternal goiter as well as stricture of the trachea can be clearly defined (Fig. 3.13). Furthermore, cancer growth that no longer respects organ limits and infiltrates into adjacent structures can be reliably evaluated (Fig. 3.14). The differentiation of small carcinomas, however, is no longer

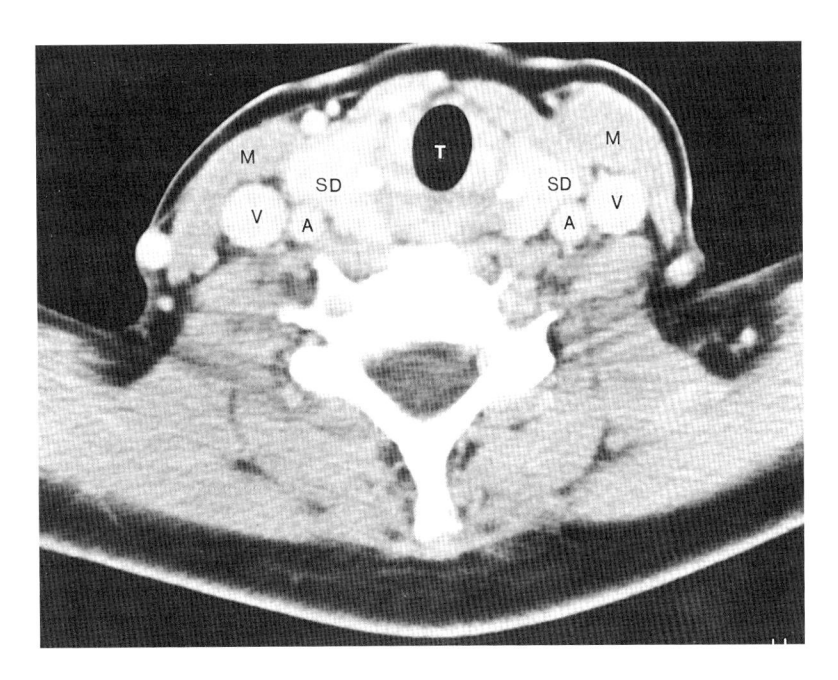

Fig. 3.12 Normal anatomy of the thyroid on a contrast-enhanced CT scan.
T = trachea,
SD = thyroid gland,
A = common carotid artery,
V = jugular vein,
M = sternocleidoid muscle

56   3 Thyroid Gland

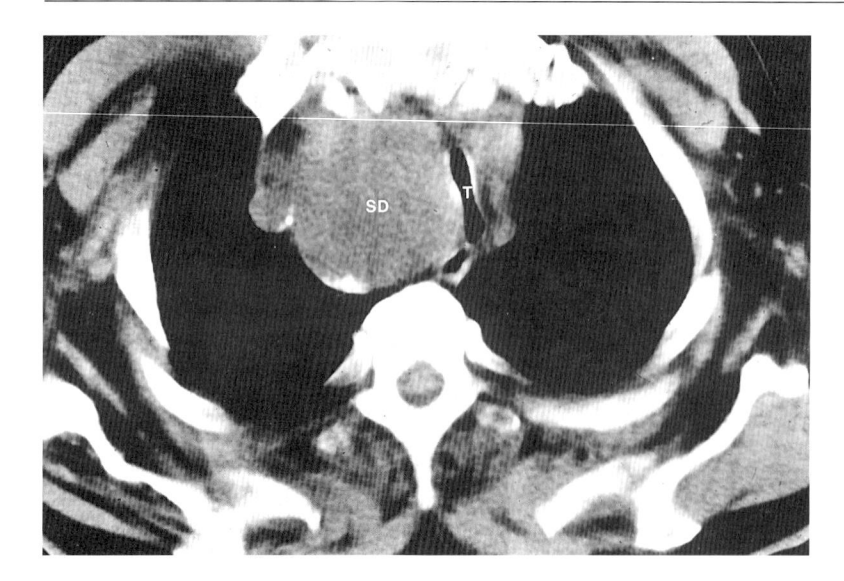

Fig. 3.**13**   Extensive retrosternal goiter (SD) with subtotal stenosis of the scabbard trachea (T)

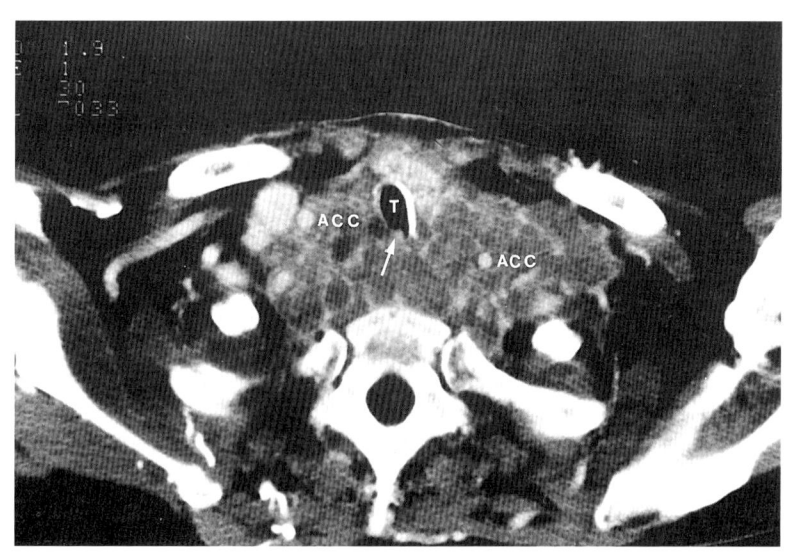

Fig. 3.**14**   Anaplastic thyroid carcinoma with infiltration of the membranous part of the trachea (arrow) and embedding of the common carotid arteries (ACC)

an indication for computed tomography because iodine contrast application prevents ^{131}I therapy.

Summary

CT plays only a very minor role in the diagnosis of thyroid diseases compared with scintigraphy, sonography, and MRI because the required contrast medium administration is frequently contraindicated (3, 5, 6). The only indications for CT are preoperative evaluation of tracheal stenosis, the retrosternal growth of goiter, and the spread of a carcinoma beyond the borders of the organ involved.

References

1 Grebe SF, Müller H. Hyperthyreose-Risiko bei Kontrastmittelverabreichung. In: Riemann HE, Kollath J. Digitale Radiographie. Konstanz: Schnetztor; 1984:339–344.

2 Lenz M, Bähren W, Haase S, Ranzinger G, Wierschien W. Beitrag der Computertomographie zur Diagnostik maligner Tumoren der Mundhöhle, des Hypopharynx und des Larynx sowie ihrer regionären Lymphknotenmetastasen. Röntgenpraxis 1983;36:333–349.

3 Pirschel J, Hübener KH. Computertomographische Diagnostik von Schilddrüsenerkrankungen unter besonderer Berücksichtigung des szintigraphisch kalten Knotens. Fortschr Röntgenstr 1979;130:175–179.

4 Rendl J, Börner W. Minderung des Risikos bei Kontrastmitteluntersuchungen. Risikogruppe Schilddrüsenerkrankungen. In: Riemann HE, Kollath J, Rienhoff O. Digitale Radiographie. Konstanz: Schnetztor; 1990:304–315.

5 Sekiya T, Tada S, Kawakami K, Kino M. Clinical applications of computed tomography of thyroid disease. Comput Tomogr 1979;3:185–193.

6 Vogl Th, Mühlig M, Mees K. Kernspintomographische Untersuchungen der Schilddrüse und Nebenschilddrüsen. Therapiewoche 1985;21:316–321.

7 Wolf BS, Nakagawa H, Yeh HC. Visualization of the thyroid gland with computed tomography. Radiology 1977;123:368–373.

MR Imaging

W. Auffermann and C. B. Higgins

MRI provides a diagnostic tool with specific advantages and disadvantages for evaluating the thyroid gland in conjunction with other modalities or, rarely, as the sole means of evaluation. Relaxation times and proton density values allow the differentiation of the thyroid from parathyroid, muscle, fat, lymph nodes, blood vessels, and salivary glands (15, 22, 27). MRI offers a detailed description of the anatomy of the normal thyroid gland on T1-weighted, proton density and on T2-weighted images. Since paramagnetic contrast agents do not contain iodine, they can even be given to patients in hyperthyroid states when iodine contrast agents are prohibited.

Technique

Different field strengths have been successfully used for thyroid gland imaging (2, 8, 14, 16, 18, 19, 24, 25). Because thin sections and high spatial resolution are required, high field strength imaging seems to be advantageous for obtaining optimal images of the thyroid. However, excellent images have also been obtained using medium and low field strength. The superficial midline location of the thyroid gland makes it an ideal target for surface coils, which optimize the filling factor between the narrow neck and the coil, resulting in improved image quality. Various surface coils have been used, from a solenoid coil, which wraps around the neck, to flat, circular, or elliptical coils, Philadelphia collar saddle-shaped coils, and Helmholtz coils specially adapted to the neck region (11).

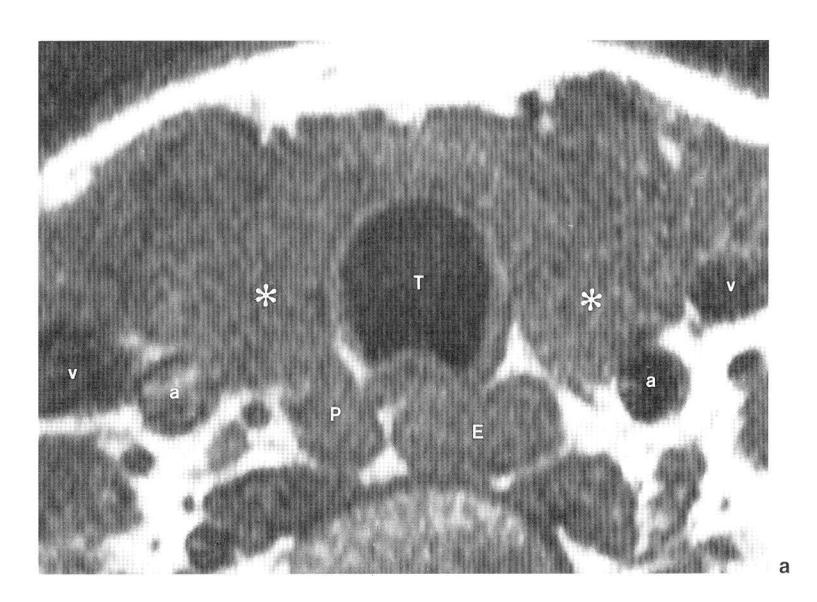

Fig. 3.**15** Transverse spin-echo (SE) images (**a**) T1-weighted image with TR = 500 msec and TE = 15 msec and (**b**) T2-weighted image with TR = 2000 msec and TE = 60 msec of the neck at the level of the thyroid gland (*). The thyroid shows lower intensity than the surrounding strap muscles (arrow) and the longus colli muscle (L) on the T1-weighted image. Note the signal within the jugular vein that is intensified on the T2-weighted image.
P = parathyroid adenoma;
T = trachea;
E = esophagus;
a = carotid artery;
v = jugular vein

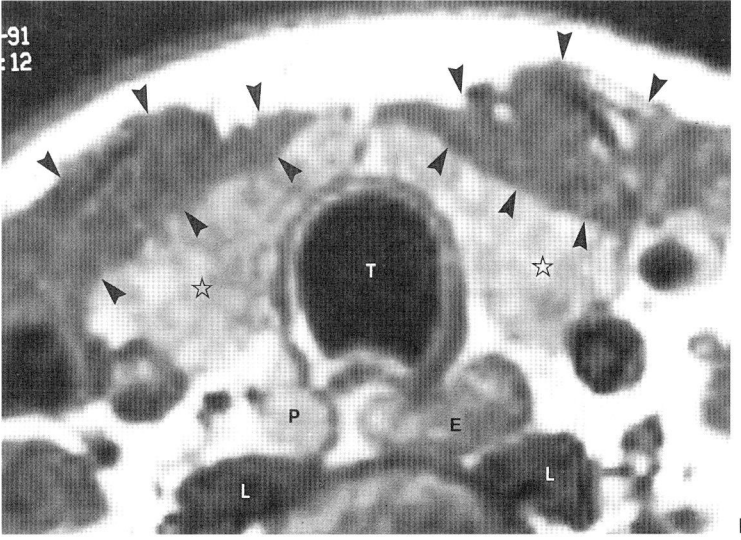

Thyroid imaging requires thin sections (less than 5 mm thick), the acquisition of both T1- and T2-weighted sequences, and paramagnetic contrast enhancement. Submillimeter spatial resolution is obtained by a small field of view (less than 16 × 16 cm) and a matrix of 512 × 512. Artifacts from blood flow, respiration, and swallowing are reduced by a presaturation pulse (applied in the z-axis) and the elimination of wraparound artifacts in the x and y direction. The transverse plane is standard and should encompass the neck from the hyoid bone down to at least the upper thoracic aperture (11).

ECG-gated chest imaging is required for diseases that extend beyond the sternoclavicular junction into the mediastinum, such as substernal goiter, recurrent thyroid carcinoma, or recurrent hyperparathyroidism. For large neck masses extending into the mediastinum, coronal views are an important complement to the routine transverse scans. Calculating T2-relaxation times and intensity ratios (to fat, muscle, or normal parenchyma) has been used for tissue characterization in MRI (3). MR contrast media have the advantage that they can be given to patients in hyperthyroid states and even to patients with documented allergy to iodine-based contrast media. The usual dose applied for Gd-DTPA is 0.1–0.2 mmol/kg body weight.

Normal Thyroid

The normal thyroid gland is located between the oblique line of the thyroid cartilage and the sixth ring of the trachea. It is surrounded by a fibrous capsule and is enclosed in a fascial compartment formed by the pretracheal fascia. The thyroid gland varies tremendously in size depending on age, sex, and nutrition (7). The normal thyroid gland, with its two lobes, surrounds the anterior and lateral circumference of the trachea and measures about 5 cm in height, 3 cm in width and 1–2 cm in depth for each lobe (Fig. 3.15). Each lobe approaches the prevertebral fascia covering the long muscle of the neck posteriorly and, the

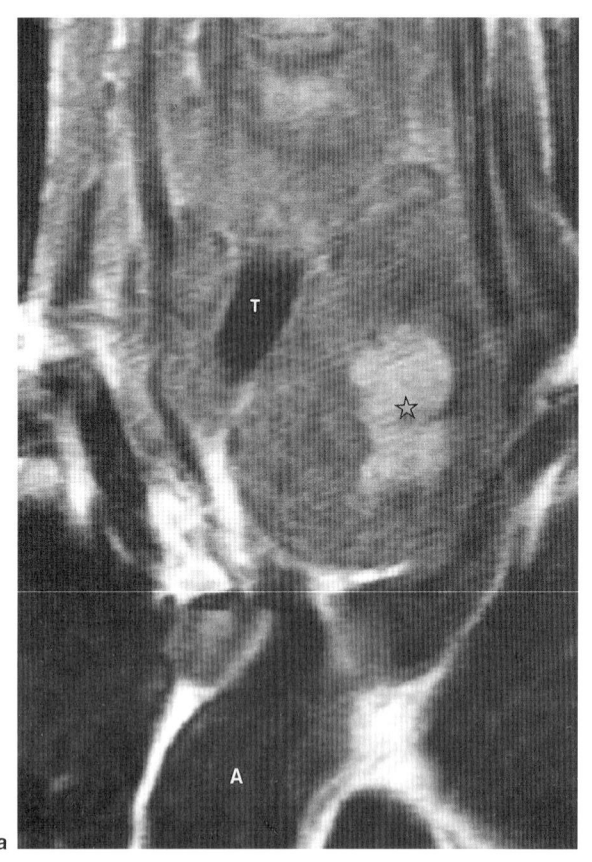

Fig. 3.**16** Multinodular goiter
a T1-weighted coronal spin-echo image, 500/15. Multinodular retrosternal goiter with almost homogeneous low intensity with a large central hyperintense protein-rich cystic follicle. Note the lateral displacement and compression of the trachea (T) and adjacent vascular structures (open arrows)

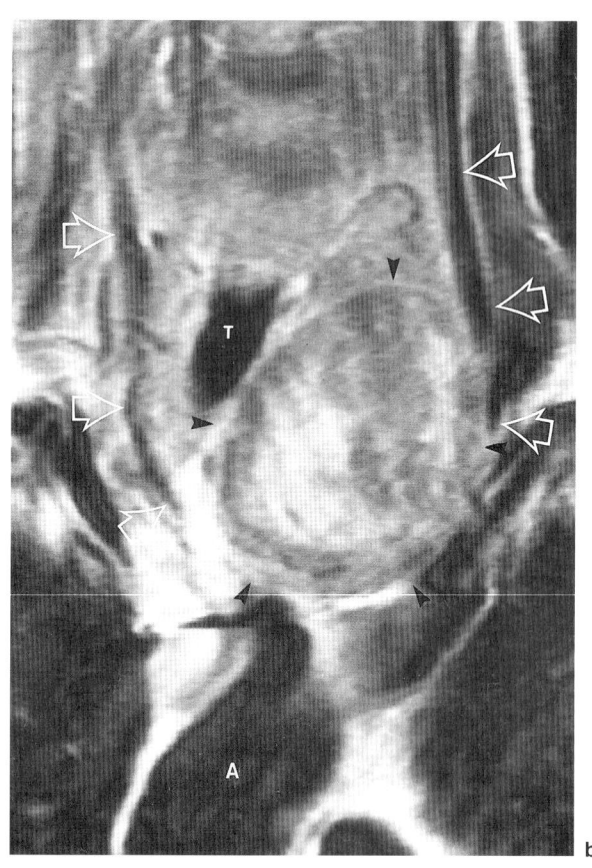

b T1-weighted coronal spin-echo image, 500/15, after Gd-DTPA. Gd-DTPA causes a more inhomogeneous MR appearance without enhancement of the central follicular part (asterix) of the goiterous nodule (arrowheads) A = Aorta

carotid sheath, laterally. At the lower pole, fat separates the gland from the longus colli muscles.

MR signal intensity of the normal thyroid is usually homogeneous on T1- and T2-weighted images. Due to their relatively low signal intensity, the strap muscles can be distinguished from the subcutaneous fat and the immediately abutting thyroid gland. T2-weighted images allow optimal contrast for the differentiation of the thyroid from the overlying sternohyoid and sternothyroid muscles anteriorly and the sternocleidoid muscles laterally. Between the two lobes, prominent veins may be seen anteriorly, representing portions of the inferior thyroid vein. Posterior to the trachea, the esophagus can be identified with its mucosal layers showing higher intensity than the muscular wall on T2-weighted images (Fig. 3.**15**).

Pathological Findings

T1- and T2-relaxation times of abnormal thyroid tissue have a large interindividual variability (6, 10, 21, 22) because of the mixed composition of colloid, fibrosis, necrosis, and hemorrhage (6) in the tissue.

Goiter

Multinodular goiters resulting from thyroid hyperplasia, asymmetrical focal involution, hemorrhage, and scarring (7) are easily identifiable due to their usually hypointense to isointense appearance on T1-weighted images, and increased intensity on T2-weighted images (Fig. 3.**16**). The nodular, inhomogeneous appearance with focal areas of high intensity

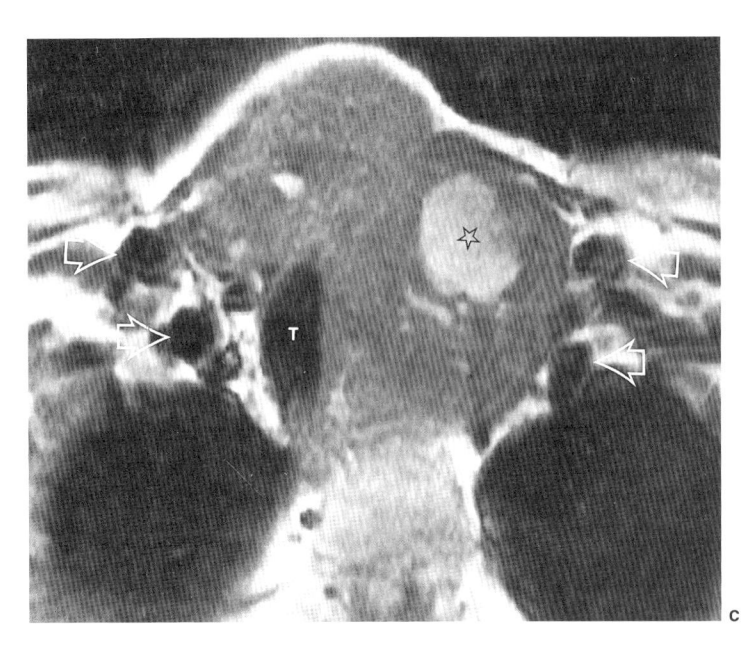

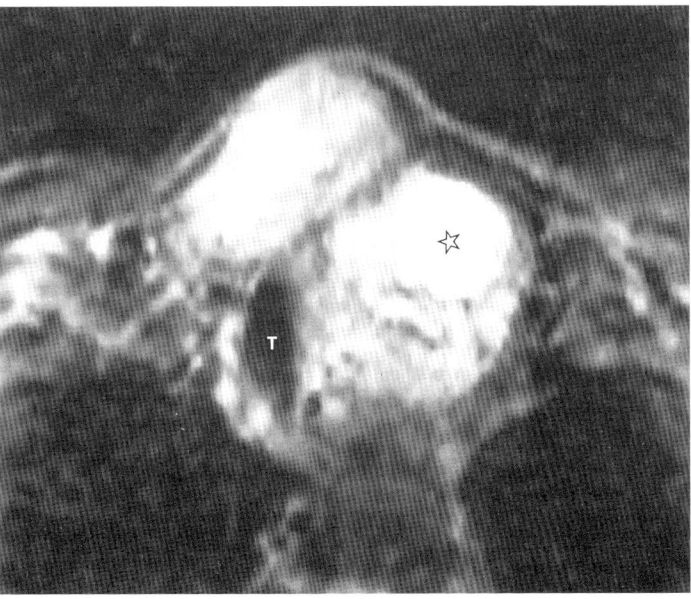

Fig. 3.**16c–d**
c T1-weighted transverse MR image, SE 500/15, precontrast
d T2-weighted transverse MR image, SE 2500/90. Heterogeneous, partly high-intensity mass with multiple nodules (Courtesy of R. Bittner, Berlin)

3 Thyroid Gland

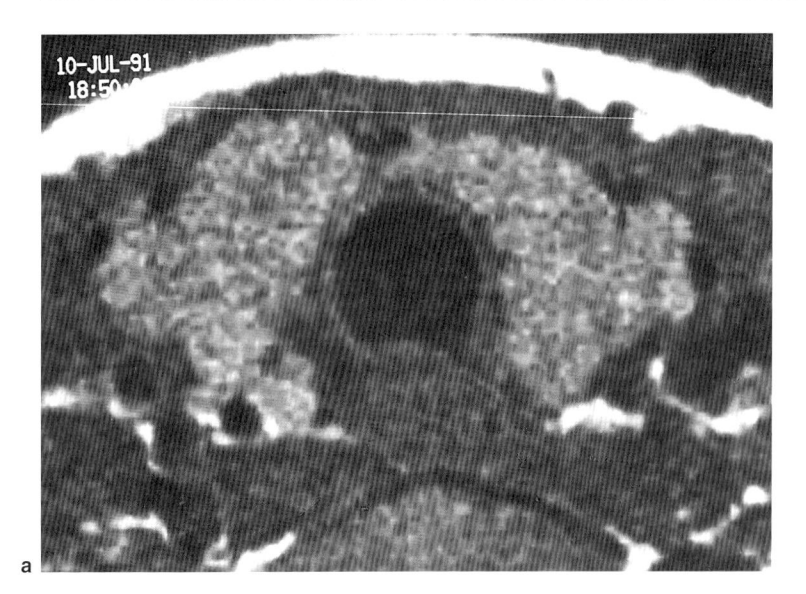

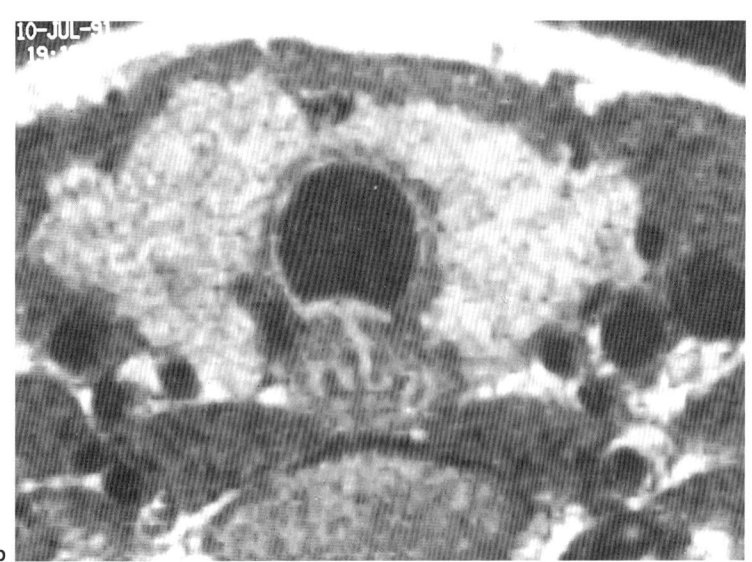

Fig. 3.**17** Graves disease in a 17-year-old woman. The thyroid shows increased signal on the T1-weighted image with further increase after Gd-DTPA. Hyperfunctioning thyroid tissue shows homogeneously high signal on the T2-weighted image
a T1-weighted transverse precontrast MR image, SE 500/15
b T1-weighted transverse Gd-enhanced MR image, SE 500/15
c T2-weighted transverse MR image, SE 2500/90
d Intensity ratios of thyroid vs. muscle on T1-weighted images show a direct linear correlation to serum thyroxine (T_4) levels in normal subjects and in patients with Graves disease (from Charkes et al., Radiology 1987)

is characteristic (4, 9, 11, 13, 18). These areas may represent colloid cysts or hemorrhagic imbibition of degenerated adenomatous or cystic debris. Cysts exhibit lower signal intensity than the residual thyroid tissue and show higher intensity than normal thyroid tissue on T2-weighted images (12). Calcified areas, which may be present (7), exhibit low signal intensity or complete signal loss on T1- as well as on T2-weighted images. Because of decreased vascularization, cystic, hemorrhagic, and calcified regions do not enhance with Gd-DTPA.

MRI is superior to other imaging modalities in the evaluation of substernal extention and vascular or tracheal compression, which often accompanies large goiters. When imaging substernal goiters, ECG gating may be useful in order to define their entire intrathoracic extent. The superiority of MRI over CT in the mediastinum is due to the large scale soft-tissue contrast in differentiating vessels from solid and cystic mediastinal masses without the need for iodine contrast agents. Another important advantage is the possibility to image in any plane. Because it provides a three-dimensional data set, MRI offers exact volume calculations and permits a quantitative assessment of the reduction in thyroid mass as a response to therapy.

Graves Disease

Several unique signal intensity patterns have been suggested on MRI in Graves disease and multinodular goiter (4, 9). Diffusely increased intensity on T1- and T2-weighted images suggests Graves disease (Fig. 3.**17**). T1-relaxation times are longer in patients with Graves disease (22). Results of another study (4) sug-

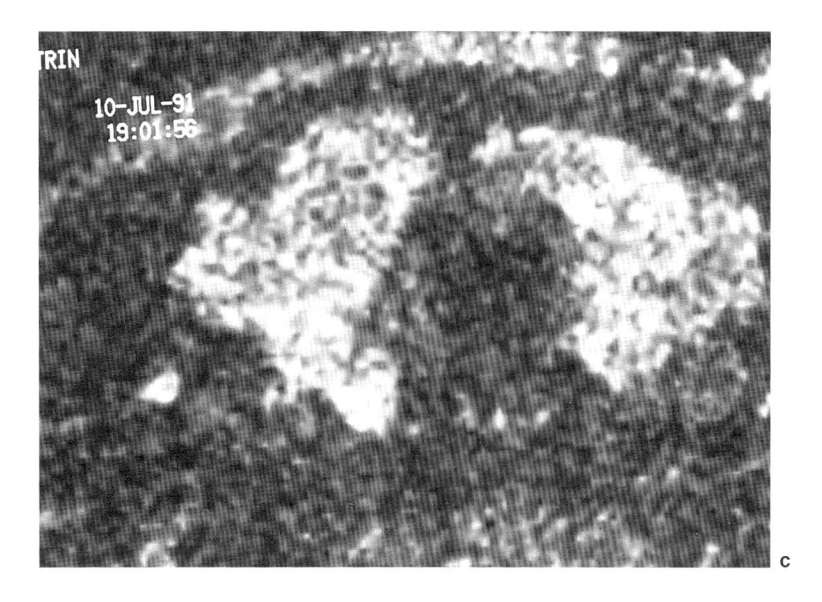

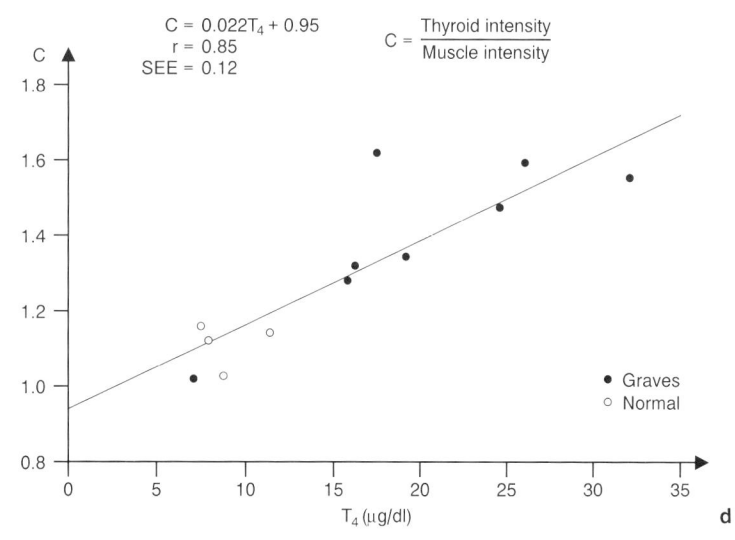

Fig. 3.**17c–d**

$$C = 0.022 T_4 + 0.95$$
$$r = 0.85$$
$$SEE = 0.12$$

$$C = \frac{\text{Thyroid intensity}}{\text{Muscle intensity}}$$

- Graves
- Normal

gest a close correlation between intensity ratios of thyroid to muscle on T1-weighted images and serum thyroxine levels. Serum thyroxine levels and 24-hour uptake of ^{123}I were significantly higher in patients with an intensity ratio of thyroid to muscle greater than 1:4 than in patients with lower intensity ratios (4). Therefore, in Graves disease, the thyroid gland presents an abnormally high signal throughout the entire thyroid parenchyma. Moreover, MR imaging in Graves disease has revealed numerous coarse, bandlike structures within the gland representing fibrous trunks around thyroid lobules, as well as multiple dilated vessels representing venous structures (17). However, in the differentiation of Graves disease from other causes of hyperthyroidism, MRI is still limited (20). Recent studies suggest an increased uptake of Gd-DTPA in hyperfunctioning thyroid tissue.

Thyroiditis

Few cases of MRI findings in thyroiditis have been reported (10, 16). Hashimoto disease has been described as a diffusely enlarged gland without distinct characteristics on T1-weighted images. The signal intensity pattern of the gland is usually heterogeneous on T2-weighted images. Substantial signal increase of the gland with low intensity stripes indicative of fibrosis have been found in some cases (17). Like scintigraphy, MRI is nonspecific in thyroiditis, and the diagnosis is based on laboratory findings.

Adenoma

The adenoma is the most common benign thyroid tumor with its criteria of complete fibrous encapsula-

62   3 Thyroid Gland

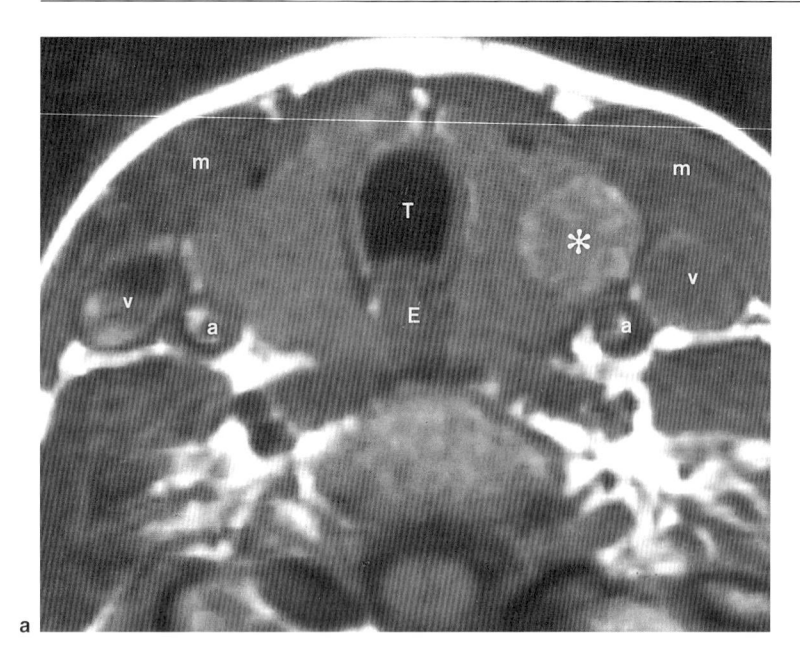

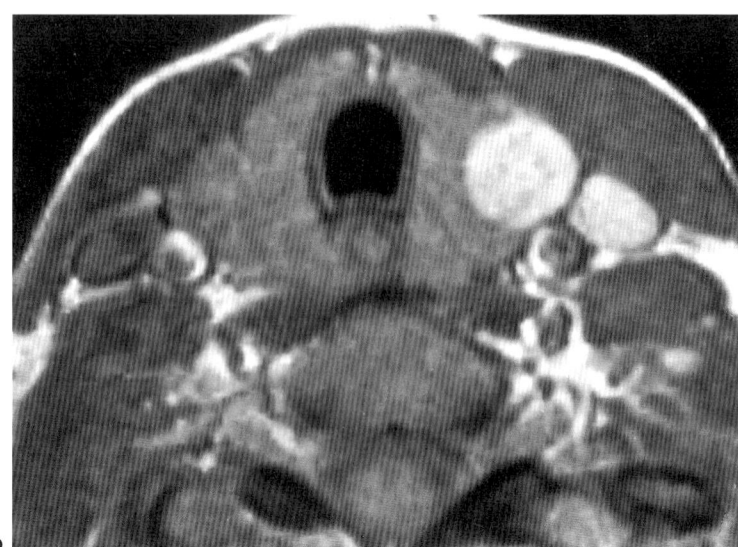

Fig. 3.**18** Hyperfunctioning follicular adenoma (*) of the left thyroid lobe in a 27-year-old woman with inhomogeneous, slightly higher intensity than the remaining thyroid tissue on T1-weighted images and homogeneously higher intensity than the thyroid on T2-weighted images. Trachea (T), esophagus (E), veins (v), arteries (a), and sternocleidomastoid muscles (m)
a T1-weighted transverse MR image, SE 500/15
b Proton density transverse MR image, SE 2500/22
c T2-weighted transverse MR image, SE 2500/90
d T1-weighted transverse MR images, SE 2500/90, post contrast, show an increased Gd enhancement in the center of the adenoma

tion, clear distinction between the architecture of the adenoma inside and outside of the capsule, a uniform histologic structure, and compression of the surrounding thyroid (7). The variable MR appearance of adenomas results from their variable histopathologic substrate (10). The MR appearance of adenomas is usually hypointense or isointense to the remaining thyroid on T1-weighted MR images, with a signal increase on T2-weighted images (Fig. 3.**18**). Therefore, adenomas may not be discernible from the surrounding tissue on T1-weighted images. Due to long T2 relaxation times of adenomas and adenomatous hyperplasia, T2-weighted images show high contrast of these lesions relative to normal thyroid tissue (10). Colloid most likely causes shortening of T1 and may account for the slightly higher signal intensity of some adenomas compared to normal thyroid tissue on T1-weighted images. Most adenomas have longer T1 and T2 relaxation times than normal thyroid tissue. The high paramagnetic contrast enhancement after Gd-DTPA is related to the high vascular density and a large extracellular space of an adenoma compared to normal thyroid tissue (Fig. 3.**18**). High intensity on T1-weighted images indicates either subacute hemorrhage within an adenoma or highly proteinaceous fluid within a colloid cyst (9, 17). However, there have been descriptions of non-hemorrhagic, solid adenomas with high signal intensity on T1-weighted images (4, 12, 17).

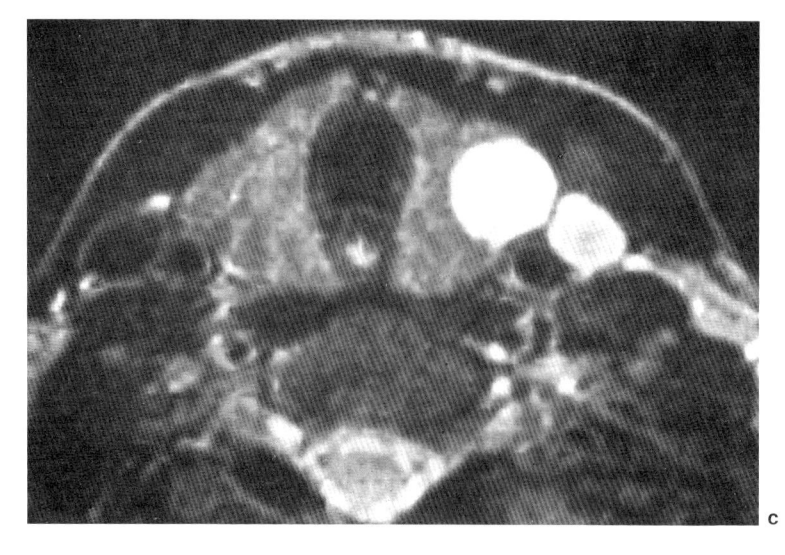

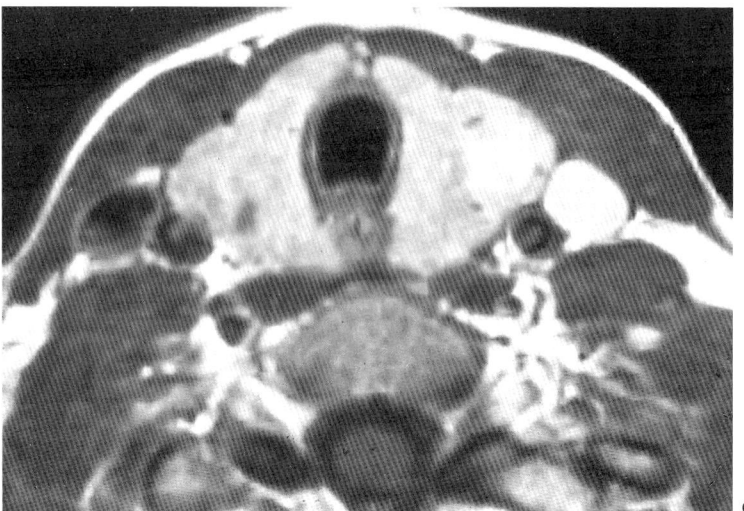

Fig. 3.**18c-d**

Cysts or Cystic Degeneration

Cysts usually have low intensity on T1-weighted images and high intensity on T2-weighted images. Cysts with either colloid or acute hemorrhagic content can show high signal on T1- and T2-weighted images (Fig. 3.**19**). If a hemorrhage is more than 14 to 21 days old, the MRI appearance may be characterized by the presence of a hemosiderin rim. As previously described with intracranial hematomas, this is seen as a low intensity rim on T2-weighted images (Fig. 3.**19**).

Carcinoma

Thyroid carcinoma occurs in different histologic forms: papillary, follicular, medullary, and anaplastic. Because of the different ways of expansion and metastasis, MRI evaluation should not only encompass the thyroid bed with short and long TR sequences as well as with paramagnetic contrast enhancement, but also study lymphatic drainage regions in the neck and chest. Like scintigraphy, MRI is nonspecific with respect to most solitary nodules and can not differentiate adenoma from carcinoma based on the signal intensity pattern alone. Although thyroid malignancies have abnormal T1 and T2 values relative to normal thyroid tissue, in no study have the patterns of signal intensities been consistently distinctive compared to those of benign adenomas and multinodular goiters.

Follicular and papillary carcinomas usually exhibit similar or slightly lower signal intensities than normal thyroid tissue on T1-weighted images and higher signal intensities than normal thyroid tissue on

64   3 Thyroid Gland

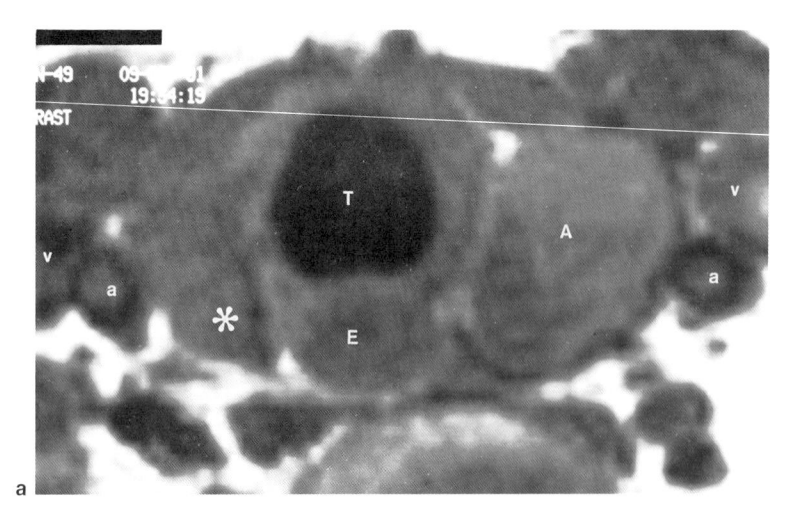

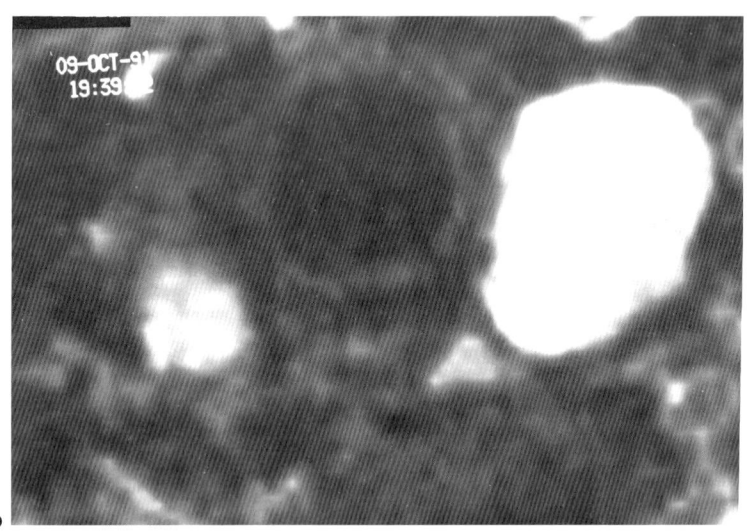

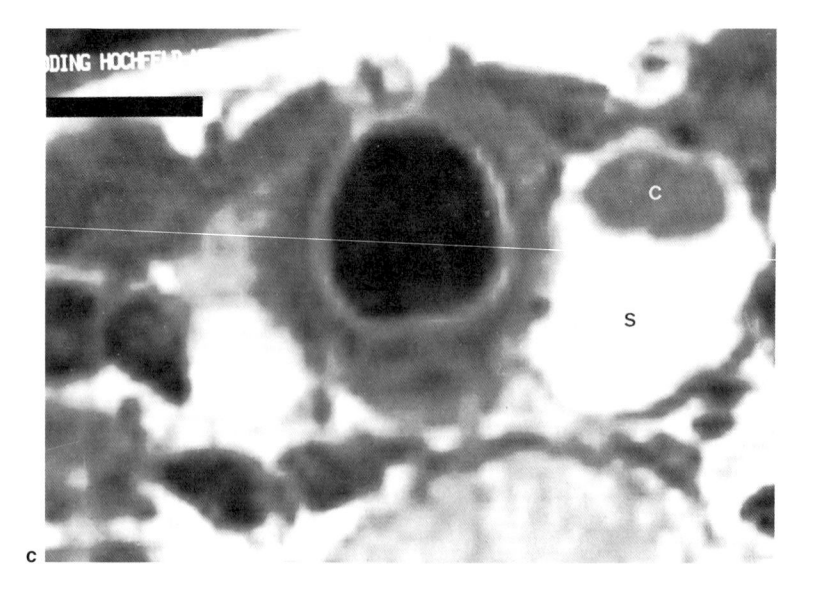

Fig. 3.**19** Partially cystic degeneration of an adenoma of the left thyroid lobe. Note a parathyroid adenoma (*) posteroinferior to the right thyroid lobe. A = adenoma, T = trachea, E = esophagus, a = carotid artery, v = jugular vein, S = solid part, and C = cystic part of the left-sided thyroid adenoma
a T1-weighted transverse MR image, SE 500/15
b T2-weighted transverse MR image, SE 2500/90
c T1-weighted transverse MR image, SE 500/15, postcontrast

T2-weighted images (Fig. 3.20). Usually, the MR intensity of those highly differentiated types is similar to that of adenomas. With its low differentiation and high invasiveness, the anaplastic type may extend beyond the thyroid bed and produce large bulky masses. MR appearance is low on T1-weighted images and high on T2-weighted images. Thyroid lymphoma shows low to medium intensity on T1-weighted images and heterogeneously high intensity on T2-weighted images (Fig. 3.21). The MR appearance of malignant thyroid tumors varies from slightly hyperintense to slightly hypointense or isointense relative to normal thyroid tissue. Tumors are generally heterogeneous with partially high intensity due to regional hemorrhage. Contrast enhancement with Gd-DTPA offers important additional information for the distinction of benign and malignant thyroid tumors (23). The infiltration of surrounding tissue layers in particular, is more clearly defined on Gd-DTPA-enhanced, T1-weighted images than on T2-weighted images because of the better image quality of the former. However, no definite distinction between inflammatory and tumorous infiltration of muscle can be made with Gd enhancement (26).

MRI is superior to other techniques in evaluating mass extention, amount of invasion, and tumor recurrence in the neck and particularly in the mediastinum. It is sensitive in the detection of muscle invasion or inflammation caused by close association of tumor to muscle. Signal intensity of muscle is altered by a number of processes, including fatty degeneration, inflammatory edema, and tumor invasion (3). The involved muscular structures show higher signal intensity than the contralateral side. Inflammation may also cause increased signal intensity, simulating tumor invasion (3). However, if disruption and invasion of normal soft-tissue planes is identified, carcinoma can be suggested on the basis of the MRI appearance. Therefore, MRI may detect early invasion of muscles, esophagus, trachea, larynx, neurovascular bundles, and other structures of the neck with a higher sensitivity than CT. Because of the high sensitivity of MRI for either edema or invasion, normal adjacent muscle (or fat) probably excludes tumor invasion. Focal signal in-

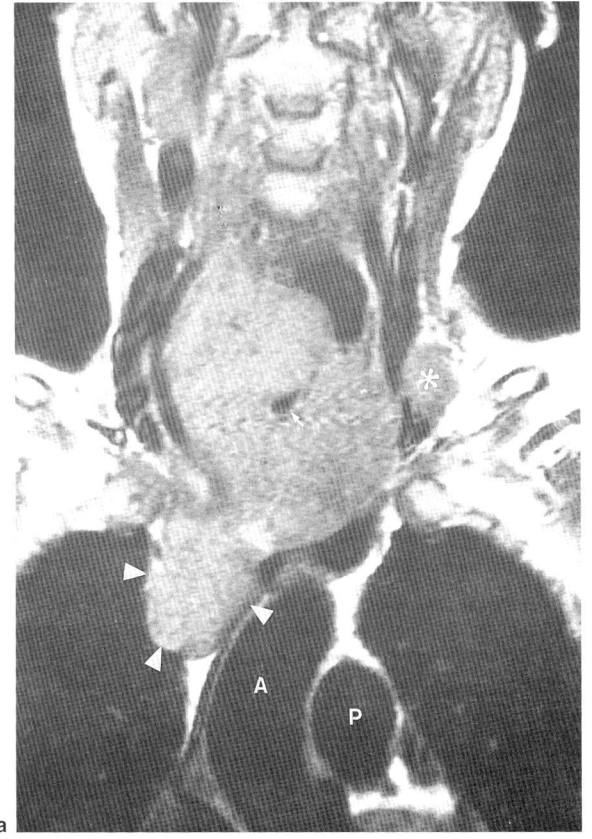

Fig. 3.20 Large thyroid carcinoma with extensive mediastinal invasion (arrowheads), tracheal (arrow), and vascular compression as well as multiple cervical nodal metastases (*). A = aorta, P = pulmonary artery, L = lung, trachea (open arrow), vessels (arrows)
a T1-weighted coronal MR image, SE 500/15
b T1-weighted coronal MR image, SE 500/15, post contrast

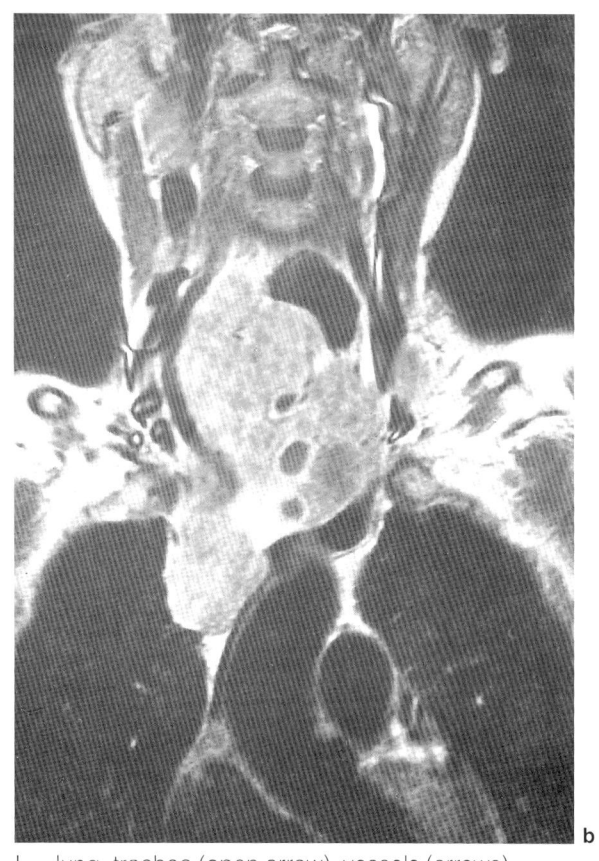

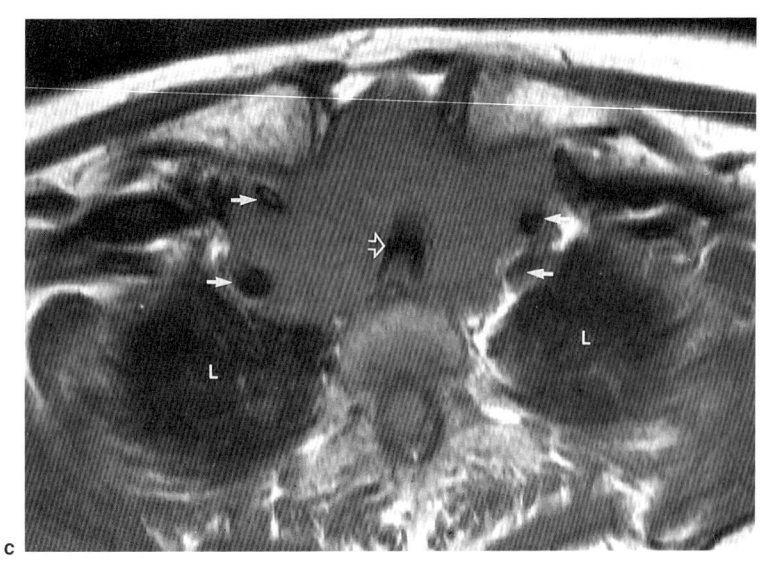

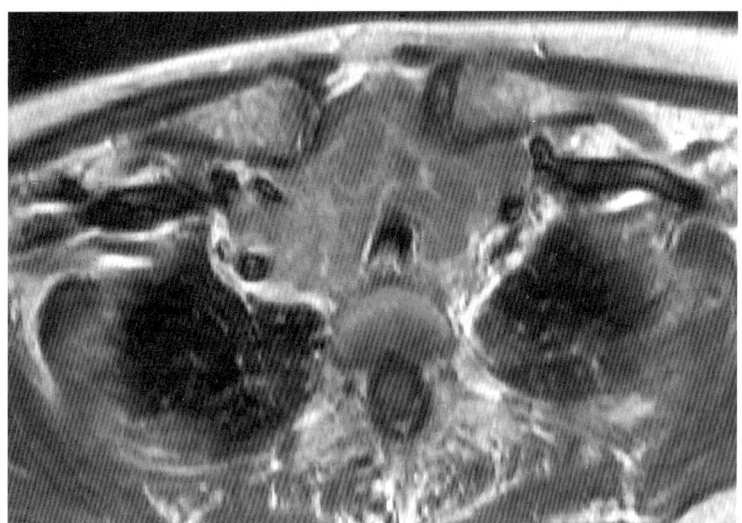

Fig. 3.**20 c–d**
c T1-weighted transverse MR image, SE 500/15
d T1-weighted transverse MR image, SE 500/15, post contrast
(Courtesy of R. Bittner, Berlin)

crease makes invasion more likely, whereas diffuse increase may be caused by either inflammation or tumor involvement. Muscle and fat layers are best distinguished on T1-weighted, spin-echo images, whereas tumorous and muscular tissue is usually well separated on T2-weighted images (Fig. 3.**22**).

MRI is particularly useful when attempting to evaluate recurrence of medullary carcinoma (3, 5) because a tumor does not accumulate ^{131}I, limiting the use of nuclear scans (1). The MR characteristics of tumor recurrence generally allow differentiation from scarring in the normal thyroid bed. Local recurrence is generally characterized by low to medium intensity on T1-weighted images, medium to high intensity on T2-weighted images, and considerable enhancement with MR contrast media (3, 26). Scar in the normal postoperative thyroid bed has low intensity on T1- and T2-weighted images, depending on the time after thyroidectomy. Postoperative edema, infection, or bleeding can be expected to produce high intensity on T2-weighted images and thereby might simulate recurrence (Fig. 3.**23**). In the early postoperative phase, MRI may not allow differentiation. However, in the later phase, MRI seems useful in defining invasion of adjacent muscles and extension into the mediastinum. Likewise, cervical nodal metastases may be seen with MRI.

MR Imaging 67

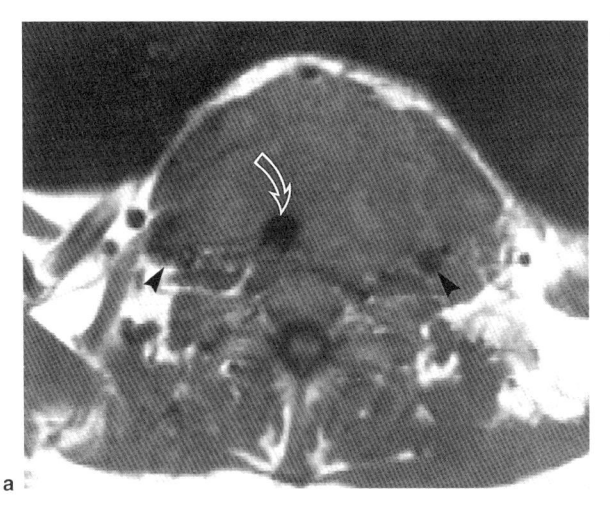

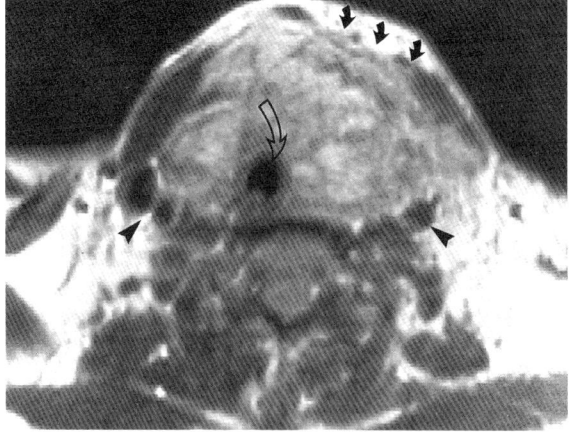

Fig. 3.**21** Thyroid Lymphoma
a T1-weighted spin-echo image, TR = 500 msec, TE = 30 msec, shows large mass of heterogeneous intensity, but most of the mass has similar intensity to and is indistinguishable from muscle
b T2-weighted spin-echo image, TR = 2000 msec, TE = 60 msec, shows high-intensity heterogeneous mass.

Note alteration of intensity of strap (closed arrows) and left sternocleidomastoid muscle on the T2-weighted image. This finding suggests invasion of muscle. Neurovascular bundles are displaced posteriorly (arrowheads). The open curved arrow points to the displaced trachea (from Higgins & Auffermann, AJR 1988)

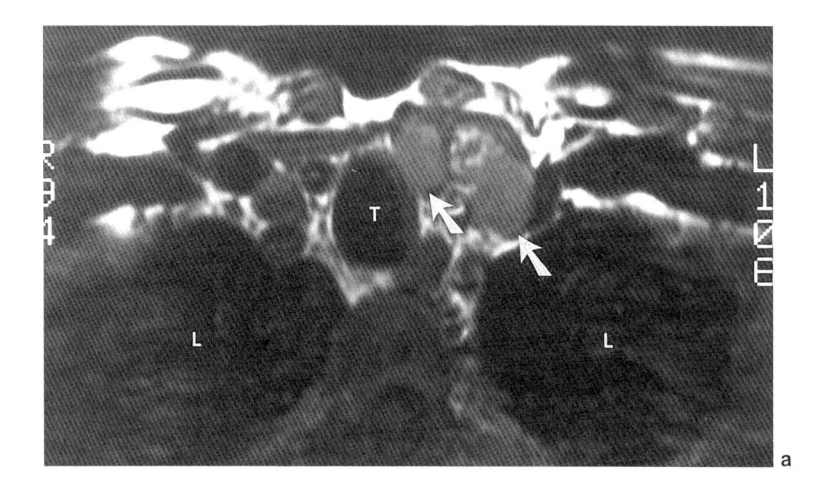

Fig. 3.**22** Recurrent thyroid carcinoma (arrows) shows high intensity on the T2-weighted image and thereby is clearly distinguishable from scar tissue. T = trachea, L = lung
a T1-weighted transverse MR image, SE 500/20
b T2-weighted transverse MR image, SE 2000/60
(from Auffermann et al., AJR 1988)

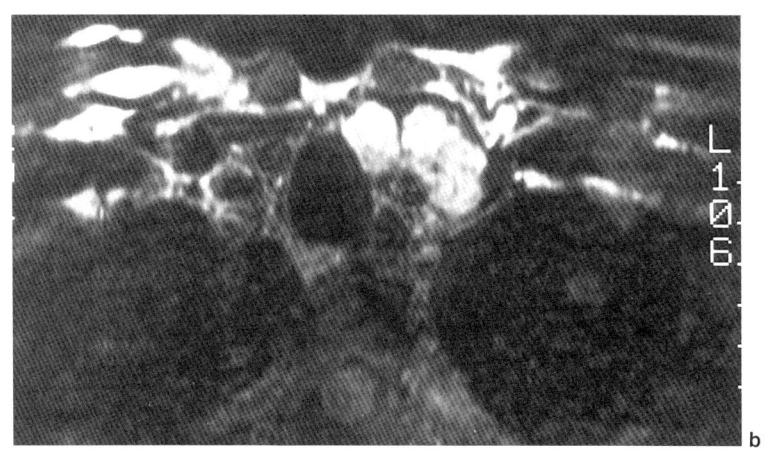

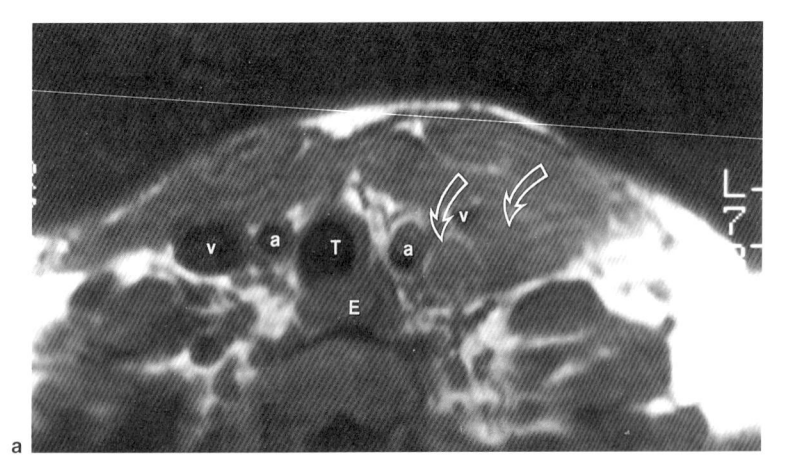

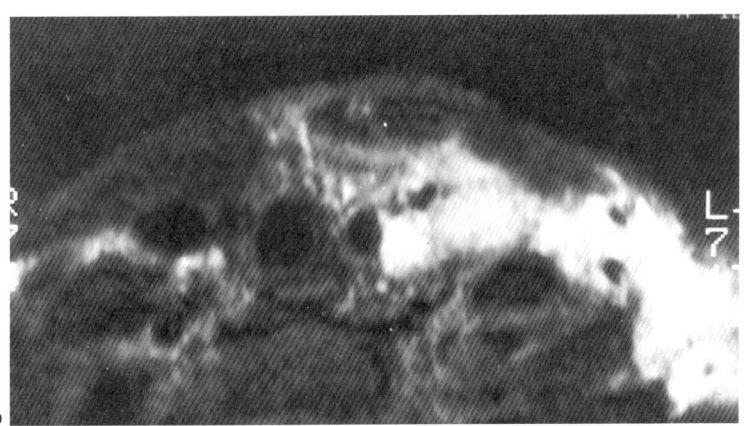

Fig. 3.**23** Inflammatory changes in the left thyroid bed and in cervical lymph nodes 6 months after total thyroidectomy for papillary thyroid carcinoma. Reactive lymphatic hyperplasia (open arrows) shows low intensity on T1-weighted images and high intensity on T2-weighted images. The left jugular vein (v) is compressed. T = trachea, E = esophagus, a = carotid artery
a T1-weighted transverse MR image, SE 500/20
b T2-weighted transverse MR image, SE 2000/60
(from Auffermann et al., AJR 1988)

References

1. Arnstein NB, Juni JE, Sisson JC, Lloyd RV, Thompson NW. Recurrent medullary carcinoma of the thyroid demonstrated by thallium-201 scintigraphy. J Nucl Med 1986;27:1564–1568.
2. Arrington EF, Eisenberg B. Magnetic resonance imaging of the thyroid. In: Eisenberg B. Imaging of the thyroid and parathyroid glands. New York: Churchill Livingstone; 1991:133–144.
3. Auffermann W, Clark OH, Thurnher S, Galante M, Higgins CB. Recurrent thyroid carcinoma. Characteristics on MR images. Radiology. 1988;168:753–757.
4. Charkes ND, Maurer AH, Siegel JA, Radecki PD, Malmud LS. MR imaging in thyroid disorders: Correlation of signal intensity with Graves disease activity. Radiology. 1987;164:491–494.
5. Crow JP, Azar-Kia B, Prinz RA. Recurrent occult medullary thyroid carcinoma detected by MR imaging. Am J Roentgenol. 1989;152:1255.
6. De Certaines J, Herry JY, Lancien G, Benoist L, Bernard AM, Le Clech G. Evaluation of human thyroid tumors by proton nuclear magnetic resonance. J Nucl Med. 1982;23:48–51
7. DeGroot LJ, ed. Endocrinology; vol 1. Philadelphia: Saunders, 1989.
8. Eisenberg B, Velchik MG, Gefter WB et al. Correlative MR and scintigraphic thyroid imaging. Am J physiol Imaging. 1990;5:9–15.
9. Gefter WB, Spritzer CE, Eisenberg B et al. Thyroid imaging with high-field-strength surface-coil MR. Radiology. 1987;164:483–490.
10. Higgins CB, McNamara MT, Fisher MR, Clark OH. MR imaging of the thyroid. Am J Roentgenol. 1985;147:1255–1261.
11. Higgins CB, Auffermann W. Normal anatomy: the neck, chest, and heart. In: Higgins CB, Hricak H, eds. Magnetic Resonance Imaging of the Body. New York: Raven; 1987:49–74.
12. Higgins CB, Fisher MR. The neck. In: Higgins CB, Hricak H, eds. Magnetic Resonance Imaging of the Body. New York: Raven; 1987:145–172.
13. Higgins CB, Auffermann W. MR imaging of the thyroid and parathyroid glands. A review of current status. Am J Roentgenol. 1988;151:1095–1106.
14. Johnson JC, Coleman LL. Magnetic resonance imaging of a lingual thyroid gland. Pediat Radiol. 1989;19:461–463.
15. Johnson M, Selinsky B, Davis M, et al. In vitro NMR evaluation of human thyroid lesions. Invest Radiol. 1989;24:666–670.
16. Mountz JM, Glazer GM, Dmuchowski C, Sisson JC. MR imaging of the thyroid. Comparison with scintigraphy in the normal and diseased gland. J Comput assist Tomogr. 1987;11:612–619.
17. Noma C, Nishimura K, Togashi K, et al. Thyroid gland. MR imaging. Radiology. 1987;164:495–499.
18. Noma W, Kanaoka M, Minami S, et al. Thyroid masses. MR imaging and pathologic correlation. Radiology. 1988;168:759–764.
19. Noma S, Konishi J, Morikawa M, et al. MR imaging of thyroid hemochromatosis. J Comput assist Tomogr. 1988;12:623–626.
20. Sandler MP, Patton JA. Multimodality imaging of the thyroid and parathyroid glands. J Nucl Med. 1987;28:122–129.
21. Schara M, Sentjurc M, Auersperg M, et al. Characterization of malignant thyroid gland tissue by magnetic resonance methods. Br J Cancer. 1974;29:483–486.
22. Sinadinovic J, Ratkovic S, Kraincanic M, et al. Relationship of biochemical and morphological changes in rat thyroid and proton spin-relaxation of the tissue water. Endokrinologie. 1977;69:55–66.
23. Smelkal A v, Kozak B, Niemeyer M, Hedde JP. Magnetic resonance imaging in therapy monitoring of well differentiated thyroid carcinoma. 8th Annual Congress of the European Society for Magnetic Resonance in Medicine and Biology. Books of Ab-

stracts. Zürich: European Society for Magnetic Resonance in Medicine and Biology; 1991:50.
24 Stark DD, Moss AA, Gamsu G, Clark OH, Gooding GAW, Webb WR. Magnetic resonance imaging of the neck. Radiology. 1984;150:455–461.
25 Takashima S, Ikezoe J, Morimoto S, et al. MR imaging of primary thyroid lymphoma. J Comput Assist Tomogr. 1989;13:517.
26 Tella S, Beomonte ZB, Datalano C, et al. MRI of thyroid gland. A comparative study. 8th Annual Congress of the European Society for Magnetic Resonance in Medicine and Biology. Book of Abstracts. Zürich: Eupean Society for Magnetic Resonance in Medicine and Biology; 1991:50.
27 Tennvall J, Björklund A, Möller T, Olsson M, Persson B, Akerman M. Studies of NMR-relaxation-times in malignant tumours and normal tissues of the human thyroid gland. Prog Nucl Med. 1984;8:142–148.

Nuclear Medicine

U. Keske

Method

Scintigraphic imaging plays a unique role in the evaluation of thyroid disease. This is explained by the fact that iodine is an essential and specific component of thyroid hormone. Thyroid scintigraphy not only enables the physician to determine thyroid size, but also to evaluate the function of thyroid nodules, to detect occult or ectopic thyroid tissue and to find metastases from thyroid carcinoma.

Radiopharmaceuticals

At first, only sodium **Iodine-131,** a nuclear reactor by-product, was available for use in thyroid scintigraphy. Because of its relatively long half-life (8.1 days) and the relatively high energy gamma radiation (364 keV) and beta radiation, it is not an ideal radionuclide for thyroid imaging and is nowadays used only for radionuclide therapy and a few clinical conditions. These include scanning for ectopic thyroid tissue or substernal goiter, whole body scintigraphy in patients with thyroid carcinoma, and determination of radioiodine uptake before radioiodine therapy. Radiation exposure to the thyroid is 1000 mGy/1.85 MBq.

Technetium-99m-pertechnetate (^{99m}Tc) is readily available in every nuclear medicine department, since it is obtained from portable Mo-99 generators. It differs from iodine in that iodine isotopes are incorporated like stable iodine and are therefore physiological tracers, whereas pertechnetate is only trapped by the thyroid, and not incorporated into thyroid hormone. Pertechnetate has largely replaced ^{131}I. Application of as much as 185–350 mBq is possible. Since the principal emission is at 140 keV, the images obtained are of higher quality. Thyroid uptake may be measured using ^{99m}Tc (15, 23) either with a scintillation camera and computer or with an uptake probe. A few reports exist about pertechnetate uptake in thyroid nodules that did not trap any iodine (14). Nevertheless, it is generally thought that pertechnetate is an appropriate radiopharmaceutical for thyroid scintigraphy. Radiation exposure to the thyroid is 3.4 mGy/37 MBq.

Iodine-123 is a cyclotron product with a relatively short half-life (13.3 hours) and a relatively low gamma energy (159 keV). It emits no beta radiation. The absorbed thyroidal radiation dose is only about one-thousandth of that from ^{131}I, which allows administration of sufficient amounts for imaging with the gamma camera. Uptake measurements are possible for up to 24 hours. Although its biological and physical characteristics make it an ideal agent for routine thyroid imaging, it has not gained wide acceptance, mostly because of its high cost. Radiation exposure to the thyroid is 100 mGy/18.5 MBq.

Thyroid Scintigraphy

It is important that the patient has not been exposed to exogenous iodine or thyroid hormone before scintigraphy, as this decreases the thyroid uptake of the radiotracer. Thyroid uptake and scintigraphy may be influenced for 2–6 weeks after application of ionic and nonionic contrast media used for angiography, computed tomography, or urography, and up to 6 months after application of biliary contrast media. After lymphography, thyroid tests may even be affected for 1.5–2 years (11). Thyroxine has to be stopped 8 days before scintigraphy. For whole-body scintigraphy in thyroid cancer, the interval has to be longer (11, see below). Potassium perchlorate given before application of the tracer will also decrease thyroid uptake and make scintigraphy impossible.

Thyroid scintigrams are currently obtained by an Anger **scintillation camera.** The images are superior to those obtained using the rectilinear scanner, which affords lower resolution and sensitivity and requires a longer imaging time. A parallel-hole or pinhole collimator may be used. Thyroid scintigraphy is performed 2 hours after i. v. administration of 18.5 MBq Na^{123}I, 20 minutes after i. v. administration of 37 MBq ^{99m}Tc-O$_4$, or 24 hours after oral or i. v. administration of 200 kBq Na^{131}I. These doses have to be fractionated for children.

Thyroid Uptake

Thyroid uptake may be measured using a gamma camera or a thyroid probe. The thyroid probe consists of a flat-field collimator, a small-diameter crystal, a single or multichannel analyzer, and a scaler. Measurements of the radionuclide syringe before and after injection of the patient are necessary. With the gamma camera, evaluation is performed within regions of interest (ROI) using a specially designed software (9).

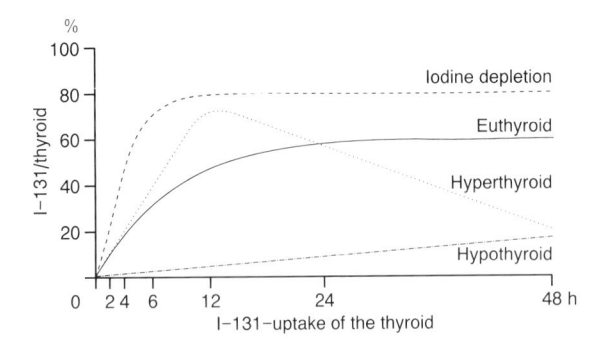

Fig. 3.24 ^{131}I uptake of the thyroid. In hyperthyroidism, a fast and high tracer accumulation within the thyroid is found, and excretion is rapid. In iodine depletion, uptake is fast, while the excretion rate is very low. In primary hypothyroidism, almost no tracer uptake within the thyroid is found (adapted from 21)

Uptake measurements are usually performed at the time of scintigraphy (see above). Normal range is 23–49% for iodine (2 hours p.i.) and 1.5–5% for pertechnetate (20 minutes p.i.). Thyroid measurements over a total period of 5–10 days reflect the endogenous iodine kinetic (Fig. 3.24). They can only be performed with ^{131}I. In hyperthyroidism, a rapid and high iodine uptake is found and excretion is fast. In hypothyroidism, initial uptake is slow and reaches a maximum only after several days. In iodine depletion, initial uptake is fast and high, but excretion is low. Determination of the biologic half-life is important for radioiodine therapy of goiter and hyperthyroidism.

Special Tests

A **suppression test** is performed if autonomous thyroid tissue is suspected. Thyroid scintigraphy is repeated after administration of 60 μg T$_3$ over at least 8 days or 200 μg T$_4$ over 14 days (17). Thyroid tissue that is still regulated by TSH will show a decreased uptake, whereas autonomous thyroid tissue will have an unchanged uptake. The test is important for detection of compensated autonomous adenomas and disseminated thyroid autonomy.

The **perchlorate discharge test** is performed in order to search for defects in organification. Two hours after administration of radioiodine, thyroid uptake is measured. Afterwards, potassium perchlorate is given orally (1 g to adults, 0.6 g to children). After 30 minutes and again, after 60 minutes, the thyroid content of iodine is measured. A decrease of more than 10% of the 2-hour value indicates an impaired organification of iodine (9).

Scintigraphic Findings

Normal Findings

The **normal thyroid scan** shows a symmetric thyroid gland with uniform activity distribution (Fig. 3.25), a mean length and width of the lobes of 5.1 ± 0.8 cm × 2.1 ± 0.3 cm (right) and 4.6 ± 0.8 cm × 2.0 ± 0.3 cm (left). The upper right pole usually lies about 0.5 cm higher than the left lobe. The long axes of the lobes converge caudally or lie parallel. Thyroid volume may be approximated by the formula length × width^2 : 2 (9).

Goiter

Goiters have to be separated into diffuse and nodular goiter. There are numerous underlying pathologies, including iodine-deficient goiter, Graves disease, and thyroid carcinoma.

Diffuse goiter is represented as a uniformly and symmetrically enlarged thyroid with homogeneous activity distribution. Radionuclide uptake may be increased in iodine deficiency (Fig. 3.26), but is mostly normal.

Multinodular goiter may be asymmetric with gross loss of normal configuration. Activity distribution is inhomogeneous (Fig. 3.27). Cold nodules may be seen, and hot nodules are a frequent finding especially in longstanding nodular goiters (Fig. 3.30). A suppression scintigram may help to detect thyroid autonomy (see below). Especially in large thyroids, tracer uptake per surface area is reduced, which results in suboptimal image quality. Injection of a double dose of radionuclide may be advantageous (14).

Scintigraphy of **substernal or intrathoracic goiter** may be difficult because the low gamma energy of ^{99m}Tc and ^{123}I may be absorbed by the sternum. But even with ^{131}I, a substernal goiter may be missed because it is typically multinodular and may contain little or no functioning tissue (9).

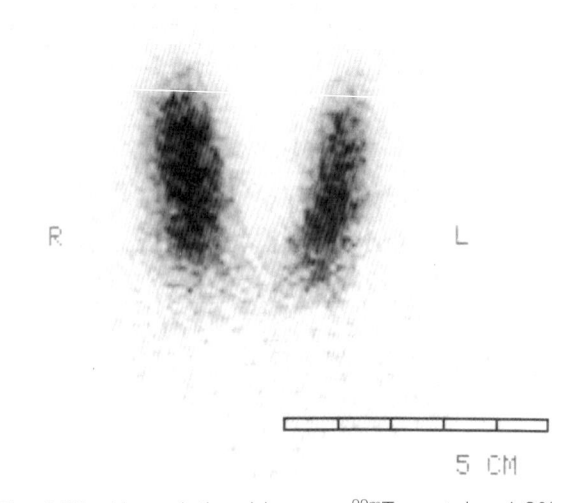

Fig. 3.25 Normal thyroid scan. ^{99m}Tc uptake 1.8% (normal 1.5–5%)

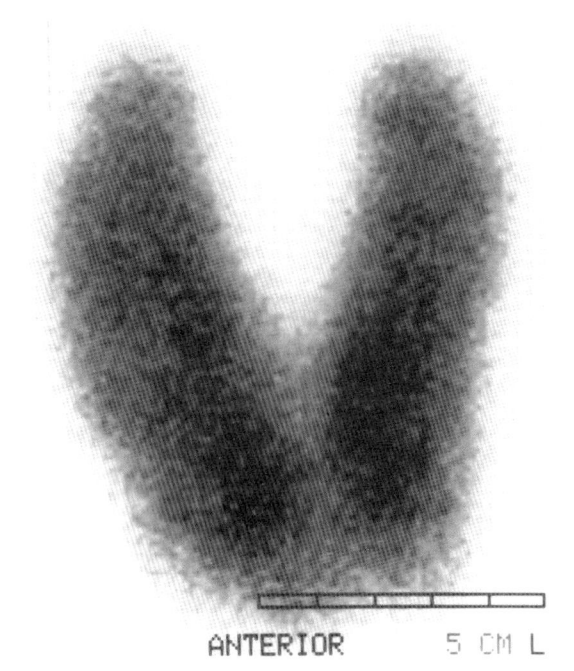

Fig. 3.**26** Diffuse goiter in a 12-year-old boy with iodine depletion. Ultrasound revealed a thyroid volume of 35 mL, no nodules were found. ^{99m}Tc uptake is increased with 36% (normal 1.5 –5%)

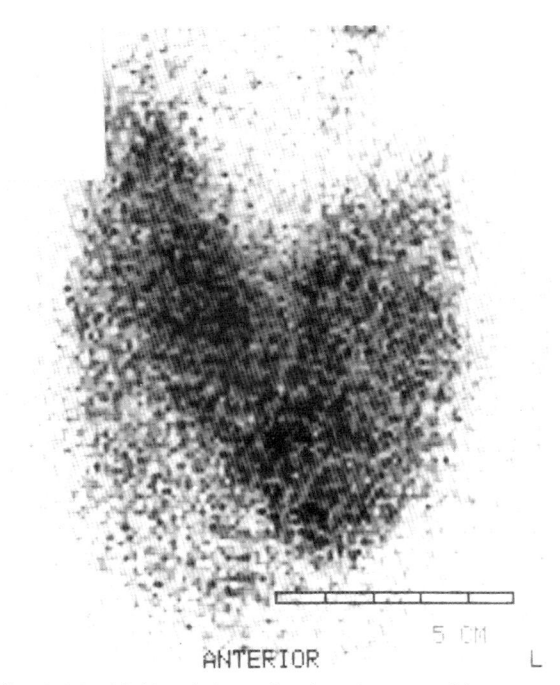

Fig. 3.**27** Multinodular goiter in a 80-year-old woman. Inhomogeneous radionuclide uptake of the thyroid, cold nodule in the lower right lobe. Ultrasound revealed a thyroid volume of 106 mL. Surgery revealed no malignancy

Thyroid Nodules

Evaluation of thyroid nodules is one of the most important tasks of thyroid scintigraphy. The relation of nodes to the thyroid and their sizes are easily determined by ultrasound. However, scintigraphic differentiation of functioning and nonfunctioning nodules (hot or cold nodules) is important for therapy.

The Nonfunctioning Nodule (Cold Nodule)

The underlying pathology of cold nodules includes regressive nodules, cysts, and carcinomas. The most frequent causes are cysts and regressive nodules. Bleeding may also present as a cold nodule. The most important differential diagnosis, however, is thyroid carcinoma (Fig. 3.**28**). Cold nodules necessitate careful management, because the therapeutic consequences are immense. Malignancy is found in 10–25% of cold thyroid nodules (11, 20). Therefore, thyroid carcinoma always needs to be ruled out. In query cases, fine needle biopsy is indicated. Scintigraphic differentiation is usually not possible. However, a large nodule that sharply imprints the lobar margin and extends laterally is usually benign (14). Note that a cold nodule may appear warm when functioning thyroid tissue is found on top of or underneath it. Areas of focally decreased uptake may also be caused by suppression of thyroid function in thyroid autonomy and are occasionally seen in thyroiditis. Extrathyroidal tumors that invade the thyroid will also present as cold lesions.

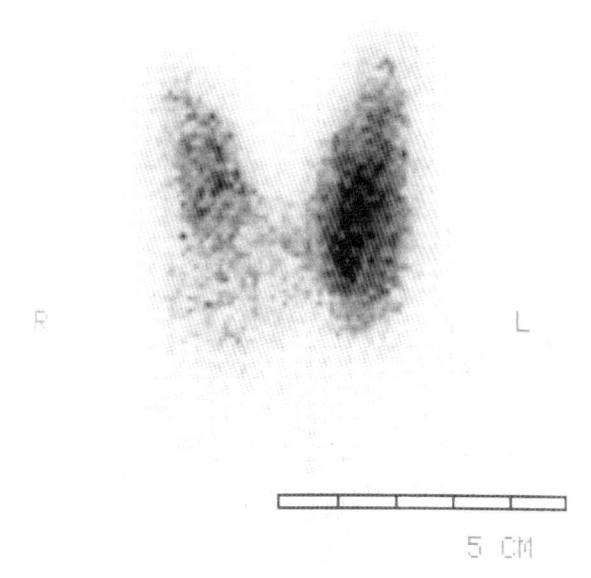

Fig. 3.**28** Cold nodule in the lower right lobe that had developed over the previous 6 months. Histological examination revealed a papillary carcinoma

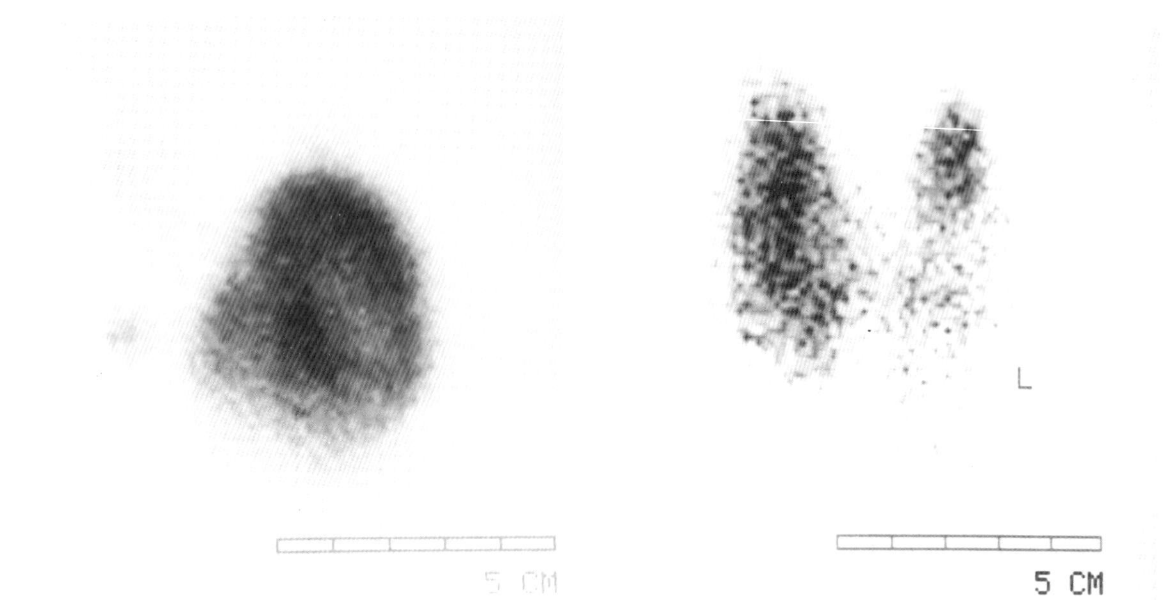

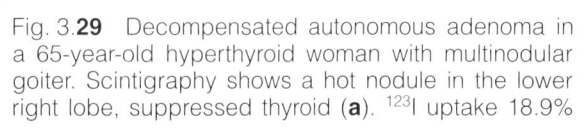

Fig. 3.**29** Decompensated autonomous adenoma in a 65-year-old hyperthyroid woman with multinodular goiter. Scintigraphy shows a hot nodule in the lower right lobe, suppressed thyroid (**a**). ^{123}I uptake 18.9% (normal 17–48%). After radioiodine therapy, complete ablation of the adenoma is found. Inhomogeneous radionuclide uptake of the thyroid due to multinodular goiter (**b**)

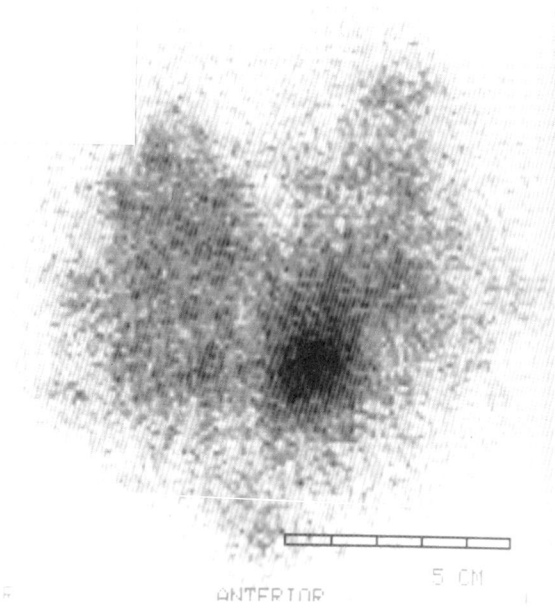

Fig. 3.**30** Partially decompensated autonomous adenoma in a multinodular goiter

The Functioning Nodule

Functioning nodules are caused by autonomous thyroid tissue, which produces thyroid hormones independently of TSH stimulation (Figs. 3.**29** and 3.**30**). Underlying pathology may be adenomatous hyperplasia, benign adenoma, or nontoxic nodular goiter. Functioning nodules may safely be regarded as benign (14). There are very few documented cases of follicular carcinoma exhibiting as a hot nodule in pertechnetate scintigraphy. This finding has not been reported for scanning with ^{131}I or ^{123}I.

It is important to differentiate nodular uptake from uptake in a single thyroid lobe. The latter may be caused by contralateral lobectomy or hemiagenesis. Focally increased uptake with visualization of the rest of the lobe may be caused by focal thickening of the lobe, underlining the necessity of an additional ultrasound examination.

Autonomous adenomas may show a focally decreased uptake in the center, which is caused by necrosis, fibrosis, or hemorrhage (Fig. 3.**29**). Scintigraphy differentiates *compensated* from *decompensated autonomous adenomas*. Decompensated autonomous adenomas present as a hot nodules, with the surrounding tissue showing little or no tracer uptake. The decreased uptake is only functional and is caused by suppression due to a reduction of the serum TSH, which occurs because of increased hormone production of the autonomous adenoma. Compensated autonomous adenomas show a tracer uptake similar to that of the surrounding thyroid. Usually, they are only detected by suppression scintigraphy, where they present as a hot nodule with a suppressed thyroid. Whereas compensated autonomous adenomas are only found in euthyroid state, decompensated autonomous adenomas may be found with normal T_4 or T_3 levels, but a negative TRH test or in hyperthyroid state.

Multifocal autonomy is caused by multiple autonomous areas throughout the thyroid (Fig. 3.**31** and

Nuclear Medicine 73

Fig. 3.**31** Autonomous adenoma (1), multifocal autonomy (2), and disseminated autonomy (3) of the thyroid (adapted from 21)

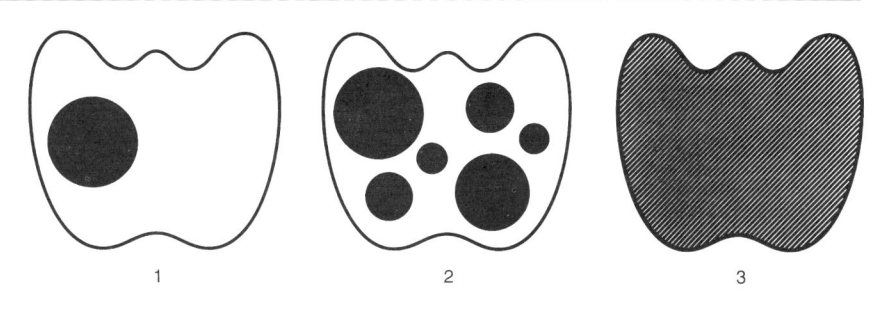

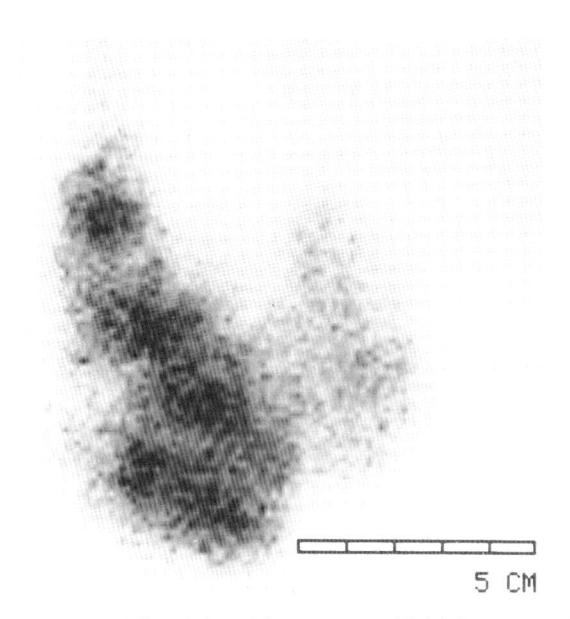

Fig. 3.**32** Multifocal thyroid autonomy. Multiple areas of increased radionuclide uptake in the right lobe

Fig. 3.**33** Graves disease in a 34-year-old woman. Note visualization of the pyramid lobe, which is a frequent finding in Graves disease. ^{99m}Tc uptake 6.2% (normal 1.5–5%)

3.**32**). Occasionally, differentiation from cold nodules may be difficult.

Disseminated autonomy causes homogeneously increased radionuclide uptake in a normal-sized or enlarged thyroid (Fig. 3.**31**), which may simulate Graves disease (see below).

Iatrogenic hyperthyroidism may be caused by excessive thyroxine medication or excessive iodine, presenting scintigraphically as a suppressed thyroid. Occasionally, thyroid autonomy is seen.

Graves Disease

Toxic diffuse goiter in Graves disease shows homogeneously increased radionuclide uptake in a well-lobulated thyroid; visualization of the pyramid lobe is a frequent finding (22, Fig. 3.**33**). The thyroid is usually moderately and symmetrically enlarged, but may also have a normal size (2, 13). An inhomogeneous radionuclide uptake and even nonfunctioning nodules may be seen. This may be caused by inflammatory infiltrates or a preexisting multinodular goiter (Fig. 3.**34**).

Thyroiditis

The term thyroiditis includes diseases of different etiology, such as acute or subacute nonsuppurative thyroiditis and autoimmune thyroiditis (Hashimoto disease). The latter is the most common cause of hypothyroidism (16). Scintigraphic findings are variable and nonspecific. Generally, the most common finding is an enlarged thyroid with an inhomogeneous uptake, which is always suggestive of thyroiditis (11). Cold nodules and asymmetry due to unilateral enlargement may be seen (Fig. 3.**35**); nonvisualization of an entire lobe may be found (14). Due to impaired tracer trapping in the inflamed thyroid tissue, areas of decreased uptake are found. Usually, thyroid uptake is low. The inflamed thyroid tissue may show tracer uptake in gallium scans.

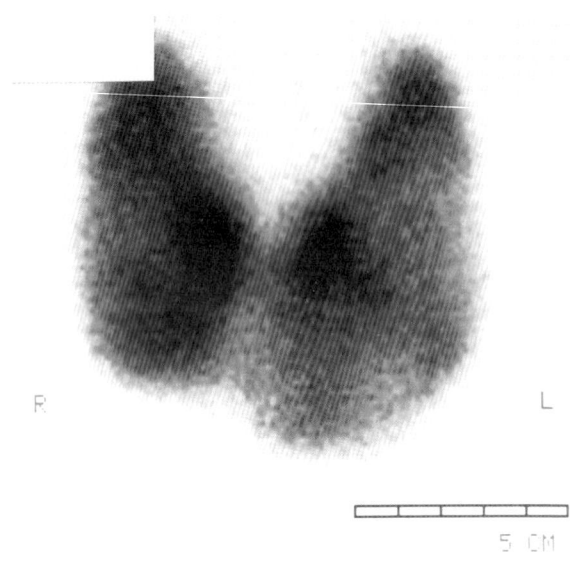

Fig. 3.**34** Graves disease in a 39-year-old female. Due to a preexistent nodular goiter, an inhomogeneous uptake is found with decreased uptake in the lateral left lobe. ^{99m}Tc uptake is increased by 31% (normal 1.5–5%)

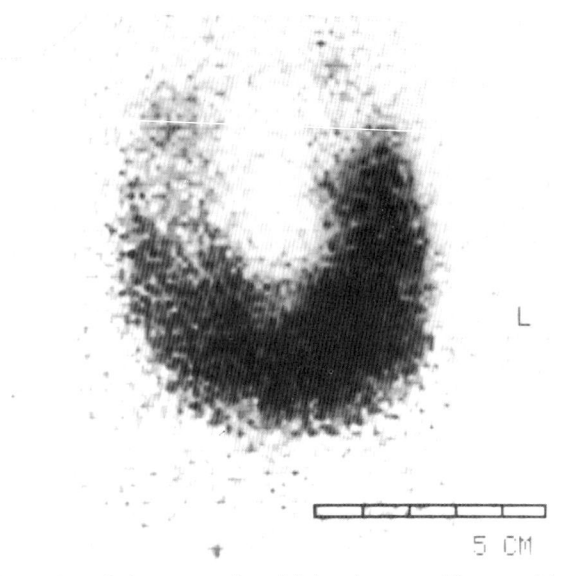

Fig. 3.**35** Subacute thyroiditis in a 46-year-old patient. Note the inhomogeneous radionuclide uptake with focally decreased uptake in the right upper lobe

Ectopic Thyroid

Ectopic thyroid tissue results from an aberrant migration of the gland. It is always found in the midline, adjacent to the thyroglossal duct, and is most frequently located in the cecal foramen, sublingually, or infrahyoidally. Thyroid tissue may be found at the very site of origin, sublingually, cervicomediastinally, or even intracardially (11). The most common thyroid rest is the pyramidal lobe, which occurs in 23–68% of patients (10). Because of the high pertechnetate uptake of the salivary glands, scintigraphy for ectopic thyroid tissue needs to be performed with iodine. The upper cervical, oropharyngeal, and thoracic regions need to be examined; lateral views of the oropharynx are necessary. An additional examination under TSH administration may be helpful (14).

Struma ovarii may show radionuclide uptake. However, it should not be regarded as ectopic thyroid tissue, because it consists of an anomalous development of thyroid tissue within a teratoma (10).

Whole Body Scintigraphy in Thyroid Carcinoma

It is a well-known fact that metastases from well-differentiated carcinoma of the thyroid show radioiodine uptake. As a consequence, radioiodine plays a major role in imaging and therapy of metastatic thyroid cancer.

Method

Whole body scintigraphy is performed with ^{131}I in patients with thyroid carcinoma; 37–74 MBq Na^{131}I-131 are given orally. Imaging is usually performed 24 hours later and is possible until 120 hours after administration. Delayed scans (>96 hours) show higher image quality (7). Scintigraphy is usually performed 5 weeks after radical removement of the thyroid in combination with radioiodine therapy (13). Thereafter, whole body scintigraphy is repeated every 12–24 months. In order to maximize the radioiodine uptake of metastatic thyroid carcinoma, whole body scanning has to be performed in a hypothyroid state. Therefore, T$_4$ has to be discontinued 5 weeks before scintigraphy. For the first 3 weeks, T$_3$ is given to maintain an euthyroid state. After this time, all thyroid medication has to be stopped for about 2 weeks, until TSH is elevated. Whenever metastasis is suggested, whole body scanning is followed by additional radioiodine therapy. Afterwards, thyroid medication is resumed.

An additional method is **Thallium-scintigraphy,** which is performed 20–60 minutes after i. v. injection of 75–110 MBq Thallium-201 (^{201}Tl). The method is helpful for differentiated thyroid carcinoma that shows no iodine uptake (6). Promising results have also been reported for scintigraphy with **^{99m}Tc-MIBI** (Tc-99m-(1)-hexakis(2-methoxyisobutyl-isonitrile), 6).

Scintigraphic Findings

Radioiodine uptake of thyroid neoplasms is significantly lower compared to that of normal thyroid tissue. Thus, the thyroid needs to be completely removed before scanning of metastases can be performed. This is usually done surgically and completed by radioiodine therapy, which removes minor remainders, which the first scintigram will usually show. Scintigraphy needs to be repeated to search for metastases.

Physiological uptake is seen in the salivary glands and saliva, gastric and nasal mucosa, the small and large intestines, the liver, the female breasts, and occasionally in the gallbladder. Confusion may be caused by saliva retention in the piriform sinuses and cervical esophagus (4, 14). Images made over a series of days may be helpful to differentiate pyhsiological from pathological uptake.

Follicular carcinomas set hematogenous metastases into the lungs and bones (Figs. 3.36 and 3.37), whereas papillary carcinomas cause lymphogenous metastases in regional lymph nodes. Metastases of anaplastic and oncocytic carcinomas usually show no radioiodine uptake (21).

Additional bone scanning may be helpful to detect skeletal metastases, especially in follicular carcinoma.

Medullary Carcinoma

Medullary thyroid cancer has its origin in the parafollicular C cells. Medullary carcinomas usually do not trap iodine. However, exceptions are noted in literature and a special "intermediate" type that offers cellular features of both follicular and medullary thyroid carcinoma has been postulated (3, 18). Preoperatively, they present as cold nodules. Postoperatively, radioiodine scintigraphy and therapy is of no help except for ablation of residual thyroid tissue after total thyroidectomy. Serum thyrocalcitonin levels are an important tumor marker for postoperative management. When levels are elevated, scintigraphy should be performed to localize the tumor tissue.

An unspecific tumor uptake is found with ^{201}Tl (3). Scintigraphy with ^{201}Tl is performed immediately after injection of 74 MBq ^{201}Tl and should focus on the neck, since metastatic lymph nodes are a common finding.

Scintigraphy may also be performed with ^{131}I- or ^{123}I-metaiodobenzylguanidine (mIBG), a guanethidine analog also used for imaging of the adrenal medullary and of carcinoids. It is bound in the chromaffin granulas, which are present in C cells. Eighteen MBq ^{131}I-mIBG or 370 MBq ^{123}I-mIBG are given intravenously. Patient preparation with Lugol's solution (strong iodine solution) (10 drops/day) or potassium perchlorate (300 mg/day) one day before

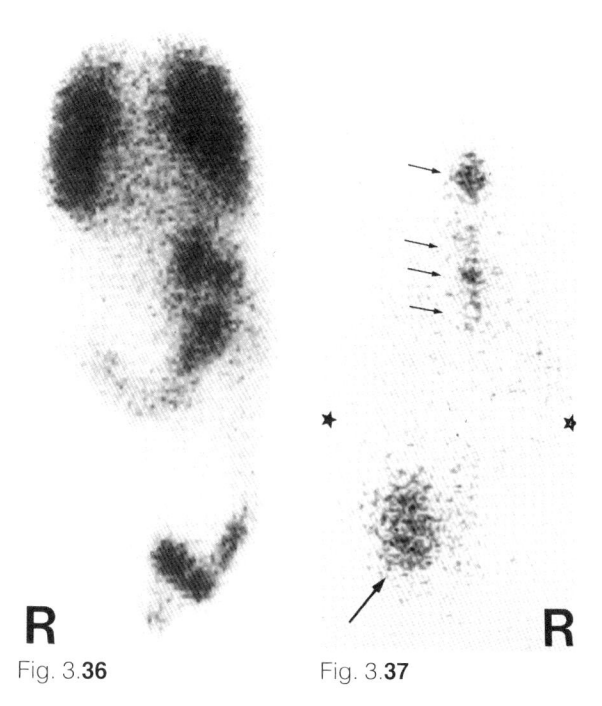

Fig. 3.36 Fig. 3.37

Fig. 3.36 23-year-old patient with metastatic papillary carcinoma of the thyroid. Whole-body ^{131}I scan shows pathologic tracer accumulation in both lungs due to disseminated pulmonary metastases, physiologic tracer accumulation in the large bowels

Fig. 3.37 Seventy-five-year-old patient with metastatic papillary carcinoma of the thyroid. ^{131}I whole-body scan shows bone metastases in the left pelvis (large arrow) and the vertebral column (small arrows). ✣ = iliac crest

and for one week after the administration of mIBG is necessary (see chapters 5 and 7 for details).

A new approach is the implementation of ^{99m}Tc-labeled pentavalent dimercaptosuccinic acid (**DMSA (V)**, 1, 8, 19). It has been reported that this radiopharmaceutical may show even very small volume disease (8, 19). The patient is injected with 555 MBq ^{99m}Tc-DMSA (V) scintigraphy is performed 1–6 hours later. Physiologic tracer uptake due to free technetium may be found in the salivary glands and the gastric mucosa. The mechanism of tracer uptake is not fully understood (1).

Another promising attempt is scintigraphy with the murine **^{99m}Tc-labeled monoclonal antibody against carcinoembryogenic antigen (CEA;** BW 431/26, Behring-Werke, Marburg, Germany, cf. 5 and 12).

Additional bone scintigraphy with ^{99m}Tc-dicarboxypropandiphosphonate (^{99m}Tc-DPD) or analogs is helpful to detect bone metastases.

References

1. Abrams MJ. Small Coordination Complexes in Tumor Imaging. J Nucl Med. 1991;32:849–850.
2. Becker DV, Hurley JR. Radioiodine Treatment of Hyperthyroidism. In: Volume 2: Gottschalk A, Hoffer PB, Potchen EH, eds. Diagnostic Nuclear Medicine. 2nd ed. Baltimore: Williams & Wilkins; 1988:778–791.
3. Becker, W. Besonderheiten bei der Nachsorge des C-Zell-Karzinoms. Der Nuklearmediziner. 1986;3/9:167–181.
4. Achong DM, Oates E, Lee SL, Doherty FJ. Gallbladder Visualization During Post-Therapy Iodine-131 Imaging of Thyroid Carcinoma. J Nucl Med. 1991;32,12:2275–2277.
5. Baew-Christow T, Baum RP, Hertel A, Lorenz M, Hör G. ^{99m}Tc-markierte monoklonale Anti-CEA Antikörper – prospektive klinische Untersuchung der Immunszintigraphie bei Patienten mit CEA-exprimierenden Tumoren. In: Höfer R, Bergmann H, Sinzinger H: Radioactive Isotope in Klinik und Forschung – Radioactive Isotopes in Clinical Medicine and Research. Stuttgart: Schattauer; 1991:467–472.
6. Briele B, Hotze A, Bockisch A, Overbeck B, Grünwald F, Kaiser W, Biersack HJ. Vergleich von ^{201}Tl und ^{99m}Tc-MIBI in der Nachsorge des differenzierten Schilddrüsenkarzinoms. Nucl Med. 1991;30:115–124.
7. Briele B, Hotze A, Grünwald F, Overbeck B, Biersack HJ. Erhöhte Sensitivität der Ganzkörperszintigraphie mit ^{131}J für den Nachweis jodspeichernder Metastasen durch spätere Aufnahme-Zeitpunkte. Nucl Med. 1990;29:264–268.
8. Castellani MR, Crippa F, Del Bo L, et al. ^{99m}Tc-DMSA(V) scintigraphy in diagnosis of occult recurrences of medullary thyroid carcinoma: preliminary results. In: Schmidt HAE, van der Schoot JB, eds. Nuclear Medicine. The State of the Art of Nuclear Medicine in Europe. Stuttgart: Schattauer; 1991:334–336.
9. Cavalieri RR. Quantitative In Vivo Tests. In: Werner SC, Ingbar SH, eds. The Thyroid. 4th ed. Hagerston: Harper & Row; 1978:284–296.
10. Feind CR. Clinical Aspects of Anomalous Development. In: Werner SC, Ingbar SH, eds. The Thyroid. 4th ed. Hagerston: Harper & Row; 1978:421–425.
11. Feine U, zum Winkel K. Nuklearmedizin-Szintigraphische Diagnostik. 2nd ed. Thieme; Stuttgart: 1980.
12. Fritsche H. Immumszintigraphischer Nachweis von Primärtumor und Metastasen beim medullären Schilddrüsenkarzinom mit Technetium-markierten nonoklonalen Antikörpern BW 431/26. In: Höfer R, Bergmann H, Sinzinger H. Radioactive Isotope in Klinik und Forschung—Radioactive Isotopes in Clinical Medicine and Research. Stuttgart: Schattauer; 1991:474–479.
13. Hurley R, Becker DV. Treatment of Thyroid Carcinoma With Radioiodine. In: Gottschalk A, Hoffer PB, Potchen EH, eds. Volume 2: Diagnostic Nuclear Medicine. 2nd ed. Baltimore: Williams & Wilkins; 1988:792–814.
14. Johnson PM. Thyroid and Whole-Body Scanning. In: Werner SC, Ingbar SH, eds. The Thyroid. 4th ed. Hagerston: Harper & Row; 1978:297–317.
15. Kreisig T, Pickardt CR, Kirsch CM, Knesewitsch P. 99mTc-Uptake der Schilddrüse (TcU) für eine verbesserte Diagnostik des Morbus Basedow. In: Höfer R, Bergmann H. Sinzinger H. Radioactive Isotope in Klinik und Forschung-Radioactive Isotopes in Clinical Medicine and Research. Stuttgart: Schattauer; 1991:520–521.
16. Lamberton P, Surks MI. Thyroiditis. In: Becker KL, ed. Principles and Practice of Endocrinology and Metabolism. Philadelphia: Lippincott; 1990:370–377.
17. Leisner B. Schilddrüse in vivo. In: Büll U, Hör G, eds. Klinische Nuklearmedizin. 1st ed. Weinheim: VCH; 1987:107–117.
18. Mazzaferri EL. Thyroid cancer. In: Becker KL, ed. Principles and Practice of Endocrinology and Metabolism. Philadelphia: Lippincott; 1990:319–331.
19. Mojiminiyi OA, Udelsman R, Soper NDW, Shepstone BJ, Dudley NE. Clinical application of [^{99m}Tc(V)] DMSA scintigraphy in patients with medullary carcinoma of the thyroid. In: Schmidt HAE, van der Schoot JB, eds. Nuclear Medicine. The State of the Art of Nuclear Medicine in Europe. Stuttgart: Schattauer; 1991:344–346.
20. Papanicolaou N, Simeone JF. Clinical Correlation of Thyroid Ultrasonography with Radionuclide Imaging. In: Gottschalk A, Hoffer PB, Potchen EH, eds. Volume 2: Diagnostic Nuclear Medicine. 2nd ed. Baltimore: Williams & Wilkins; 1988:769–777.
21. Pfannenstiel P. Schilddrüsenkrankheiten-Diagnose und Therapie. Berlin: Grosse; 1985.
22. Sarkar SD. In Vivo Thyroid Studies. In: Gottschalk A, Hoffer PB, Potchen EH, eds. Volume 2: Diagnostic Nuclear Medicine. 2nd ed. Baltimore: Williams & Wilkins; 1988:756–768.
23. Vosberg H, Szabo Z, Larraß R. Untersuchungen der Pertechnetatkinetik in der Schilddrüse mittels Dekonvolutionsanalyse. In: Höfer R, Bergmann H, Sinzinger H. Radioactive Isotope in Klinik und Forschung-Radioactive Isotopes in Clinical Medicine and Research. Stuttgart: Schattauer; 1991:333–336.

Diagnostic Imaging in Graves Ophthalmopathy

N. Hosten

Graves ophthalmopathy is an inflammatory alteration of the eye frequently observed in conjunction with autoimmune thyroiditis (1). Because this condition is often resistant to therapy, appropriate diagnosis and therapy require close cooperation between internists, ophthalmologists, and radiologists. This overview discusses the role of diagnostic imaging in the differential diagnosis, the evaluation of local pathology, and the establishment of indications for potential therapeutic intervention.

Clinical Presentation and Pathophysiology

Graves ophthalmopathy presents as an inflammatory alteration of various parts of the eye: retrobulbar adipose tissue, extracular eye muscle, and lids may be affected to differing degrees. In the early stage of the disease, histologic examination of affected tissue reveals an increase in acidic mucopolysaccharides produced by fibroblasts. This substance is highly hygroscopic, causing edema and, consequently volume increase of the tissue in which it is deposited. Accordingly, the early clinical presentation of Graves ophthalmopathy is characterized by conspicuous lid edema and a feeling of increased pressure behind the eyes, caused by an increase in volume of the retrobulbar adipose tissue and eye muscles. The role of diagnostic imaging is to evaluate the extraocular eye muscles for signs of increased diameter; often, increased volume of the retrobulbar adipose tissue can be documented as well. In the majority of patients, edematous changes in affected tissue return to normal after a course of variable length. In more severe cases, the disease may enter a residual stage with fatty or fibrotic degeneration of the eye muscles.

During the edema stage, immune-suppressive measures (glucocorticoids, cyclosporine, or percutaneous radiation of the orbits) are appropriate means of treatment. Residual alterations may require any of several operative procedures in order to relieve retro-

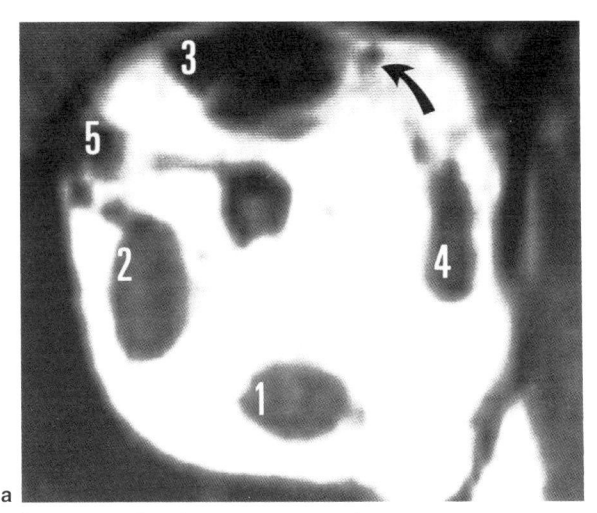

Fig. 3.**38** Sectional anatomy of structures important in the differential diagnosis of Graves ophthalmopathy in two coronary MR images (female patient with Graves ophthalmopathy; surface coil to reduce partial volume effects is placed over the eye)
a Coronary T$_1$-weighted image through the retrobulbar space, directly posterior to the globe. Slight thickening of the eye muscles in the region of tendon insertion. Unremarkable representation of orbital vasculature

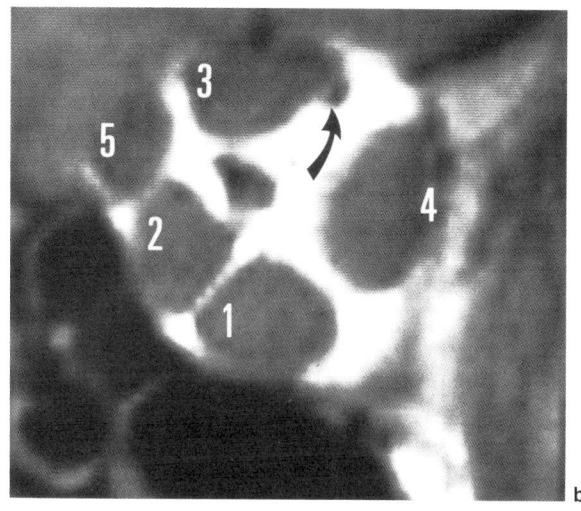

b Coronary T$_1$-weighted image through the dorsal portion of the orbit. Marked thickening of all straight eye muscles and the superior oblique muscle is apparent
1. Inferior rectus muscle
2. Medial rectus muscle
3. Superior rectus muscle
4. Lateral rectus muscle
5. Superior oblique muscle; superior ophthalmic vein (arrow)

bulbar pressure (removal of retrobulbar adipose tissue via rostral approach, fenestration of the neighboring walls of the ethmoid cells or upper maxillary sinus, 6).

Examination Technique and Diagnostic Criteria

Imaging modalities—CT and MRI—are useful primarily in evaluating the diameter of the extraocular eye muscles. Evaluation of the muscles may be difficult due to the convergence of the orbital apices superiorly and medially, necessarily resulting in diagonal sections of the muscles. Partial volume effects may thus falsely exaggerate muscle size. Axial and coronary sections should be obtained with both modalities. While images in both orientations can be acquired effortlessly in MRI, CT requires reconstruction of coronary images from axial sections, or an additional examination to obtain direct coronary sections with the patient's head hyperextended. Slice thickness should be limited (12) to minimize factitious enlargement of the eye muscles (2 mm in CT; 5 mm or, if possible, 3 mm in MRI). The diameter of the four rectus eye muscles (inferior, medial, lateral, and superior; the superior rectus muscle can often not be distinguished from the levator palpebrae muscle lying just above) as well as the superior oblique muscles (Fig. 3.**38**) are determined. The inferior oblique muscle, running caudad to the globe in the frontal plane, is rarely seen. Bilateral comparison of the muscle cross sections reveals enlarged muscles by their asymmetry; when muscles are symmetrically affected, the rule of thumb is that all straight muscles should appear approximately equal in diameter, not exceeding a size of 4–5 by 8 mm (bilateral and cephalocaudal cross-sectional diameters, respectively). The size of the medial and lateral rectus muscles is best determined in axial sections; that of the inferior and superior recti in coronary sections. These orientations help to minimize partial volume effects (Fig. 3.**39**).

MRI should be performed using T$_1$ and T$_2$-weighted spin-echo sequences to allow assessment of subtle tissue changes. The intramuscular edema predominant in the early stages is only revealed in MR images (Fig. 3.**40 a, b**), and is seen in highly T$_2$-weighted coronal images as areas of hyperintensity (7). In calculating purely T$_2$-weighted images, measurements of the T$_2$ relaxation time can provide a means of quantifying changes resulting from therapy during the course of follow-up (8). The normal range of T$_2$ relaxation times, as reported by a number of authors, naturally varies due to hardware differences. Nevertheless, if the white matter of the frontal brain is used as a reference and has a T$_2$ time of 80 ms, a T$_2$ time of greater than 100 ms for the eye muscles, when enlarged, can be considered pathological. Fatty degeneration of the eye muscles may also be revealed in CT, seen here as small, circumscribed areas of hy-

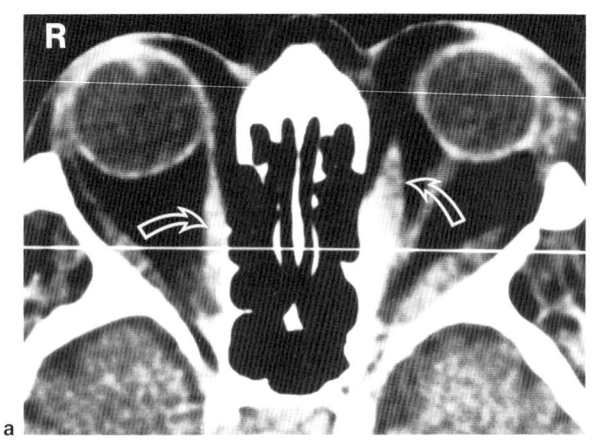

78   3 Thyroid Gland

Fig. 3.**39**   CT appearance of Graves ophthalmopathy
a In plain, axial CT image, the size of the lateral and medial rectus muscles (arrows) can be evaluated well. Normal diameter of the right lateral rectus; thickening of the left lateral rectus muscle
b Coronary reconstruction at the level of the horizontal line in (**a**). Both inferior rectus muscles are thickened; marked thickening of the left rectus superior muscle as well (arrow, bilateral asymmetry!)
c Direct coronary CT in another patient with Graves ophthalmopathy. Image quality considerably improved over the reconstruction (**b**). Slight thickening of the medial rectus muscles is apparent

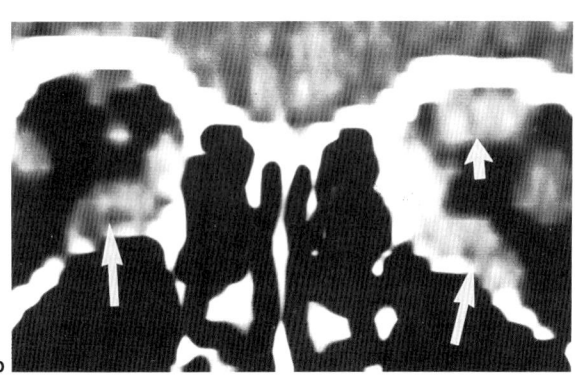

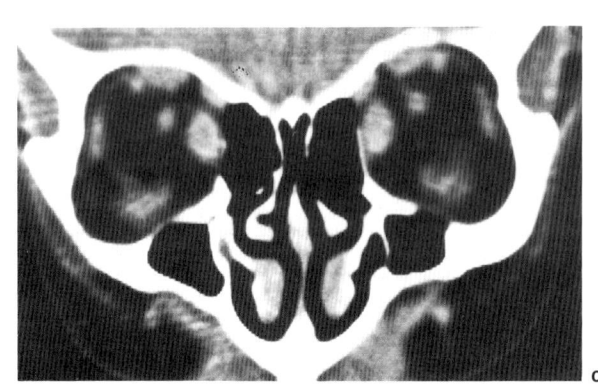

podensity within a thickened muscle. In MR imaging, these small inclusions are seen with high signal intensity in T_1-weighted images. Fibrosis of the eye muscles cannot be recognized in CT; however, MR occasionally reveals fibrosis as regions of marked signal attenuation in the affected muscles (Fig. 3.**40b**). Measured T_2 relaxation times are then often greatly reduced, typically, to well under 75 ms.

Both CT and MR are often unsatisfactory when evaluating marked proptosis in the absence of thickened eye muscles. In such cases, proptosis is due solely to the increased volume of the retrobulbar adipose tissues. Both imaging modalities can, however, reveal typical, indirect signs. Increased retrobulbar pressure causes deformation of two structures that offer low resistance: the lamina papyracea and the orbital septum. Deformation of the lamina papyracea is recognized by change seen in the ethmoid labyrinth. Whereas the labyrinth is normally seen as a more or less rectangular structure, or at most with a slight convergence in the occipital direction, increased retrobulbar volume displaces the medial orbital walls, lending a bottle-like shape to the labyrinth (the so-called "Coca-Cola sign"). The orbital septum, continuous with the orbital periosteum (periorbita), originates from the equator of the globe, attaching the globe to the bony orbital wall. When there is increased fat tissue volume in the orbit, the medial and lateral septa are typically displaced superiorly (Fig. 3.**40c**).

Differential Diagnosis

In differentiating between the diseases that may cause thickening of the extraocular muscles, Graves ophthalmopathy is the most common cause of changes such as the following:

- usually causes thickening of the inferior rectus muscles;
- when other muscles are affected, the inferior rectus muscles are as a rule affected;
- muscle thickening involves almost exclusively the belly of the muscle, sparing the tendon.

Diseases that must be differentiated from Graves ophthalmopathy include particularly the myositis of inflammatory pseudotumor, lymphoma of the eye muscle, and changes secondary to carotid-cavernous sinus fistula.

The most important of these differential diagnostic possibilities is the myositis of inflammatory pseudotumor (3, 4). Histologic findings may reveal signs of inflammation with a low cell count. Clinically there is a sudden painful onset, with similarly abrupt improvement in symptoms follwing cortisone therapy.

Diagnostic Imaging in Graves Ophthalmopathy

Fig. 3.40 Appearance of Graves ophthalmopathy in MR imaging: muscular type (**a**, **b**) and adipose type (**c**)
a Graves ophthalmopathy, muscular type. Coronary T_1-weighted image (spin-echo, TR = 400 ms, TE = 30 ms). Enormous thickening of the left inferior rectus muscle (straight arrow), slight thickening of the right inferior rectus muscle (curved arrow)
b Coronary T_2-weighted image, same patient as in (**a**). Markedly increased signal intensity from the left superior rectus muscle (straight arrow) is a sign of edematous change during the acute, inflammatory stage (T_2time: 145 ms). The right inferior rectus muscle (curved arrow) shows low signal intensity; T_2time at 68 ms was substantially below the normal range, an indication of fibrosis. Clinically there was a year-long history of Graves ophthalmopathy with acute involvement of the left eye and chronic involvement of the right eye
c Graves ophthalmopathy, adipose type; axial T_1-weighted image. Marked exophthalmos, but unremarkable size of the extraocular eye muscles. Increased volume of adipose tissue can be documented as the cause of the protrusion rostrally (solid arrow) and medially (open arrow). The ethmoid labyrinth has assumed the shape of a bottle

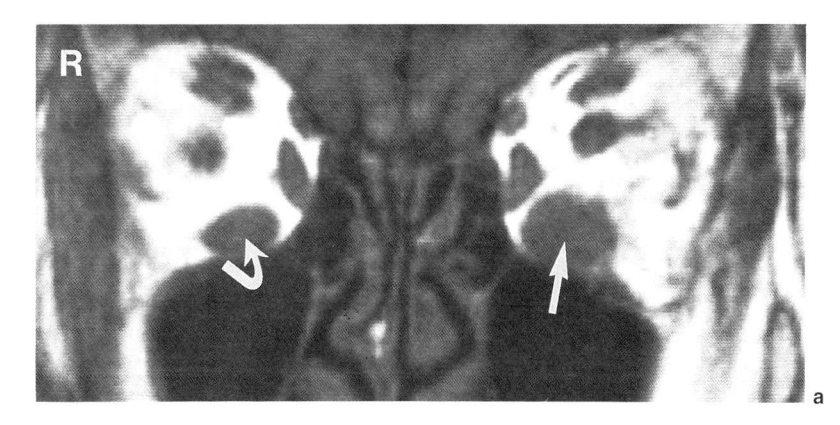

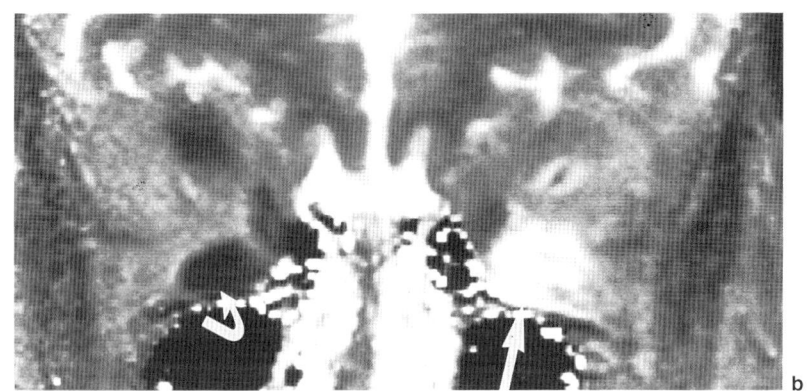

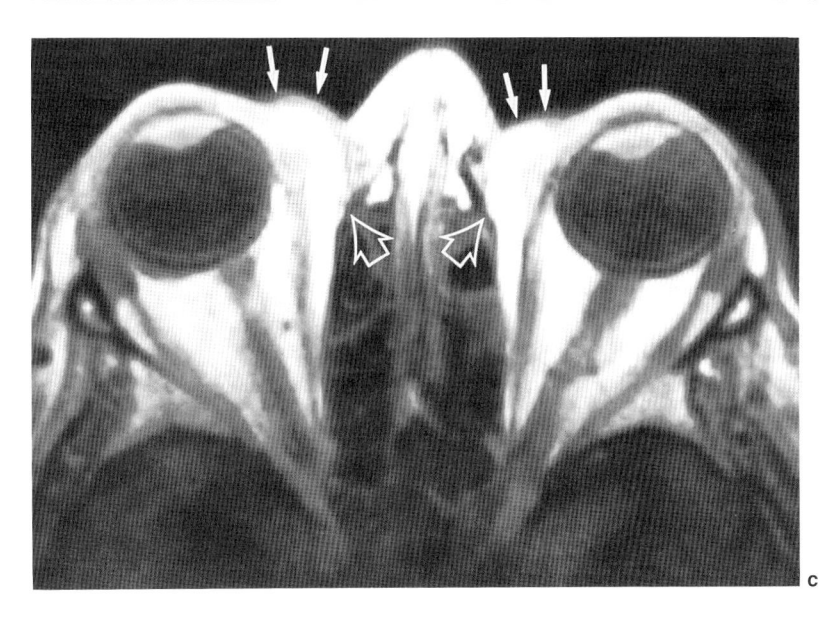

Sectional imaging methods generally reveal multifocal orbit involvement, manifesting as perineuritis (mass surrounding the optical nerve), periscleritis (mass contiguous with the posterior wall of the globe), and myositis (thickening of the eye muscles). As a rule, the tendons of the eye muscles are thickened as well.

Lymphoma can develop in any of the eye muscles; there is no predilection for the inferior rectus. Thickening is usually seen in the anterior portion of the eye muscle, and continues into the lids (5). Optimum MR examination technique may reveal that the mass is not located in the eye muscle itself, but rather, adjoins it (Fig. 3.**41**).

The carotid-cavernous sinus fistula causes thickening of *all* eye muscles, due to venous stasis in the

80   3 Thyroid Gland

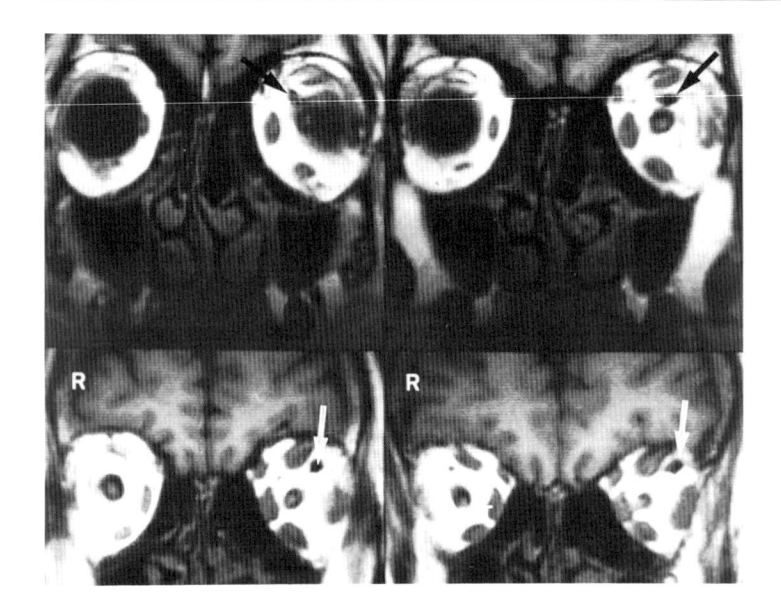

Fig. 3.**41** Carotid-cavernous sinus fistula, clinically presenting with left-sided exophthalmos. Coronary T$_1$-weighted MR image. Clockwise, beginning above left, localization from rostral to occipital. Diagnostic landmark is the increased caliber of the superior ophthalmic vein (arrow), due to venous stasis. Uniform, moderate, and bilaterally asymmetric thickening of all left extraocular muscles

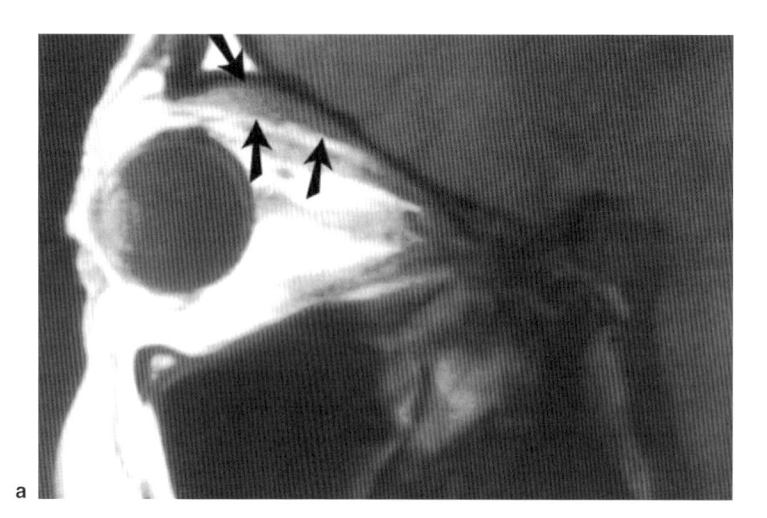

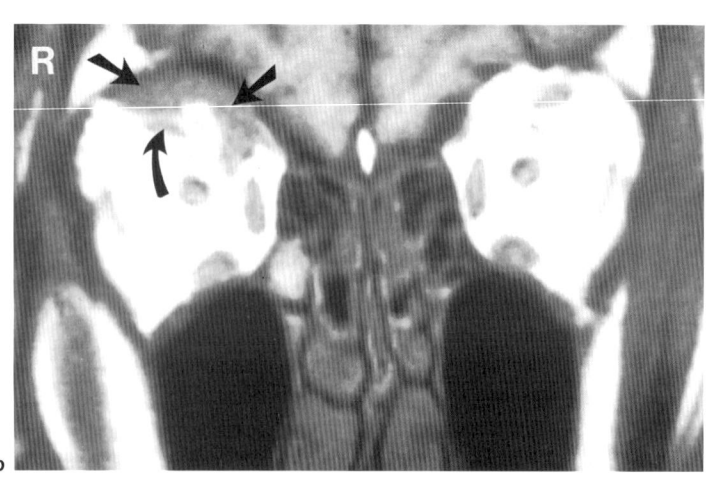

Fig. 3.**42** Orbital lymphoma in a patient clinically presenting with right-sided exophthalmos; there was no evidence of extraocular lymphoma
a Parasagittal, T$_1$-weighted image shows a mass hypointense to the retrobulbar fat tissues, below the orbital roof; the mass can be delineated from the superior rectus muscle (arrow). No deformity of the muscle or the bony orbital walls
b In the coronary T$_1$-weighted image, the mass (straight arrow) can not be clearly delineated from the levator palpebrae muscle (curved arrow)

muscle interstitium (9). When symptoms are not typical (i.e., history of trauma, pulsating exophthalmos, visible conjunctival injection), differentiation from Graves ophthalmopathy may require sectional imaging. The presence of uniform but mild thickening of all muscles suggests the diagnosis.

A large number of other, much rarer causes of thickening of the extraocular eye muscles is not discussed here; the interested reader is invited to turn to the original literature (2, 10, 11).

References

1. Char, DH. Thyroid eye disease. 1st ed. Philadelphia: Williams & Wilkins; 1985.
2. Dal Pozzo, G, Boschi MC. Extraocular muscle enlargement in acromegaly. J Comp Assist Tomogr. 1982;6:706–707.
3. Dresner, SC, Rothfus WE, Slamovits TL, et al. Computed tomography of orbital myositis. AJR. 1984;143:671–676.
4. Enzman, D, Donaldson SS, Marshall WH, Kriss JP. Computed tomography in orbital pseudotumor (Idiopathic orbital inflammation). Radiology. 1976;120:597–601.
5. Flanders, AE, Espinosa GA, Markiewicz DA, Howell DD. Orbital Lymphoma, role of CT and MRI. Radiol Clin North Am 1987;25:601–613.
6. Gorman, CA, DeSanto LW, MacCarthy CS, et al. Optic Neuropathy of Graves' disease. Treatment by transantral and transfrontal orbital decompression. N Engl J Med. 1974;290:70–75.
7. Hosten, N, Sander B, Cordes M, et al. Graves' ophthalmopathy: MR imaging of the orbits. Radiology. 172 (1989) 759–762
8. Just, M, Kahaly G, Higer HP, et al. Graves' ophthalmopathy: Role of MR imaging in radiation therapy. Radiology. 1991;179:187–190.
9. Merlis, AL, Schaiberger CL, Adler R. External carotid-cavernous sinus fistula simulating unilateral Graves' ophthalmopathy. J Comput Assist Tomogr. 1982;6:1006–1009.
10. Rothfus, WE, Curtin HD. Extraocular muscle enlargement: a CT review. Radiology. 1984;151:677–681.
11. Trokel, SL, Hilal SK. Recognition and differential diagnosis of enlarged extraocular muscles in computed tomography. Am J Ophthalmol. 1979;87:503–512.
12. Zonneveld, F, Koornneef L, Hillen B, de Slegte RGM. Normal direct multiplanar CT anatomy of the orbit with correlative anatomic cryosections. Radiol Clin N Amer. 1987;15:381–408.

A Surgeon's View

T. Steinmüller

Apart from patient history, clinical symptoms, and laboratory findings, the obligatory diagnostic repertoire of all surgically relevant diseases of the thyroid includes ultrasound as the first diagnostic measure of choice. Ultrasound is helpful in deciding on the next diagnostic methods or steps. It provides the surgeon with important information on size and tissue properties and enables an objective postoperative follow-up.

In the following, the extent to which other imaging procedures in thyroid diagnostics influence the indication for surgery or postoperative procedures is discussed. An overview of indications for preoperative imaging from a surgical point of view is given in Table 3.7.

Multinodular Goiter

If multinodular goiter leads to significant mechanical obstruction because of the size of the goiter (tracheal stenosis, displacement of the esophagus, superior vena cava obstruction), and if corresponding clinical symptoms are present, surgical treatment is indicated. This also applies to cases in which conservative treatment has not been effective. In such patients, imaging beyond ultrasound does not provide any further useful information for the surgeon, because it modifies neither the indication nor the operational procedure. In particular, in regions with iodine deficiency there is no qualitative difference between euthyroid and "toxic" multinodular goiter, only a difference in quantity, which merely comprises the extent of autonomic hormone secretion, autonomic growth, and autonomic function coexistence. In the surgical concept of subtotal resection, the nodules are completely removed, and intact thyroid tissue is left. Thyroidectomy in benign disease has not gained general acceptance.

Scintigraphic indications of autonomous and cold areas do not allow the surgeon to remove all nodules, but require intraoperative and perhaps histologic evaluation. The autonomous, hormone-secreting follicles are not always identical to nodule topography. Preoperative scintigraphy is not absolutely necessary, but may have surgical relevance in special constellations (see Table 3.7).

For the differential diagnosis of solitary thyroid nodules, scintigraphy is essential and provides an important contribution to the diagnostic and therapeutic algorithm. Solitary, scintigraphically cold nodules urgently require further investigation. Warm or hot nodules usually correspond to adenomas, but do not, however, exclude malignancy (see below).

In cases of retrosternal and intrathoracic processes, the scintigraphic proof of iodine storing tissue is relevant to surgical strategy; a cervical approach can be applied for most retrosternal goiters (16). If the nodules are large, computed tomography may also be helpful (17, 18). With goiters in the anterior mediastinum, there may be "genuine" goiter supplied by thoracic vessels, which always requires thoracotomy.

In the case of recurrent goiter, the significantly higher surgical risk requires information about the location of iodinestoring tissue in order to consider the therapeutic options (operation, radioactive iodine treatment) and to plan the surgical management (unilateral intervention) (19, 20, 21).

Hyperthyroidism

If there is immune hyperthyroidism corresponding to Graves disease, and if the decision to operate has been made, medication is administered in order to achieve

Table 3.7 Overview of indications for preoperative imaging

Clinical Findings	Ultrasound	Scintigraphy	Other Imaging Procedures
Normothyroid			
Multinodular goiter WHO Grade II–III	Size of thyroid gland, detection, evaluation and localization of nodes	Preoperatively dispensable from a surgeon's view	dispensable
Uninodular goiter	idem	required for differential diagnosis	dispensable
Recurrent goiter	idem	required for surgical planning	dispensable
Restrosternal of intrathoracic goiter	idem (fails retrosternally)	required for surgical planning	CT in extensive masses
Suggestion of malignancy	idem	useful for surgical planning	CT (or MR) for demonstration of tumor size, infiltration, metastatic involvement of cervical and mediastinal lymph nodes, etc.
Hyperthyroid			
Graves disease	idem	preoperatively dispensable from a surgeon's view	dispensable
Multifocal autonomy in multinodular goiter	idem	preoperatively dispensable from a surgeon's view	dispensable
Uninodular goiter with suggestion of autonomous adenoma	idem	required for differential diagnosis	dispensable

an euthyroid state. Then, an extensive subtotal resection is performed, leaving a small remainder of parenchyma weighing only a few grams. For surgical purposes, only preoperative ultrasonic imaging is required, although in the course of the disease numerous scintigraphic investigations will have already been carried out. Hyperthyroidism in multinodular autonomy (Plummer disease) has already been mentioned; in this disease there is nodular goiter, and it is important to gain information on the extent of the disseminated autonomous areas. With respect to surgery, the same procedure as for nodular goiter is applied (subtotal resection with removal of all nodules) (5, 6). Preoperative ultrasound is necessary for surgical planning.

Scintigraphy is not absolutely necessary, but has usually already been carried out. If there is a solitary nodule in a hyperthyroid situation, a scintigram is necessary for differential diagnosis and also for surgical planning (partial thyroid resection). In the rare cases of iodine-induced hyperthyroidism, scintigraphic investigation should take place in spite of decreased radioiodine uptake.

Malignancies

The differentiated thyroid carcinomas comprise the papillary, follicular, and oncocytic forms, which all share a comparatively favorable prognosis. Suggestion of a differentiated thyroid carcinoma justifies operative histologic investigation. If it is confirmed, thyroidectomy is indicated. In cases of "occult" papillary carcinoma in young patients, restriction to lobectomy is currently being discusssed.

The patient's fairly unspecific history and clinical symptoms underline the importance of preoperative thyroid diagnostics, which are sonography, scintigraphy, and in particular, needle biopsy. Differentiated thyroid carcinomas can store iodine, but appear as cold nodules in primary diagnostics. The cold nodule, however, is neither a sensitive nor a specific characteristic of thyroid carcinoma (30). Freitag et al. mention a proportion of 6% warm and 10% hot nodules in differentiated thyroid malignancies. In general, the diagnostic usefulness of preoperative scintigraphy can be questioned (32, 33, 34, 35). Nevertheless, the demonstration or the exclusion of restrosternal and ectopic thyroid tissue is relevant for the surgeon. The main contribution of scintigraphy, however, lies in the identification of carcinoma metastases *after* thyroidectomy.

Plain films, CT, or MRI are of limited value in the assessment of malignancy. They are, however, of importance in excluding lung metastases, in demonstrating displacement or compression of the trachea, and in the assessment of regional tumor extension. Particularly in the differentiated iodine-storing thyroid carcinoma, MRI should be considered because it may demonstrate the extension of the tumor without administering iodine-containing contrast media (30).

In the rare medullary thyroid carcinoma ("C cell carcinoma"), thyroidectomy with extensive lymphadenectomy is indicated (36, 37, 38); in the familiar form it must always be carried out bilaterally and, depending on the findings, may involve the anterior mediastinum (39). Lymph node metastases are common and are of special prognostic relevance (40). In this situation, CT gains a special significance in the evaluation of the neck and upper mediastinum. The tumor marker calcitonin, if necessary after stimulation with pentagastrin, is indicative for the diagnosis and follow-up. The differentiation of the familiar and the sporadic form of medullary cancer is of great clinical importance; if there is a MEN syndrome type IIa or IIb, a pheochromocytoma must be excluded preoperatively via ^{131}I-mIBG scintigraphy. In the familiar forms, family screening is necessary (41).

Patient history and findings are often so typical in undifferentiated thyroid malignancies that a clinical diagnosis is usually already possible at this stage. The tumors are aggressive and at the time of diagnosis already at an advanced stage with poor prognosis. The value of surgery is controversial; there is, however, no primary alternative therapy. Although surgery only serves palliative purposes, more recent studies seem to show that a multimodality treatment scheme (42) or radical surgical intervention with conventional radiation (43, 44) hold some promise. Either way, the demonstration of cervical and mediastinal tumor extension with the help of imaging procedures is of great significance for planning therapy.

References

1. Pfannenstiel P, Cordes M. The Place of Ultrasound in the Diagnosis and Treatment of Thyroid Diseases. Prog Surg. 1988;19:21–29
2. Bay V. Struma mit Euthyreose. Langenbecks Arch Chir. Suppl II, Kongressbericht 1990.
3. Dralle H. Operationsindikation und operative Verfahrenswahl bei Schilddrüsenerkrankungen. Internist. 1988;29:570–576.
4. Ladurner D. Das Schilddrüsenszintigramm. Chirurg. 1990;61:647–650.
5. Studer H, Ramelli F. Simple goiter and its variants: Euthyroid and hyperthyroid multinodular goiters. Endocr Rev. 1982;3:40.
6. Teuscher J, Petre HJ, Gerber H, Berchthold R, Studer H. Pathogenesis of nodular goiter and its implication for surgical management. Surgery 1988;103(1):87–93.
7. Röher HD. Endokrine Chirurgie. Stuttgart: Thieme; 1987.
8. Gemsenjäger E, Heitz PU, Staub J, Girard J, Barthe P, Benz UF. Surgical aspects of thyroid autonomy in multinodular goiter. World J Surg. 1983;7:363.
9. Reeve TS, Delbridge L, Cohen A, Crummer P. Total Thyroidectomy. Ann. Surg. 1987;206(6):782–786.
10. Clark OH. Letter to the editor. Ann Surg. 1987;208(2):244–245.
11. Studer H, Peter HJ, Gerber H. Morphologic and functional changes in developing goiters. In: Hall R, Köbberling J, eds. Thyroid disorders Associated with Iodine Deficiency and Excess. New York: Raven Press; 1985:227–241.
12. Rothmund M, Zielke A. Der solitäre Schilddrüsenknoten – befundgerechte Operation. Chirurg 1991;62:162–168.
13. Boeckl O, Pimpl W, Galvan G, et al. Wann Lappenteilresektion, wann Hemithyreoidektomie bei der Operation des isolierten Schilddrüsenknotens? Panel Discussion. Langenbecks Arch Chir 1990;375:318–323.
14. Wheeler MH. Indications and Strategy for Surgery of Thyroid Nodules. In: Prog Surg. 1988;19:1–20.
15. Wahl RA, Goretzki P, Meybier H, Nitschke J, Linder MM, Röher HD. Coexistence of hyperparathyroidism and thyroid cancer. World J Surg. 1982;6:385.
16. Röher HD, Goretzki PE, Wahl RA, Frilling A. Intrathorakale Struma. Chirurg 1989;60:384.
17. Cooper JC, Nakielny R, Talbot CH. The use of computed tomography in the evaluation of large multinodular goiters. Ann R Coll Surg Engl. 1991;73(1):32–35.
18. Maruotti RA, Zannini P, Viani MP. Surgical treatment of substernal goiters. Int Surg 1991;76(1):12–17.
19. Schicha H. Die Rezidivstruma. Medwelt 1990;41:525–533.
20. Bay V, Engel U, Zornig C. Technik und Komplikationen bei Rezidiveingriffen an der Schilddrüse. Wien Klin Woschr. 1988;100(11):352–354.
21. Dralle H, Pichlmayr R. Risikominderung bei Rezidiveingriffen wegen benigner Struma. Chirurg. 1991;62:169–175.
22. Röher HD, Horster FA, Frilling A, Goretzki PE. Morphologie und funktionsgerechte Chirurgie verschiedener Hyperthyreoseformen. Chirurg. 1991;62:176–181.
23. Goretzki, Frilling A, Grussendorf M, Röher HD. Chirurgische Therapie der Hyperthyreose. Akt Chir. 1989;24:47–52.
24. Dralle H, Lang W, Pretschner DP, Pichlmayer R, Hesch RD. Operationsindikation und chirurgisches Vorgehen bei jodinduzierten Hyperthyreosen. Langenbecks Arch Chir. 1985;365:79–89.
25. Clark OH, Levin K, Zeng QH, Greenspan FS, Siperstein A. Thyroid cancer: the case for total thyroidectomy. Eur J Cancer Clin Oncol. 1988;24(2):305–313.
26. Demeure MJ, Clark OH. Surgery in treatment of thyroid cancer. Endocrinol Metab Clin North Am. 1990;19(3):663–83.
27. Rossi R, Cady B, Silverman M, Wool M, Horner T. Current Results of Conservative Surgery of Differentiated Thyroid Carcinoma. World J Surg. 1986;10:612–22.
28. Hay ID, Grant CS, Taylor WF, McConahey WM. Ipsilateral lobectomy versus bilateral lobar resection in papillary thyroid carcinoma. Surgery. 1987;102(6):1088–95.
29. Schröder DM, Chambors A, France ChJ. Operative Strategy for Thyroid Cancer. Cancer. 1986;58:2320–28.
30. Börner W, Becker W, Reiners Chr, Müller H-A. Diagnostik der differenzierten Karzinome der Thyreozyten. In: W. Börner ed. Schildddrüsenmalignome. Stuttgart: Schattauer; 1987.
31. Freitas J, Gross M, Ripley S, Shapiro B. Radionuclide diagnosis and therapy of thyroid carcinoma: current status report. Sem Nucl Med. 1985;15:106–31.
32. Smeds S, Madsen M, Lennquist S. Evaluation of preoperative diagnosis and surgical management of thyroid tumors. Acta Chir Scand. 1984;115:513.
33. Lennquist S. Surgical Strategy in Thyroid Carcinoma: A Clinical Review. Acta Chir Scand. 1986;152:321–338.
34. Wheeler MH. Indications and Strategy for Surgery of Thyroid Nodules. Prog Surg. 1988;19:1–20.
35. Clark KC, Moffat FL, Ketcham AS, Legaspi A, Robinson DS. Nonoperative techniques for tissue diagnosis in the management of thyroid nodules and goiters. Semin Surg Oncol. 1991;7(2).76–80.
36. Duh QY, Sancho JJ, Greenspan FS, et al. Medullary Thyroid Carcinoma. Arch Surg. 1989;124(10):1206–1210.

37 Tisell LE, Hansson G, Jansson S, Salander H. Reoperations in the treatment of symptomatic metastasizing medullary thyroid carcinoma. Surgery. 1986;99:60.
38 Bottger T, Klupp J, Sorger K, Junginger T. Therapie and prognosis of medullary thyroid cancer. Med Klin. 1991;86(1):8–14.
39 Laimore TC, Wells SA Jr. Medullary Carcinoma of the thyroid: current diagnosis and treatment. Semin Surg Oncol 1991;7(2):92–99.
40 Wahl RA, Brabscheid D, Goretzki PE, Röher HD. Chirurgische Therapie des C-Zell-Karzinoms. In: W. Börner, ed. Schilddrüsenmalignome. Stuttgart: Schattauer; 1987.
41 Spelsberg F, Müller OA. Die multiplen endokrinen Neoplasien. In: Röher HD, ed. Endokrine Chirurgie. Stuttgart: Thieme; 1987.
42 Werner B, Abela J, Alveryd A, et al. Multimodal therapy in anaplastic giant cell thyroid carcinoma. World J Surg. 1984;8(1):64.
43 Scheumann GF, Wegener G, Dralle H. Radikale chirurgische Intervention mit konventioneller Radiatio versus multimodalem Therapieschema beim undifferenzierten Schilddrüsenkarzinom. Wien Klin Woschr. 1990;102(9):271–273.
44 Scheumann GF, Wegener G, Kemnitz J, Dralle H. Undifferentiated thyroid cancer: improved therapeutic results following initial radical intervention and early postoperative radiotherapy. Helv Chir Acta. 1990;57(1):57–60.

4 Parathyroid Gland

Anatomy

J. Staudt

The epithelial corpora or parathyroid glands are represented by four lens-shaped organs, normally located at the posterior face or within the fibrous capsule of both thyroid lobes. They have a red-brown color, measure about 6 mm in length, 3–4 mm in width, and 0.2–2 mm in depth and weigh around 35 mg each. They are usually located in the area near the entrance of one of the large thyroid arteries (Fig. 4.**1**). Embryologically, they originate from the third and fourth pharyngeal pouches. The inferior glands rise from the third pharyngeal pouch and descend together with the thymus. This explains their frequently ectopic position within the mediastinum in up to 10% of humans. The upper glands, arising from the posterior portion of the fourth branchial pouch migrate a lesser distance together with the thyroid.

Endocrinology

K.-J. Gräf

Physiology

The parathyroid glands, usually four, but occasionally six to eight epithelial bodies, play a central role in the regulation of calcium metabolism because of the production of parathyroid hormone (PTH) (see also Chapter 11). Together with calcitriol and calcitonin, calcium homeostasis is regulated above all by PTH. PTH increases calcium resorption in the distal tubule of the kidneys, while simultaneously promoting phosphaturia. In bones, PTH stimulates osteoblast and osteoclast activity. In addition, PTH leads to the production of $1\alpha,25$-dehydroxy vitamin D_3 in the kidney which, in turn, promotes the synthesis of calcium-binding proteins of the small bowel mucosa and, hence, intestinal calcium absorption.

Hypoparathyroidism

Hypoparathyroidism is defined as reduced or absent PTH secretion. This disease is clinically relevant because of hypocalcemia and hyperphosphatemia. With a few rare exceptions (e.g., due to infiltrative or autoimmune disease), hypoparathyreoidism occurs most commonly iatrogenically, (usually postoperatively secondary to bilateral thyroidectomy), which can be either permanent (average 1–3% in experienced surgical centers, or transient. The main clinical symptoms of hypoparathyroidism are summarized in Table 4.**1**. The condition of pseudohypoparathyroidism (resistance to PTH) is characterized by the clinical symptoms of hypocalcemia also. A defect in the second messenger system (cAMP) is one of several causal factors of this disease.

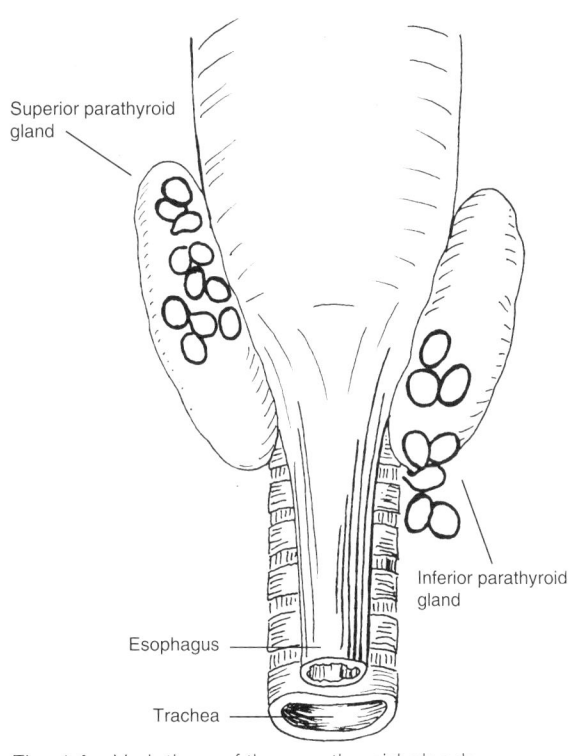

Fig. 4.**1** Variations of the parathyroid glands

Hyperparathyroidism

Hyperparathyroidism results from the increased secretion of PTH due to hyperplasia, adenomas, or carcinomas (very rare). The symptomatology is deter-

Table 4.1 Symptoms of hypoparathyroidism/hypocalcemia

Increased neuromuscular excitability
– carbopedal spasms, paresthesias, tetany
basal ganglia calcification (Fahr syndrome)
Increase of bone density
Formation of cataracts
Psychic symptoms
– Anxiety, psychosis, depression
Prolongation of the QT time, increase of T wave
ECG changes

Table 4.2 Clinical symptoms of hyperparathyroidism with hypercalcemia

Tiredness, lethargy
Drowsiness, psychosis, depression
Polyuria, nocturia, polydipsia
Inappetence, nausea, vomiting, constipation
Myasthenia, myopathia
Arthralgia
ECG changes, QT time shortening, tachycardiac arrhythmias, hypertension, hypersensitivity to digitalis
Nephrolithiasis
Promotion of ulcers
Skeletal changes (osteolysis generalized osteitis fibrosa cystica, Recklingshausen disease)

mined by the sequelae of the hypercalcemia (see Table 4.2). The main diagnostic measures in hyperparathyroidism are, if necessary, multiple determination of the serum concentrations of PTH, calcium, and phosphate. Imaging procedures such as ultrasound, CT, MRI, and scintigraphy are helpful in the individual case, but their sensitivity is low.

The therapy of hyperparathyroidism depends largely on the clinical symptomatology. A low-calcium diet with adequate fluid intake is sufficient in mild cases, while surgical exploration and, if applicable, tumor excision are required in severe forms, e.g., in recurrent nephrolithiasis, a history of ulcers, psychic symptomatology, etc. If necessary the operation should be done even in cases of negative preoperative localization.

The most important complication of hyperparathyroidism is a hypercalcemic crisis. This is characterized by neurological symptoms such as stupor, somnolence or coma, hypotension, exsiccosis, tachycardiac arrhythmias, and hypercalcemia, usually above 3.5 mmol/L.

Apart from treating the exsiccosis, intensive medical care is aimed mainly at reducing the serum calcium concentration by means of calciuric drugs such as furosemide or corticosteroids, calcitonin, mithramycin, or biphosphonates. After initial therapy of the hypercalcemic syndrome, treatment of the underlying disease—in hyperparathyroidism, surgical intervention—is the therapy of choice.

Ultrasound

G. A. W. Gooding

Ultrasound of the neck offers a wealth of information about the carotid arteries,[1, 2] the jugular veins, cervical adenopathy,[3] salivary,[4] thyroid, and parathyroid glands.

For a noninvasive study of parathyroid disease, ultrasound is the first imaging step.

Ultrasound Imaging Technique

Ultrasound of the thyroid and parathyroid is technique and operator dependent. The examination is less costly than other imaging studies, requires no contrast injection, and is biologically safe.

The anatomy of the neck is superficial and therefore requires high-resolution 5–10 MHz transducers to image appropriately. Linear array transducers are the current choice, primarily because the near field is so well seen. Sector transducers have a poor near field of view and must be used with a water path interface to focus the acoustic beam in the near field.

Initially, the thyroid and parathyroid areas are scanned with the highest transducer frequency available, preferably a 10 MHz transducer. A 10 MHz transducer generates an image only 4–5 cm deep and a few centimeters wide. If that examination does not identify an abnormality, a lower frequency, 7.5 or 5 MHz transducer is employed, because it is possible to miss a large posterior lesion with 10 MHz due to inadequate depth penetration. However, using a 5 MHz transducer as the only one is fraught with difficulties because a small parathyroid adenoma of less than a centimeter may be easily overlooked.

For the ultrasound of the neck, no preparation is necessary. The patient lies supine with a pillow under the shoulders to accentuate hyperextension of the neck. If the patient can not hyperextend the neck, as in ankylosing spondylitis, the lower thyroid and the lower parathyroid glands can be completely missed, tucked down as they are behind the clavicle in the superior mediastinum. Swallowing may transiently elevate this area back up into the neck.

An aqueous gel is spread over the area to be scanned to make an air tight seal between the transducer and the skin.

The patient's neck is then scanned in two planes at right angles to one another: 1. a transverse plane that extends from the hyoid bone to the sternal notch craniocaudally, and laterally extends beyond the jugular vein; as well as 2. longitudinal scans that are carried out in the same defined area.

Scans are carried out just lateral to the jugular vein, because a few (1.6%) parathyroid adenomas lie in the carotid sheath[5]. Masses lateral to the jugular are much more likely to be lymph nodes than parathyroid lesions.

Most ectopic parathyroid glands (13%), lie in the thymus of the anterior mediastinum, not amenable to sonographic detection.

Duplex and color-coded phased array transducers also offer the option of flow characterization. With these instruments, the superior and inferior thyroidal arteries can be appreciated and the vascularity of identified masses can be assessed. Experience with angiography has shown that parathyroid tumors are highly vascular. The experience with color-coded Doppler demonstrates that vascularity is primarily a function of size. Parathyroid tumors 1 cm or less tend to be avascular (Fig. 4.**2**); most of those 2 cm or greater are vascular (Fig. 4.**3**)[6]. Thyroid lesions are more likely to be vascular when only 0.5 cm in size.

Ralls, et al., have shown that hyperfunction of the thyroid gland in Graves disease causes a marked increase in vascularity noted by color-coding as an "inferno" effect of increased pixels of color representing hypervascularity [7]. This is one area in which ultrasound can indicate a functional state. Ordinarily, sonography defines anatomy and morphologic changes, not, as in scintigraphy, the functional status of the thyroid or parathyroid, although enlargement of the parathyroid gland is synonymous with hyperfunction.

Normal Findings

In sonography, the thyroid gland is homogeneous, hyperechoic, easily recognized, and differentiated from the adjacent soft tissues of the neck. The salivary glands have a similar hyperechoic appearance but are at some distance from the thyroid and are not confused with it.

The esophagus is usually seen medial to the thyroid posterior on the left side. On transverse scan, it appears as concentric rings, which, with swallowing, sparkle transiently with air or saliva. On longitudinal scans, the esophagus is seen posterior to the thyroid medially, as linear parallel echoes typical of bowel that move with peristalsis when the patient swallows. Saliva is noted as a bright reflector and air in the esophagus causes transient acoustic scattering.

The recurrent laryngeal nerve is occasionally noted on both transverse and longitudinal sonograms next to the carotid sheath as a tiny hypoechoic tube with hyperechoic walls.

Adenopathy, when it is present, tends to be superior or inferior to the thyroid, rather than interposing between the thyroid and the adjacent carotid artery. Masses in that interposition location are typical for parathyroid or thyroid in origin. Single nodes, typically inferior to the thyroid when they are about 1 cm in size, can be confused with parathyroid adenoma because the size and shape are similar and the same hypoechoic texture may be present, although some benign nodes can have a hyperechoic center that parathyroid glands do not have.

The longus colli is a consistent marker of the posterior extent of the thyroid gland. Posterior to the carotid artery, on transverse scan it tends to extend bilaterally medially as a kind of triangle with the base lateral and the apex medial. This muscle tends to be quite hypoechoic or anechoic and is larger in men than women. It can occasionally be confused with a long linear variant of parathyroid adenoma (Fig. 4.**4**). When parathyroid adenomas are adjacent to the longus colli muscle, which they frequently are, they tend to appear immediately anterior to the muscle. On transverse scans, these parathyroid adenomas are rounded, while the longus colli is more triangular in shape and immediately posterior to the parathyroid.

The musculature anterior to the thyroid is skeletal and by sonography has a hypoechoic pattern interrupted by striations, caused by the muscle bundles. The largest of these is the sternocleidomastoid muscle, which extends out laterally anterior to the carotid artery and jugular veins. This muscle is much larger in males than females. The strap muscles overlying the thyroid gland may or may not be distinguished from each other, depending on the resolution of the transducers used. A 10 MHz transducer can usually define a fine slip of platysma muscle just beneath the skin surface of the neck.

Pathologic Findings

In 1978, the first examples of parathyroid adenomas identified by grey scale sonography were published by Sample and his associates[8]. In 1981, the technique was used to do a biopsy of a suspected parathyroid adenoma in a patient with recurrent disease[9].

The classic appearance of a parathyroid adenoma on a sonographic image is a lesion of about 1 cm, a hypoechoic or anechoic oval mass, oriented craniocaudally, posterior to the thyroid, and often adjacent and medial to the carotid artery[10, 11].

As a rule, hyperechoic lesions are not parathyroid in origin, but usually, not always, benign thyroid lesions.

There are usually four normal parathyroid glands, two superior and two inferior, often posterior, and adjacent to the thyroid gland. While the classic dictum is that the parathyroids number four (84%), some patients have only three (3%), and a few patients have multiple glands numbering five or more (13%)[12]. In sonography, the normal glands are usually not identified because they are small, flat, and blend with the soft tissues. Normal glands are usually only a few millimeters wide and less than 1.5 cm long. As the glands begin to enlarge, they become apparent by sonogra-

88 4 Parathyroid Gland

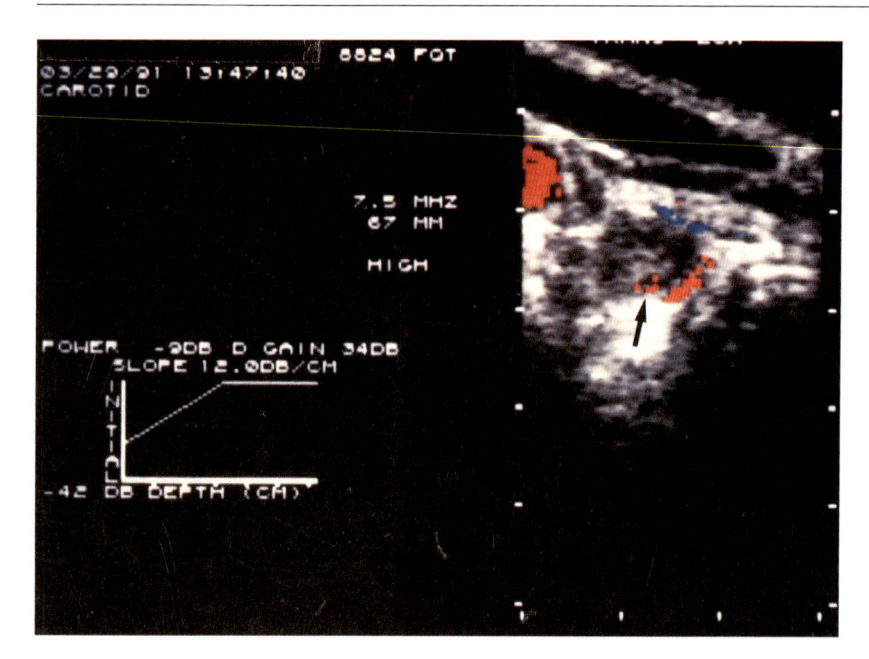

Fig. 4.2 A transverse color-coded sonogram of the right thyroid lobe shows a small parathyroid adenoma (arrow) with a vascular rim medially

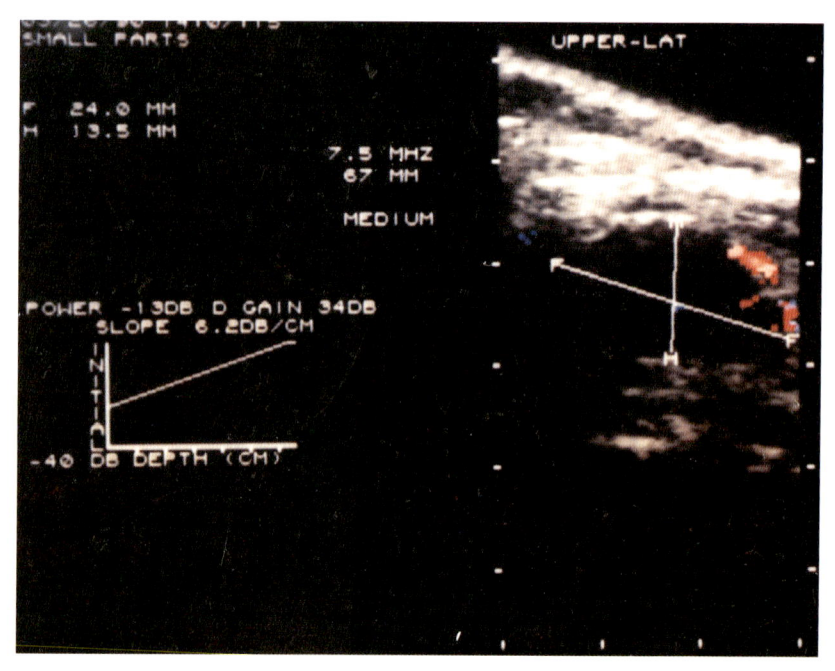

Fig. 4.3 A longitudinal color-coded sonogram shows a large posterior parathyroid adenoma with an inferior vascular rim

phy, usually rounding up in contour at 3–4 mm when they are recognized. As the abnormal glands enlarge, they take on a typical oval appearance, with craniocaudal orientation. Usually hypoechoic or anechoic, these parathyroid tumors do not demonstrate through transmission the way a cyst would be expected to behave. Of course, as the parathyroid neoplasms become larger, they exhibit characteristics of any large mass and can develop cystic areas from necrosis or hemorrhage[13].

A common location for the parathyroid adenoma is immediately medial to the carotid artery at the level of the thyroid gland.

While most parathyroid lesions are posterior to the thyroid, many are not (Fig. 4.5). Some are quite anterior in position, and a few are intrathyroidal (Fig. 4.6)[14]. As embryonic derivatives of the fourth branchial pouch, superior glands tend to be positioned posteriorly, and are therefore likely responsible for the aberrant positions that are retroesophageal or in the carotid sheath (1.6%), as well as the ectopic parathyroid lesions in the posterior mediastinum[15].

The lower parathyroid glands lie just posterior or inferior to the thyroid and can, upon enlargement, be found actually quite anterior in position (Fig. 4.5). The migratory path of the inferior lesions is this ven-

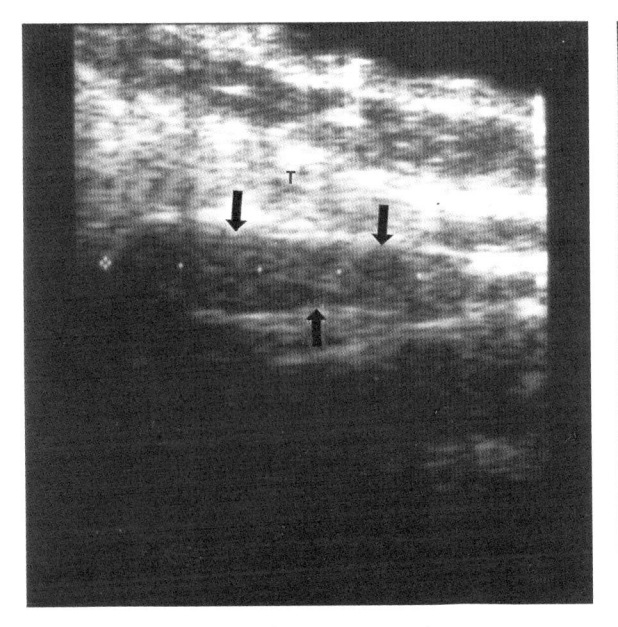

Fig. 4.4 A longitudinal sonogram demonstrates a long tubular parathyroid adenoma (arrows), which has the possibility of being misconstrued as a longus colli muscle. T = Thyroid

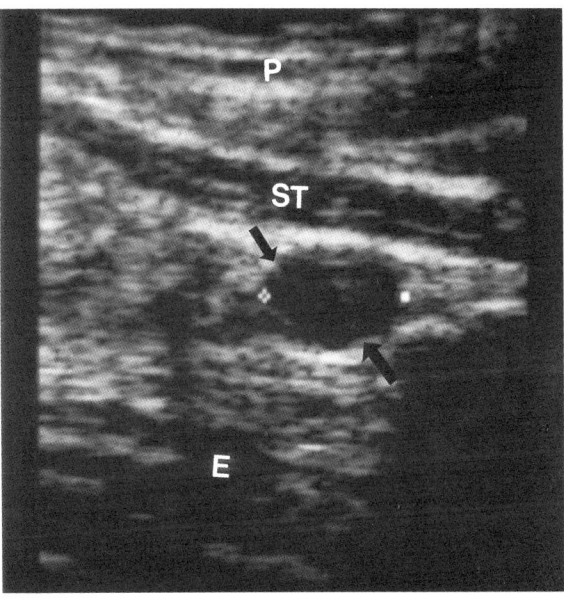

Fig. 4.5 A longitudinal sonogram demonstrates an anterior inferior small parathyroid adenoma (arrows) anterior to the esophagus (E). ST = Strap muscle, P = Platysma muscle

tral route. The inferior parathyroid glands, which are embryonic derivatives of the third branchial pouch as is the thymus, find their way to ectopic positions in the anterior mediastinum (10–13%)[16]. These inferior lesions are supplied by the inferior thyroidal arteries, which, along with the superior thyroidal arteries, can be specifically seen using ultrasound, especially with color-coded Doppler, as branches from the external carotid artery.

Parathyroid Cysts

Classic cystic lesions can be thyroid or parathyroid in origin. Thyroid cysts tend to be in some stage of degeneration of adenomatous hyperplasia and can, on aspiration biopsy, have bloody fluid, chocolate-colored fluid, or xanthochromic fluid depending upon the stage of hemorrhagic evolution. Parathyroid cysts, on the other hand, tend to contain clear fluid (Fig. 4.7)[17]. Parathyroid cysts usually do not cause hyperparathyroidism, even though the cyst fluid has an elevated parathormone level, but a number of cases of hyperparathyroidism have been reported on the basis of a parathyroid cyst[17–20].

Pitfalls

In the assessment of parathyroid disease using ultrasound, there are certain inherent limitations of which

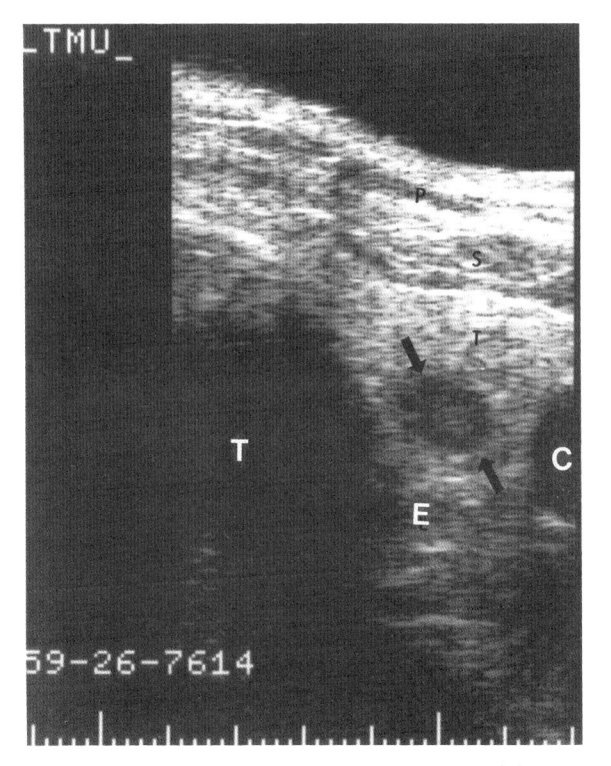

Fig. 4.6 A transverse scan of the left thyroid (T) demonstrates an intrathyroidal parathyroid adenoma (arrows). C = Carotid artery, T = Trachea, E = Esophagus, S = Strap muscle, P = Platysma

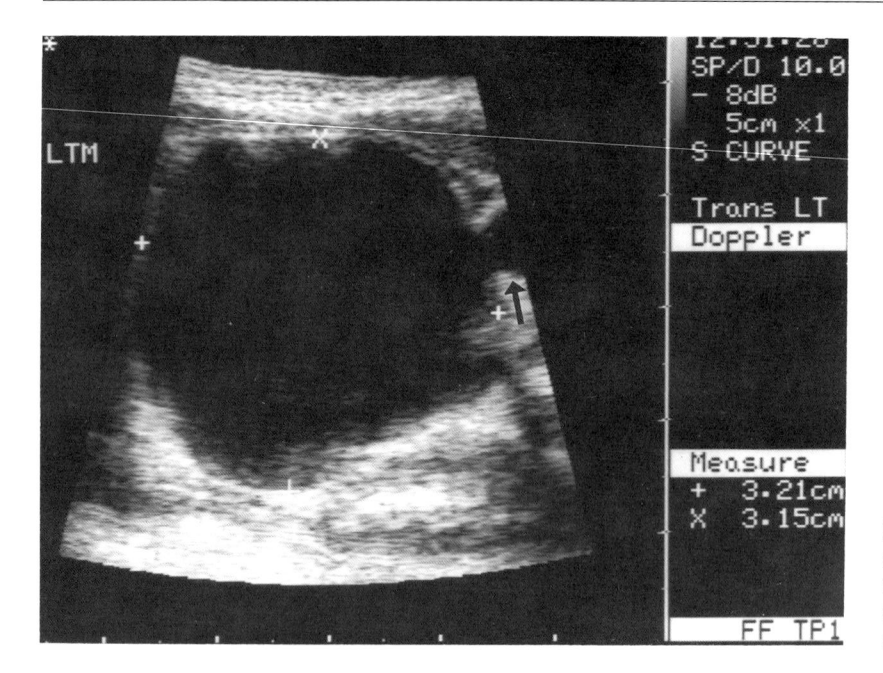

Fig. 4.7 A transverse scan demonstrates a large cyst demarcated by markers immediately medial to the carotid artery (arrow)

the examiner should be aware. First of all, normal glands are not ordinarily seen. Secondly, parathyroid tumors in the mediastinum or the pericardium are not amenable to sonographic visualization because of the obscuring bony thorax and air-filled lung. Some parathyroid tumors in the neck will also be obscured, particularly those behind the air-filled esophagus or trachea, the rare pharyngeal implant, or those lesions directly behind the thyroid cartilages which absorb sound, casting acoustic shadows that also obscure.

An elongated tubular parathyroid variant can be confused with the hypoechoic posterior longus coli muscle (Fig. 4.4).

A parathyroid tumor medial to one of the lobes of the thyroid can be missed when the overlying air in the trachea obscures it.

Parathyroid glands superior to the thyroid gland seem to be most easily missed, which may be related to the thyroid cartilage that casts a prominent acoustic shadow in the area.

Clumps of metallic surgical clips are another source of obscuration, but not usually of such magnitude to actually obscure an underlying mass.

In a hyperparathyroid patient who has had a thyroidectomy for thyroid cancer, and has a hypoechoic mass in the thyroid bed, recurrent thyroid cancer or parathyroid adenoma are suggested. Aspiration biopsy is indicated to differentiate the two.

A cluster of small nodes in the lower neck inferior to the thyroid gland can mask a parathyroid adenoma, since it can appear similar sonographically. Larger nodes often have a hilar distribution of vascularity on color-coded Doppler, and large parathyroids develop rim or scattered vascularity.

A large goiter can obscure a small parathyroid adenoma. A diffusely hypoechoic thyroid gland, typical for Hashimoto's disease, can make delineation of a small hypoechoic parathyroid adenoma more difficult.

Hashimoto disease tends to produce a nodular, strikingly hypoechoic thyroid. Since parathyroid lesions tend to be hypoechoic, concomitant disease can be missed or obscured.

Because of the lack of an acoustic window, ultrasound can fail to detect inferior parathyroid lesions when the thyroid gland normally extends inferiorly into the mediastinum.

Multiple focal thyroid lesions can also mask a small parathyroid adenoma. In such a situation, an intrathyroidal parathyroid adenoma may not be recognized.

Multiple thyroid nodules in an enlarged thyroid gland may obscure small hyperplastic parathyroid lesions.

Clinical Setting

The patient, who is typically an adult, and predominantly female (3 to 1), comes to sonography with a diagnosis of hyperparathyroidism already at hand. What has set off this cascade of endocrinologic abnormalities is unknown.

Unless it is giant, the parathyroid lesion is not palpable. Ultrasound is not used as a screening test for the disease before biochemical evidence of elevated serum calcium and elevated PTH levels have been established, although, on occasion in our practice, a clinically unsuspected parathyroid adenoma has been

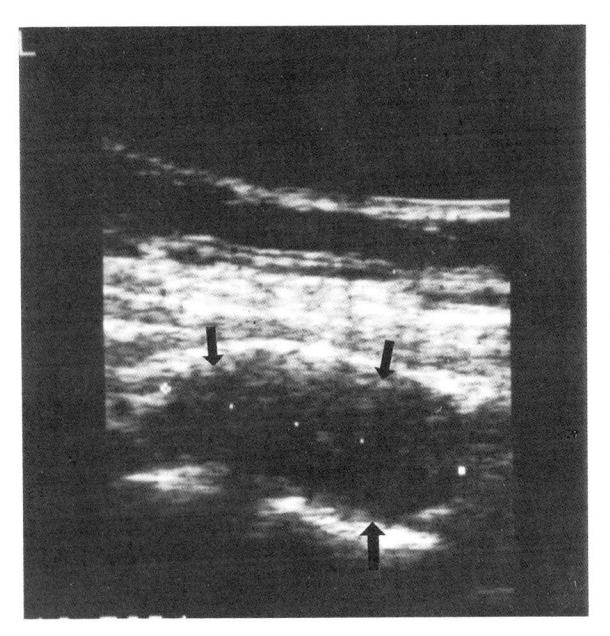

Fig. 4.**8** A longitudinal sonogram demonstrates a large anechoic parathyroid adenoma posterior in the lower neck (arrows)

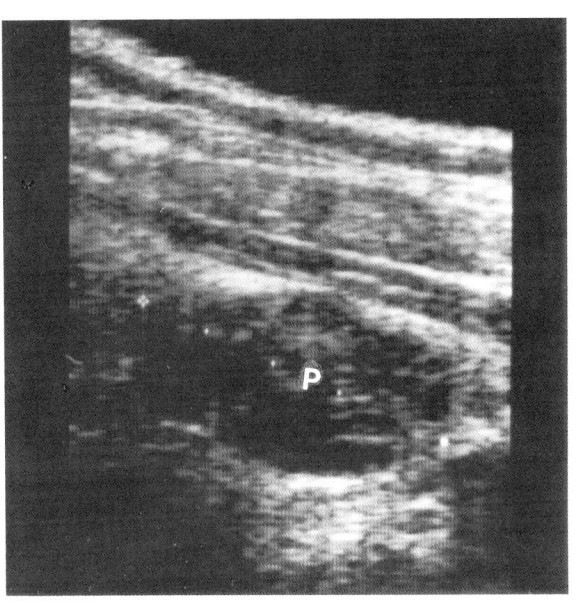

Fig. 4.**9** A longitudinal scan of the lower neck demonstrates an irregular, both hypoechoic and anechoic, parathyroid adenoma with cystic degeneration. (P)

detected when the patient was referred to us for a sonogram of the neck for a different problem.

If the patient is suggestive of primary hyperparathyroidism, a single parathyroid adenoma is by far the most likely situation (80%) (Fig. 4.**8**). These can usually be defined by sonography in about 76% of all cases [21]. About 12% of patients will manifest this disease by developing primary parathyroid hyperplasia [13]. In these instances, detection by ultrasound or any other imaging modality, is less likely to be fully successful (less than 50% detection). These parathyroid glands are variable in size; some may be quite small and easily missed. About 3% of patients with primary hyperparathyroidism present with multiple enlarged parathyroid glands, and a few have parathyroid cancer or a parathyroid cyst that explains the abnormal biochemical profile.

Variants

Hyperechogenicity of a parathyroid lesion has been reported in the rare case of parathyroid lipoadenoma,[22] which can produce hyperparathyroidism. Other sonographic variations from the norm include lobular configuration, cystic degeneration, calcification, and giant size (Fig. 4.**9**)[12].

Recurrent or persistent hyperparathyroidism is a particularly common problem in patients with multiple endocrine neoplasia or familial hyperparathyroidism[13].

Secondary Hyperparathyroidism

Patients with secondary hyperparathyroidism have variably sized parathyroid adenomas. Some may have small parathyroid glands of different sized glands, and others may have four large glands (Fig. 4.**10**). Usually, the enlarged glands differ in size, from each other and are of such a dimension that sonography is used to detect them in about 76% of cases [23, 24].

Treatment is directed toward medical therapy, rather than surgery, unless in the few instances in which marked hypercalcemia or bone loss develops, in which case surgery is recommended[25].

Familial Hyperparathyroidism

When patients have a family history of parathyroid disease, other family members may wish to be screened with sonography for the detection of parathyroid adenoma, since this is an autosomal dominant disease that produces parathyroid hyperplasia.

Multiple Endocrine Neoplasia (MEN)

Both the thyroid and the parathyroid glands are affected in this autosomal dominant group of diseases. Type I refers to Wermer syndrome which encompasses parathyroid adenomas or hyperplasia and differentiated thyroid cancer, as well as endocrine tumors of the pancreas, the pituitary, the adrenal cortex and ovary. It also conprises bronchial carcinoid,[26] bronchial adenomas, melanoma, and

4 Parathyroid Gland

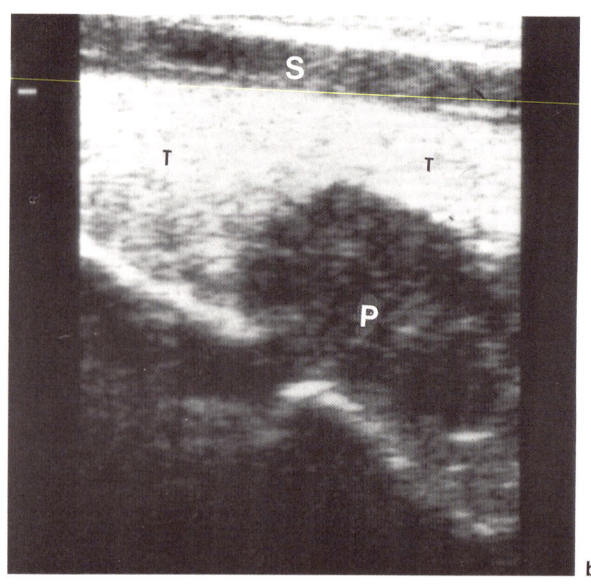

Fig. 4.**10a** A surgical specimen demonstrates four large hyperplastic parathyroid glands in a patient with secondary hyperparathyroidism. Note that the gland at the lower right (arrow) is smaller than the others (from Dr. Orlo Clark, Department of Surgery, University of California, San Francisco)

b A longitudinal sonogram of the thyroid (T) shows one of the hyperplastic parathyroid glands (P). S = Strap muscle

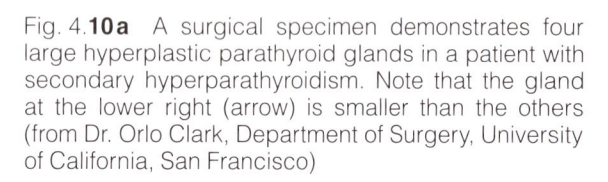

gastrointestinal ulcers, most of which are associated with Zollinger–Ellison syndrome [27].

Patients with multiple endocrine neoplasia, which is inherited as an autosomal dominant, develop hyperplasia of all the parathyroid glands and tend to develop recurrent or persistent parathyroid disease after surgical therapy [13]. At times, normal-sized glands can be hyperplastic, as determined through surgery, but will not be readily identified by ultrasound. Over time, multiple hyperplastic parathyroid glands may develop in a single patient. Some patients have continued to develop additional tumors after several parathyroidectomies, one in our experience, 16 to date.

Because parathyroid hyperplasia, parathyroid adenoma, medullary thyroid carcinoma, and pheochromocytoma are all components of MEN type II, sonography of the neck fulfills two goals: a search for parathyroid disease, and for medullary thyroid carcinoma. In some instances of medullary thyroid carcinoma, large clumps of calcification are noted in the thyroidal mass [28, 29]. Metastatic adenopathy of the neck from medullary thyroid cancer is also associated with clumps of calcification within the lymph nodes. Ultrasound basically defines the thyroid mass and the nature of its consistency, which is solid, fluid-filled or a combination of the two; it cannot be used to specifically determine the thyroid pathology without a biopsy.

MEN type III refers to those patients affected with medullary thyroid carcinoma, pheochromocytoma, mucosal neuromas, and ganglioneuromatosis or all four [13]. These patients do not usually have parathyroid disease [27].

Risk Factors

Oral lithium therapy appears to precipitate hyperparathyroidism in some patients [30].

Patients who have had low-dose radiation to the neck are also more susceptible to developing hyperparathyroidism; these patients also have an acceleration of carotid atherosclerosis in the neck and an increased risk of thyroid carcinoma [31].

Parathyroid Biopsy

On aspiration biopsy, thyroid and parathyroid cells have similarities [9, 32–37]. The greatest difference is the increased size and colloid of the thyroid epithelial cells. To differentiate thyroid from parathyroid and to confirm the parathyroid origin of the lesion, special staining such as the immunoperoxidase technique may be in order [35]. Another way to determine the parathyroid origin of the aspirated sample is to do a bioassay of the material.

The technique of parathyroid biopsy is as follows: The patient lies supine with the neck hyperextended and with a pillow between the shoulder blades. The lesion is identified in both the longitudinal and transverse planes and the skin is marked with an indelible marker or with the temporary mark from the end of a wooden stick pushed into the skin over the lesion. A sterile field is prepared with an iodine solution. A local injection of anesthetic is injected under the skin. Then the lesion is marked by sonography in centimeters from the skin to the anterior wall of the parathyroid. The 22-gauge needle is marked for proper depth, attached to a 10 ml syringe, and inserted into the lesion, where suction is applied as the needle is moved up and down in the lesion (Fig. 4.**11**). Then, suction is released and the aspirated specimen is put on a slide, smeared, and prepared by the pathologist with both air dry techniques and alcohol fixation.

One of several of the needle aspirates is put in saline solution for bioassay of PTH as another confirmation of the origin of the lesion.

Parathyroid Variants

The classic parathyroid is homogenously hypoechoic or anechoic and discrete, an appearance probably related to the encapsulation of sheets of chief cells seen on pathological examination. As the lesion enlarges, it may become lobular (2%) and more echo producing (Fig. 4.**12**)[12]. Areas of hemorrhage and fatty infiltration contribute to this heterogeneous appearance. Cystic degeneration can occur (3.8%) (Fig. 4.**13**)[12]. Giant lesions, greater than 3 cm (4.6%), can distort the local anatomy and cause mass effects (Fig. 4.**14**)[12]. Larger lesions tend to have greater biochemical elevations of calcium and PTH, but this is not an absolutely linear relationship[38].

Calcifications are not the norm in parathyroid lesions, occurring in only about (2.5%)[12]. On the other hand, calcifications are common in both benign and malignant thyroid masses. Fine, sonographically detected microcalcifications have been reported in 62% of thyroid malignancies but are uncommon in benign disease[39].

Patients with primary hyperparathyroidism also exhibit soft tissue calcifications, including those of the heart, particularly in the interventricular septum, the myocardium, and the aortic and mitral valves, all detectable by ECG [40].

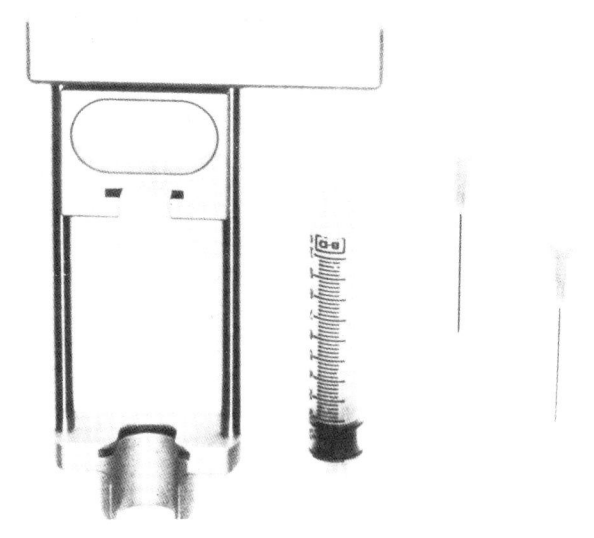

Fig. 4.**11** Photograph of the aspiration cytology device. The syringe fits into the device and suction is easily developed once the needle has been placed within the lesion

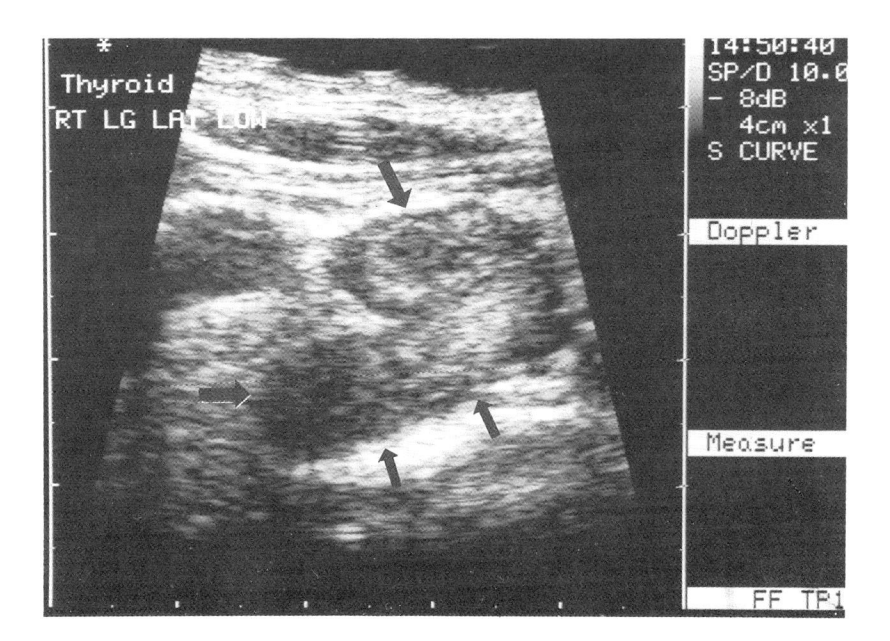

Fig. 4.**12** A longitudinal lateral transverse scan of the lower neck demonstrates a multilobulated large parathyroid adenoma in a patient with multiple endocrine neoplasia. She also had a thyroid lesion (not shown on this image)

94   4 Parathyroid Gland

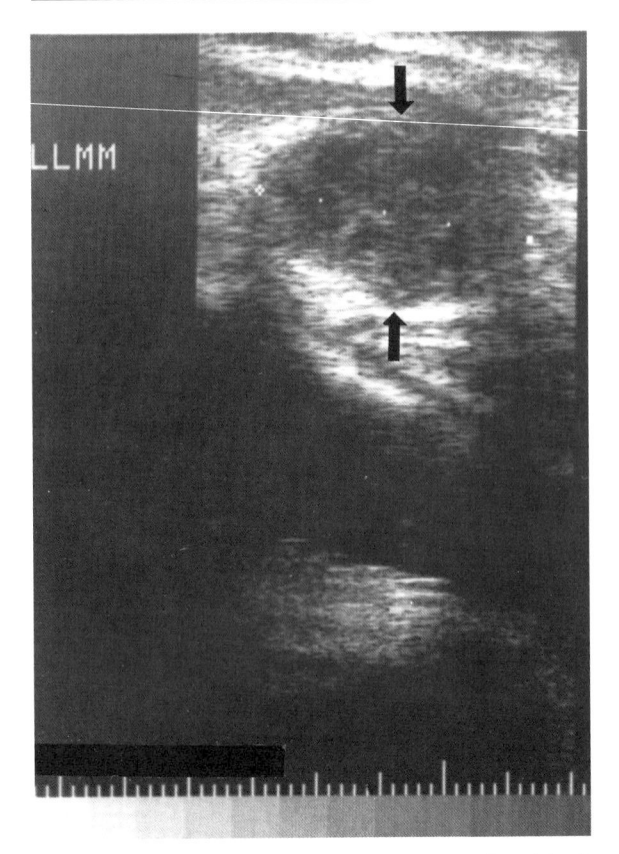

Fig. 4.13 A longitudinal scan shows a parathyroid adenoma with several anechoic areas, some of which slightly enhance; at pathology, this represented cystic degeneration

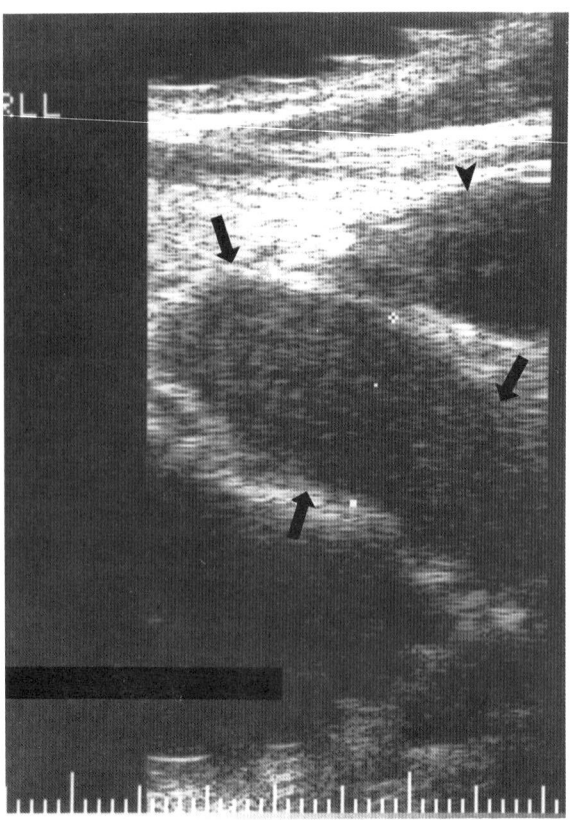

Fig. 4.14 A longitudinal sonogram (10 MHz) shows a giant parathyroid adenoma (arrows) posterior to the jugular vein, low in the neck (arrowhead)

Parathyroid Hyperplasia

Primary parathyroid hyperplasia can not be as successfully imaged as parathyroid adenoma by either ultrasound, [41] CT, scintigraphy, or MRI [42]. In some cases the glands are small, in others the glands are of low weight, less than 200 mg (Fig. 4.15). In primary hyperparathyroidism, when the radiologist detects a classic dominant lesion, he or she may be less attuned to other small subtle abnormalities that may represent examples of parathyroid hyperplasia and may erroneously consider them to be of thyroid origin and of no consequence.

Hyperplasia of the parathyroids, whether primary or secondary, is treated surgically by subtotal resection [43].

Posterior parathyroid adenomas, as they enlarge, tend to bulge into the thyroid parenchyma. About 1% of parathyroid adenomas will be completely surrounded by thyroid tissue, that is, intrathyroidal [13]. When these parathyroid tumors are large, discrete, oval, and hypoechoic, they can be easily recognized, since thyroid lesions in general tend to be rounded and more echoic or complex than parathyroid masses. Nevertheless, small parathyroid adenomas are often rounded hypoechoic lesions that intrathyroidally, cannot be distinguished from the thyroid without aspiration biopsy and bioassay of hormone.

Parathyroid Cancer

In a sonographic image, parathyroid cancer can appear similar to a parathyroid adenoma and have calcium elevations just above the norm as is typical of those with primary hyperparathyroidism from a parathyroid adenoma.

Some patients with parathyroid cancer do show signs of aggressive invasion of the lesion into the adjacent soft tissues, including the strap muscles (Fig. 4.16) [44, 45]. With these lesions, it may not be possible to distinguish a thyroid malignancy from a parathyroid one, although a number of patients with parathyroid cancer have markedly elevated levels of serum calcium. Patients can have parathyroid cancer in addition to other benign parathyroid or thyroid pathology.

Thyroid disease, benign and malignant, is relatively common, as is primary hyperparathyroidism, which occurs in about 1 in 700 people.

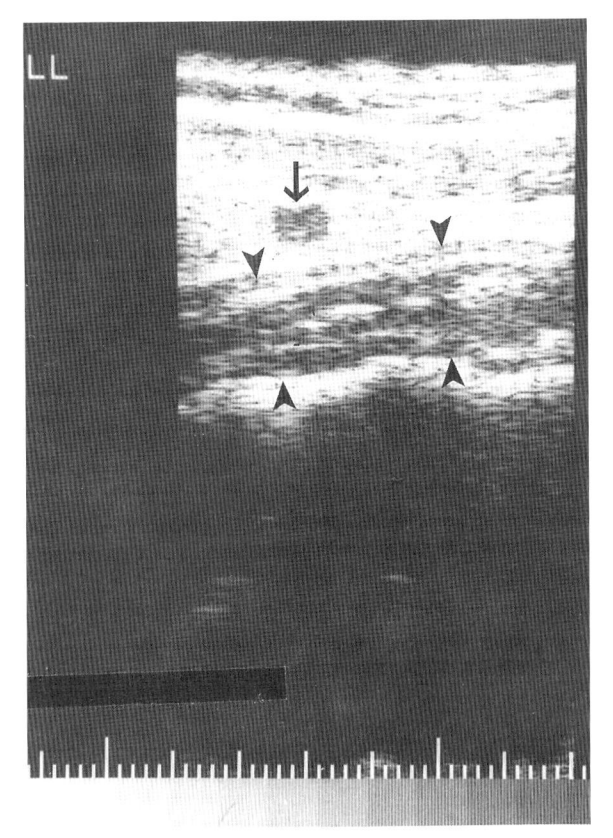

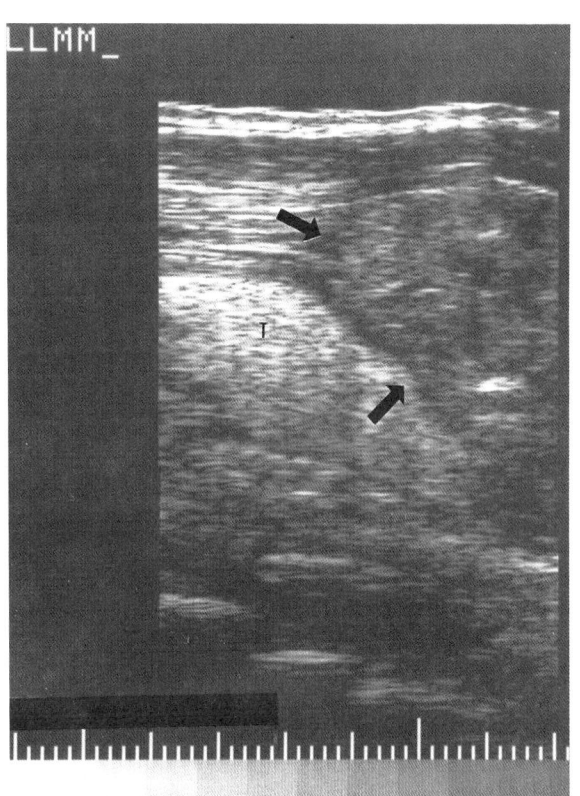

Fig. 4.15 A longitudinal scan demonstrates a small hyperplastic parathyroid gland (arrow) within the thyroid, anterior to the esophagus (arrowheads)

Fig. 4.16 A longitudinal sonogram (10 MHz) shows carcinoma of the parathyroid invading the strap muscles (arrows). T = thyroid

It stands to reason therefore that both thyroid and parathyroid pathology would occur concomitantly and they do. In fact, thyroid masses are present in almost half of those examined for parathyroid disease by sonography[46] and, specifically, thyroid malignancy noted by sonography occurs in about 6–11%[47,48] of patients with parathyroid pathology.

Treatment

Surgical resection is the traditional way to treat primary hyperparathyroidism. Many surgeons are content to go directly to surgery without preliminary localizing techniques for a virgin case of hyperparathyroidism because of the high likelihood of detecting and resecting the parathyroid neoplasm. Others are strong proponents of imaging before surgical resection, particularly in cases of recurrent or persistent disease, because the surgical success rate drops dramatically in these situations[49].

The operative field is more complicated by anatomic distortion and scarring if some resection has occurred, the extent of which is not always known at the time of surgery. Negative results from ultrasound of the neck are one indication that the lesion may be ectopic, or that perhaps this patient has parathyroid hyperplasia. Positive results immediately direct the surgeon to the appropriate side and the particular site. Sonography has the potential to suggest complicating factors before surgery when the patient is found to have a thyroid lesion suggestive of medullary thyroid carcinoma, or significant adenopathy in the neck with calcifications in addition to the parathyroid pathology, or a lesion that appears aggressive.

Intraoperative localization of parathyroid adenoma[50,51] has the potential to become viable as sonographic units become easier to use, near field resolution improves, and small transducers of high resolution specifically designed for a small field become available.

Intraoperative use of ultrasound involves cleaning the entire unit before taking it to the operating room. Then, sterile acoustic gel is applied to the transducer of choice. After this, a sterile sheath encompasses the transducer and cord and any air bubbles are effaced from the transducer surface to avoid artifacts. The operative field is bathed with saline as a couplant, and scanning proceeds. Intrathyroidal localization of parathyroid adenoma is also possible at the time of surgery with this technique. An intrathyroidal parathyroid gland can not be detected visually by the surgeon unless the thyroid is dissected.

Confirmation that the lesion has been resected is another advantage of intraoperative sonography, because at times in persistent disease, sonograms after surgery have revealed that the parathyroid tumor is still present at the previously identified site.

Following surgical resection, the pathologist and the surgeon work in concert to make a correct diagnosis, because the sheets of chief cells may not always be distinguishable; adenoma versus hyperplasia, normal from abnormal. The color and texture of the parathyroid tumor in the neck may help make the distinction.

Surgery is the definitive therapy for primary hyperparathyroidism, but embolization techniques have been used in the mediastinum to infarct the offending gland [52-54]. Another alternative experimental approach is to destroy the enlarged gland by ethanol injection of the parathyroid tumor. Localization for ethanol treatment takes place under the guidance of ultrasound, which is used to direct the needle accurately to its destination if the patient can not tolerate surgery or has severe hypercalcemia [54, 55]. This innovative treatment may be associated with recurrence. In a small series this procedure has been associated with vocal cord paralysis in a few instances when the recurrent laryngeal nerve has been injured [54, 55], and the paralysis has been both transient and permanent.

Embolization by interventional radiography has been successful for the ablation of parathyroid adenoma, particularly when obscure mediastinal disease is suspected.

Future Considerations

Perhaps the introduction of intravenous or oral contrast agents for ultrasound, which are in the developmental stages, will enhance the vascular signal on duplex or color-flow Doppler in such a way that subtle parathyroid masses will stand out from the adjacent soft tissues.

Perspectives in Imaging

Localization of a parathyroid tumor prior to surgery has several potential benefits [56, 57]. It may reduce the time of the surgical procedure and allow the surgeon the luxury of knowing whether or not a mediastinal approach will be necessary or likely. It gives the patient some assurance that a lesion consistent with parathyroid has been located. In selected instances, a unilateral dissection may be considered [58].

Without preoperative imaging, surgeons are quite successful (95%) in resecting the abnormal parathyroid gland [43].

Patients with hereditary susceptibility and patients with persistent or recurrent parathyroid disease probably have the most to gain from preoperative localization procedures of parathyroid disease (Fig. 4.**17**). Reoperation for parathyroid disease before these methods existed was successful in only 65% of all cases [49].

Ultrasound, CT, scintigraphy, and MRI all offer ways to define the parathyroid prior to surgery [43, 59]. The choice depends on what instrumentation is available, the experience of both the examiners and the interpreters of the examinations, and where the lesion is most likely to be. For instrumentation, high-resolution transducers are necessary for ultrasound. In MRI, the proper neck coil is important. CT requires a positioning device to avoid artifacts produced by the shoulders which obscure the lower neck. With dual tracer scintigraphy using ^{201}Tl and ^{99m}Tc, color is important.

Sonography as a first choice for parathyroid detection is appropriate. It is not invasive, is the least expensive, and, when combined with biopsy localization, can provide a definitive answer. Studies relating sensitivities of ultrasound vary considerably (38% to nearly 100%) [42, 60-62]. Ultrasound can not detect parathyroid disease in every case. Mediastinal disease cannot be defined by ultrasound. Retroesophageal or retrotracheal parathyroid disease is obscured. Parathyroids nestled behind cartilage or bone, i.e., beneath the clavicle, are not noted. Hyperplastic glands less than 250 mg are missed [41, 42]. Our experience to date

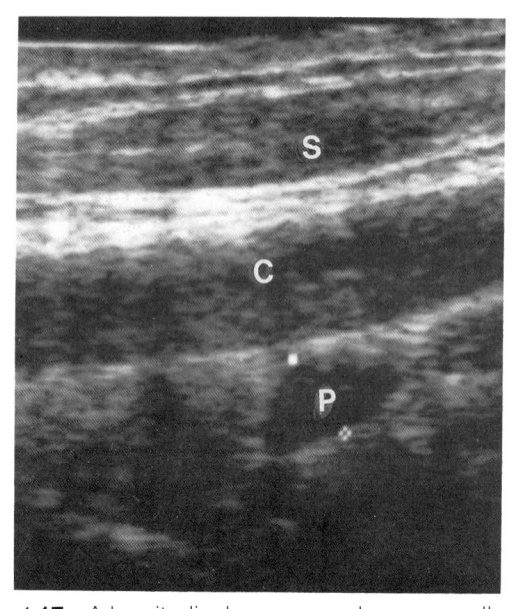

Fig. 4.**17** A longitudinal sonogram shows a small parathyroid adenoma (P) behind the carotid artery (C) and the strap muscle (S) in a patient with recurrent hyperparathyroidism

in detecting parathyroid disease prospectively has ranged from 48% to 82%, the former in primary parathyroid hyperplasia and the latter in parathyroid adenoma[21]. Specificities have been uniformly high (86–91%).

However, when the information is not conclusive or the results are equivocal, another modality can be chosen. Two different modalities in combination can increase the sensitivity of detection[11,41,63–66].

Naturally, the experience in each institution will vary according to the patient population, the instrumentation available, and the experience of the radiologists and technicians[66].

In one group of 100 patients, the sensitivity of detection of parathyroid disease was 55% with sonography, 57% with MRI, 68% with CT, and 73% with dual tracer scintigraphy[42]. In this series, specificities were high, 87% or greater[42]. In another group of 33 patients with parathyroid adenoma, there was a 77% sensitivity for ultrasound, 81% for MRI, 76% for CT, and 65% for scintigraphy[67]. In another, dual tracer scintigraphy and ultrasound in combination resulted in 91% sensitivity of detection[68]. MRI used together with sonography detected 86% of parathyroid lesions prospectively and a higher percentage retrospectively [63]. Specificities are uniformly high with any of the major imaging modalities[69].

For mediastinal disease detection in a large series of 192 patients, ultrasound had a sensitivity of detection of 87%, CT of 56%, and thallium technetium scintigraphy of 71%[70]. Not without risk, DSA has largely been supplanted by these other imaging modalities[71]. Selective venous catheterization and venous sampling, which is an expensive, invasive procedure, is reserved for difficult cases in which information from prior studies is equivocal, contradictory, negative, or particularly when recurrent or persistent disease is documented.

Patients with typical parathyroid adenomas in an otherwise normal neck are relatively easy to diagnose correctly by any modality. More difficult for all modalities are small hyperplastic parathyroid lesions. Also, situations such as thyroid enlargement or nodules, adenopathy, or other concomitant pathologic lesions in the neck can make a correct diagnosis more problematic.

References

1 Caroll B. Carotid sonography. Radiology. 1991;178:303.
2 Gooding GAW, Langman AW, Dillon WP, Kaplan MJ. Malignant carotid artery invasion: sonographic detection. Radiology. 1989;171:435.
3 van den Brekel MWM, Castelijns JA, Stel HV, et al. Occult metastatic neck disease: detection with US and US-guided fineneedle aspiration cytology. Radiology. 1991;180:457.
4 Gooding GAW, Sooy CD, Hybarger CP. Ultrasound of cystic parotid lesions in HIV infection: similarity of sonographic appearance with Sjögren's syndrome. J Ultrasound Med. 1992;II:35–39.
5 Goldman L, Gordan GS, Roof BS. The parathyroids: progress, problems and practice. Curr Probl Surg. 171;8:1.
6 Gooding GAW, Clark OH. Use of Color Doppler imaging in the distinction between thyroid and parathyroid lesions. Am J Surg. 1992;64:51–56.
7 Ralls PW, Mayekawa DS, Lee KP, et al. Color-flow Doppler sonography in Graves disease: "thyroid inferno". Am J Roentgenol. 1899;150:781.
8 Sample FW, Mitchell SP, Bledsoe RC. Parathyroid ultrasonography. Radiology. 1978;127:485.
9 Clark OH, Gooding GAW, Ljung BM: Locating a parathyroid adenoma by ultrasonography and aspiration biopsy cytology. West J Med. 1981;135:154.
10 Simeone JF, Mueller PR, Ferucci JT, et al. High-resolution realtime sonography of the parathyroid. Radiology. 1981;141:745.
11 Stark DD, Gooding GAW, Clark OH. Noninvasive parathyroid imaging. Sem Ultrasound, CT, MR. 1985;6:310.
12 Akerstrom G, Malmaeus J, Bergstrom R. Surgical anatomy of human parathyroid glands. Surgery. 1984;95:14.
13 Randel SB, Gooding GAW, Clark OH, et al. Parathyroid variants, US evaluation. Radiology. 1987;165:191.
14 Clark OH: Hyperparathyroidism. In: Endocrine Surgery of the Thyroid and Parathyroid Glands. Mosby; St. Louis: pp. 172–240, 1985.
15 Smoker WRK, Harnsberger Hr. The neck. In: Head and Neck Imaging. Sorn PM, Bergeron (eds), Mosby Year Book, St. Louis p. 500, 1991.
16 Gooding GAW. Localization of a parathyroid adenoma. In: Margulis AR, Gooding CA, eds. Diagnostic Radiology. San Francisco Department of Radiology, University of California; 1983:315–321.
17 Krudy AG, Doppman JL, Shawker TH, et al. Hyperfunctioning cystic parathyroid glands: CT and sonographic findings. Am J Roentgenol. 1984;142:175.
18 Clark OH: Parathyroid cysts. Am J Surg. 1978;135:395.
19 Calandra DB, Shah KH, Prinz RA, et al. Parathyroid cysts: a report of eleven cases including two associated with hyperparathyroid crisis. Surgery. 1983;94:887.
20 Clark OH, Okerlund MD, Cavalieri RR, Greenspan FS. Diagnosis and treatment of thyroid, parathyroid and thyroglossal duct cysts. J Clin Endocr Metab. 1979;48:983.
21 Gooding GAW, Okerlund MD, Stark DD, Clark OH. Parathyroid imaging: comparison of double tracer (Thallium-201 Technetium-99m) scintigraphy and high resolution sonography. Radiology. 1986;161:57.
22 Obara T, Fujimoto Y, Ito Y, et al. Functioning parathyroid lipoadenoma – report of four cases: clinicopathological and ultrasonographic features. Endo Japonica 1989;36:135.
23 Clark OH, Stark DD, Duh D, Arnaud CD, Gooding GA. Value of high resolution real-time ultrasonography in secondary hyperparathyroidism. Am J Surg. 1985;150:9.
24 Takebayashi S, Matsui K, Onohara Y, Hidai H: Sonography for early diagnosis of enlarged parathyroid glands in patients with secondary hyperparathyroidism. Am J Roentgenol. 1987;148:911.
25 Clark OH: Secondary Hyperparathyroidism. In: Endocrine Surgery of the Thyroid and Parathyroid Glands. St. Louis: Mosby; 1985:241–255.
26 Duh Q-Y, Hybarger CP, Geist R, et al. Carcinoids with multiple endocrine neoplasia syndroms. Amer J. Surg. 1987;154:142.
27 Demos TC, Blonder J, Schey WL, et al. Multiple endocrine neoplasia (MEN) syndrome. Type IIB: Gastrointestinal manifestations. Am J Roentgenol. 1983;140:73.
28 Gorman B, Charboneau JW, James EM, et al. Medullary thyroid carcinoma: role of high-resolution US. Radiology. 1987;162:147.
29 Sutton RT, Reading CC, Charboneau JW, James EM, Grant CS, Hay ID. US-guided biopsy of neck masses in postoperative management of patients with thyroid cancer. Radiology. 1988;168:769.
30 Braunwald EE, Isselbacher KJ, Petersdorf RG, et al. Diseases of the parathyroid gland and other hyper- and hypocalcemic disorders. In: Potts, JT Jr, ed. Harrison's Principles of Internal Medicine. New York: McGraw-Hill; 1988:1870–1888.
31 Prinz RA, et al: Radiation-associated hyperparathyroidism: a new syndrome? Surgery. 1977;82:296.
32 Karstrup S, Glenthoj A, Hainau B, et al. Ultrasoundguided, histological, fine-needle biopsy from suspect parathyroid tumours: success-rate and reliability of histological diagnosis. Br J Radiol. 1989;62:981.

33 Kahaly G, Krause U, Dienes HP, et al. Fine-needle biopsy of parathyroid adenomas. Klin Wochenschr. 1986;64:1176.
34 Solbiati L, Montali G, Croce, et al. Parathyroid tumors detected by fine needle aspiration biopsy under ultrasonic guidance. Radiology. 1983;148:793.
35 Winkler V, Gooding GAW, Montgomery CK, et al. Immunoperoxidase confirmation of parathyroid origin of ultrasound-guided fine needle aspirates of the parathyroid glands. Acta Cytol. 1987;31:40.
36 Karstrup S, Glenthoj A, Hainau B, et al. Ultrasound-guided, histological, fine-needle biopsy from suspect parathyroid tumours: success-rate and reliability of histological diagnosis. Br J Radiol. 1989;62:981.
37 Karstrup S, Glenthoj A, Torp-Pederson S, et al. Ultrasonically guided fine needle aspiration of suggested enlarged parathyroid glands. Acta Radiol. 1988;29:213.
38 Reading CC, Charboneau JW, James EM, et al. High resolution parathyroid sonography. Am J Roentgenol. 1982;139:539.
39 Solbiati L, Ballarati E, Cioffi V, et al. Microcalcifications: A clue in the diagnosis of thyroid malignancies. Radiology. 1990;177(P):140
40 Niederle B, Stefenelli T, Glogar D, Woloszczuk W, Roka R, Mayr H. Cardiac calcific deposits in patients with primary hyperparathyroidism: preliminary results of a prospective echocardiographic study. Surgery. 1990;108:1052.
41 Stein BL, Wexler MJ. Preoperative parathyroid localization: a prospective evaluation of ultrasonography and thallium-technetium scintigraphy in hyperparathyroidism. Can J Surg. 1990;33:175.
42 Krubsack AJ, Wilson SD, Lawson TL, et al. Prospective comparison of radionuclide, computed tomographic, sonographic, and magnetic resonance localization of parathyroid tumors. Surgery. 1989;106:639.
43 Clark OH, Duh QY. Primary hyperparathyroidism. A surgical perspective. Endocrin Metab Clin N Am. 1989;18:701.
44 Edmonson GR, Charboneau JW, James EM, et al. Parathyroid carcinoma: high-frequency sonographic features. Radiology. 1986;161:65.
45 Daly BD, Coffey SL, Behan M. Ultrasonographic appearances of parathyroid carcinoma. Br J Radiol. 1989;62:1017.
46 Stark DD, Clark OH, Gooding GAW, Moss AA. High resolution ultrasound and computerized tomography of thyroid lesions in patients with hyperparathyroidism. Surgery. 1983;94:863.
47 Prinz RA, Barbato AL, Braithwaite SS, et al. Simultaneous primary hyperparathyroidism and nodular thyroid disease. Surgery. 1982;92:454.
48 LiVolsi VA, Feind CR. Parathyroid adenoma and nonmedullary thyroid carcinoma. Cancer. 1976;38:1391.
49 Satava RM Jr., Beahrs HO, Scholz DA. Success rate of cervical exploration for hyperparathyroidism. Arch Surg. 1975;10:625.
50 Miller DL, Doppman JL, Krudy AG, et al. Localization of parathyroid adenomas in patients who have undergone surgery. Part II. Invasive Procedures. Radiology. 1987;162:138.
51 Sigel B, Kraft AR, Nyhus LM, et al. Identification of a parathyroid adenoma by operative ultrasonography. Arch Surg. 1981;116:234.
52 Geelhoed GW, Krudy AG, Doppman JL. Long-term follow-up of patients with hyperparathyroidism treated by transcatheter staining with contrast agent. Surgery. 1983;94:849.
53 Doppman JL, Marx SJ, Spiegel AM, et al. Treatment of hyperparathyroidism by percutaneous embolization of a mediastinal adenoma. Radiology. 1975;115:37.
54 Karstrup S, Transbol I, Holm HH, et al. Ultrasound-guided chemical parathyroidectomy in patients with primary hyperparathyroidism: a prospective study. Br J Radiol. 1989;62:1037.
55 Karstrup S, Holm HH, Glenthoj A, Hegedus L. Nonsurgical treatment of primary hyperparathyroidism with sonographically guided percutaneous injection of ethanol: results in a selected series of patients. Am J Roentgenol. 1990;154:1087–1090.
56 Summers GW, Dodge DL, Kammer H. Accuracy and costeffectiveness of preoperative isotope and ultrasound imaging in primary hyperparathyroidism. Otolaryngol Head Neck Surg. 1989;100:210.
57 Clark OH, Stark DD, Gooding GA, et al. Localization procedures in patients requiring reoperation for hyperparathyroidism. World J Surg. 1984;8:509.
58 Lucas RJ, Welsh RJ, Glover JL. Unilateral neck exploration for primary hyperparathyroidism. Arch Surg. 1990;125:982.
59 Eisenberg H, Pallotta J, Sacks B, Brickman AS. Parathyroid localization, three-dimensional modeling, and percutaneous ablation techniques. Endocr Metab Clin North Am. 1989;18:659.
60 Uden P, Aspelin P, Berglund J, et al. Preoperative localization in unilateral parathyroid surgery. A cost benefit study on ultrasound, computed tomography, and scintigraphy. Acta Chir Scand. 1990;156:29.
61 Miller DL, Doppman JL, Shawker TH, et al. Localization of parathyroid adenomas in patients who have undergone surgery. Part I. Noninvasive imaging methods. Radiology. 1987;162:133.
62 Moreau JF, Chigot JP, De Feraudy MN, et al. Preoperative parathyroid ultrasonography. 45 recent verified cases. Presse Med. 1987;16:804.
63 Auffermann W, Gooding GAW, Okerlund MD, et al. Diagnosis of recurrent hyper-parathyroidism: comparison of MR to other imaging techniques. Am J Roentgenol. 1988;150:1027.
64 Levin KE, Gooding GAW, Okerlund MD, et al. Localizing studies in patients with persistent or recurrent hyperparathyroidism. Surgery. 1987;102:917.
65 Erdman WA, Breslau NA, Weinreb JC, et al. Noninvasive localization of parathyroid adenomas; a comparison of X-ray computerized tomography, ultrasound, scintigraphy, and MRI. Magnet Reson Imag 1989;7:187.
66 Lloyd MN, Lees WR, Milroy EJ. Pre-operative localization in primary hyperparathyroidism. Clin Radiol. 1990;41:239.
67 Erdman WA, Breslau NA, Weinreb JC, et al. Noninvasive localization of parathyroid adenomas: a comparison of X-ray computerized tomography, ultrasound, scintigraphy, and MR. Magn Reson Imaging. 1989;7:187.
68 Winzelberg GG, Hydrovitz JD, O'Hara KR, et al. Parathyroid adenomas evaluated by Tl/201/Tc-99m pertechnetate subtraction scintigraphy and high-resolution ultrasonography. Radiology. 1985;155:231.
69 Attie JN, Khan A, Rumancik WM, et al. Preoperative localization of parathyroid adenomas. Am J Surg. 1988;156:323.
70 Grant CS, Charboneau JW, James EM, Reading CC. Reoperative parathyroid surgery. Wiener Klin Wochenschr. 1988;100:360.
71 Miller DL, Chang R, Doppman JL, Norton JA. Localization of parathyroid adenomas: superselective arterial DSA versus superselective conventional angiography. Radiology. 1989;170:1003.

Computed Tomography

B. P. Kreft and D. D. Stark

Hyperthyroidism is increasingly being recognized because of the widespread use of multiphasic screening for hypercalcemia. Approximately 100 000 new cases develop each year in the United States; women are affected twice as often as men, and the incidence of hyperparathyroidism increases with age (1–3). A Swedish autopsy study revealed parathyroid adenoma in 2.4% and hyperplasia in another 7% of people without signs of renal impairment (3), indicating a high prevalence of subclinical parathyroid disease.

The clinical diagnosis of hyperparathyroidism is established by persistent hypercalcemia and an elevated serum parathyroid hormone concentration (1, 2). Untreated hyperparathyroidism can lead to organ deterioration, such as bone loss, renal impairment, or hypertension, and might cause psychiatric problems, however, presentation with bone disease, which is evident from standard radiography or from the presence of nephrolithiasis or other complications, is uncommon today (1).

The treatment of choice for hyperparathyroidism is surgery, and it is highly successful when done by an experienced surgeon. The success rate is greater than 90%, with a low mortality and a persisting cure in many cases (1–3).

The use of noninvasive imaging procedures, such as ultrasound and CT, before a first operation is still controversial (1). Some surgeons do not use preoperative imaging because of the high success rate for the operative exploration of the neck. Others find it helpful in planning the sequence of an operation, and it has been shown that in some cases correct preoperative localization of an adenoma can permit unilateral parathyroidectomy, reducing the time needed for surgery and anesthesia (4).

Contrary localizing studies are strongly recommended in patients with persistent or recurrent hyperparathyroidism, who undergo a second neck exploration, and CT has proven helpful, especially if parathyroid tumors are in ectopic locations (5–11).

Technique

The diagnostic accuracy of conventional parathyroid CT scanning can be limited by shoulder-streak artifacts, poor spatial resolution and section registration, and image unsharpness due to magnification (5). Tortuous vessels, a collapsed esophagus, thyroid masses, and lymph nodes may be mistaken for enlarged parathyroid glands, and additionally, the relative positions and configurations of these soft tissues can change with neck position and swallowing (5, 12, 13).

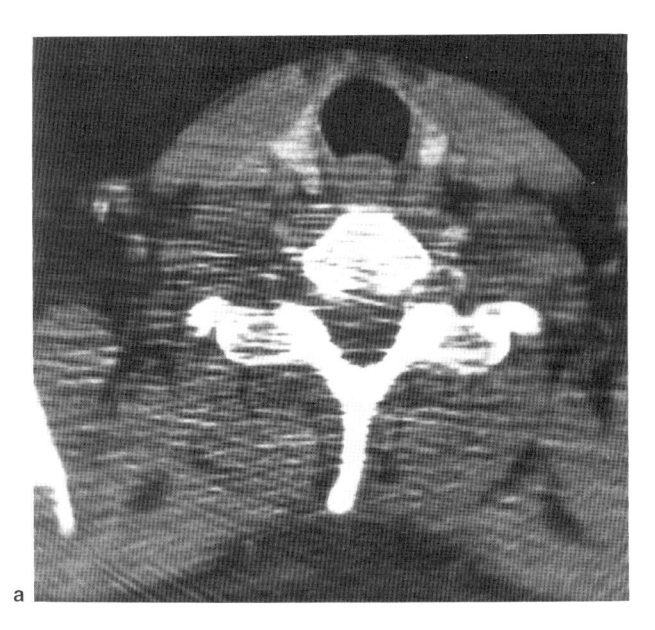

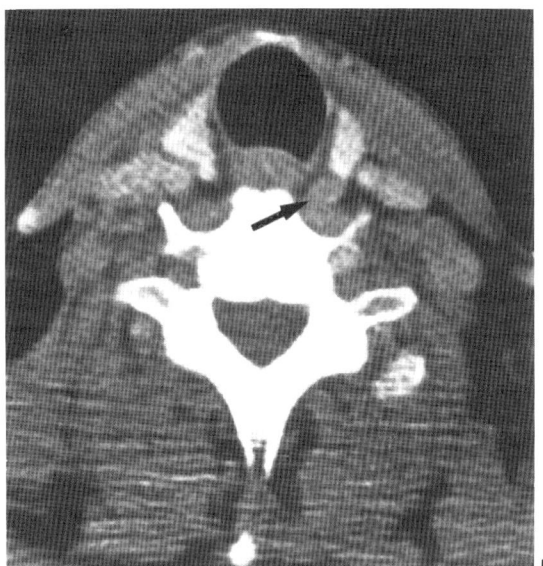

Fig. 4.**18** Scans without (**a**) and with (**b**) the patient positioning device. The elimination of shoulder-streak artifacts results in better definition of a retrothyroidal parathyroid adenoma (arrow). The drawing (**c**) contains labels corresponding to (**b**). C = carotid artery, E = esophagus, EJ = external jugular vein, IJ = internal jugular vein, LC = longus colli muscle, P = parathyroid adenoma, SCM = sternocleidomastoid muscle, SHM = sternohyoid muscle, Th = thyroid, and Tr = trachea

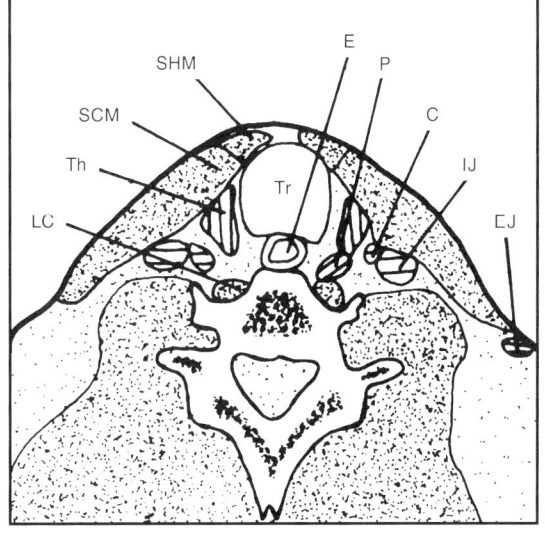

By proper positioning using a specially designed device that immobilizes the shoulders and fixes the neck in hyperextension, streak artifacts related to shoulder position and mobility can be eliminated or displaced posteriorly (Fig. 4.**18**). Additionally, due to hyperextension of the neck, the thyroid, parathyroid glands, and parts of the thymus are elevated, and vessels are straightened and therefore more easily identified.

Dynamic scanning and the intravenous administration of a bolus of contrast media lead to easy differentiation of vessels from nonvascular masses. Enhanced tumors, due to their asymmetry, lack continuity on adjacent sections, and sometimes incomplete or irregular enhancement can also be distinguished from vessels (Fig. 4.**19**) (5).

After positioning, the patient should be instructed to breathe quietly and avoid swallowing. A scout view (four 5 mm axial sextions) is used to locate the cricoid cartilage and the arch of the left innominate vein. Iodinated contrast media (i.e., 120 mL of 60% meglumine diatrizoate) should be administered by intravenous bolus during dynamic scanning, with table incrementation of 3–4 mm between sequential scans and contiguous 3–4 mm sections should be obtained from the cricoid cartilage to the left innominate vein. Patients who had previous parathyroid surgery should also be scanned from the left innominate vein to the tracheal carina using 1 cm sections (5, 6). If neccessary, selected sections can be obtained again following swallows of saliva or methylglucamine diatrizoate (Gastrografin) by the patient if the esophagus was not delineated clearly.

Normal Anatomy

The normal parathyroid glands lie in 80% symmetrically in characteristic upper and lower positions behind the thyroid gland and are too small to be visualized by CT. The most difficult area to evaluate by CT scans is immediately below the thyroid gland because of the complex anatomy and the numerous vessels passing through the superior thoracic aperture (12). Criteria such as asymmetry, continuity on adjacent slices, and dense opacification after contrast bolus administration help to differentiate vessels from other structures (6).

The thyroid gland is the orientation mark for parathyroid imaging. Without contrast media, normal thyroid tissue is usually slightly hyperdense to other soft tissues in this region (50–85 H) and enhances to 90–110 H after contrast media administration (12). Structures that can be confused with parathyroid adenoma are thyroid nodules adjacent to the posterior surface of the thyroid, neck muscles, such as the longus colli or scalene, which show minimal or no postcontrast enhancement (12). The esophagus may also migrate from behind the trachea, rarely to the right, more commonly to the left, and this may mimic a parathyroid adenoma (13). However, after oral contrast media administration the esophagus can usually be identified (5).

Pathology

Parathyroid Hyperplasia

Any asymmetry in the fascial planes posterior to the thyroid suggests the presence and side of enlarged

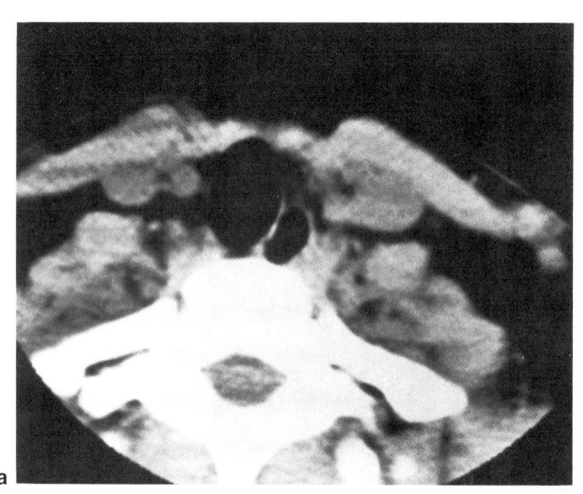

Fig. 4.**19** Parathyroid adenoma. (**a**) Localizing section below the level of the thyroid, obtained without contrast material. (**b**) Same section as (**a**). Dynamic sequence images were obtained after administration of a bolus of contrast material. An incompletely enhanced parathyroid adenoma (arrow) and associated vessel (arrowhead) are now apparent. c = carotid artery, J = jugular vein, and L = longus colli muscle

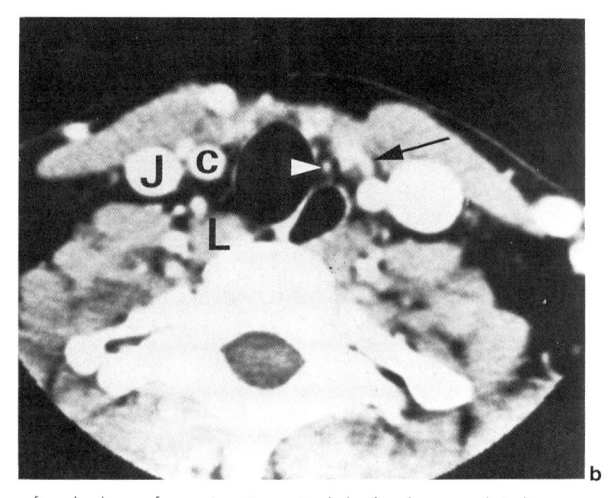

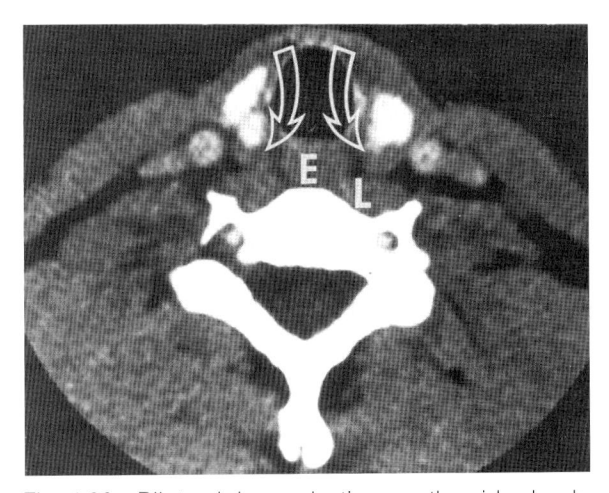

Fig. 4.**20** Bilateral hyperplastic parathyroid glands (arrows) at upper pole of thyroid gland in patient with chronic renal failure. Right gland measured 17 × 11 × 5 mm and left gland 20 × 12 × 6 mm at surgery. E = esophagus, L = longus colli muscle

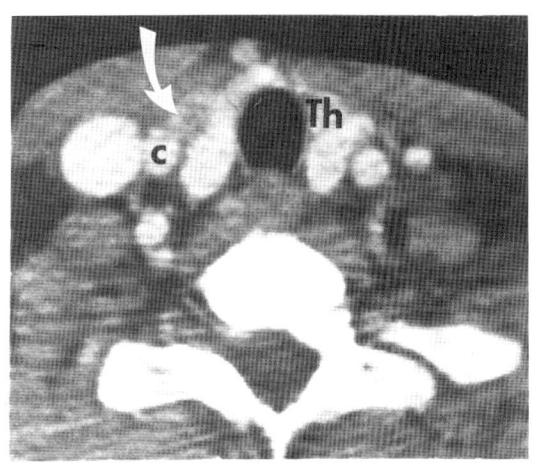

Fig. 4.**21** CT scan of an ectopic hyperplastic parathyroid gland. Mild contrast enhancement of the parathyroid gland (arrow), localized in front of the thyroid (Th) and carotid artery (c)

parathyroid glands, and the finding of more than one enlarged gland strongly indicates secondary hyperparathyroidism (Fig. 4.**20**) (14, 15). Prior to intravenous contrast media administration, hyperplastic glands are similar in attenuation to parathyroid adenomas and muscle tissue (6, 13).

Contrast enhancement, usually homogeneous, is seen in approximately 25% and related to size; large hyperplastic glands are more likely to enhance than small hyperplastic glands (Fig. 4.**21**) (6). The detection of hyperplastic glands is strongly size related with a sensitivity of 33% in pathological glands smaller than 500 mg, and of 88% for larger hyperplastic glands (6, 15). If multinodular goiter is present, it might be even more difficult to differentiate small hyperplastic glands from thyroid nodules (16).

Parathyroid Adenoma

Parathyroid adenomas usually lie medial to the vascular bundle and lateral to the esophagus and trachea. Adenomas of the superior glands are imaged posterior to the mid or lower portion of the tyhroid, and adenomas of the inferior glands are imaged just inferior to the thyroid (13). The most typical CT appearance is a round or ovoid soft tissue mass only seen on one or two sections. A thin, fat plane between the adenoma and the thyroid gland or the esophagus is useful for diagnosis (Fig. 4.**22**) (13).

Prior to contrast media administration, the attenuation of adenomas is similar to that of muscles (35–45 HU) (8). After contrast media administration adenomas enhance in about 25%, with large adenomas more likely to enhance than small adenomas (6). The enhancement of adenomas is usually homogeneous with attenuation coefficients of 65–80 H and lower compared to the enhancement of normal thyroid tissue (Fig. 4.**23**) (12).

Atypical appearances include calcified adenomas (13), cystic components or hemorrhage in the adenoma, and ring enhancement of the adenoma. The sensitivity of high-resolution CT for detecting parathyroid adenomas ranges from 70% to 81% and the specificity from 92% to 96% (5, 6, 12, 13, 16).

Ectopic Parathyroid Adenomas

Ectopic glands may be found in approximately 10% to 20% of cases, anywhere from the midline to lateral to the carotid sheath, from the anterior thyroid margin

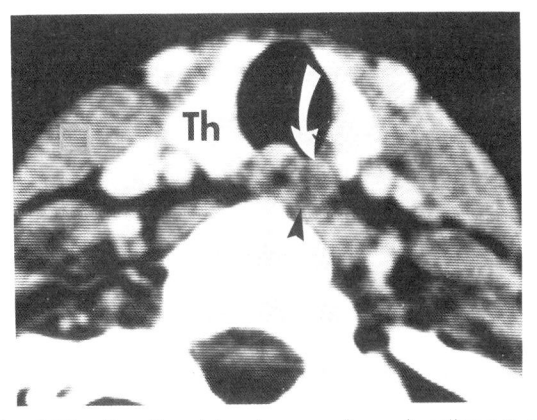

Fig. 4.**22** Parathyroid adenoma (arrow) adjacent to the esophagus. CT diagnosis based on tissue plane delineating the wall of esophagus (arrowhead). Adenoma measured 12 × 6 × 4 mm at surgery. Th = Thyroid

102   4 Parathyroid Gland

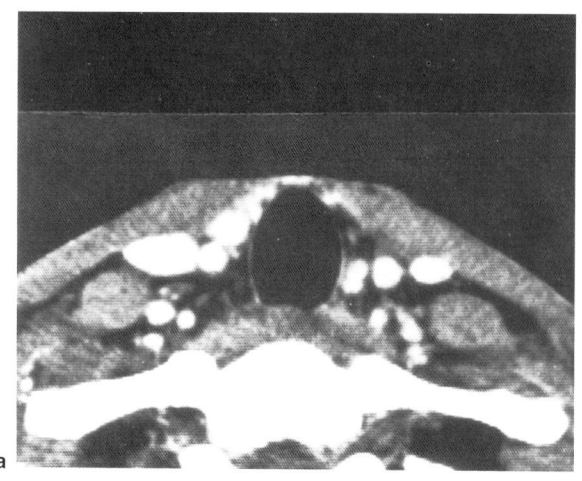

Fig. 4.23 Contrast-enhancing parathyroid adenoma. (a) Axial CT section with tumor at left lower pole of thyroid gland. At operation, adenoma measured 20 × 9 × 5 mm. (b) The drawing contains labels corresponding to (a) VA,V = vertebral artery, vein; IJ = internal jugular vein; Th = thyroid gland; Tr = trachea; E = esophagus; P = parathyroid adenoma; C = carotid artery; LC = longus colli muscle

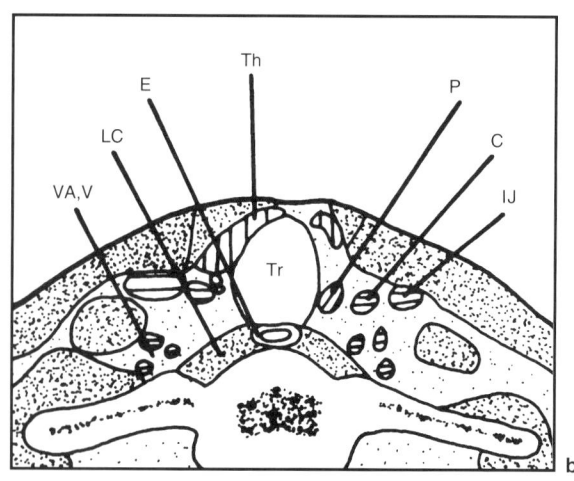

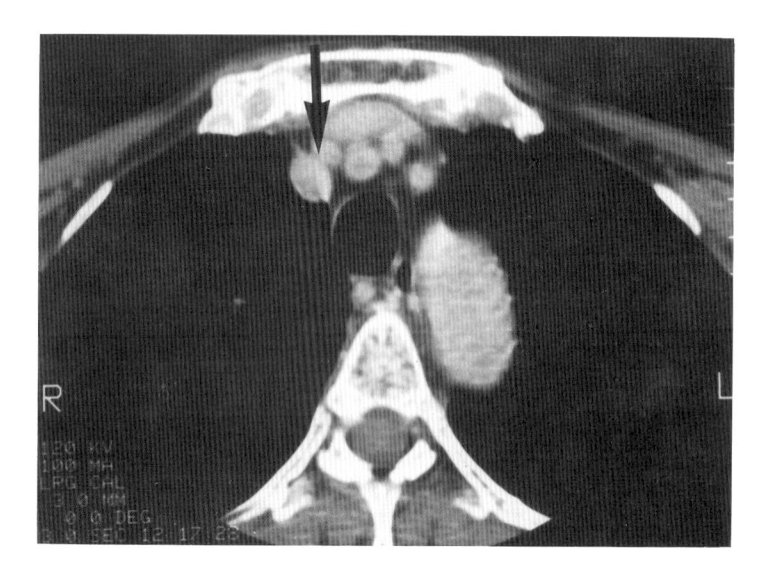

Fig. 4.24 Ectopic parathyroid adenoma. A contrast enhancing adenoma (arrow) is seen on the right border of the anterior mediastinum just below the level of the aortic arch

to posterior to the esophagus, and from the mandibular angle to the aortic root (17). The larger an adenoma, the higher the likelihood that it is ectopic (18). About 20% are located substernally within the thymus, 5% lie intrathyroidally, 5–10% are in the posterior mediastinum, 1–2% are in the anterior mediastinum, and 1% are in the carotid sheath (18). The CT appearance of ectopic adenomas does not differ from that of adenomas in the usual position.

CT is especially helpful in localizing adenomas in retrosternal and mediastinal positions (Fig. 4.24), but it is inferior to ultrasound in detecting intrathyroidal adenomas (19, 20).

Detectability by CT depends not only on lesion size but on location. A small lesion surrounded by mediastinal fat may be clearly evident, whereas the same lesion closely adjacent to normal mediastinal structures will not be visible. Additionally, thymic tissue in a younger patient can easily obscure small adenomas (21).

Persistent or Recurrent Hyperparathyroidism

Preoperative localization studies are essential for patients who have undergone previous parathyroid operations. This is because the remaining parathyroid glands are more difficult to identify during surgery because of increased scarring with loss of tissue planes and because the remaining abnormal parathyroid tissue is more likely to be situated in an ectopic posi-

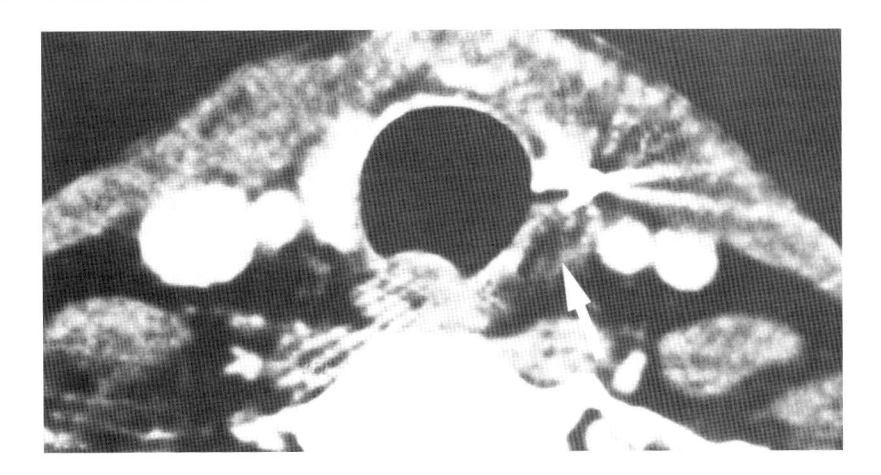

Fig. 4.**25** Persistend hyperparathyroidism. CT demonstrates parathyroid adenoma (arrow) posterior to surgical clip. At operation a 15 × 12 × 10 mm parathyroid adenoma was removed

tion (7). Despite scarring and surgical clips, CT is able to locate tumors in areas of prior surgery with a sensitivity of 44–63% and a specificity of 88–94% (6–8). Fortunately, surgical clips usually mark areas that were carefully explored during the previous operation, and these areas are usually free of tumor on reexploration (Fig. 4.**25**) (2).

Parathyroid Carcinoma

Primary hyperthyroidism can also be caused by carcinomas of the parathyroid with an incidence of 1–4% (17, 22, 23). Local recurrence occurs in about 30% of the cases. Metastatic spread, which also occurs in about 30% of the cases, is usually late and to regional lymph nodes, lungs, liver, and bone (22). Parathyroid carcinoma can not be differentiated from adenoma by CT. In the later stage, associated enlargement of cervical lymph nodes or metastases elsewhere in the body might suggest the presence of a carcinoma (24).

Summary

CT complements other imaging techniques for preoperative localization of enlarged parathyroid glands. CT is strongly indicated if ectopic parathyroid adenomas are suggested or in patients with persistent or recurrent hyperparathyroidism, who undergo a second neck exploration.

References

1. NIH Conference, Diagnosis and Management of Asymptomatic Primary Hyperparathyroidism: Consensus Develpment Conference Statement. Ann Int Med. 1991;114:593–597.
2. Potts JT Jr. Clinical Review 9, Management of Asymptomatic Hyperparathyroidism. JCE & M 1990;70:1489–1493
3. Akerstroem G, Rastad J, Ljunghall S, Johannson H. Clinical and experimental Advances in sporadic primary hyperparathyroidism. Acta Chir Scand 1990;156:23–28.
4. Uden P, Aspelin P, Berglund J, et al. Preoperative localization in unilateral parathyroid surgery. Acta Chir Scand. 1990;156:29–35.
5. Stark DD, Moss AA, Gooding GAW, et al. Parathyroid scanning by computed tomography. Radiology. 1983;148:297–299.
6. Stark DD, Gooding GAW, Moss AA, et al. Parathyroid imaging: Comparison of High-Resolution CT and High-Resolution Sonography. AJR. 1983;141:633–638.
7. Clark OH, Okerlund MD, Moss AA, et al. Localization studies in patients with persistent or recurrent hyperparathyroidism. Surgery. 1985;98:1083–1094.
8. Clark OH, Stark DD, Gooding GAW, et al. Localization procedures in patients requiring reoperation for hyperparathyroidism. World J Surg. 1984;8:509–521.
9. Krubsack AJ, Wilson SD, Lawson TL, et al. Prospective comparison of radionuclide, computed tomographic, sonographic, and magnetic resonance localization of parathyroid tumors. Surgery. 1989;106:639–644.
10. Miller DL, Doppmann JL, Shawker TH, et al. Localization of parathyroid adenomas in patients who have undergone surgery. Part I. Noninvasive imaging methods. Radiology. 1987;162:133–137.
11. Ovenfors CO, Stark DD, Moss AA, et al. Localization of parathyroid adenoma by computed tomography. J Comp Assist Tomogr. 1982;6:1094–1098.
12. Sommer B, Welter HF, Spelsberg F, et al. Computed tomography for localizing enlarged parathyroid glands in primary hyperparathyroidism. J Comp Assist Tomogr. 1982;6:521–526.
13. Cates JD, Thorsen MK, Lawson TL, et al. CT evaluation of parathyroid adenomas: Diagnostic criteria and pitfalls. J Comp Assist Tomogr. 1988;12:626–629.
14. Whitley NO, Bohlman M, Connor TB, et al. Computed tomography for localization of Parathyroid adenomas. J Comput Assist Tomogr. 1981;5:812–817.
15. Takagi H, Tominaga Y, Uchida K, et al. Preoperative diagnosis of secondary hyperparathyroidism using computed tomography. J Comput Assist Tomogr. 1982;6:527–528.
16. Carmalt HL, Gillet DJ, Chu J, et al. Prospective comparison of radionuclide, ultrasound, and computed tomography in the preoperative localization of parathyroid glands. World J Surg. 1988;12:830–834.
17. Lloyd MN, Less WR, Milroy EJ. Pre-operative localization in primary hyperparathyroidism. Clin Radiol. 1990;41:239–243.
18. Thompson NW, Eckhauser FE, Harness JK. The anatomy of primary hyperparatyhroidism. Surgery. 1982;92:814–821.
19. Doppman JL, Shawker TH, Krudy AG, et al. Parathymic parathyroid: CT, US, and angiographic findings. Radiology. 1985;157:419–423.
20. Stark DD, Clark OH, Goding GAW, et al. High-resolution ultrasonography and computed tomography of thyroid lesions in patients with hyperparathyroidism. Surgery. 1983;94:863–868.
21. Krudy AG, Doppman JL, Brennan MF, et al. The detection of mediastinal parathyroid glands by computed tomography, selective arteriography, and venous sampling. Radiology. 1981; 140:739–744.
22. Schantz A, Castleman B. Parathyroid carcinoma. Cancer. 1972;31:600–605.

23 Heerden JA van, Weiland LH, ReMine WH, et al. Cancer of the parathyroid glands. Arch Surg. 1979;114:475–480.
24 Krudy AG, Doppman JL, Marx SJ, et al. Radiographic findings in recurrent parathyroid carcinoma. Radiology. 1982; 142:625–629.

MR Imaging

C. B. Higgins and W. Auffermann

MRI is now being used extensively and is generally recognized as an effective imaging technique for the diagnosis of abnormalities of the parathyroid glands (1–9). The evaluation of a patient with hyperparathyroidism prior to the initial operation is usually by high-resolution ultrasound. For the patient with persistent or recurrent hyperparathyroidism after surgery, MRI and other imaging modalities are used.

The major indications for MRI of parathyroid disease are as follows:

1. Recurrent or persistent hyperparathyroidism after surgery
2. Suspected ectopic location of an adenoma prior to surgery

If the high-resolution ultrasound scan does not identify an enlarged gland in the parathyroid vicinity, an ectopic location should be considered and the use of MRI considered preoperatively.

Technique

MRI of the parathyroid has been effective using imagers of both medium and high magnetic field strength. One advantage of high field strength is the possibility of acquiring thin sections (3–5 mm) with high spatial resolution in a short imaging period (two excitations). However, adequate studies have been done using lower field strength imagers (0.35–0.50 T). Surface coils and various specially shaped coils that optimize the "filling factor" between the narrow neck and the coil can substantially increase image quality. Because of the small diameter of the neck, a smaller coil can be used compared to that needed for imaging of the remainder of the body. Consequently, there is less tissue bulk in the coil, which can produce noise. The decrease in noise associated with the use of a smaller receiver coil causes an improvement in the signal-to-noise ratio.

The recommended protocol for imaging of the neck consists of thin (3–5 mm) transaxial T1- and T2-weighted images. A sagittal localizer image is obtained initially, 700/20 (TR/TE), with one or two excitations, in order to prescribe the location of the transaxial images. Submillimeter resolution (0.6 × 0.6 mm) can be achieved by using a 16 cm field of view and 256 × 192 matrix in the transaxial images. Artifacts from blood flow, respiration, and swallowing are reduced by using a presaturation pulse (applied in the z-axis), and elimination of wraparound artifacts in the x- and y-axes. T1-weighted sequences 700/20 (TR/TE) and T2-weighted sequences 2000/20,70 in the transaxial plane are used in most patients. The fast spin-echo technique with a 16 echo train using 3000/85–102 is now preferred in order to diminish motion artifacts. With this sequence the time required to produce T2-weighted spin-echo images is less than 5 minutes. The imaging volume extends from the hyoid bone to the lung apex. For evaluation of persistent or recurrent hyperparathyroidism (HPT), additional ECG-gated transaxial scans of the upper chest and mediastinum are done. The coronal plane is used for the evaluation of large neck masses that extend below the cervicothoracic junction, such as substernal goiters.

In many instances contrast-enhanced T1-weighted images are done after intravenous administration of Gd-DTPA. This MR contrast medium causes considerable enhancement of enlarged parathyroid glands (adenomas or hyperplastic glands) and lymph nodes (10). The signal intensity of these structures is augmented to an extent similar to that observed on nonenhanced T2-weighted images. Because standard T2-weighted images are prone to considerable degradation by swallowing and patient motion, it is useful in some patients to use Gd-DTPA-enhanced T1-weighted images in order to obviate the need for T2-weighted sequences. This approach is attractive in situations in which the quality of the initial T1-weighted images is considered borderlined, or in patients in whom one can predict that the T2-weighted image will likely be of poor quality.

Fat suppression techniques used with Gd-DTPA should also be considered for the neck. Suppression of the fat signal with these techniques combined with enhanced signal of the thyroid and especially enlarged parathyroid glands, renders considerable conspicuity for abnormalities of the thyroid and parathyroid glands.

Anatomy

The superior parathyroid glands are usually attached to the posterior aspect of the middle of the thyroid gland. They are not normally visible on MR images. The inferior parathyroid glands usually are located at the lower poles of the thyroid gland. High-quality images at this site display the vascular components of the minor neurovascular bundle (inferior thyroid artery and vein) lying within high-intensity fat (Fig. 4.**26**). In nearly all individuals there is a substantial layer of fat between the lower pole of the thyroid lobes and the longus colli muscle, where the inferior parathyroid glands are located. The recurrent laryn-

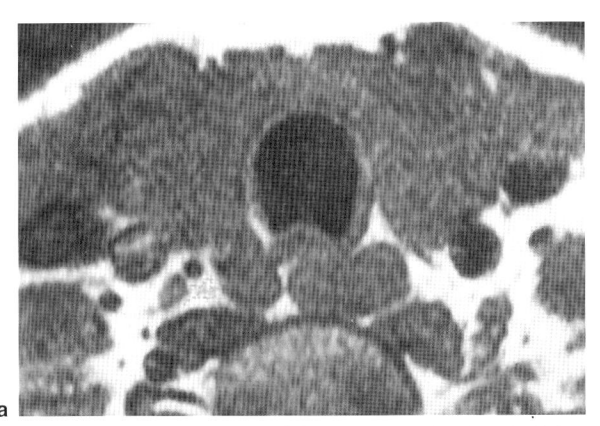

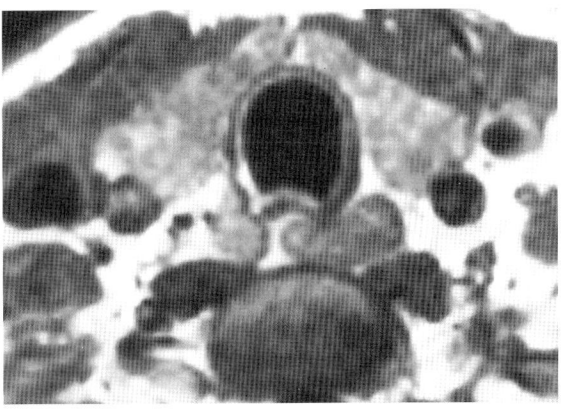

Fig. 4.**26** T1 (**a**) and T2 (**b**) images at the level of the thyroid gland. The thyroid gland increases in signal intensity on the T2-weighted compared to the T1-weighted image. There is a thin layer of fat between the dorsal aspect of the thyroid gland and the longus colli muscle. The inferior parathyroid glands are located within this layer of fat. The parathyroid glands are frequently located at the level of the minor neurovascular bundle, which is shown at the dorsal aspect of the right lobe of the thyroid on the T1-weighted image. The minor neurovascular bundle consists of the inferior thyroid artery and vein, which may be visible, and the recurrent laryngeal nerve, which is not visible on MR images

geal nerve is not visible on standard images. The small vessels of the minor neurovascular bundle may be seen in the fat located between the posterior aspect of the thyroidal poles and the longus colli muscles. The normal-sized parathyroid glands are located here, but usually are too small to identify.

Most humans (89–97%) have four parathyroid glands, although the number of glands may vary from two to six or even more (11). The normal paired superior and inferior glands average $5 \times 3 \times 1$ mm and weigh approximately 40 mg each. The superior parathyroid glands arise from the 4th brachial cleft pouch, along with the thyroid. Because only minimal migration from this area occurs in fetal development, the superior parathyroid glands usually lie dorsal to the upper pole of the thyroid gland, cephalad to where the recurrent laryngeal nerve and inferior thyroid artery cross. Other locations for aberrant superior parathyroid glands are within the thyroid (1–3%), retroesophageal (1%), within the carotid sheath (1%), or in the posterior mediastinum (5%). The inferior parathyroid glands arise from the third brachial cleft pouch with the ipsilateral thymic lobe. Both the inferior parathyroid gland and the thymus migrate together down the neck. Although the inferior parathyroid glands are most often located inferior, posterior, or lateral to the lower thyroid lobe, they can be located anywhere from the angle of the jaw to the pericardium. The most common ectopic location is in the perithymic tissues or thyrothymic ligament (10–15%) (11). The undescended inferior parathyroid glands, or "parathymic parathyroids," remain at the position of the third pharyngeal pouch at the level of the hyoid bone, anterior to the internal carotid artery.

Hyperparathyroidism

Primary HPT is a generalized disorder of calcium, phosphate, and bone metabolism that results from an increased secretion of PTH (12). It occurs in approximately 1 in 700 people and is the most frequent cause of hypercalcemia (13, 14). It is more common in women than in men, with a peak incidence between the third and fifth decades.

Eighty-five percent of patients with primary HPT have a solitary parathyroid adenoma, 10% have diffuse hyperplasia, 4% have multiple adenomas, and 1% have carcinoma, although the incidence of carcinoma has been reported to range from 0.5% to 5% (15). Other rare causes of HPT include parathyroid carcinoma, lipoadenoma (16), parathyroid cysts (17), and lipohyperplasia (18). Hyperparathyroidism may be familial and occurs in patients with MEN type I, MEN type II, familial hypocalciuric hypercalcemia, and neurofibromatosis (12, 19). Patients who have received low-dose radiation therapy to the neck also have an increased incidence of HPT. Secondary HPT is due to excessive production of PTH in patients with renal failure or in patients who have partial resistance to the metabolic action of the hormone and thus, hypocalcemia.

Although half of patients with HPT are asymptomatic, others show signs or symptoms of hypercalcemia, the most common manifestation. Hypercalcemia may be either sustained or intermittent, and is due to a cause other than HPT or malignancy less than 10% of the time (12). Immunoreactive PTH levels may be used to diagnose HPT; they are either elevated or inappropriately normal for the degree of hypercalcemia. Other serologic abnormalities associated with

HPT include hypercalciuria, hypophosphatemia, and elevated nephrogenous cAMP.

Once HPT has been correctly diagnosed, the disorder may be treated either medically or surgically. Medical treatment entails administation of diuretics to increase urinary excretion of calcium and oral phosphates to decrease serum calcium levels. Surgical treatment consists of gland resection and is advocated by those who cite a 95% success rate for primary cervical operations (20). Currently, there is general agreement that surgery should be performed in patients with symptomatic HPT, and in asymptomatic patients with a serum level of 1 mg/dL above normal. It is known that some complications of hyperparathyroidism will develop in about 50% of asymptomatic patients within 10 years of diagnosis if surgical extirpation of the abnormal parathyroid gland(s) is not accomplished (21). Consequently, the need for identification of the abnormal gland is apparent for all patients with hyperparathyroidism.

Preoperative Localization of Abnormal Parathyroid Glands

Preoperative localization of abnormal parathyroid glands in patients with HPT who have not had prior surgery may not be performed routinely, due to the high surgical success rate (95%) on initial cervical exploration (20). If a preoperative localization study is used, ultrasound is usually selected. In patients with persistent or recurrent HPT, however, surgical success rates range from 62% to 90%, depending on whether or not preoperative localization studies are performed (22, 23). In 12–18% of patients, reexploration requires a median sternotomy (22, 24). It is in this group of patients with persistent or recurrent HPT that preoperative imaging studies have been most efficacious. Noninvasive and invasive radiologic modalities used to localize abnormal parathyroid glands have included high-resolution sonography, contrast-enhanced CT, technetium-thallium scintigraphy, MRI, selective arteriography, and selective venous sampling.

Even prior to the initial surgery, MR should be applied in circumstances in which an ectopic location is more likely than usual. Such a circumstance exists if an initial high-resolution ultrasound study does not reveal an abnormal gland.

Imaging Characteristics of Parathyroid Disorders

Due to their small size (average 5 × 3 × 1 mm) normal parathyroid glands are difficult to detect using current MRI techniques. Abnormal parathyroid glands, including those with enlargement due to either hyperplasia or adenoma, have shown variable appearance on T1- and T2-weighted images. The most common pattern is an intermediate signal intensity nodule that is similar in intensity to that of muscle or thyroid on T1-weighted images, and with signal intensity greater than or isointense with fat on T2-weighted images (2, 25) (Fig. 4.26).

However, not all adenomas demonstrate this pattern. Hemorrhage into an adenoma may cause high signal intensity on both T1- and T2-weighted images (Fig. 4.27), and some adenomas may have low signal intensity on both T1- and T2-weighted images (Fig. 4.27). In a study of ten patients that attempted to correlate the MR appearance of parathyroid adenomas with their histologic characteristics, the adenomas were divided into groups (25). Group I consisted of adenomas that had low signal intensity on T1-weighted

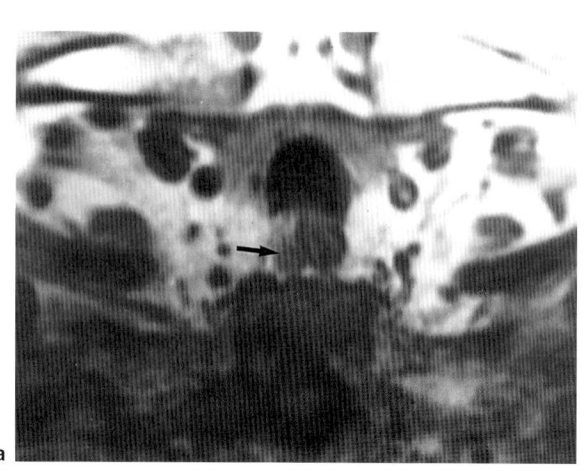

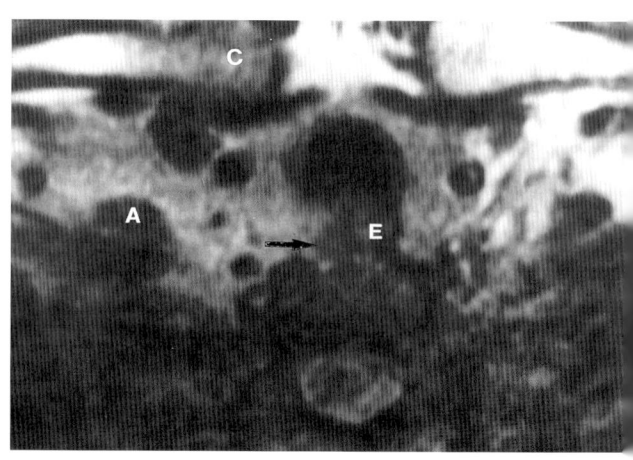

Fig. 4.27 T1- (a) and T2- (b) weighted images demonstrate an abnormal parathyroid gland in the right paraesophageal region (arrow), wich shows low signal intensity on both T1- and T2-weighted images. A = anterior scalene muscle; C = clavicular heads; E = esophagus

images and high signal intensity on T2-weighted images, which corresponded histologically with high cellularity without degeneration or fibrosis. Group II adenomas had low signal intensity on both T1- and T2-weighted images, which corresponded with cellular degenerative changes, old hemorrhage with hemosiderin-containing macrophages, and fibrosis, or both. Group III adenomas showed high signal intensity on both T1-weighted and T2-weighted images.

Histologically, group III adenomas showed evidence of subacute hemorrhage without degenerative or fibrotic changes.

As a consequence of the variability in signal intensity that has been reported with parathyroid adenomas, it follows that these adenomas may mimic the signal intensity of adjacent structures such as lymph nodes and hyperplastic nodules projecting off the back of the thyroid gland and thereby escape detec-

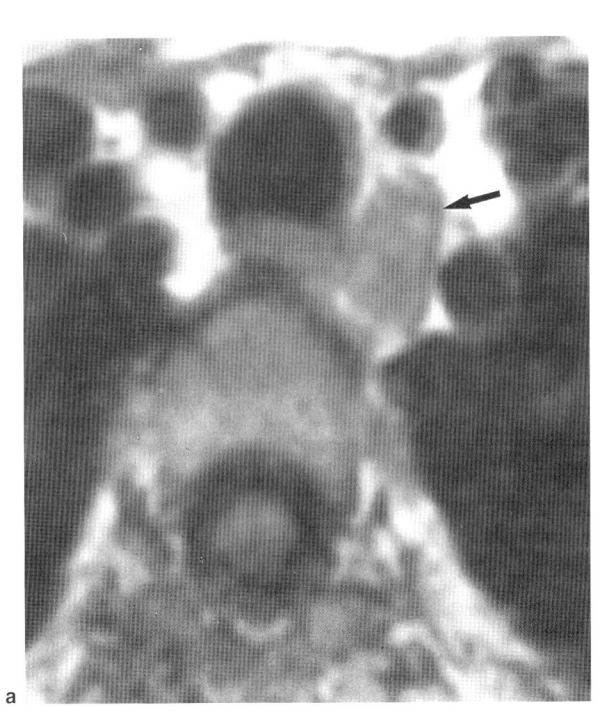

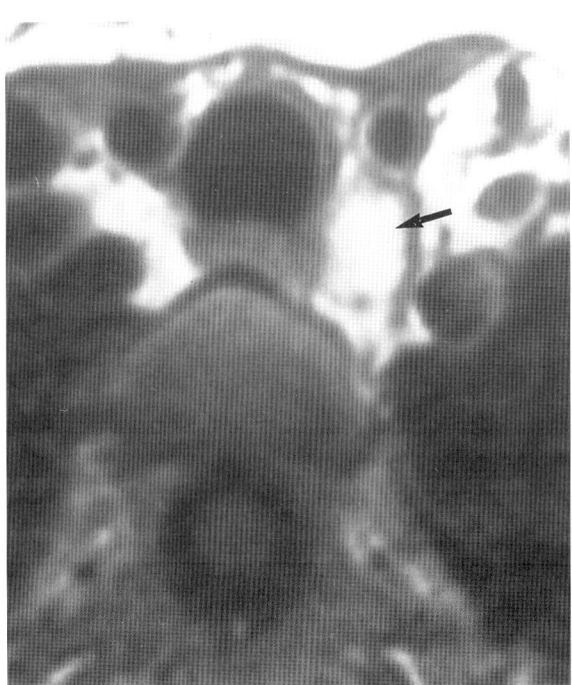

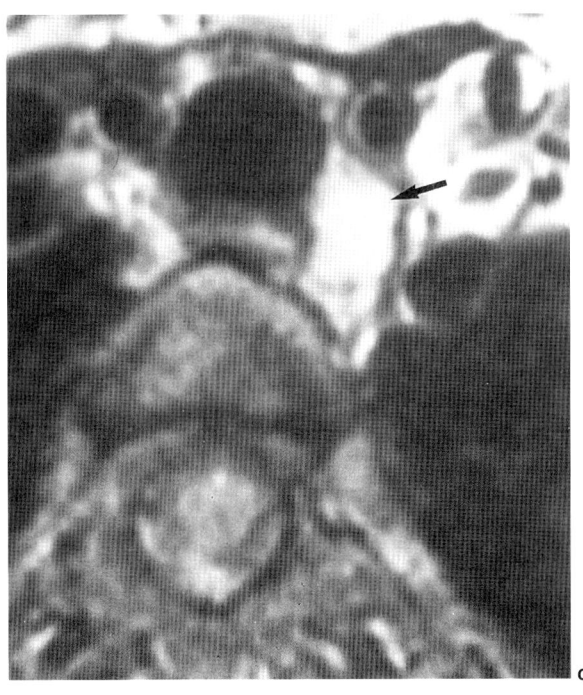

Fig. 4.**28** T1-weighted images before (**a**) and after (**b**) the administration of Gd-DTPA, and a T2-weighted image (**c**) in a patient with a large parathyroid adenoma. Prior to the administration of gadolinium, the adenoma has medium signal intensity on the T1-weighted image. After administration of gadolinium there is substantial enhancement of the adenoma, causing it to have a high signal intensity. It becomes isointense with surrounding fat. This adenoma also produces high signal intensity on the T2-weighted image. The appearance on the gadolinium-enhanced T1-weighted image is similar to the appearance on the T2-weighted image

108   4 Parathyroid Gland

tion. Distortion of cervical anatomy by a goiter or large thyroid adenoma may also complicate interpretation.

Differentiation of abnormal parathyroid glands from surrounding vascular structures may be accomplished either with presaturation pulses applied to tissue on the boundary of the multislice imaging volume to effect a flow void, or with an additional gradient-refocused echo sequence intended to highlight blood vessels. Intravenous administration of the MR contrast agent Gd-DTPA may be effective in identifying abnormal parathyroid glands (10) (Fig. 4.28).

The usual location of the parathyroid glands is adjacent to the dorsal aspect of the thyroid gland or just caudal to the lower poles of the thyroid gland. At these sites the enlarged parathyroid glands lie within fat and can usually be recognized as low signal nodules on T1-weighted images (Figure 4.26). Signal intensity may become nearly isointense with fat on T2-weighted images but usually shows higher intensity than fat on images with TE exceeding 60 ms (Figs. 4.26, 4.29). All of the various ectopic locations can be examined using MR images. These include the carotid sheath (Fig. 4.30); base of the neck in remnant thymic tissues (Fig. 4.31); and in the paraesophageal region (Fig. 4.32). The most rare ectopic site in the neck is parapharyngeal. These glands are situated at the level of the hyoid bone; they represent unmigrated glands lying in their embryonic position at the level of the fourth pharyngeal pouch.

Ectopic locations in the thorax are demonstrated

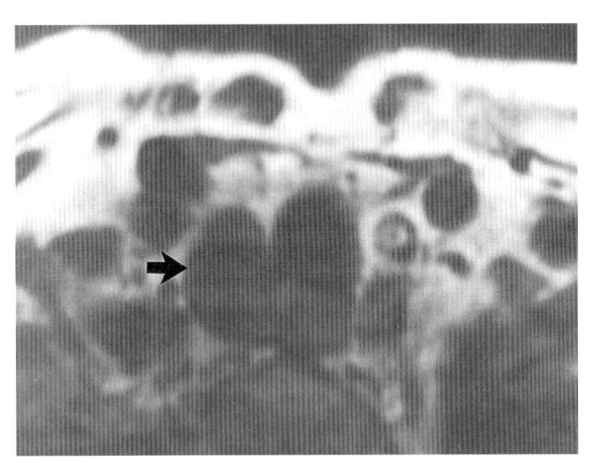

Fig. 4.29 T1- (a) and T2- (b) weighted images in a patient with a large parathyroid adenoma. This parathyroid adenoma (arrow) is located caudal to the thyroid gland at the cervicothoracic junction. The adenoma shows characteristic signal intensities features, which are low to medium signal intensity on the T1-weighted image and high signal intensity on the T2-weighted image

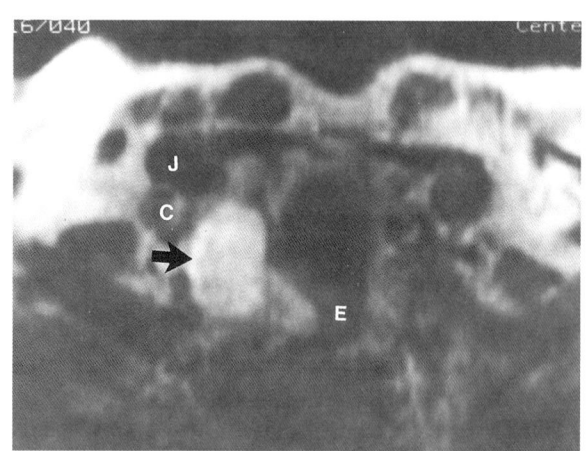

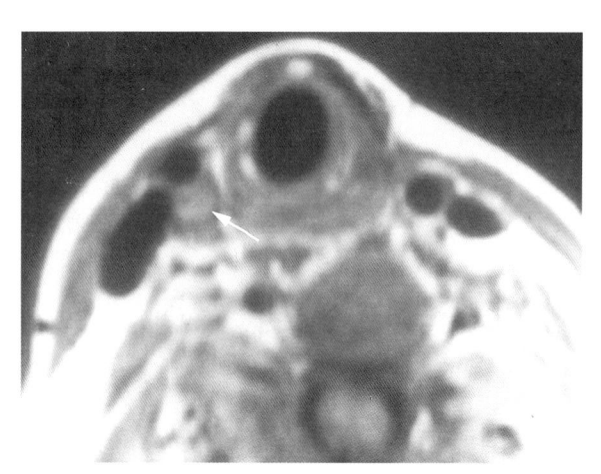

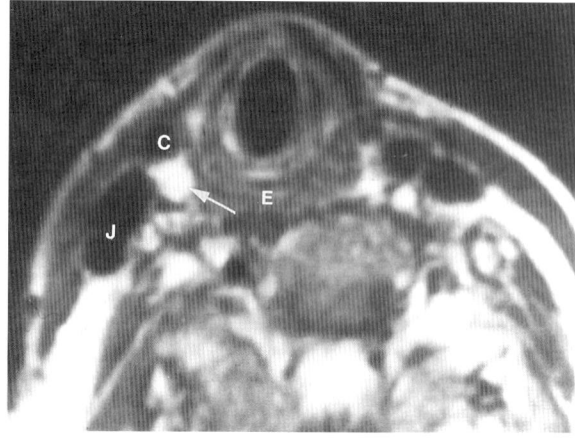

Fig. 4.30 T1- (a) and T2- (b) weighted images in a patient with a parathyroid adenoma in the right carotid sheath. The abnormal parathyroid gland (arrow) is located directly dorsal to the right common carotid artery. The abnormal parathyroid gland has medium signal intensity on the T1-weighted image and high signal intensity on the T2-weighted image

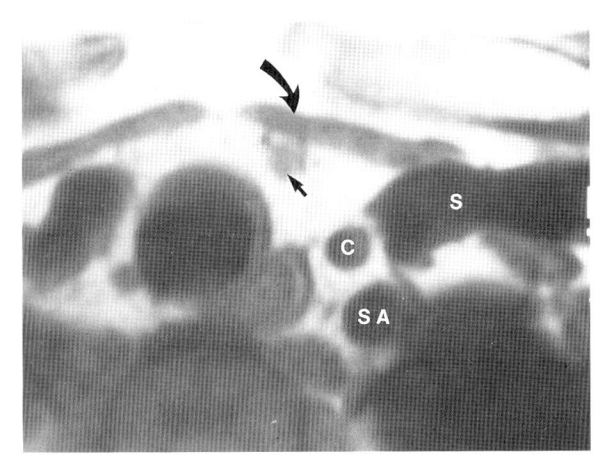

Fig. 4.**31** T1-weighted image below the cervicothoracic junction demonstrates an ectopic parathyroid gland. The moderately enlarged gland (arrow) is located directly dorsal to the sternothyroid-sternohyoid muscles (curved arrows). C = carotid artery; S = subclavian vein; SA = subclavian artery

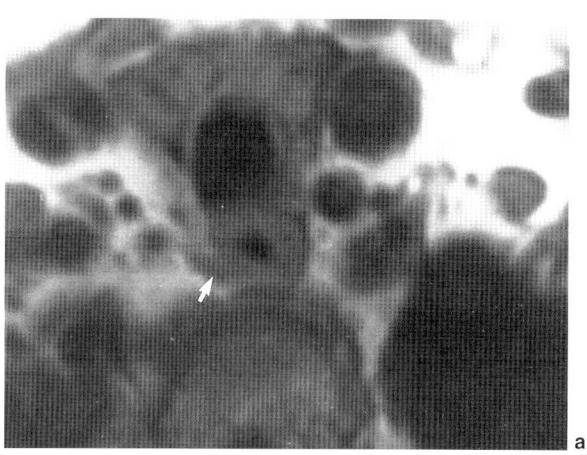

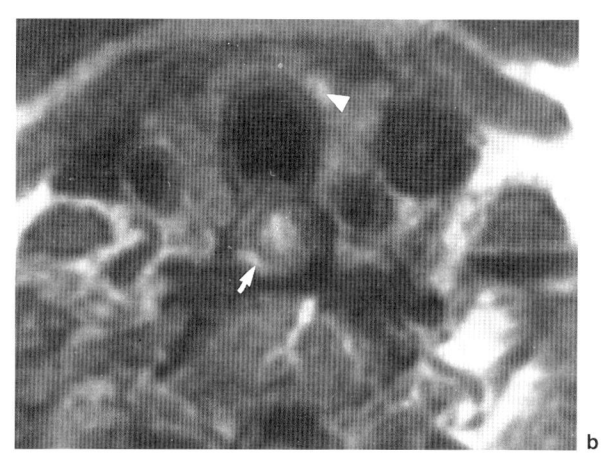

Fig. 4.**32** T1- (**a**) and T2- (**b**) weighted images at the base of the neck demonstrate a paraesophageal location of an ectopic parathyroid gland. The moderately enlarged gland (arrow) has a low signal intensity on the T1-weighted image; its signal intensity is similar to the wall of the esophagus. The parathyroid gland demonstrates high signal intensity on the T2-weighted image. There is also a high signal intensity focus (arrowhead) within the left lobe of the thyroid gland. Since ectopic parathyroid glands can reside within the thyroid gland, it is not possible to exclude an ectopic parathyroid gland lying within the thyroid lobe

using ECG-gated images in the transverse and coronal planes. Any location from the cervicothoracic junction to the diaphragm may be possible as the ectopic parathyroid follows the caudal migration of the thymus. However, the most frequent sites are in the retrosternal region lying just ventral to the left brachiocephalic vein (Fig. 4.**33**) or within the prevascular space of the mediastinum (Fig. 4.**34**).

Pitfalls in the Detection of Abnormal Parathyroid Glands by MRI

Several pitfalls exist in the imaging of abnormal parathyroid glands. The typical signal intensities of abnormal parathyroid glands on T1- and T2-weighted MR images are no different from those observed with cervical lymph nodes. Consequently, MRI can differentiate between enlarged glands and nodes only on the basis of location and shape of the structures. A location medial to the carotid sheath is expected for the enlarged glands, while the nodes are most frequently situated around or lateral to the sheath. The enlarged parathyroid glands are considered to have an elliptical or oblong configuration while the lymph nodes tend to be spherical.

Enlarged glands must also be distinguished from other structures in the neck, including large cervical ganglia (Fig. 4.**35**). These structures also show low intensity on T1-weighted and high signal on T2-weighted images.

One of the ectopic locations of parathyroid glands is within the thyroid glands. At this site they can be recognized by their high signal intensity on T2-weighted images. A problem in this regard is that about 40% of thyroid glands show high signal intensity foci on T2-weighted images in subjects with no known thyroid disease (Fig. 4.**36**) (26).

An additional dilemma is recognizing more than one abnormal site on both sides of the neck, or in the neck and mediastinum. This causes confusion in directing the surgical approach. In some instances one of the sites has indeed proven to be the adenoma, whereas the other site has represented fibrosis around sutures or metal clips implanted at a prior unsuccessful surgery.

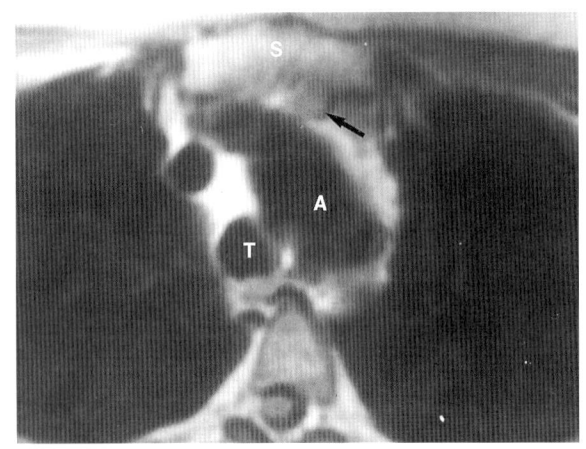

110   4 Parathyroid Gland

Fig. 4.**33** The ECG-gated, T1-weighted image demonstrates an ectopic parathyroid gland (arrow) situated directly dorsal to the sternum. The gland is located immediately ventral to the crossing left brachiocephalic vein. A = aortic arch; S = sternum; T = trachea

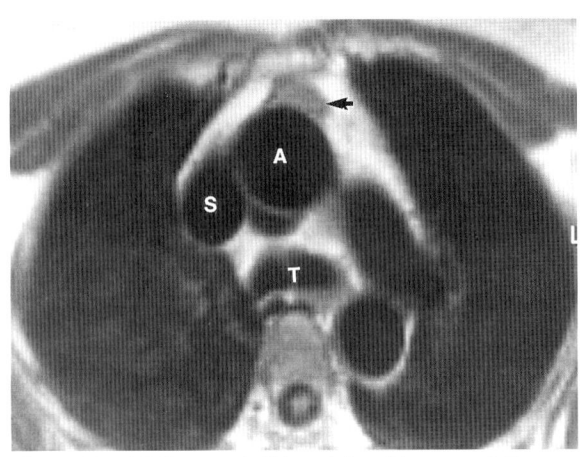

Fig. 4.**34** ECG-gated, T1-weighted image of the superior mediastinum demonstrates an ectopic parathyroid gland (arrow) situated within the fat of the anterior mediastinum. A = ascending aorta; S = superior vena cava; T = tracheal carina

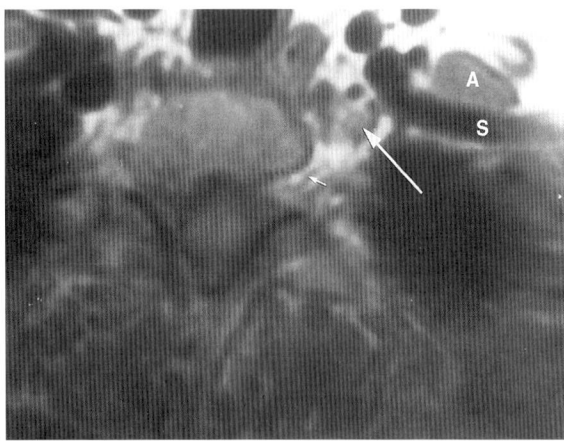

Fig. 4.**35** T1- (**a**) and T2- (**b**) weighted transaxial images at the cervicothoracic junction demonstrate a spherical structure (arrow) located directly adjacent to the subclavian artery. This structure was shown to represent an enlarged cervical ganglion at the time of surgery. It is possible to recognize a nerve root (small arrow) coursing towards the ganglion. There are several high signal intensity nodules within the lower portion of the thyroid gland. A = anterior scalene muscle; S = subclavian artery

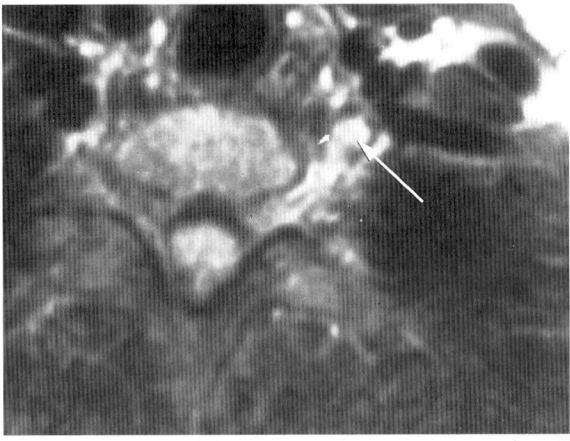

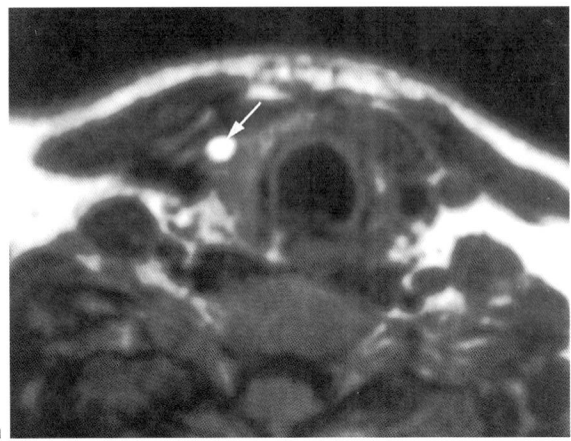

Fig. 4.**36** T2-weighted images in two patients demonstrate in each a nodule of high signal intensity in the thyroid gland. One represented a thyroid nodule (**a**) and the other (**b**) represented an ectopic intrathyroidal parathyroid adenoma

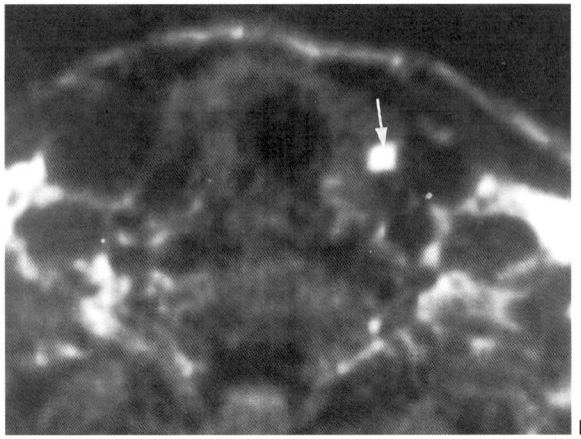

MR Contrast Media: Effect on Signal Intensity of Abnormal Parathyroid Glands

The relative enhancement of muscle, fat, thyroid, and abnormal parathyroid glands on T1-weighted images after the intravenous administration of Gd-DTPA has been determined (10). Gd-DTPA produces substantially greater enhancement of the abnormal parathyroid gland and moderately greater enhancement of the thyroid gland compared to skeletal muscle (Fig. 4.**28**). This causes the gland to be nearly isointense with fat on T1-weighted images. However, fat suppression sequences employed with Gd-DTPA may improve conspicuity of the gland.

The relative intensity (relative to muscle) of abnormal parathyroid glands on Gd-enhanced T1-weighted images was 118%, which compared with 18% on nonenhanced T1-weighted images. On the other hand, the relative increase in signal intensity of the abnormal glands on T2-weighted images was 285%. This observation indicates that the Gd-DTPA does not increase the conspicuity of the abnormal gland in relation to nonenhanced T2-weighted images. However, in some circumstances the diagnostic quality of T2-weighted images is inadequate due to swallowing and patient motion. In this situation, Gd-DTPA can be used to cause bright signal of the abnormal glands and produce an appearance similar to that observed on T2-weighted images. This approach may obviate the need for T2-weighted images in the uncooperative patient.

Results Using MRI for Preoperative Localization in Recurrent or Persistent Hyperparathyroidism

Investigations using MR as a noninvasive preoperative localization technique in patients with persistent or recurrent HPT have yielded success rates comparable or better than other noninvasive imaging modalities. Miller et al. (4) compared ultrasound, CT, thallium scintigraphy and MRI in 53 patients with proved parathyroid adenomas and previous unsuccessful parathyroid surgery. Although MR was performed in only 16 patients, it had the highest detection rate (50%) compared with 47% for CT, 36% for ultrasound, and 27% for scintigraphy. Levin et al. (3) performed a similar study comparing the same four noninvasive imaging modalities in 59 consecutive patients undergoing reoperation for persistent or recurrent HPT. MR was performed in only 17 patients, but had the highest accurate localization rate (65%) compared with 56% for ultrasound, 46% for CT, and 49% for thallium scintigraphy. One or more of these noninvasive tests was positive in 78% of the cases; however, the false-positive rate ranged from 13–23%.

Auffermann et al. (2) compared the prospective accuracy of MR to that of high-resolution sonography and thallium scintigraphy in 30 patients with recurrent or persistent HPT after surgery. CT was not included in the study. Twenty-three and 26 patients also had high-resolution sonography and thallium scintigraphy, respectively. MR accurately localized abnormal parathyroid glands in 75% evaluated prospectively, whereas scintigraphy localized 64% prospectively and sonography detected 57%. MR imaging detected three out of four mediastinal adenomas prospectively. Each of the three tests gave one false-positive result. Comparison of the detection rate among studies showed a statistically significant difference between MR and sonography only.

A study of 47 patients with hyperparathyroidism, of which nearly all patients had recurrent signs after surgery, showed that MRI provided preoperative localization of the abnormal gland in 75% of patients (26A). A recent preliminary report (26B) of 25 patients with abnormal glands in the mediastinum indicated that MRI identified the abnormal gland in 88% of patients.

Recently, Erdman et al. (27) evaluated 32 patients with hyperparathyroidism with a combination of CT, ultrasound, thallium scintigraphy, and MRI. Seventeen of these patients had prior surgery for the treatment of hyperparathyroidism. Of the patients with prior surgery who were imaged by all four modalities, the respective sensitivities were as follows: MR 70%, thallium scintigraphy 75%, CT 55%, and ultrasound 55%. They found that as gland size decreased to below 500 mg, MR and ultrasound maintained accuracy, while scintigraphy performed poorly. However, most of the postoperative neck patients (11 of 17) had large glands ranging from 650 to 4700 mg.

A combination of preoperative localization procedures increases the sensitivity for detection of abnormal parathyroid glands (2, 3, 4, 27). Auffermann et al. (2) reported a detection rate of 84% for the combination of MR and thallium scintigraphy, 86% for the combination of MR and sonography, and 80% for the combination of sonography and thallium scintigraphy. In patients who underwent all three examinations before surgery, the detection rate was 90% prospectively. Erdman et al. (27) calculated the sensitivity and true-positive ratio (patients with a positive test and disease specifically at the location indicated divided by all the patients with a positive test for multiple imaging modalities (CT, ultrasound, scintigraphy, MR) in 32 patients with primary hyperparathyroidism both with and without prior surgery. With multiple techniques considered as a single test (i.e., a positive localization required two or more tests to be positive at the same location), sensitivity for a two-study combination was 79% and the true-positive ratio was 86%. Sensitivity and true-positive ratio for a three-study combination were 63% and 92%, respectively, while sensitivity and true-positive ratio for a combination of all four modalities were 40% and 10%, respectively. The authors found no significant difference in the various combinations of techniques employed (i.e., CT and ultrasound, ultrasound and MR, MR and scintigraphy), although when only two modalities were used, the combination of MR and thallium scintigraphy had the highest true-positive ratio (100%) with no false-positives in the 12 patients imaged.

Comparison of Diagnostic Techniques in Hyperparathyroidism

Multiple noninvasive and invasive modalities are currently employed in the preoperative localization of abnormal parathyroid glands in patients with HPT, including sonography (2, 27, 28–35), CT (3, 4, 27, 34–39), scintigraphy (2–4, 6, 7, 27, 29, 30, 31, 34, 35, 40–42), MR (2–9, 27), venous sampling (3, 20, 32, 43, 44), and arteriography (44). Ultrasonic detection of parathyroid hyperplasia ranges from 43–69%. Sonography is limited in the localization of adenomas in the mediastinum because of the lack of an acoustic window and difficult visualization behind the trachea or esophagus.

CT has a sensitivity of 50–87%. CT has been shown to be superior to sonography in patients who have had neck surgery, but has difficulty detecting glandular hyperplasia (33). The sensitivity of thallium scintigraphy ranges from 60–87%. It is limited because thalium chloride accumulates in both normal and abnormal thyroid tissues, carcinomatous metastases, as well as parathyroid glands, thereby limiting parathyroid detectability.

MRI is the newest modality that has been used to evaluate abnormal parathyroid glands. Although the total number of patients imaged thus far is less than that with any of the other noninvasive imaging modalities, the prospective sensitivity thus far has been reported as approximately 65–80% in patients with and without prior surgery. The accuracy in the detection of intrathoracic glands has recently been reported to be 88% (26B). In studies of the same patients in which MR has been directly compared with other imaging modalities, its sensitivity has been either equal to or greater than that of CT, sonography, or scintigraphy with the exception of one study, in which the sensitivity of scintigraphy was slightly greater than that of MR. The sensitivity in detecting abnormal parathyroid glands in patients who have had prior surgery varies depending on the modality used and has been reported to be in the range of 47–82% for ultrasound, 44–66% for CT, and 50–75% for MRI.

References

1. Higgins CB, Auffermann WA. MR imaging of thyroid and parathyroid glands: A review of current status. AJR. 1988;151:1095.
2. Auffermann W, Gooding GAW, Okerlund MD, et al. Diagnosis of recurrent hyperparathyroidism: comparison of MR imaging and other imaging techniques. AJR. 1988;150:1027–1033.
3. Levin KE, Gooding GAW, Okerlund MD, et al. Localizing studies in patients with persistent or recurrent hyperparathyroidism. Surgery. 1987;102:917–925.
4. Miller DL, Doppman JL, Shawker TH, et al. Localization of parathyroid adenomas in patients who have undergone surgery. Part I. Noninvasive imaging methods. Radiology. 1987;162:133–137.
5. Vogl T, Hefele B, Hahn D, Nieden Z, Muhlig HP. Results of a comparative study of MR. CT and sonography of patients with primary hyperparathyroidism. ROFO. 1986;145:167–172.
6. Peck WW, Higgins CB, Fisher MR, Ling M, Okerlund MD, Clark OH. Hyperparathyroidism: comparison of MR imaging with radionuclide scanning. Radiology. 1987;163:415–420.
7. Kneeland JB, Krubsack AJ, Lawson TL, et al. Enlarged parathyroid glands: high-resolution local coil MR imaging. Radiology. 1987;162:143–146.
8. Spritzer CE, Gefter WB, Hamilton R, Greenberg BM, Axel L, Kressel HY. Abnormal parathyroid glands: high-resolution MR imaging. Radiology. 1987;162:487–491.
9. Kier R, Herfkens RJ, Blinder RA, et al. MR with surface coils for parathyroid tumors: preliminary investigation. AJR. 1986;147:497–500.
10. Seelos KC, DeMarco R, Clark OH, Higgins CB. Persistent and recurrent hyperparathyroidism: assessment with gadopentetate dimeglumine-enhanced MR imaging. Radiology. 1990;177:373–378.
11. Akerstrom G, Malmaeus J, Bergstrom R. Surgical anatomy of human parathyroid glands. Surgery. 1984;95:14–21.
12. Potts JT. Diseases of the parathyroid gland and other hyper- and hypocalcemic disorders. In: Braunwald E, Isselbacher KJ, Petersdorf RG, Wilson JD, Martin JB, and Fauci AS, eds. Harrison's Principles of Internal Medicine, 11th ed. New York: McGraw-Hill; 1987:1870–1889.
13. Clark OH. Hyperparathyroidism. In: Current Surgical Therapy, Grand Junction, CO: Decker; 1986:306–310.
14. Clark OH. Management of primary hyperparathyroidism. In: Najarian JS, Delaney JP, eds. Advances in Breast and Endocrine Surgery. Chicago: Yearbook Medical Publishers; 1986:385–390.
15. Cohn K, Silverman M, Corrado J, Sedgewick C. Parathyroid carcinoma: The Lahey Clinic experience. Surgery. 1985;98:1095–1098.
16. Obara T, Fujimoto Y, Ito Y. Functioning parathyroid lipoadenoma – Report of four cases: Clinicopathological and ultrasonographic features. Endocrinol Jpn. 1989;36(1):135–145.
17. Clark OH. Parathyroid cysts. Am J Surg. 1978;135:395–402.
18. Straus FH II, Kaplan EL, Nishiyama RH, Bigos ST. Five cases of parathyroid lipohyperplasia. Surgery. 1983;94:901–905.
19. Vogelzang PJ, Oates E, Bankoff MS. Parathyroid adenoma associated with neurofibromatosis: Correlative scintigraphic and magnetic resonance imaging. Clin Nucl Med. 1989;14:168–170.
20. Satava RM Jr, Beahrs OH, Scholz DA. Success rate of cervical exploration for hyperparathyroidism. Arch Surg 1975;110:625–628.
21. Scholz DA, Purnell DC. Asymptomatic primary hyperparathyroidism. Mayo Clin Proc. 1981;56:473.
22. Wang C, Gaz RD, Moncure AC. Mediastinal parathyroid exploration: A clinical and pathologic study of 47 cases. World J Surg. 1986;10:687–695.
23. Cheung PSY, Borgstrom A, Thompson NW. Strategy in reoperative surgery for hyperparathyroidism. Arch Surg. 1989;124:676–680.
24. Brennan MF, Norton JA. Reoperation for persistent and recurrent hyperparathyroidism. Ann Surg. 1985;40–44.
25. Auffermann W, Guis M, Tavares NJ, Clark OH, Higgins CB. MR signal intensity of parathyroid adenomas: Correlation with histopathology. AJR. 1989;153:873–876.
26. Funari M, Campos Z, Gooding GAW, Higgins CB. Detection of asymptomatic thyroid nodules in hyperparathyroidism by MRI and high resolution ultrasound. J Comput Assist Tomogr. [In press].
26A. Stevens S, Chang J-M, Clark OH, Chang PJ, Higgins CB. Magnetic resonance imaging of hyperparathyroidism at 1.5T: Prospective and retrospective assessment. AJR, 1992 (submitted).
26B. Kang Y, Rosen K, Clark O, Higgins CB. MR imaging for preoperative localization of mediastinal parathyroid adenomas. Program of 78th Scientific Session of the RSNA. RSNA: 1992.

27. Erdman WA, Breslau NA, Weinreb JC, et al. Noninvasive localization of parathyroid adenomas: A comparison of x-ray computerized tomography, ultrasound, scintigraphy and MRI. Magn Reson Imaging. 1989;7:187–194.
28. Takebayashi S, Matsui K, Onohara Y, Hidai H. Sonography for early diagnosis of enlarged parathyroid glands in patients with secondary hyperparathyroidism. AJR. 1987;148:911–914.
29. Gooding GAW, Okerlund MD, Stark DD, Clark OH. Parathyroid imaging: Comparison of double-tracer (T1-201, Tc-99m) scintigraphy and high-resolution US. Radiology. 1986;161:57–64.
30. Clark OH, Okerlund MD, Moss AA, et al. Localization studies in patients with persistent or recurrent hyperparathyroidism. Surgery. 1985;98:1083–1094.
31. Reading CC, Charboneau JW, James EM, et al. Postoperative parathyroid highfrequency sonography: evaluation of persistent or recurrent hyperparathyroidism. AJR. 1985;144:399–402.
32. Winzelberg GG, Hydovitz JD, O'Hara KR. Parathyroid adenomas evaluated by T1-201/Tc-99m pertechnetate subtraction scintigraphy and high-resolution ultrasonography. Radiology. 1985;155:231–235.
33. Stark DD, Gooding GAW, Moss AA, Clark OH, Ovenfors C-O. Parathyroid imaging: Comparison of high-resolution CT and high-resolution sonography. AJR. 1983;141:633–638.
34. Roses DF, Sudarsky LA, Sanger J, Raghavendra BN, Reede DL, Blum M. The use of preoperative localization of adenomas of the parathyroid glands by thallium-technetium subtraction scintigraphy, high-resolution ultrasonography and computed tomography. Surgery. 1989;168:99–106.
35. Krubsack HJ, Wilson SD, Lawson TL, Collier BD, Hellman HS, Isitman AT. Prospective comparison of radionuclide, computed tomographic, and sonographic localization of parathyroid tumors. World J Surg. 1986;10:579–585.
36. Takagi H, Tominaga Y, Uchida K, et al. Preoperative diagnosis of secondary hyperparathyroidism using computed tomography. J Comput Assist Tomogr. 1982;6:527–528.
37. Doppman JL, Krudy AG, Brennan MF, Schneider P, Lasker RD, Marx SJ. CT appearance of enlarged parathyroid glands in the posterior superior mediastinum. J Comput Assist Tomogr. 1982;6:1099–1102.
38. Ovenfors C-O, Stark D, Moss A, Goldberg H, Clark O, Galante M. Localization of parathyroid adenoma by computed tomography. J Comput Assist Tomogr. 1982;6:1094–1098.
39. Sommer B, Welter HF, Spelsberg F, Scherer U, Lissner J. Computed tomography for localizing enlarged parathyroid glands in primary hyperparathyroidism. J Comput Assist Tomogr. 1982;6:521–526.
40. Borsato N, Zanco P, Camerani M, Saitta B, Ferlin G. Scintigraphy of the parathyroid glands with [201]Tl: Experience with 250 operated patients. Nuklearmed. 1989;28:26–28.
41. Zwas ST, Czerniak A, Boruchowsky S, Avigad I, Wolfstein I. Preoperative parathyroid localization by superimposed iodine-131 toluidine blue and technetium-99m pertechnetate imaging. J Nucl Med. 1987;28:298–307.
42. Skibber JM, Reynolds JC, Spiegel AM, et al. Computerized technetium/thallium scans and parathyroid reoperation. Surgery. 1985;98:1077–1082.
43. Brennan MF, Doppman JL, Kurdy AG, Marx SJ, Spiegel AM, Aurbach GD. Assessment of techniques for preoperative parathyroid gland localization in patients undergoing reoperation for hyperparathyroidism. Surgery. 1982;91:6–11.
44. Winzelberg GG. Parathyroid imaging. Ann Intern Med. 1987;107:64–70.

Angiography and Venous Sampling

R. Sörensen

Primary hyperparathyroidism can be cured surgically by parathyroidectomy in 95% of patients (Fig. 4.**37**; 1, 2, 3). In recurrent or persistent disease (15%) reoperation has to be performed which is less successful and

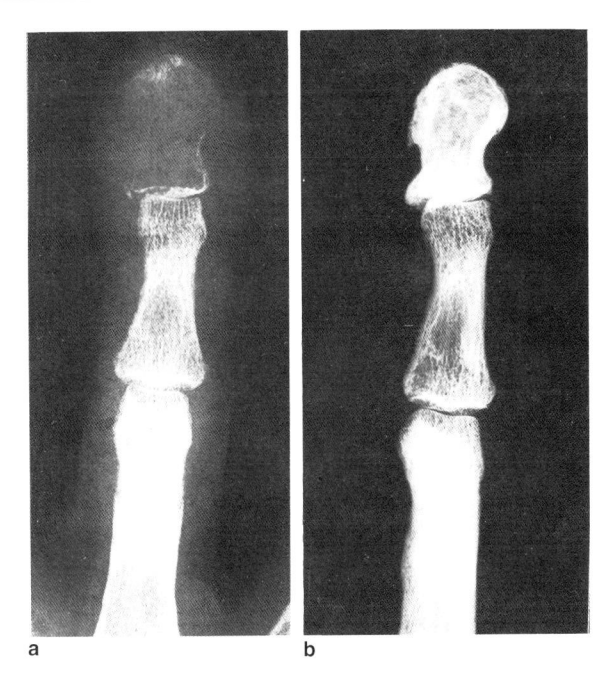

Fig. 4.**37** Primary hyperparathyroidism before and after surgical treatment of a parathyroid adenoma
a Destruction cortical bony structures by a brown tumor of the distal phalanx of the third finger
b Recalcification 6 weeks after surgery

has a higher morbidity rate (4, 5). In those cases, catheterization and venous sampling is necessary to locate the remaining or ectopic parathyroid tissue (4, 6, 7, 8, 9). Ectopic tissue is usually found in the mediastinum. If hypercalcemia is again present following surgery, and noninvasive imaging has failed to locate the excess hormone production, selective venous sampling is the method of choice.

Parathyroid Veins

Human parathyroid tissue is divided in two to six portions. There are usually four glands (10, 11, 12, 13, 14). PTH is secreted by parathyroid glands or by ectopic parathyroid tissue. The physician should be familiar with the potential locations ectopic tissue before the invasive procedure is started (Fig. 4.**38**).

The parathyroid glands drain into the ipsilateral inferior thyroid veins. They join to form a common inferior thyroid vein before entering the left innominate vein (Fig. 4.**39**, Fig. 4.**40**; 14, 15, 16, 17). The jugular and brachiocephalic veins drain the superior, middle, and inferior thyroid veins (Fig. 4.**39**, Fig. 4.**40**; 14, 15). The inferior thyroid veins empty into a trunk that drains into the left brachiocephalic vein at its superior wall (Fig. 4.**41**). Ectopic glands are drained by the thymic veins, which enter the left brachiocephalic vein (Fig. 4.**42**, Fig. 4.**43**) opposite to the thyroid trunk. The thymic vein of Keynes empties into the left

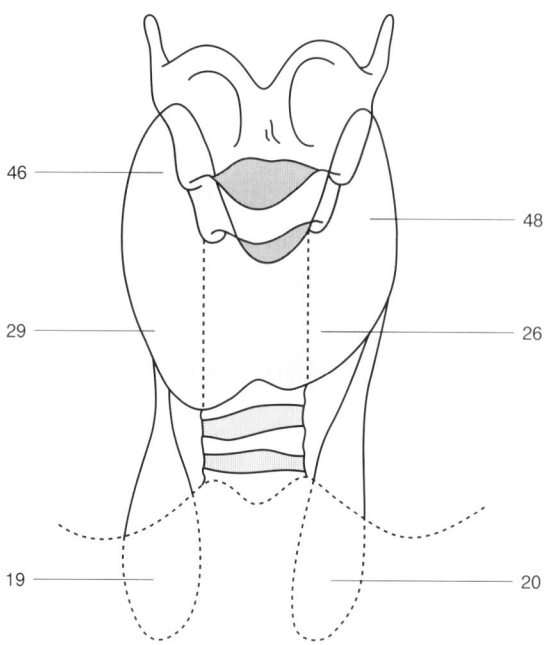

Fig. 4.**38** Location of normal (superimposed on the thyroid gland; 46, 48, 29, 26) and ectopic parathyroid glands (distal to the thyroid gland; 19, 20) in 47 postmortem cases according to Nathaniels. The drawing demonstrates the number of glands identified

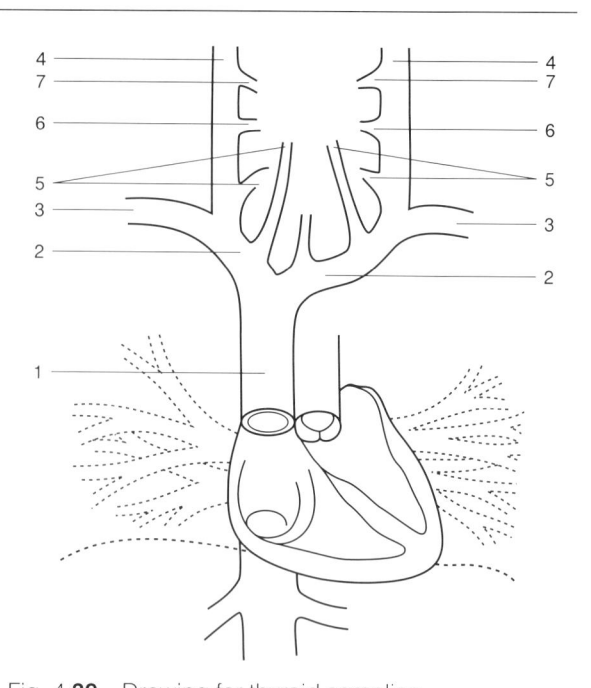

Fig. 4.**39** Drawing for thyroid sampling.
1. Superior vena cava; 2. Brachiocephalic veins; 3. Subclavian veins; 4. Internal jugular veins; 5. Inferior thyroid veins, isthmic veins; 6. Middle thyroid veins; 7. Superior thyroid veins

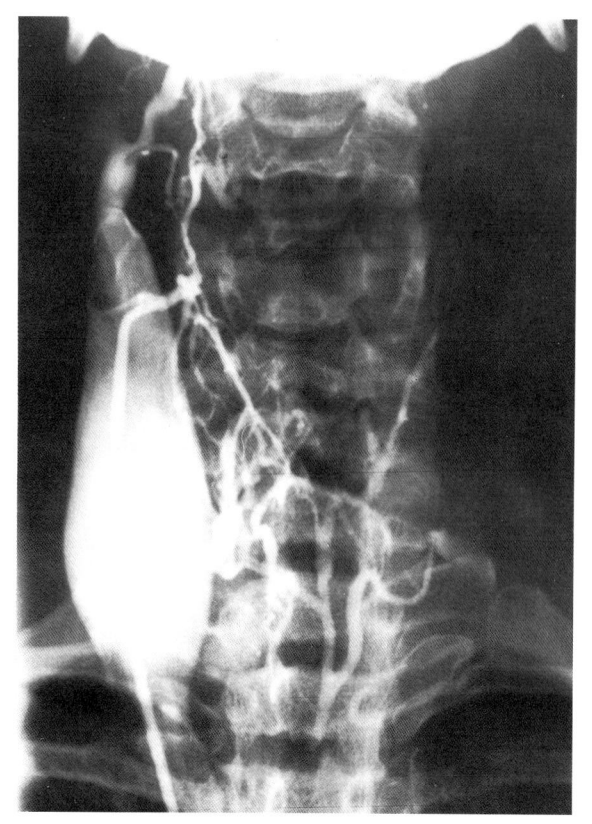

Fig. 4.**40** Dilatation of the right internal jugular vein which is opacified by an retrograde injection into the right middle thyroid vein

innominate vein at its inferior margin. An elevated plasma PTH level in this vein suggests an adenoma in the anterior mediastinum. The azygos vein is found at the posterior wall of the superior vena cava (Fig. 4.**44**); it drains the right superior intercostal vein and the mediastinal veins (Fig. 4.**45**).

Variations in venous anatomy are common, especially accessory inferior thyroid veins on the left side. Because venous sampling is performed following parathyroid surgery, the inferior thyroid veins are distorted or ligated (Fig. 4.**46**). For this reason, a road map of the venous drainage pattern after an arterial injection into the thyrocervical trunk and delayed radiographs showing the venous phase can be helpful. Samples from the middle and superior thyroid veins are usually not valuable for localizing hormone excess unless the inferior veins have been ligated, and venous flow from the thyroid lobes is draining from the upper portion of the glands.

Catherization has to be selective within the draining vein to obtain good samples. Parathyroid glands always drain into the thyroid veins descending along the lateral margin of the thyroid lobe (16; Fig. 4.**39**); it must be stressed that samples from the medial lobar and the isthmic veins are of little value. The vertebral veins may serve as collaterals and can have elevated PTH levels if the adenoma is in the neck or in the posterior superior mediastinum.

Angiography and Venous Sampling 115

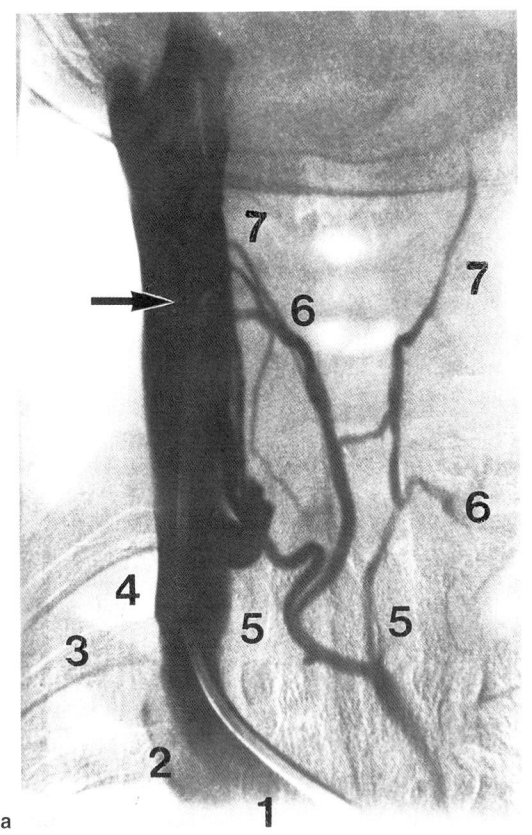

Fig. 4.**41** Major veins of the thyroid glands following retrograde venography with an injection into the superior thyroid vein (arrow) with (**a**) and without (**b**) phototechnical subtraction. Interconnections of thyroid veins 1. Superior vena cava; 2. Right brachiocephalic vein; 3. Right subclavian vein; 4. Internal jugular veins; 5. Inferior thyroid veins, isthmic veins; 6. Middle thyroid veins; 7. Superior thyroid veins

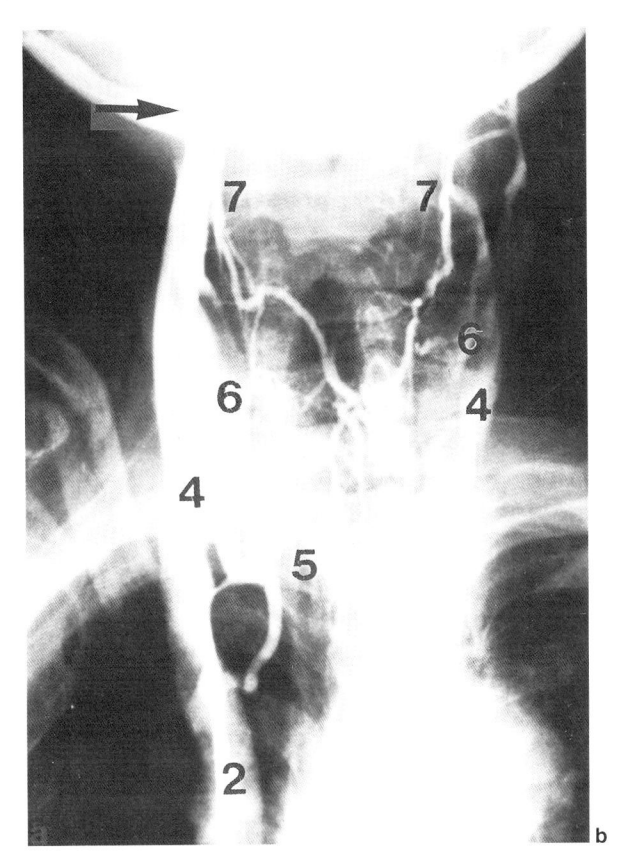

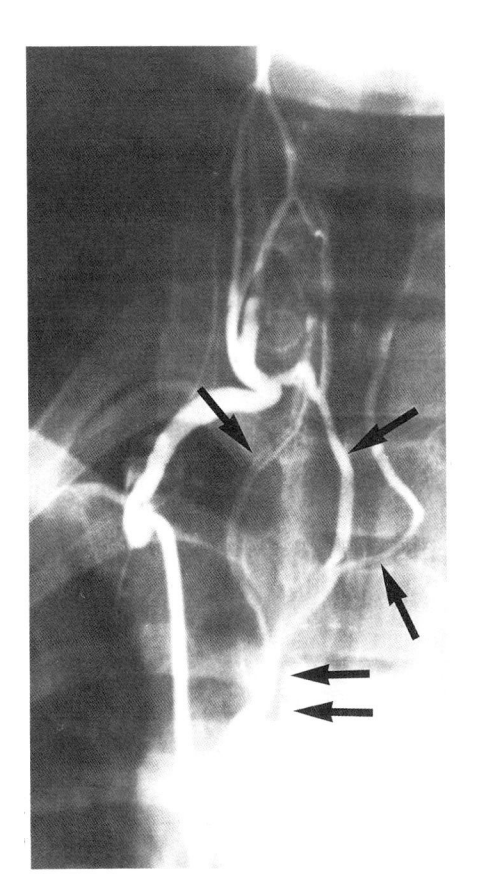

Fig. 4.**42** Inferior thyroid trunc (double arrow) The catheter is introduced by the right femoral approach into an aberrant inferior thyroid vein. Retrograde contrast media injection of the aberrant inferior thyroid vein shows filling of one left and two additional right inferior thyroidal veins as well faint opacification of the right internal jugular vein

116   4 Parathyroid Gland

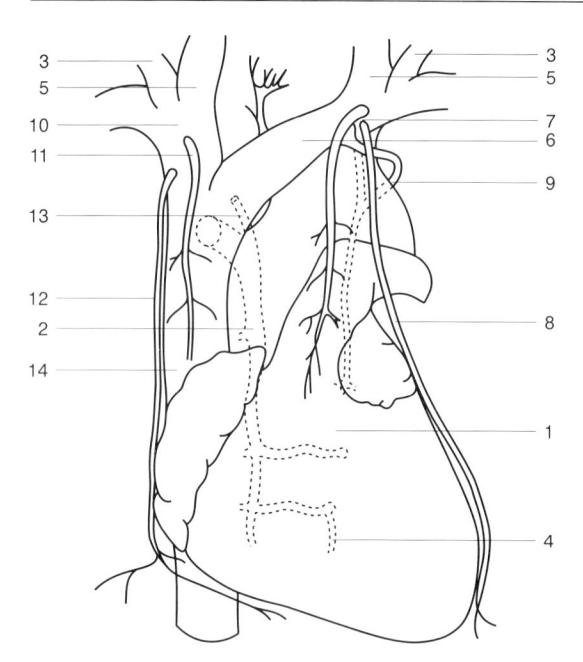

Fig. 4.**43**   Thoracic veins, anterior-posterior position
1. Accessory hemiazygos vein; 2. Azygos vein; 3. External jugular vein; 4. Hemiazygos vein; 5. Internal jugular vein; 6. Left brachiocephalic vein; 7. Internal thoracic vein; 8. Left pericardiophrenic vein; 9. Left superior intercostal vein; 10. Right brachiocephalic vein; 11. Right internal thoracic vein; 12. Right pericardiophrenic vein; 13. Right superior intercostal vein 14. Superior vena cava (from Godwin AJR 1986;147:674–684)

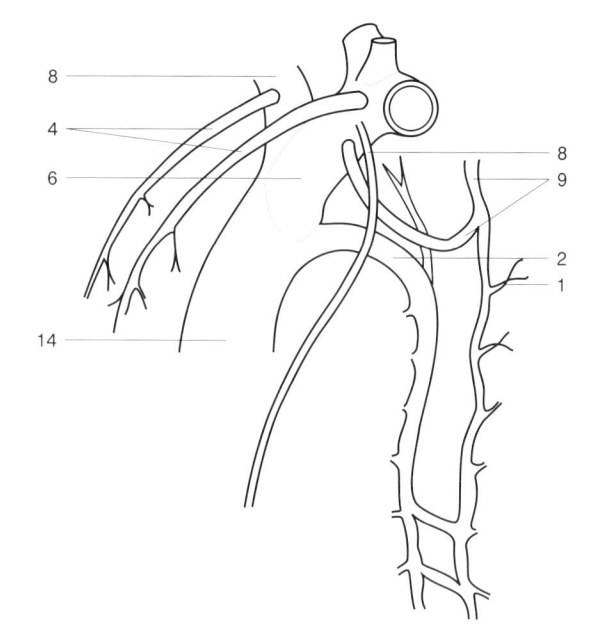

Fig. 4.**44**   Thoracic veins, lateral position
1. Accessory hemiazygos vein; 2. Azygos vein; 3. External jugular vein; 4. Hemiazygos vein; 5. Internal jugular vein; 6. Left brachiocephalic vein; 7. Internal thoracic vein; 8. Left pericardiophrenic vein; 9. Left superior intercostal vein; 10. Right brachiocephalic vein; 11. Right internal thoracic vein; 12. Right pericardiophrenic vein; 13. Right superior intercostal vein; 14. Superior vena cava (from Godwin AJR 1986; 147:674–684)

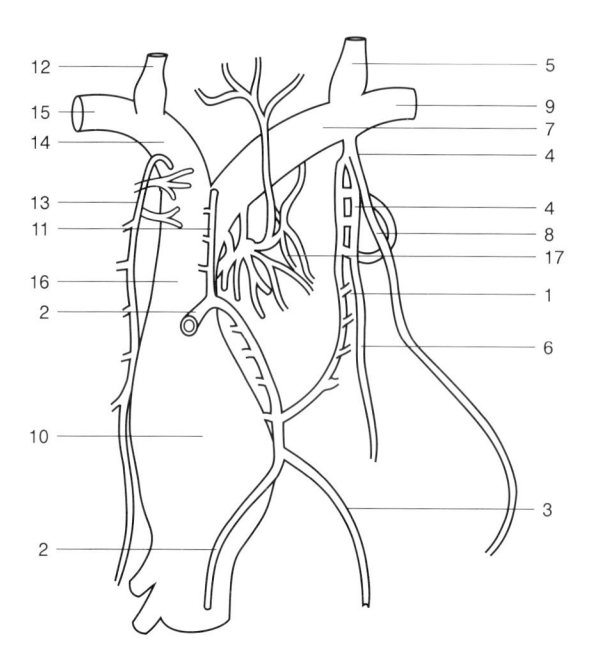

Fig. 4.**45**   Mediastinal veins
Schematic drawing of normal venous structures of the mediastinum.
1. Accessory hemiazygos vein; 2. Azygos vein; 3. Hemiazygos vein; 4. Left highest intercostal vein; 5. Left internal jugular vein; 6. Left internal mammary vein; 7. Left innominate vein; 8. Lateral mediastinal-phrenic vein; 9. Left subclavian vein; 10. Right atrium; 11. Right highest intercostal vein; 12. Right internal jugular vein; 13. Right internal mammary vein; 14. Right innominate vein; 15. Right subclavian vein; Superior vena cava; 17. Thymic vein (according to Yune, Radiology 1972;105:285)

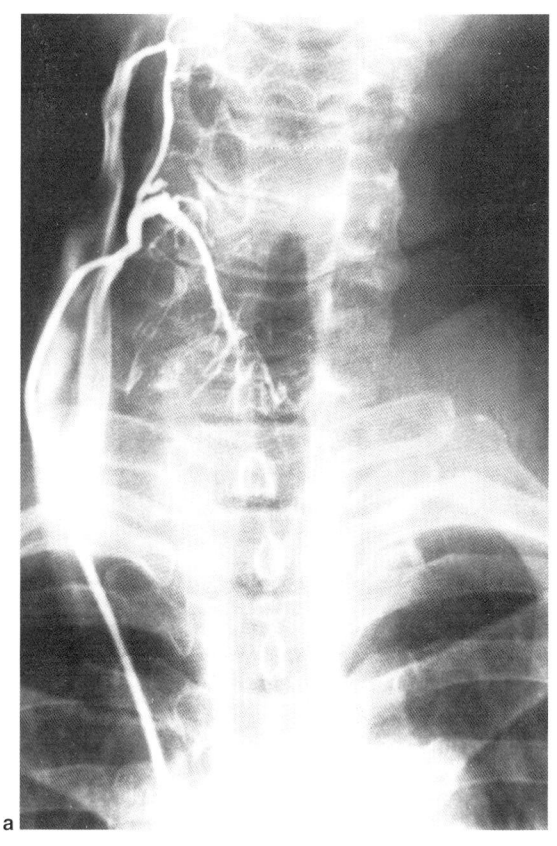

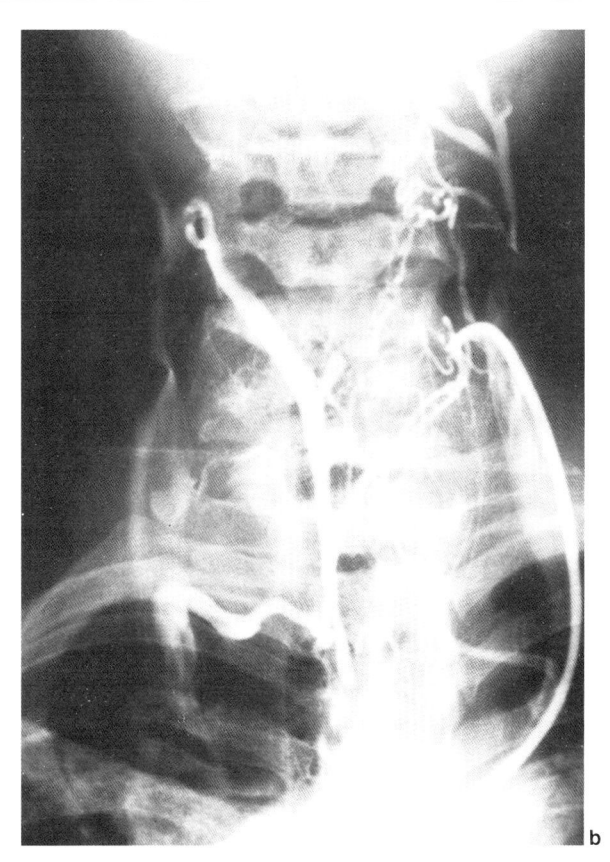

Fig. 4.**46** Distorted venous anatomy following partial thyroidectomy

Venous sampling from large vessels (jugular veins, innominate veins, superior vena cava) is not helpful (18). Elevation of PTH levels in these veins is difficult to interpret in comparison to the gradients in selective veins. Interpretation of gradients in the left innominate vein is particularly difficult because the mediastinum and both sides of the neck drain into this vessel. Looking for peripheral PTH gradients following unilateral neck massage is also of no value in this group of patients (19, 20, 21, 22).

Anastomoses between the inferior thyroid and the thymic veins are common, especially on the left side. Doppman (23, 24, 25) has found increased PTH levels in the thymic veins with cervical adenomas as well as in cervical veins with mediastinal adenomas.

Demonstration of the venous phase following and arterial study before sampling usually eases sampling.

Autotransplanted Parathyroid Tissue

Special attention should be given to parathyroid autografts performed for treatment of postoperative hypoparathyroidism. Parathyroid tissue is usually transplanted into the forearm. One complication of long-term autotransplanted grafts is recurrence of the clinical signs of hyperparathyroidism due to proliferation of the transplant (26, 27, 28, 29, 30).

Venous Sampling Technique

Venous sampling is performed under local anesthesia by the transfemoral approach (31). A vascular sheath helps to ease the exchange of catheters. A 5/7 french catheter (headhunter 1, cobra shape, length 100 cm) is suitable to catheterize the left and right jugular veins and its tributaries (Fig. 4.**47a**; 5, 6, 7). Sampling is easier if one or two sideholes are drilled close to the tip of the catheter (Fig. 4.**47b**). The catheter is advanced through the right atrium into the brachiocephalic and jugular veins under fluoroscopic control. The patients should be monitored during the procedure by ECG.

Jugular veins have venous valves, which are often difficult to pass. The valvular leaflets cannot be deliberately perforated with catheters or wires without the risk of perforation of the vessel itself. Steerable guide wires and specially coated wires (Terumo guides) usually lead the catheter tip through the valves (Fig. 4.**48**). When veins are tortuous, especially in elderly patients, swallowing of water will momentarily straighten them as the thyroid gland as-

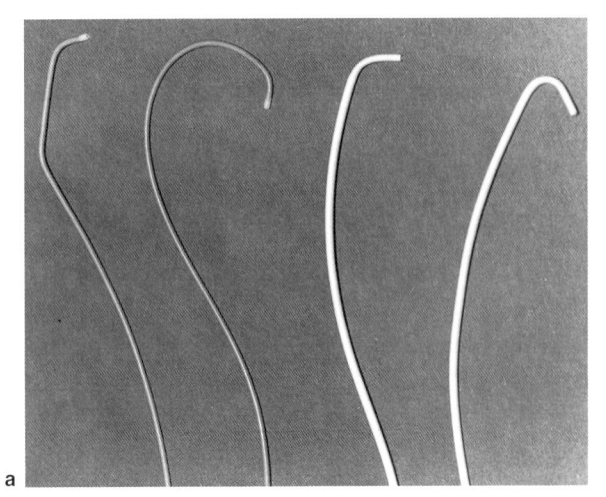

Fig. 4.**47** Shapes of catheters for parathyroid sampling
All catheters should have one or two sideholes as close as possible to the catheter tip

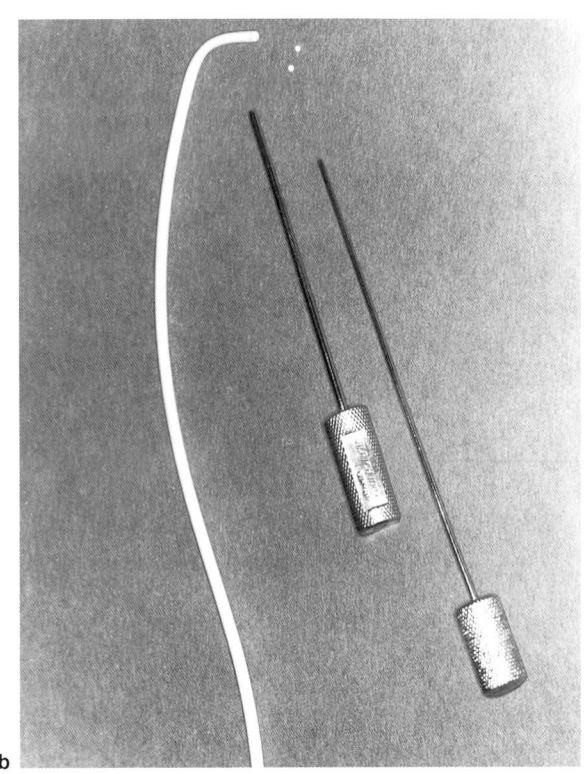

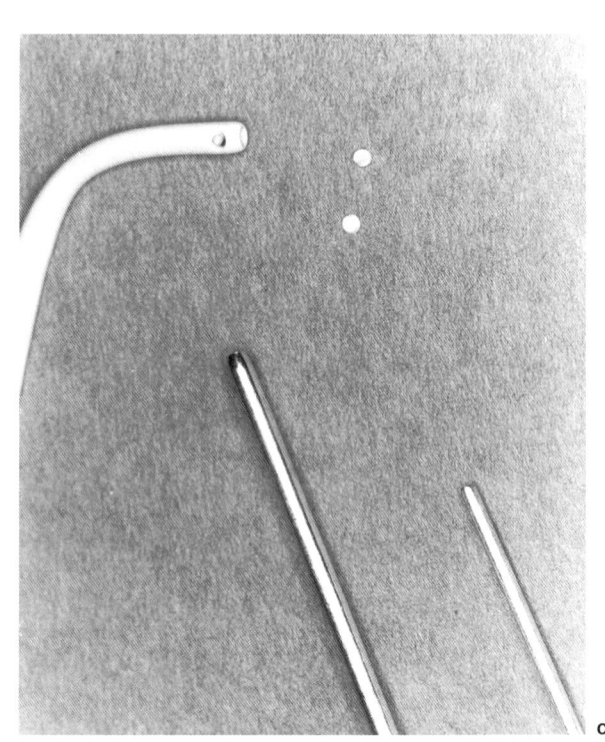

cends and may permit the catheter to be advanced. Aspiration of the blood sample can be equally frustrating. Gentle suction to avoid venous collapse, turning of the head, having the patient perform a Valsalva maneuver, as well as siphonage may be helpful.

In the presence of an extremely dilated jugular vein (Fig. 4.**49**) catheterization can be a problem. Catheters with different shapes must be available (Fig. 4.**47**). A large amount of PTH will be in the ipsilateral venous sampling in the presence of an adenoma on this side. Comparison to the PTH content in peripheral blood and the blood samples of the opposite side is necessary, and gradients should be calculated (8, 15, 32). Samples from the inferior thyroid vein on the other side are at background levels because the remaining normal parathyroid glands are suppressed by the high PTH production of an adenoma. Primary hyperplasia results in bilateral, unequally elevated PTH gradients because hyperplasia is generally an asymmetric process. If PTH levels are more than two times the background (inferior vena cava, peripheral blood) they are considered to be significantly elevated (33).

Road-mapping of Sampling

Radiographs should only be taken to "road-map" the anatomy. A retrograde venogram will display the complete thyroid venous bed and ease the catheteriza-

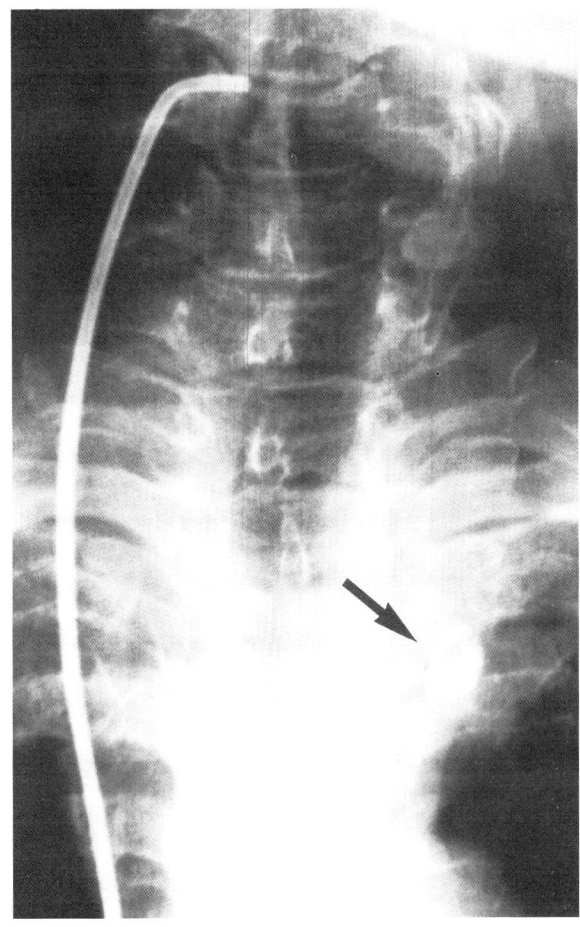

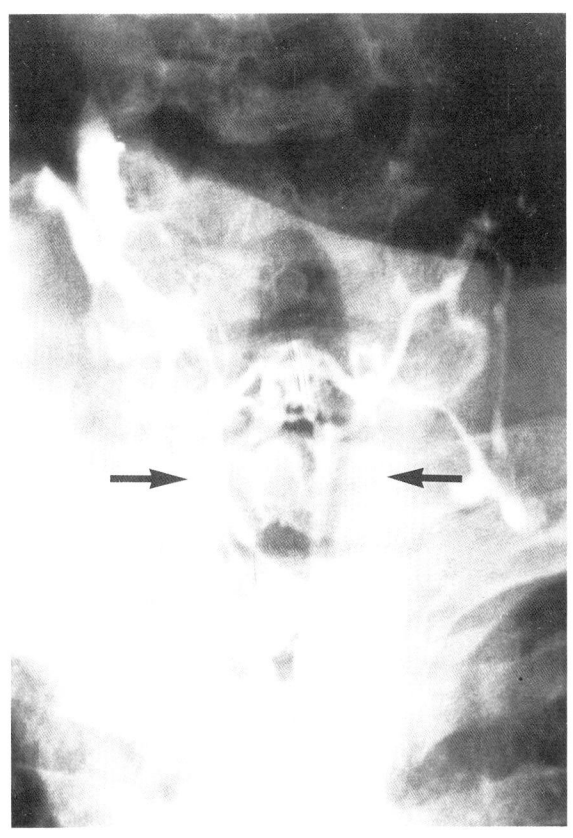

Fig. 4.**48** Catheters for venous sampling in the upper part of the right jugular vein. Opacification of a venous valve of the orifice of the left jugular vein from a previous injection (arrow)

Fig. 4.**49** Displacement of thyroid veins by a large parathyroid tumor of the left lower parathyroid gland (arrows)

tion procedure (Fig. 4.**40**). Catheter position should be marked for each blood sample (Fig. 4.**41**). Doppman (14) feels that unsuccessful surgery should be followed by parathyroid arteriography, venous sampling and CT of the mediastinum (34, 35); and parathyroid arteriography should be followed by venous sampling. The venous phase of the arteriogram provides useful information on whether veins are still intact and able to to drain the parathyroid glands or not. Some authors follow a different approach and sample before arteriography (36, 37).

Sometimes adenomas are stained by forceful retrograde contrast media injections or are seen displacing vascular structures (Fig. 4.**49**). Demonstration of a capsular or circumscribing vein surrounding the adenoma (38) is also helpful.

There are technical difficulties in sampling (aberrant parathyroid tissue, postoperative anatomy); still, venous sampling remains the method of choice for localizing a parathyroid adenoma. Mediastinal parathyroid tissue occurs in about 20% of cases examined for hyperparathyroidism (6).

Sampling Results

The accuracy of the sampling technique in predicting the site of hormone excess ranges from 50% to 90%, according to the literature (1, 8, 25, 36, 39). The sensitivity of selective thyroid and thymic venous sampling is decreased when there are thyroid–thymic vein connections and distortion of the venous anatomy by previous surgical procedures (5, 16, 40, 41). The detection rate of venous sampling increases when sampling is performed in combination with arteriography (43, 44, 45).

A review of Doppmans last 75 patients with one to four previous unsuccessful surgical explorations shows that positive arteriographicvenographic localization was achieved in 50% and useful information was provided in 77% of cases. False-positive localiza-

120   4 Parathyroid Gland

tions are rare. Failure generally occurs in patients who have had thyroidectomies, complete or subtotal. Thyroid veins become extremely small and difficult to sample after surgery; catheter access to the parathyroid vascular system is feasible only because the parathyroid glands share the larger thyroid vessels. Intrathyroid parathyroid glands (the surgeon's justification for resection of the thyroid gland) are extremely rare (46). Doppman found only six and all were correctly predicted by arteriography (20, 22).

Surgeons failing to identify disease during the initial neck exploration must be urged not to perform thyreoidectomies before localizing studies are performed.

Parathyroid Arteries

Normal parathyroid glands are 1–2 mm in diameter and are never visualized arteriographically. Enlarged glands appear as oval or rounded areas of diffuse stain superimposed upon or lying below the thyroid lobes (31, 36, 45).

Blood supply to a mediastinal adenoma may arise proximaly to the inferior thyroid artery or to the thyrocervical trunk and may be missed by an injection distally. With the new highflow thin-wall catheters and the tracker catheter coaxial systems, selectivity of very small vessels is easy.

The inferior thyroid artery may supply a contralateral parathyroid adenoma (Fig. 4.**50**), especially if the contralateral inferior thyroid artery has been ligated. The internal mammary artery may originate from a common trunk with the thyrocervical trunk.

Multiple anterior intercostal arteries arise from the medial margin of the internal mammary artery (Fig. 4.**50**) to supply the anterior intercostal spaces. A pericardiophrenic branch of the internal mammary artery can also be present. It is important that these vessels are identified and not mistaken for thymic branches. They

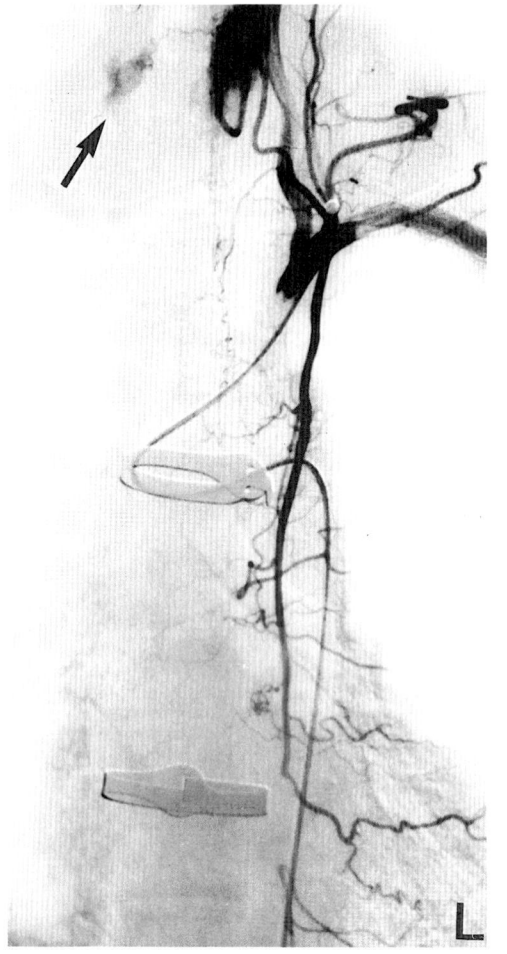

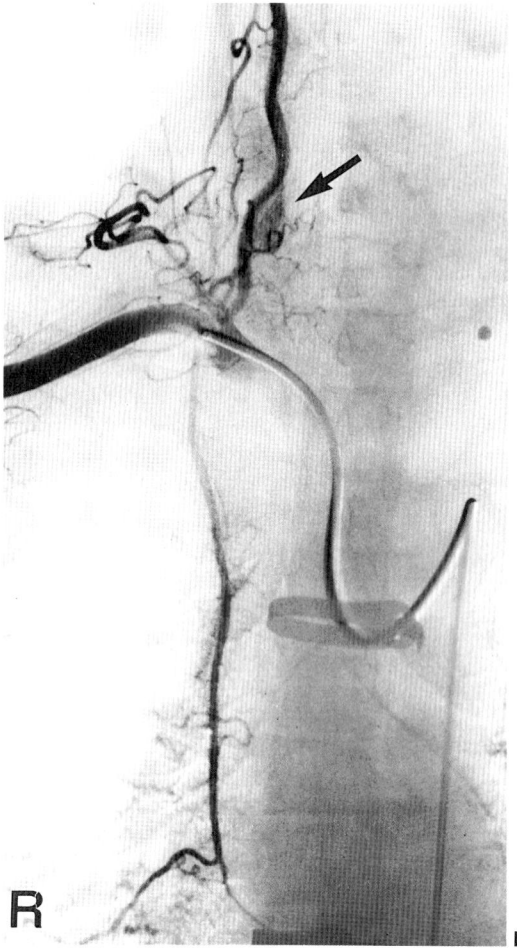

Fig. 4.**50** Subtraction arteriography of the right and left subclavian arteries in a patient with recurrent hyperparathyroidism after right thyroidectomy. There is a small adenoma on the right side which is supplied from both sides (arrow). The left lobe of the thyroid is well opacified. Normal internal mammary arteries

arise as second branches from the internal mammary artery and may supply intrathymic parathyroid adenomas of the anterior mediastinum (24, 47, 48, 49).

An artery supplying a mediastinal adenoma enlarges, easing the prodecure of selective catherization. The normal thymic gland stains following contrast media injection, especially in patients less than 20 years of age. The stain, however, does not show the discrete margins of a parathyroid adenoma. If the inferior thyroid artery is small or the thyroid lobe is not stained by either the inferior thyroid artery injection, superior thyroid artery injection, or both, a thyroid ima artery may be present (43, 44). This artery arises from the superior margin of the innominate artery and supplies the thyroid isthmus and the medial portions of both thyroid lobes. This vessel enlarges if the normal thyroid blood supply has been interrupted by surgery. Doppman (14) has detected four parathyroid adenomas supplied by this vessel only.

Selective superior thyroid artery injections rarely show pathologic parathyroid unless the ipsilateral inferior thyroid artery has been ligated. A proximally arising branch of the superior thyroid artery passes medially to supply the endolarynx and vocal cords. These show dense opacification. The normal stain must not be mistaken for ectopic, so-called parathymic parathyroid glands (49, 50). These are undescended inferior glands above the upper pole of the thyroid.

Intra-arterial Digital Subtraction Angiography

Arterial DSA of the parathyroid glands is invasive and there should be strong indications. Selective studies are necessary if patients have recurrent hypercalcemia following parathyreoidectomy and if results of noninvasive imaging techniques are inconclusive.

The most accurate method for localization of remaining parathyroid tissue is parathyroid arteriography (49, 52).

Intraarterial DSA can either be performed by nonselective injection into the aortic arch or by selective injection into the brachiocephalic arteries (45) (44% were localized by aortic injection in 16 cases, 45). The sensitivity of i.v. DSA is 31%. Miller (52) reported 49% of adenomas located by arterial DSA accurately with one false-positive finding. The sensitivity for selective parathyroid DSA was 60%. Intra-arterial DSA, selective arteriography, parathyroid venous sampling, and intraoperative sonography permits a localization of adenomas in 95% of the cases. According to Lacombe (53), it was apparant that intra-arterial DSA of the brachiocephalic vessels could locate most of the remaining abnormal cervical or mediastinal glands. Arterial DSA has a sensitivity of 81% (48, 49, 53). In the neck and mediastinum the sensitivities are 73% and 90%, respectively. Selective catheterization of the thyrocervical trunk, the internal mammary artery, and the superior thyroid artery is performed by the femoral approach (7, 16, 43, 44, 45, 54). An nonionic contrast medium is used because the injection of conventional contrast agents into small vessels is painful. Using DSA, contrast media can be diluted 1:2 to 1:4 and will still create enough staining to diagnose disease. Patients with hyperparathyroidism frequently have impaired renal function and should be well-hydrated before the procedure. If vascular anatomy prevents selective catheterization, venous sampling still can be performed.

If the catheter is in a wedged position, extensive staining may obscure pathologic lesions of the parathyroid glands. Oblique radiographs may be necessary to demonstrate the lesion. The frequency of films should be 1/s for 15 seconds to obtain arterial, capillary, and venous phases. This is also helpful in planning subsequent venous sampling (15). Enlarged glands of 4 to 5 mm can be seen on well-collimated, optimal exposed films. AP and oblique projections (25–30 degrees) are obtained on all inferior thyroid artery injections. These will demonstrate posterior adenomas obscured by opacification of thyroid tissue. When an adenoma is demonstrated in the mediastinum, a steep oblique or lateral radiograph should be obtained to distinguish anterior from posterior locations. Because of areas of faint staining, a lesion can be obscured by the overlying cervical spine. Subtraction studies should be routine.

Parathyroid arteriography should be an indication after unsuccessful surgical treatment. Venous sampling, however, with calculation of gradients is much more successful than arteriography. Still, the physician should insist that arteriography with the attempt to visualize the adenoma is an important part of the localization procedure.

Complications

Spinal cord damage with quadriplegia may occur following the injection of excessive quantities of contrast material selectively into the costocervical trunk, which commonly provides a major radiculomedullary branch to the anterior spinal artery at the cervicothoracic level. Occlusion by the catheter of this small artery is difficult to avoid, and injection of even small amounts of contrast medium is especially likely to damage the cord. The thyrocervical trunk, however, rarely supplies vessels to the cord. In more than 1000 thyrocervical trunk injections, subtracted and examined for spinal cord blood supply, Doppman found only 3 cases. However the costocervical trunk may be mistaken for the thyrocervical trunk on anteroposterior fluoroscopy, especially when the inferior thyroid artery has been ligated during the initial operation. In Doppmans broad experience with parathyroid arteriography there was no spinal complication (48, 49).

Cortical blindness complicating parathyroid arteriography has been reported, but vision always returned to normal within 48 hours. This complication is the result of a multiple, forceful injection of contrast material into the vertebral artery while searching for the thoracocervical and internal mammary trunks. Multiple endocrine adenomatosis, insulin, or epinephrine-secreting tumors, and occult pheochromocytomas (in multiple endocrine adenomatosis type II) may complicate arteriography. These risk factors should be ruled out prior to arteriography.

Treatment

Surgery is the treatment of hyperparathyroidism if the patient has symptoms, and the disease is progressive. The success of surgery depends on the removal of functioning tissue. Patients with mild, asymptomatic primary HPT should be managed conservatively if their hypercalcemia is not progressing and if there are no complications related to the disease. The elevated serum calcium level returns to normal within 24 to 48 hours following surgery. In patients with servere osteitis fibrosa, prolonged symptomatic hypocalcemia may occur and require large doses of calcium together with vitamin D, usually for 1–3 months.

There is the possibility of transcatheter ablation (16, 48, 49, 52, 56) of parathyroid adenomas, if the supplying artery is selectivly catheterized. Nonoperative ablation of parathyroid adenomas by ultrasound-guided percutaneous direct injection of ethanol (96%) into the the tumor in patients with uremia and secondary hyperparathyroidism has been performed (55, 56, 57). This treatment can be done with a fine needle under local anesthesia and an injection of ethanol (58). A decrease in PTH and ionized calcium serum levels is observed immediately (58). Complications of this therapy have not been described yet, however, small areas of hemorrhage and necrosis were found (57, 59), and theoretically, damage to the recurrent laryngeal nerve is possible (58).

References

1. Satava RM, Beahres OH, Scholz DA. Success rate of cervical exploration for hyperparathyroidism. Arch. Surg. 1975;110:625–628.
2. Dubost CI, Boucaut PH. Hyperparathyroide primaire: ètude rétropective de 500 cas. Presse Med. 1982;11:443–446.
3. Brennan MF, Norton JA. Reoperation for persistent and recurrent hyperparathyroidism. Ann Surg. 1985;201:40–44.
4. Sörensen R. Selective venous sampling for parathyroid hormone excess. In: Uflacker/Sörensen, eds. Percutaneous venous blood sampling in endocrine disease. New York: Springer; 1992;125–150.
5. Wang CA. Parathyroid re-exploration. A clinical and pathological study of 112 cases. Ann Surg. 1977;186:140–145.
6. Nathaniels EK, Nathaniels AM, Wang C. Mediastinal parathyroid tumors; a clinical and pathological study of 84 cases. Ann Surg. 1970;171:165–170.
7. Doppman JL. Parathyroid localisation: arteriography and venous sampling. Radiol Clin North Am. 1976;46:403–418.
8. O'Riordan JLH, Kendall BE, Woodhead JS. Preoperative localisation of parathyroid tumors. Lancet. 1971;2:1172–1175.
9. Levin KE, Gooding GAW, Okerlund M, Higgins CB, et al. Localization studies in patients with persistent or recurrent hyperparathyroidism. Surgery. 1987;102:917–925.
10. Akerström G, Malmaeus J, Bergström R. Surgical anatomy of the human parathyroid glands. Surgery. 1984;95:14–21.
11. Wang CA, Mahaffey J, Axelrod L, Perlman JA. Hyperfunctioning supernumerary parathyroid glands. Surg Gynecol Obstet. 1979;148:711–714.
12. Thompson NW, Eckhauser FE, Harness JH. The anatomy of primary hyperparathyroidism. Surgery. 1982;92:814–821.
13. Doppman JL. Parathyroid angiography In: Abrams HL, ed. Abrams Angiography. Boston: Little, Brown; 1983;977–999.
14. Doppman JL, Hammond WG. The anatomic basis of parathyroid venous sampling. Radiology. 1970;95:603–610.
15. Doppman JL, Hammond WG, Melson GI, Evens RG, Ketcham AS. Staining of parathyroid andenomas by selective arteriography. Radiology. 1969;92:527–530.
16. Shimkin PM, Doppman JL, Pearson KD, Powell D. Anatomic considerations in parathyroid venous sampling. AJR. 1973;118:654–662.
17. Doppman JL, Melson GL, Evens RG, Hammond WG. Selective superior and inferior thyroid vein catheterization. Invest Radiol. 1969;4:97–366.
18. Reitz RE, Pollard JJ, Wang CA, et al. Localization of parathyroid adenomas by selective venous catheterization and radioimmunoassay. New Engl J Med. 1969;281:348–351.
19. Reiss E, Canterbury JM. Primary hyperparathyreoidism: Application of radioimmunoassay in differentiation of adenoma and hyperplasia and preoperative localization of hyperfunctioning parathyroid glands. New Engl J Med. 1969;280:1381–1385.
20. Spiegel AM, Marx SJ, Doppman JL, et al. Intrathyroidal parathyroid adenoma or hyperplasia. An occasional overlooked cause of surgical failure in primary hyperparathyroidism JAMA. 1975;234:1029–1033.
21. Spiegel AM, Doppman JL, Marx SJ, et al. Preoperative localization of abnormal parathyroids: Neck massage vs. arteriography and selective venous sampling. Ann Intern Med. 1978;89:935–936.
22. Spiegel AM, Adamson RH, Mallette LE, et al. Intrathyroid parathyroid tumors: A seldom recognized cause of surgical failure in primary hyperparathyroidism. JAMA. 1975;234:1029–1033.
23. Offermann G, Opitz A, Sörensen R. Localization of parathyroid adenomas in primary hyperparathyroidism. Dtsch Med Wschr. 1974;99:1308–1312.
24. Doppman JL, Mallette LE, Marx S, et al. The localization of abnormal mediastinal parathyroid glands. Radiology. 1975;115:31–34.
25. Doppman JL, Brennan MF, Brown EM. Tracheal overlap: Arteriographic sign of parathyroid adenomas in the posterior superior mediastinum. AJR. 1978;130:1197–1199.
26. Brennan MF, Doppman JL, Marx SJ, Spiegel AM, Brown EM, Aurbach GD. Reoperative parathyroid surgery for persistent hyperparathyroidism. Surgery. 1978;83:669–676.
27. Brennan MF, Brown EM, Spiegel AM, et al. Autotransplantation of cryopreserved parathyroid tissue in man. Ann Surg. 1979;189:139–142.
28. Brennan MF, Brown EM, Marx SJ, et al. Recurrent hyperparathyroidism from an autotransplanted parathyroid adenoma. New Engl J Med. 1978;299:1057–1059.
29. Haase GM, Luce JM, Lock JP, Hammond WS, Penn I. Hyperparathyroidism following parathyroid autotransplantation. Surgery. 1979;86:694–697.
30. Wells SA jr., Ellis JG, Gunnels JC, Schneider AB, Sherwood LM. Parathyroid autotransplantation in primary parathyroid hyperplasia. N Engl J Med. 1976;295:57–62.
31. Seldinger SI. Localization of parathyroid adenomata by arteriography. Acta Radiol Stockh. 1954;42:353–366.
32. Hjern B, Almquiost S, Granberg PO, Lindvall N, Wästhed B. Preoperative localization of parathyroid tissue by selective neck vein catheterization and radioimmunoassay of parathyroid hormone. Acta Chir Scand. 1975;141:31–39.
33. Powell D, Shimkin PM, Wells S, Aurbach GD, Marx SJ, Kecham AS, Potts JT jr. Primary hyperparathyroidism: Preoperative tumor localization and differentiation between adenoma and hyperplasia. N Engl J Med. 1972;286:1169–1175.

34. Bilezikian JP, Doppman JL, Shimkin PM, et al. Preoperative localisation of abnormal parathyroid tissue: Cumulative experience with venous sampling and arteriography. Am J Med. 1973;55:505–514.
35. Doppman JL, Wells SA, Shimkin PM, et al. Parathyroid localization by angiographic techniques in patients with previous neck surgery. Br J Radiol. 1973;46:403–418.
36. Eisenberg H, Pallotta J, Sherwood LM. Selective arteriography, venography and venous hormone assay in diagnosis and localisation of parathyroid lesions. Am J Med. 1974;56:810–820.
37. Newton TH, Eisenberg E. Angiography of parathyroid adenomas. Radiology. 1966;86:843–850.
38. Doppman JL, Brennan MF, Kahn CR, Marx SJ. The circumscribing or per-adenomal vessel: A helpful angiographic finding in certain islet cell and parathyroid adenomas. AJR. 1981;136:163–165.
39. Godwin JD, Chen JTT. Thoracic venous anatomy. AJR. 1986;147:674–684.
40. Clark OH, Okerlund MD, Moss AA, et al. Localization studies in patients with persistent or recurrent hyperparathyroidism. Surgery. 1985;98:1083–1094.
41. Brennan MF, Doppman JL, Kurdy AG, Marx SJ, Spiegel AM, Aurbach GD. Assessment of techniques for preoperative parathyroid gland localization in patients undergoing reoperation for hyperparathyroidism. Surgery. 1982;91:6–12.
42. Clark OH, Okerlund MD, Moss AA, et al. Localization studies in patients with persistent or recurrent hyperparathyroidism. Surgery. 1985;98:1083–1094.
43. Krudy A, Doppman JL, Brennan MF. The significance of the thyreoidea ima artery in arteriographic localization of parathyroid adenomas. Radiology. 1980;136:51–55.
44. Krudy AG, Doppman JL, Brennan MF, Saxe AW, Marx SJ. Arteriographic localization of parathyroid adenoma in the presence of lingual thyroid. AJR. 1981;136:1127–1230.
45. Krudy AG, Doppman JL, Miller DL, et al. Work in progress – abnormal parathyroid glands: comparison of nonselective arterial digital subtraction arteriography, selective parathyroid arteriography, and venous digital arteriography as methods of detection. Radiology. 1983;148:23–29.
46. Al-Suhaili AR, Lynn J, Lavender JP. Intrathyroidal parathyroid adenoma: preoperative identification and localization by parathyroid imaging. Clin Nucl Med. 1988;13:512–515.
47. Doppman JL, Marx SJ, Brennan MF, Beazly RM, Geelhoed G, Aurbach GD. The blood supply of mediastinal parathyroid adenomas. Ann Surg. 1977;185:488–490.
48. Doppman JL, Marx SJ, Spiegel A, et al. Treatment of hyperparathyroidism by percutaneous embolization of a mediastinal adenoma. Radiology. 1975;115:37–42.
49. Doppman JL, Brown EM, Brennan MF, Spiegel A, Marx SJ, Aurbach GD. Angiographic ablation of parathyroid adenomas. Radiology. 1979;130:577–582.
50. Edis AJ, Purnell DC, Van Heerden JA. The undescended "parathymus": An occasional cause of failed neck exploration in hyperparathyroidism. Ann Surg. 1979;190:64–68.
51. Krudy AG, Doppman JL, Brennan MF, et al. The detection of mediastinal parathyroid glands by computed tomography, selective arteriography, and venous sampling. Radiology. 1981;140:739–744.
52. Miller DL, Doppman JL, Chang R, et al. Angiographic ablation of parathyroid adenomas: lessons from a 10 year experience. Radiology. 1987;165:601–606.
53. Lacombe P, Foster D, Dubost C, et al. Selective intraarterial DSA of the parathyroid glands in patients with hyperparathyroidism after parathyroidectomy. AJR. 1987;149:479–483.
54. Rossi P, Carillo FJ, Johnston B. Angiography in the diagnosis of parathyroid carcinoma. New Engl J Med. 1971;284:198–201.
55. Solbiati G, Montali G, Croce F, Belloti E, Giangrande A, Ravetto C. Parathyroid tumors detected by fine-needle aspiration biopsy under ultrasonic guidance. Radiology. 1983;148:793–797.
56. Doppman JL, Adrian GK, Stephan JM, et al. Aspiration of enlarged parathyroid glands for hormone assay. Radiology. 148:31–39.
57. Solbiati L, Giangrande A, De Pra L, et al. Percutaneous ethanol injection of parathyroid tumors under ultrasound guidance. Treatment for secondary hyperparathyroidism. Radiology. 1985;155:607–611.
58. Karstrup S, Holm HH, Torp-Pedersen S. Ultrasonically guided inactivation of parathyroid tumors. Br J Radiol. 1987;60:667–670.
59. Doppman JL, Shawker TH, Krudy AG. The parathymic parathyroid: CT, US, and angiographic findings. Radiology. 1985;157:268–281.

Nuclear Medicine

U. Keske

^{201}Tl is taken up by the parathyroids more than by normal thyroid tissue, while pertechnetate is taken up only by normal thyroid tissue. It is possible to visualize these uptake differences by thallium-technetium subtraction scintigraphy (2, 4, 7). This method has replaced scintigraphy with ^{75}Se, which has been a less reliable technique (7).

The mechanism of thallium accumulation in the thyroid and parathyroid is not fully understood. It seems to be related to total thyroidal blood flow or to the sodium–potassium ATPase system, since thallium is a potassium analogue (7). It has also been suggested that it is dependent on the presence of mitochondria-rich oxyphil cells (5).

Imaging Technique

Imaging can only be performed with a digital gamma camera. A pinhole- or special thyroid-collimator is advantageous. The patient is placed in a comfortable position underneath the collimator, it is important that he or she doesn't move for the whole examination (approximately 45 minutes). ^{99m}Tc pertechnetate (74 MBq) is injected intravenously. Twenty minutes later, thyroid scintigraphy is performed with a window setting of 140 KeV (technetium photopeak) and afterwards a window setting of 70–80 KeV (^{201}Tl photopeak, technetium scatter image). This is followed by an injection of ^{201}Tl chloride (74 MBq). Immediately afterwards, thyroid imaging is repeated with the ^{201}Tl window setting.

During postprocessing, the thallium image is cleared from the technetium scatter by substraction of the technetium scatter image. Afterwards, the technetium image is normalized and substracted from the cleared thallium image (Fig. 4.**51**). The subtracted image then shows all regions with an excessive thallium uptake (2, 7). The opposite procedure (subtraction of a pertechnetate image from a thallium image) is also possible (1).

Radiation exposure is 24 mGy for the thyroid, 30 mGy for the kidneys, 11 mGy for the gonads, 7 mGy for the bone marrow, and 5 mGy for the whole body (3).

TC TL KORRIGIERT SUBTRAKTION

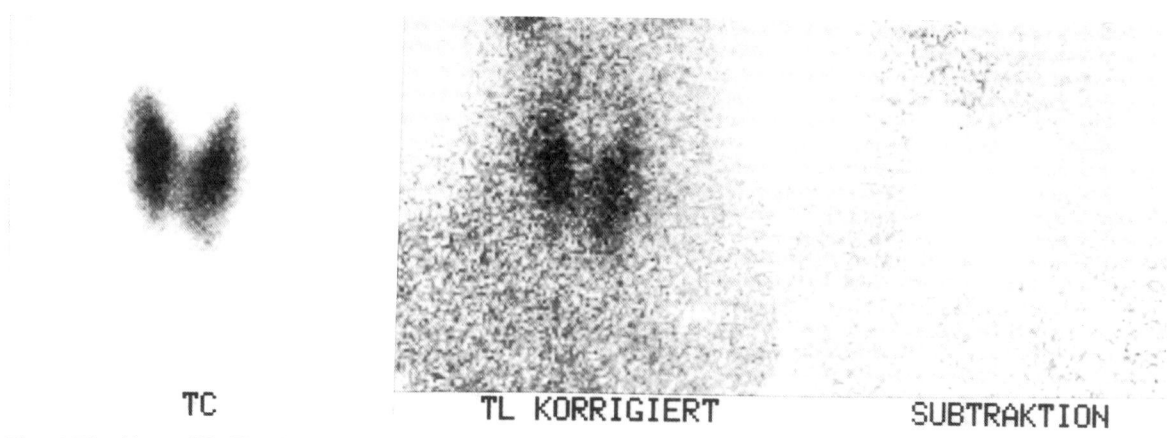

Fig. 4.**51** Normal Tc-Tl subtraction scan. Normal-sized thyroid in the Tc image (left) and the Tl scan (middle). The subtraction image (right) shows no excessive Tl uptake.

Scintigraphic Findings

In hyperparathyroidism, a solitary adenoma of one of the four parathyroids is found in 80% of patients. In 15%, more than two parathyroids are involved (9). A positive scintigraphic finding is characteristic of parathyroid adenomas, parathyroid carcinomas, or hyperplasia (7).

Parathyroid adenomas may be located completely or partially contiguous to the thyroid, extrathyroidal, or even substernal and mediastinal. Four pathologic scintigraphic patterns should be differentiated (1):
- ectopic thallium uptake,
- thallium accumulation completely or partially outside the thyroid,
- thallium accumulation corresponding to a cold or cool area in the technetium image (Fig. 4.**52**), and
- relatively high thallium uptake in an area of normal technetium uptake.

Scintigraphy makes it possible to visualize ectopic glands or glands that are completely or partially outside the thyroid. For these cases, the subtraction image is not needed. Glands that lie posterior to the thyroid are difficult to find, especially if they are small. In these cases, subtraction images remain especially useful (1).

The scintigraphic image of more than one abnormal thallium accumulation is suggestive of parathyroid hyperplasia or, less likely, multiple adenomas (7). However, imaging of hyperplastic glands still remains difficult (1, 6).

Lesions smaller than 0.5–0.8 cm are mostly undetectable (1, 4). Sensitivity is reported to be 82–90%, specicifity 98% and accuracy 98% (1, 4). Combination with ultrasound increases accuracy to 96% (4). Sensitivity is higher for primary hyperparathyroidism than for secondary hyperparathyroidism (1) and is very low for hyperplasia (44%, 8).

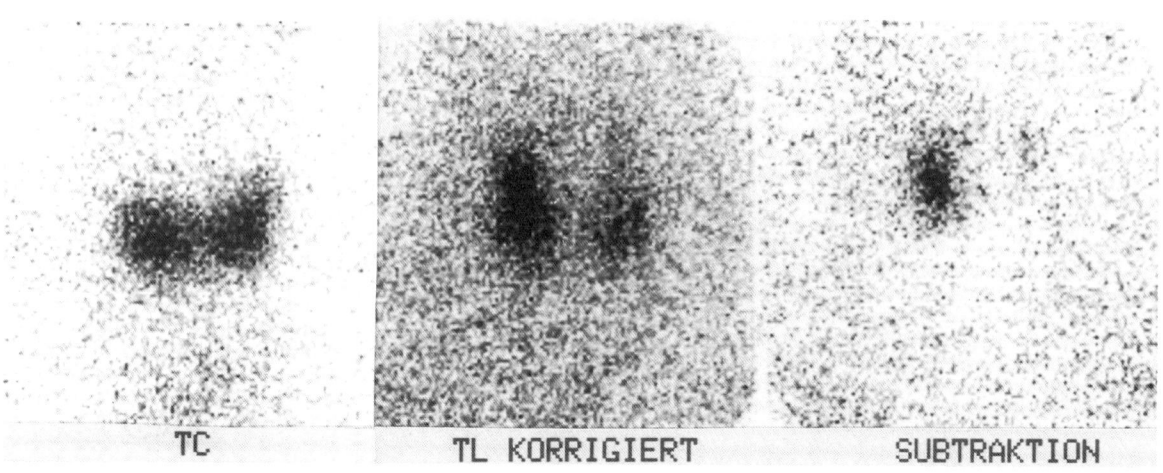

TC TL KORRIGIERT SUBTRAKTION

Fig. 4.**52** Tc-Tl subtraction scan in a patient with histologically proven parathyroid adenoma in the upper right lobe of the thyroid. The Tc scan shows a decreased tracer uptake in the upper right lobe (left). Tl uptake in this area is increased (middle). The subtraction image shows excessive Tl uptake in the upper right lobe (right).

False-positive results are known from thyroid carcinoma, adenomatous goiter, chronic thyroiditis, malignant lymphomas, swollen lymph nodes, and metastases to the neck. These lesions show a thallium uptake, but no pertechnetate or iodine uptake (1, 7).

References

1. Borsato N, Zanco P, Camerani M, Saitta B, Ferlin G. Scintigraphy of the Parathyroid Glands with ^{201}Tl: Experience with 250 Operated Patients. J. Nucl Med. 1989;29:26–28.
2. Ferlin G, Borsato N, Camerani M, Conte N, Zotti D. New perspectives in localizing enlarged parathyroids by technetium-thallium subtraction scan. J Nucl Med. 1983;24:438–441.
3. Montz R. Nebennieren und Nebenschilddrüse. In: Büll U, Hör G, eds. Klinische Nuklearmedizin. 1st ed. Weinheim: VCH; 1987:125–132.
4. Müller-Gärtner HW, Montz R, Schneider C, Kruse HP, Dietel M, Schumpelick V: Lokalisationsdiagnostik vergrößerter Nebenschilddrüsen: die 201Tl-99mTc-Subtraktionsszintigraphie im Vergleich zur 5-MHz-Sonographie. Fortschr Röntgenstr 1985;142(5):543–547.
5. Sandrock D, Merino MJ, Norton JA, Miller DL, Neumann RD. Ultrastructural Pathology Explains Results of ^{201}Tl/^{99m}Tc Parathyroid Subtraction Scintigraphy. In: Höfer R, Bergmann H, Sinzinger H. Radioactive Isotope in Klinik und Forschung – Radioactive Isotopes in Clinical Medicine and Research. Stuttgart: Schattauer; 1991:328–330.
6. van der Pompe WB, Delhez H, Savelkoul TJF. Scintigraphy of the thyroid, parathyroid and adrenal gland. In: van Rijk PP, ed. Nuclear Techniques in Diagnostic Medicine Norwell: Kluwer Academic; 1986:413–457.
7. Winzelberg G, Hydovitz JD. Radionuclide Imaging of Parathyroid Tumors: Historical Perspective and Newer Techniques. Semin Nucl Med. 1985;XV(2):161–170.
8. Young AE, Gaunt JI, Croft DN, Collins REC, Wells CP, Coakley AJ. Location of parathyroid adenomas by ^{201}thallium and ^{99m}technetium subtraction scanning. Br Med J. 1983;286:1384–1386.
9. zum Winkel K. Nuklearmedizin. 2nd ed. Berlin: Springer; 1990.

A Radiologist's View

W. Auffermann

Noninvasive imaging techniques have improved significantly in the past decade and have become part of routine preoperative evaluation for the localization of parathyroid adenomas in primary hyperparathyroidism (3, 5, 7, 8, 14, 21, 23, 50, 52). Preoperative imaging localization may avoid bilateral exploration, optimize the individual surgical strategy, shorten operation time, reduce complication rate, and reduce early hypocalcemia (8, 23, 52).

Recurrent or Persistent Hyperparathyroidism

Depending on the operation statistics, recurrent or persistent parathyroid adenomas occur in 5 to 25% of patients with prior surgery for primary hyperparathyroidism (11, 23). Most surgeons favor a radical local second resection because every other operation becomes more difficult and has a lower success rate (5, 6, 8). The remaining parathyroid tissue is more difficult to localize surgically due to scarring and fibrosis (13). Moreover, recurrent adenomas occur more often in ectopic locations. Whereas the success rate in patients without prior surgery is higher than 90%, it falls to less than 60% in patients with prior surgery, when no preoperative localization is done (10). With preoperative localization, the success rate of reoperation may be better than 90% (23).

The choice of the optimal imaging technique for localization of recurrent adenomas continues to be a difficult issue for the referring physician. In a previous study comparing various noninvasive imaging techniques (sonography, CT, scintigraphy, and MRI), none of the techniques identified more than 50% of the enlarged glands (25). In our own studies of 70 patients with hyperparathyroidism, comparing high-resolution sonography, substraction scintigraphy, and MRI, prospective localization rates were 57%, 64%, and 75% respectively (1, 2). Figure 4.**30** shows a recurrent parathyroid adenoma that is visualized with different imaging techniques. Combination of sonography or scintigraphy with MRI increases the accuracy in preoperated patients from 60% to about 90% (1, 2). Moreover, combination of these techniques can reduce the rate of false-positive diagnoses, which can be as high as 13% or even 23% depending on the individual technique used (19, 23).

Ectopic Adenomas

Mediastinal parathyroid adenomas are found in 12 to 19% of patients with hyperparathyroidism (6, 9, 10, 45, 51). Two-thirds of these adenomas may be resected by cervical incision. Median sternotomy is required in about one-third of these patients. Mediastinal exploration is associated with an increased operation morbidity and lethality (10). Hypoparathyroidism is another late complication (10 to 20%), which, however, can be successfully treated by cryoconservation of parathyroid tissue with the possibility of later autotransplantation. A study by the National Institutes of Health showed that mediastinal exploration was negative in one-third of patients because a cervical adenoma had been missed (29).

The risk of mediastinal exploration stresses the importance of preoperative localization when an ectopic parathyroid adenoma is suspected. In the search for mediastinal adenomas, MRI is clearly superior to other imaging techniques with an accuracy rate of about 78% (Table 4.**3**). Even angiography identifies only 50% maximally of those adenomas (29). A recent study using MRI, scintigraphy, and sonography allowed accurate localization of ectopic adenomas in 88%, 52%, and 13%, respectively (17).

Although with each single imaging technique, only up to two-thirds of parathyroid adenomas (14)

Table 4.3 Prospective Accuracies of Preoperative Localization of Parathyroid Adenomas

Parathyroid Adenoma – Imaging Technique	Localization Rate Median and Range 1980–1993, in %	Reference Number
Primary Hyperparathyroidism		
Sonography (5–7.5 MHz)	59 (41–82)	[18, 20, 21, 26, 28, 32, 33, 42, 48, 50]
Sonography (10 MHz)	75 (65–88)	[7, 12, 16, 26, 37, 39, 40, 44, 47, 49, 53, 55]
Thallium Scintigraphy	73 (60–90)	[4, 12, 15, 20, 21, 24, 30, 34–36, 54]
CT	72 (50–87)	[16, 20, 21, 31, 42, 44, 46, 47, 50, 54]
MRI	76 (64–79)	[2, 20, 34, 43, 50]
Ectopic Adenomas		
Sonography (7.5–10 MHz)	8 (0–20)	[1, 9, 17, 23, 25, 47]
Thallium Scintigraphy	30 (0–52)	[1, 9, 17, 23, 25, 34]
CT	41 (20–75)	[9, 23, 25, 42, 51]
MRI	78 (71–100)	[0, 17, 23, 43]
Recurrent Hyperparathyroidism		
Sonography (5–7.5 MHz)	50 (32–67)	[8, 21, 22, 25, 50]
Songraphy (10 MHz)	65 (47–82)	[1, 12, 13, 23, 38, 44, 55]
Thallium Scintigraphy	60 (27–86)	[1, 8, 12, 21, 23–25, 30, 41]
CT	57 (44–66)	[8, 13, 21, 23, 25, 44, 50]
MRI	66 (50–75)	[1, 23, 25, 50]

are identified, and, depending on the investigator and the technique, false-positive results are in the order of 13–23% (23), a combined approach of several complementary techniques may increase the accuracy of preoperative localization to about 90% (1, 2, 19, 23, 24).

References

1. Auffermann, W, Clark, OH, Gooding, GAW, et al. Diagnosis of recurrent hyperparathyroidism: comparison of magnetic resonance with other imaging modalities. Am J Roentgenol. 1988;150:1027–1033.
2. Auffermann, W, Guis, M, Tavares, NJ, Clark OH, Higgins, CB. MR imaging of hyperparathyroidism. Results in 70 patients with histopathologic correlation of MR signal intensity patterns. Radiology. 1988;169:304.
3. Auffermann, W, Higgins, CB. Hyperparathyreoidismus. Nichtinvasive Diagnostik. Dtsh. Ärztebl. 1991;88:A558–566.
4. Blake, GM, Percival, RC, Kanis, JA. Thallium-pertechnetate subtraction scintigraphy: a quantitative comparison between adenomatous and hyperplastic parathyroid glands. Eur J Nucl Med. 1986;12:31–36.
5. Brennan, MF, Doppman, H, Krudy, AG, Marx, SJ, Spiegel, AM, Aurbach, GD. Assessment of techniques for preoperative parathyroid localization in patients undergoing surgery for hyperparathyroidism. Surgery. 1982;91:6–11.
6. Brennan, MF, Norton, JA. Reoperation for persistent and recurrent hyperparathyroidism. Ann Surg. 1985;201:40–44.
7. Buchwach, KA, Mangum, WB, Hahn, FW jr. Preoperative localization of parathyroid adenomas. Laryngoscope. 1987;97:13–15.
8. Clark, OH, Okerlund, MD, Moss, AA, et al. Localization studies in patients with persistent or recurrent hyperparathyroidism. Surgery. 1985;98:1083–1094.
9. Doppman, JL, Shawker, TH, Krudy, AG, et al. Parathymic parathyroid: CT, US, and angiographic findings. Radiology. 1985;157:419–423.
10. Edis, AJ, Beahrs, OH, Sheddy. Reoperation for hyperparathyroidism. World J Surg. 1977;1:731–738.
11. Friedrichs, R, Behrendt, U, Gräf, K, Christians, T, Borgmann, V, Nagel, R. Primärer Hyperparathyreoidismus: Untersuchungen bei 4000 mit der ESWL behandelten Harnsteinpatienten. Helv Chir Acta. 1991;58:327–330.
12. Gooding, GAW, Okerlund, MD, Stark, DD, Clark, OH. Parathyroid imaging: comparison of double tracer (Tl-201, Tc-99m) scintigraphy and high resolution US. Radiology. 1986;161:57–64.
13. Grant, CS, van Heerden, JA, Charboneau, JW, James, EM, Reading, CC. Clinical management of persistent and/or recurrent primary hyperparathyroidism. World J Surg. 1986;10:555–565.
14. Higgins, CB, Auffermann, W. MR imaging of thyroid and parathyroid glands: A review of current status. Am J Roentgenol. 1988;151:1095–1106.
15. Itoh, K. Study of localization of hyperfunctioning parathyroid glands by ^{201}Tl-^{99}mTc subtraction scintigraphy. Hokkaido Igaku Zasshi. 1984;59:701–720.
16. Jarhult, J, Kristoffersson, A, Lundstrom, B, Oberg, L. Comparison of ultrasonography and computed tomography in preoperative location of parathyroid adenomas. Acta Chir Scand. 1985;151:583–587.
17. Kang, YS, Rosen, K, Clark, O, Higgins, CB. MR imaging for preoperative localization of mediastinal parathyroid adenomas. Radiology. 1992;185P:119.
18. Karstrup, S, Hegedus, L. Concomitant thyroid disease in hyperparathyroidism: reasons for unsatisfactory ultrasonographical localization of parathyroid glands. Eur J Radiol. 1986;6:149–152.
19. Kim, EE, Abello, R, Haynie, TP, Lamki, LM, Podoloff, DA. Complementary roles of radionuclide scintigraphy and magnetic resonance imaging in evaluating parathyroid adenomas and paragangliomas. J Nucl Med. 1988;29:277.
20. Kneeland, JB, Krubsack, AJ, Lawson, TL, et al. Enlarged parathyroid glands: high resolution local coil MR imaging. Radiology. 1987;162:143–146.
21. Krubsack, AJ, Wilson, SD, Lawson, TL, Collier, BD, Hellman, RS, Isitman, AT. Prospective comparison of radionuclide, computed tomographic, and sonographic localization of parathyroid tumors. World J Surg. 1986;10:579–585.
22. Krudy, AG, Shawker, TH, Doppman, JL, et al. Ultrasonic parathyroid localization in previously operated patients. Clin Radiol. 1984;35:113–118.

23. Levin, KD, Gooding, GAW, Okerlund, MD, et al. Localizing studies in patients with persistent or recurrent hyperparathyroidism. Surgery. 1987;102:917–925.
24. Manni, A, Basarab, RM, Plourde, PV, Koivunen, D, Harrison, TS, Santen, RJ. Thallium-technetium parathyroid scan: a useful noninvasive technique for localization of abnormal parathyroid tissue. Arch Intern Med. 1986;146:1077–1080.
25. Miller, DL, Doppman JL, Shawker, TH, et al. Localization of parathyroid adenomas in patients who have undergone surgery. Part 1. Noninvasive imaging methods, Radiology. 1987; 162:133–137.
26. Mohr, R, Graif, M, Itzchak, Y, et al. Parathyroid localization. Sonographic-surgical correlation. Am Surg. 1985;51:286–290.
27. Moreau, JF, Dubost, C, Buy, JN, Ferry, J. Pre-operative detection of parathyroid adenomas with ultrasound echography. Nouv Presse Med. 1981;10:1923–1927.
28. Müller, HW, Montz, R, Schneider, C, Kruse, HP, Dietel, M, Schumpelick, V. Lokalisationsdiagnostik vergrößerter Nebenschilddrüsen: Die ^{201}Tc-^{99m}Tc-Subtraktionsszintigraphie im Vergleich zur 5-MHz-Sonographie. RÖFO. 1985;142:543–547.
29. Norton, JA, Shawker, TH, Jones, BL, et al. Intraoperative ultrasound and reoperative parathyroid surgery: an initial evaluation. World J Surg. 1986;10:631–639.
30. Okerlund, MD, Sheldon, K, Corpuz, S, et al. A new method with high sensitivity and specificity for localization of abnormal parathyroid glands. Ann Surg. 1984;200:388.
31. Ovenfors, C-O, Stark, D, Moss, A, Goldberg, H, Clark, O, Galante, M. Localization of parathyroid adenoma by computed tomography. J Comput Assist Tomogr. 1982;6:1094–1098.
32. Parr, JH, Tarkunde, I, Ramsay, I. The use of ultrasound in the localization of parathyroid glands in parathyroid disorders. Clin Radiology. 1983;34:395–400.
33. Parrott, NR, Rose, PG, Farndon, JR, Johnston, ID. Pre-operative localization of parathyroid tumors using static B scan ultrasonography. Br J Surg. 1984;71:856–858.
34. Peck, WW, Higgins, CB, Fisher, MR, Ling, M, Okerlund, MD, Clark, OH. Hyperparathyroidism: Comparison of MR imaging with radionuclide scanning. Radiology. 1987;163:415–420.
35. Percival, RC, Blake, GM, Urwin, GH, Talbot, CH, Williams, JL, Kanis, JA. Assessment of thallium-pertechnetate subtraction scintigraphy in hyperparathyroidism. Br J Radiol. 1985;58:131–135.
36. Picard, D, D'Amour, P, Carrier, L, Chartrand, R, Poisson, R. Localization of abnormal parathyroid gland(s) using thallium-201/iodine-123 subtraction scintigraphy in patients with primary hyperparathyroidism. Clin Nucl Med. 1987;12:61–64.
37. Reading, CC, Charboneau, JW, James, EM, et al. High-resolution parathyroid sonography. Am J Roentgenol. 1982;139:539–546.
38. Reading, CC, Charboneau, JW, James, EM, et al. Postoperative parathyroid highfrequency sonography: evaluation of persistent or recurrent hyperparathyroidism. Am J Roentgenol. 1985;144:399–402.
39. Scheible, W, Deutsch, AL, Leopold, GR. Parathyroid adenoma: accuracy of preoperative location by high-resolution real-time sonography. J Clin Ultrasound. 1981;9:325–330.
40. Simeone, JF, Daniels, GH, Mueller, PR, et al. High resolution real time sonography of the thyroid. Radiology. 1982;45:431–435.
41. Skibber, JM, Reynolds, JC, Spiegel, AM, et al. Computerized technetium/thallium scans and parathyroid reoperation. Surgery. 1985;98:1077–1082.
42. Sommer, B, Welter, HF, Spelsberg, F, Scherer, U, Lissner, J. Computed tomography for localizing enlarged parathyroid glands in primary hyperparathyroidism. J Comput Assist Tomogr. 1982;6:521–526.
43. Spritzer, CE, Gefter, WB, Hamilton, R, Greenberg, BM, Axel, L, Kressel, HY. Abnormal parathyroid glands: high-resolution MR imaging. Radiology. 1987;162:487–491.
44. Stark, DD, Gooding, GAW, Moss, AA, Clark, OH, Ovenfors, C-O. Parathyroid imaging: comparison of high-resolution CT and high-resolution sonography. Am J Roentgenol. 1983;141:633–638.
45. Stevens, S, Chang, JM, Clark, OH, Chang, PJ, Higgins, CB. Magnetic resonance imaging of hyperparathyroidism at 1.5T: Prospective and retrospective assessment. Am J Roentgenol. 1993;160:607.
46. Takagi, H, Tominaga, Y, Uchida, K, et al. Preoperative diagnosis of secondary hyperparathyroidism using computed tomography. J Comput Assist Tomogr. 1982;6:527–528.
47. Takebayashi, S, Matsui, K, Onohara, Y, Hidai, H. Sonography for early diagnosis of enlarged parathyroid glands in patients with secondary hyperparathyroiddism. Am J Roentgenol. 1987;148:911–914.
48. Tüngerthal, S, Braulke, P, Lang, J, Scheuermann, L. Darstellung vergrößerter Nebenschilddrüsen mit digitaler Subtraktionsangiographie bei 22 Patienten mit primärem oder sekundärem Hyperparathyreoidismus. Digitale Bilddiagn. 1985;5:40–47.
49. van Heerden, JA, James, EM, Karsell, PR, Charboneau, JW, Grant, CS, Purnell, DC. Small-part ultrasonography in primary hyperparathyroidism: initial experience. Ann Surg. 1982;195:774–780.
50. Vogl, T, Hefele, B, Hahn, D, Nieden, Z, Muhlig, HP. Results of a comparative study of MR, CT and sonography of patients with primary hyperparathyroidism. RÖFO. 1986;145:167–172.
51. Wang, C, Gaz, RD, Moncure, AC. Mediastinal parathyroid exploration: a clinical and pathologic study of 47 cases. World J Surg. 1986;10:687–695.
52. Welter, G, Welter, HF, Spelsberg, F. Präoperative sonographische Lokalisationsdiagnostik vergrößerter Nebenschilddrüsen bei Verdacht auf Hyperparathyreoidismus. Chirurg. 1981;52:385–388.
53. Whitley, NO, Bohlman, M, Connor, TB, McCrea, ES, Mason, GR, Whitley, JE. Computed tomography for localization of parathyroid adenomas. J Comput Assist Tomogr. 1981;6:812–817.
54. Winzelberg, GG, Hydowitz, JD, O'Hara, KR, et al. Parathyroid adenomas evaluated by Tl-201/Tc-99m pertechnetate subtraction scintigraphy and high resolution ultrasonography. Radiology. 1985;155:231–235.
55. Zocholl, G, Kuhn, FP, Kraus, WG, Wagner, P. High-resolution 7.5/10-MHz B-scan sonography for the localization of hyperparathyroid tumors. RÖFO. 1986;144:422–427.

A Surgeon's View

O. H. Clark

Numerous articles have been written describing the results of noninvasive studies to identify parathyroid tumors in patients with primary hyperparathyroidism. These studies include ultrasonography, thallium-technetium scanning, CT scanning, MRI scanning, and other procedures. Most patients, (approximately 80%), with primary hyperparathyroidism have a solitary adenoma. Such patients have about 75% of their parathyroid adenomas successfully identified by experienced radiologists when noninvasive localizing studies are performed using state-of-the-art equipment (1). In patients with hyperplasia, which occurs in about 15 % of patients on multiple adenomas, which occurs in approximately 4% of patients, localizing studies are only effective in approximately 30% of these patients (2). In such patients, surgeons who use a unilateral approach based on one or more localizing study may be led astray when more than one abnormal parathyroid gland is actually present. These patients will have persistent hyperparathyroidism. Thus, parathyroid localization tests can be both helpful, by directing a surgeon to the abnormal parathyroid gland, and misleading by giving a false sense of confidence leading to a "failed" operation because of not identifying and resecting enough of the abnormal parathyroid gland tissue.

When noninvasive localizing studies are used in combination, such as ultrasonography with MRI, or ultrasonography and thallium-technetium scanning, up to 90% of the parathyroid tumors can be identified (3). Although I am an advocate of using localizing studies in patients who have not had previous neck surgery and have primary hyperparathyroidism, I currently only use ultrasonography because this is the least expensive procedure. Prospective studies by Dr. Wilson's group in Wisconsin (4) have suggested that localizing studies do not improve the overall results of parathyroid operations and do not decrease the time required for the operation. In my experience, however, time is saved in the operating room when a tumor is identified by the localizing study. I explore the side where the tumor has been identified first, and once I see the abnormal parathyroid gland as well as a normal parathyroid gland, I remove the abnormal gland. During the time required to process and interpret the suspected abnormal parathyroid gland by frozen section, I explore the other side, saving 20–30 minutes, which are generally required for frozen section examination. The parathyroid operation is usually completed before the frozen section results return. Localizing studies, I believe, are also helpful for high-risk patients who have not had previous neck operations as localization studies sometimes expedite the procedure and should therefore be advantageous for critically ill patients. Parathyroid localization tests also occasionally identify parathyroid tumors situated in ectopic positions.

Localizing studies are most useful, however, in patients who have had failed parathyroid operations or previous thyroid surgery because the normal tissue layers are often ablated because of scar formation. Also, many of these patients may have one or more parathyroid tumors situated in an ectopic position. In the latter group of patients with recurrent or persistent hyperthyroidism, I usually first perform ultrasound, thallium-technetium scanning, and MRI scanning (Sestimibi scanning has now replaced thallium-technetium scanning). These procedures complement each other. Ultrasound is best for lesions immediately adjacent to the thyroid or within the thyroid gland. Thallium-technetium or Sestimibi scanning is quite good for parathyroid tumors situated in ectopic positions although it occasionally misses large tumors. CT and MRI scanning are excellent for identifying large lesions and lesions in the superior mediastinum (5). When these studies are negative, in conflict, or equivocal, I do highly selective venous catheterization for PTH assay. The results of this study, when combined with the equivocal noninvasive localizing studies, have proved to be the most sensitive localization test. Percutaneous aspiration biopsy under ultrasonographic guidance for cytological examination and PTH assay is also valuable in patients who have had failed parathyroid operations.

The marked improvement and success rate reported in patients requiring reoperation for hyperparathyroidism is in great part due to the tremendous help in tumor identification we receive from these localizing studies. I might add that in reoperative surgery, in contrast to initial operative procedures, I usually do not reexplore the entire neck and upper mediastinum for fear of injuring normal parathyroid glands. Also, in patients requiring reoperation, one can, in general, determine whether a patient will have just one or several abnormal glands based on the previous operative note(s), pathology report(s), and localization studies (5). In this latter group of patients, intraoperative PTH determination is useful for documenting successful completion of the operation, although a false sense of security is occasionally obtained (6).

When a multidisciplinary approach is used involving radiologists, endocrinologists, nuclear medicine physicians, and surgeons to treat patients with persistent or recurrent hyperparathyroidism, more patients seem to benefit and success rates are higher than 90%. In conclusion, although an experienced endocrine surgeon can identify the abnormal parathyroid gland(s) in about 98% of patients who have not had previous parathyroid or thyroid surgery, localization tests are very helpful and can expedite the operation procedure. They are essential for patients requiring parathyroid reoperation.

References

1 Clark, OH, Duh, QY. Primary hyperparathyroidism: A surgical perspective. Endocriol Metab Clin North Am. 1989;18(3):701–714.
2 Duh, QY, Sancho, JJ, Clark, OH. Parathyroid localization. Acta Chir Scand. 1987;153:241–254.
3 Gooding, GAW, Okerlund, MD, Stark, DD, Clark, OH. Parathyroid imaging: Comparison of double tracer (T1-201-Tc^{99m}). Scintigraphy and high resolution sonography. Radiology. 1986;10:787–796.
4 Krubsack, AJ, Wilson, SD, Lawson, TL, et al. Prospective comparison of radionucleide, computed tomographic sonographic and magnetic resonance localization of parathyroid tumors. Surgery. 1989;106(4):639–644.
5 Levin, KE, Gooding, GAW, Okerlund, MD, et al. Advances in localizing studies (MRI, ultrasound, CT, Thallium-technetium scanning) in patients with persistent and recurrent hyperparathyroidism. Surgery. 1987;102:915–917.
6 Proye, CAG, Goropoulos, A, Tranz, C, et al. Usefulness and limits of quick intraoperative measurements of intact (I-84) parathyroid hormone in the surgical management of hyperparathyroidism: Sequential measurements in patients with multiglandular disease. Surgery. 1991;110(6):1035–1042.

5 Adrenal Gland

Anatomy

J. Staudt

The retroperitoneally located, paired adrenal glands are embedded in an adipose capsule at the upper renal pole. The right adrenal gland is flat and triangular, whereas the left adrenal gland usually has a more rounded shape. The posterior face neighbors the lumbar part of the diaphragm and borders ventrally the intraperitoneal organs at the level of the 11th thoracic vertebral body. Their location is often at the same level as the upper pole of the kidney. The adrenal

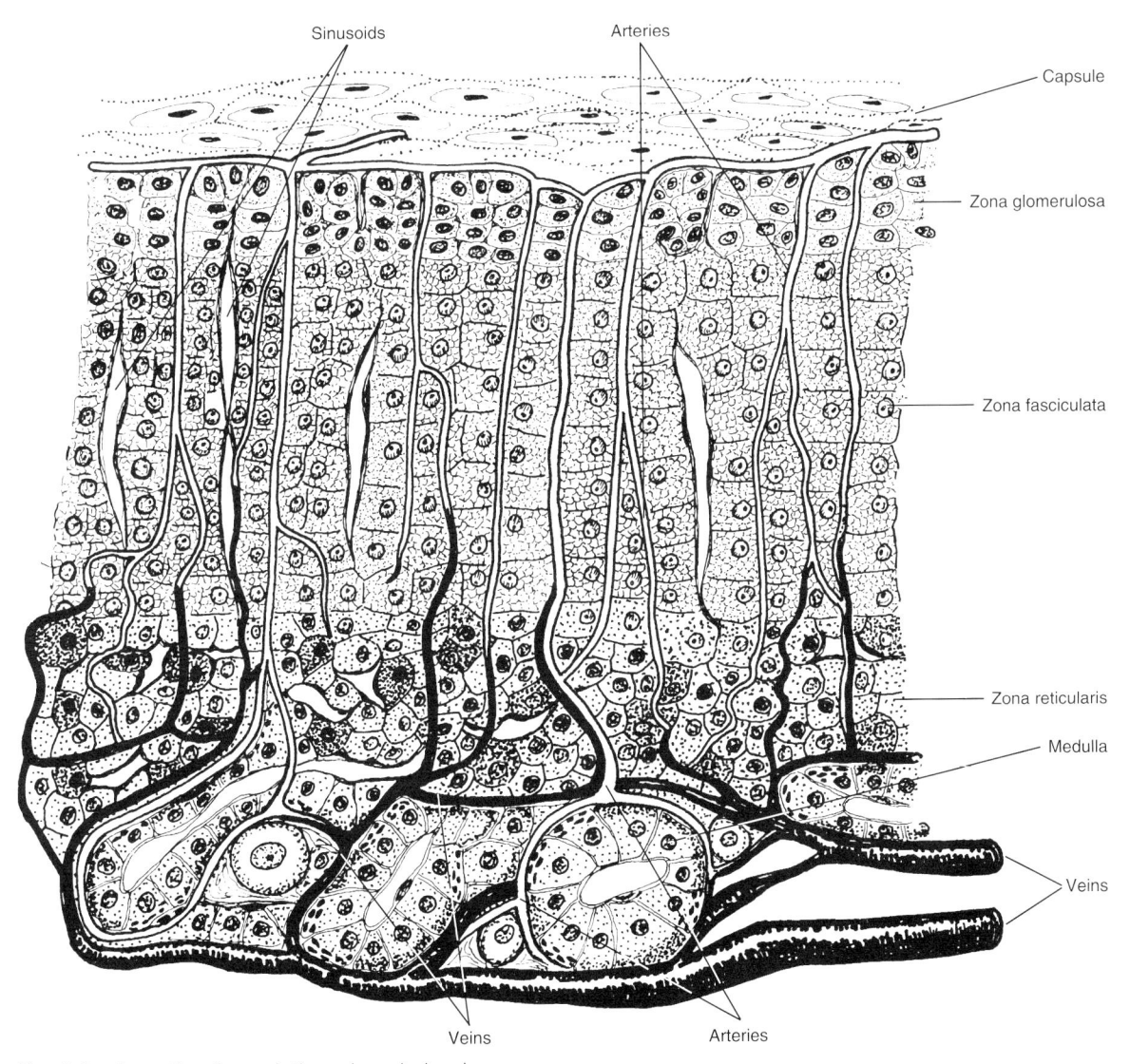

Fig. 5.1 A section through the adrenal gland

gland measures 4–6 cm in length, 2–3 cm in width and 1–3 cm in depth. Its weight is about 10 g. In the section, the cortex fills 90% of the area and can be differentiated from the medulla, which occupies only 10% of the sectional area.

Embryologically, the cortex originates from the gonadal anlage, separates early, but remains in its original retroperitoneal position. The medulla, however, develops from the ectodermal sympathetic anlage with chromaffinoblastic cells, which migrate into the adrenal cortex. If they do not reach the adrenal gland, sympathic retroperitoneal paraganglia develop. The difference between these two, apparently merged organs is most obviously manifested in their microscopic architecture. There is an additional remodeling of the adrenal cortex during its lifetime. The typical three-fold stratification is reached in puberty, and is then followed by the domination of the middle zone after the age of 50. The parenchyma of the adrenal cortex consists of regular, yellow, epithelial columns. The zona glomerulosa lies subcapsular and contains typical clues of acidophil cells, which produce the mineralocorticoid hormones. The space between the densely packed glandular cells is filled with wide sinusoid capillaries (Fig. 5.1).

The middle zone is the widest of the three layers and consists of parallel cellular columns that are perpendicular to the organ surface. The mature, yellow color is most prominent in this zone where glucocorticoid and, in smaller amounts, sexual hormones are produced. The reticular zone lies more centrally, where small cellular columns are connected like a network. Epithelial cells are smaller and contain pigmented granula with older age. Hormone production of the zona reticularis equals that of the zona fasciculata.

The medulla contains epinephrine- and adrenaline-producing cells that exhibit a chromaffin reaction. The medulla is characterized by wide capillaries and multiple, multipolar gangliocytes originating from the splanchnic nerve. Each adrenal gland is supplied by three groups of arteries: the superior adrenal arteries (up to 30) from the posterior division of the inferior phrenic artery, the medial adrenal artery from the suprarenal part of the abdominal aorta (usually a single artery), and the inferior adrenal artery from the proximal renal artery. There are multiple variants of arterial supply (Fig. 5.2). All three groups of arteries form a subcapsular vascular plexus of around 50 branches, which run from the cortex to the medulla. The cortical arterial branches form sinusoids that flow into the venous system at the level of the corticomedullary border. Therefore, the cortex does not contain veins. The arterial branches arrive via the septa directly at the medulla, where they embrace the chromaffin cells and arbitrate. Within the medulla, all veins unite into a single central vein, which exits the hilum as the suprarenal vein. The right suprarenal vein drains directly into the inferior vena cava, whereas the left suprarenal vein flows first into the left renal vein.

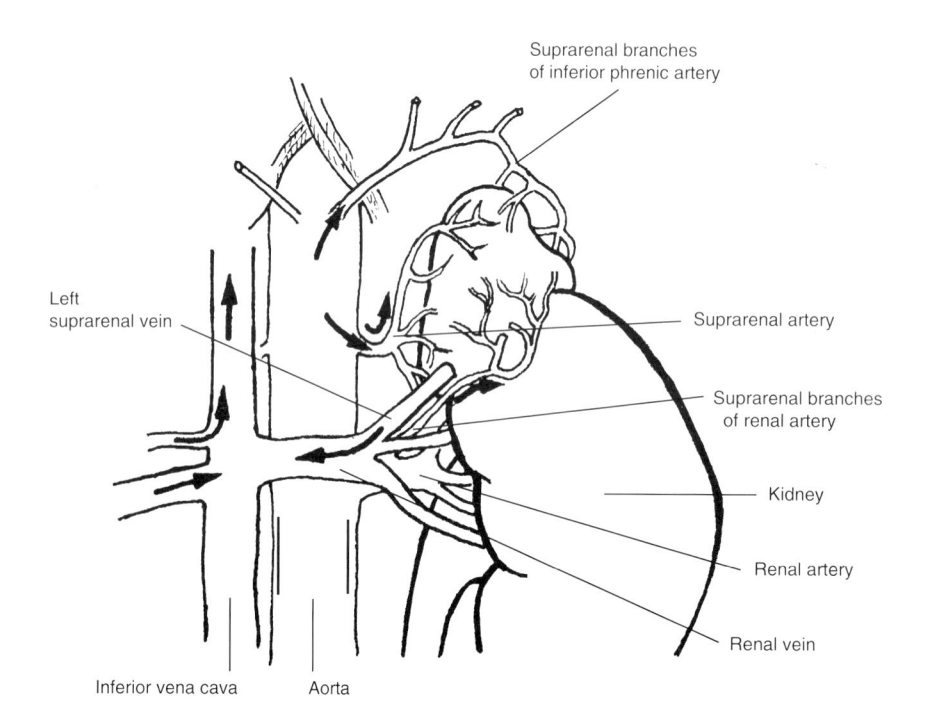

Fig. 5.2 Blood vessels of the suprarenal gland

Endocrinology

K.-J. Gräf

Physiology

Like that of the ovaries, the testes, and the thyroid, the secretion of hormones by the adrenal cortex is subject to the complex mechanisms of the hypothalamic–pituitary regulatory axis (see Fig. 2.**2**; Chapter 2). The mineralocorticoids, the main representative of which is aldosterone, are synthesized and secreted in the glomerular zone, while the synthesis and secretion of glucocorticoid steroids and androgens take place in the zona fasciculata and reticularis.

Mineralocorticoid synthesis is stimulated mainly by angiotensin II and, to a lesser extent, by ACTH, potassium, and serotonin. Dopamine inhibits aldosterone synthesis and secretion. The secretion of angiotensin II is regulated by the renin system (Fig. 5.**3**).

The biosynthesis and secretion of the glucocorticoids and androgenic steroids of the adrenal cortex are regulated primarily by ACTH (Fig. 2.**4**, Chapter 3, and Fig. 5.**4**).

The main effects of the mineralocorticoids are summarized in Table 5.**1** (see also Chapter 3).

The chromaffin cells of the adrenal medulla synthesize, store, and secrete the catecholamines adrenaline and noradrenaline. They also produce opioid peptides, e.g., enkephalins. The synthesis of catecholamines is regulated by cortical steroids and other, still unknown substances of which the secretion is mainly under the control of sympathetic nerves.

Table 5.**1** Symptomatology of hyperaldosteronism

Arterial hypertension
Hypokalemia (not obligatory)
Myasthenia
Tiredness
Proteinuria
Hyposthenuria
Polyuria, polydipsia
ECG changes
Hypernatremia
Headache
Cardiomegaly

Hyperaldosteronism

Primary hyperaldosteronism is defined as the increased autonomous production of aldosterone (Conn syndrome), usually due to adenomatous changes but, very rarely, to carcinomas as well.

So-called idiopathic hyperaldosteronism is caused by bilateral hyperplasia of the adrenal cortex, the

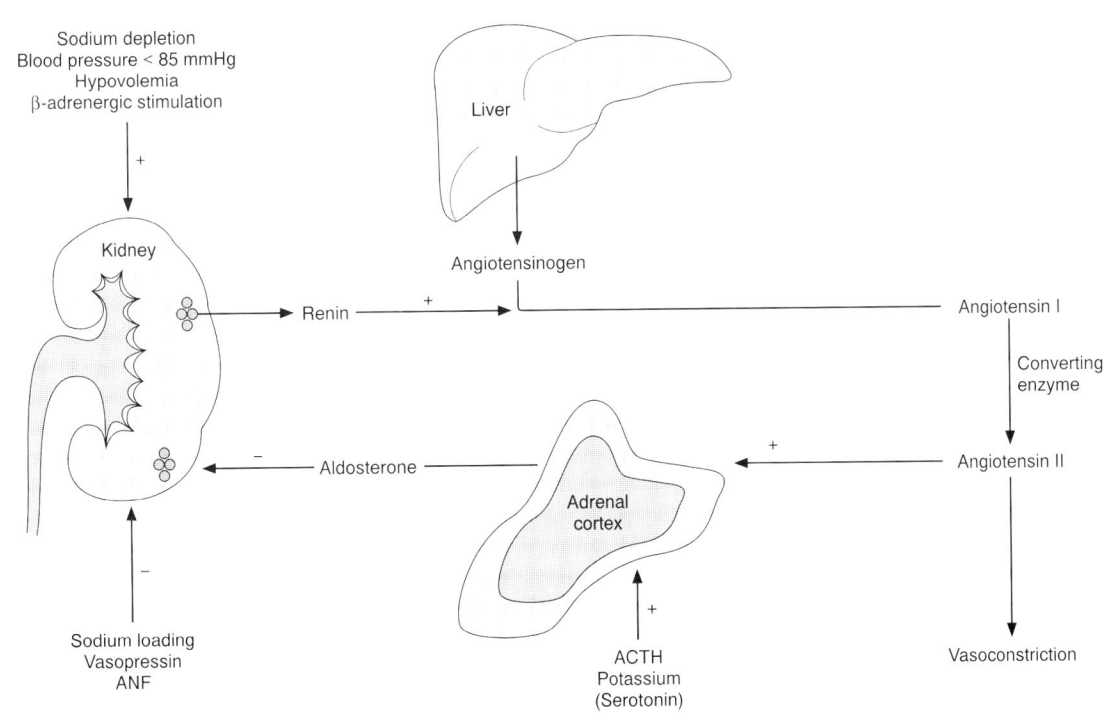

Fig. 5.**3** Mineralocorticoid synthesis

cause of which is still unclear. Secondary hyperaldosteronism is caused by increased production of renin angiotensin and is therefore not a primary disease of the adrenal cortex itself.

The symptomatology of hyperaldosteronism is characterized by arterial hypertension and the usually present hypokalamia (see Table 5.1). A diagnostic pointer, apart from the arterial hypertension and non-obligatory hypokalemia together with resulting metabolic alkalosis is the combination of the endocrinological findings of an increased aldosterone concentration with simultaneous suppression of plasma renin activity (important differentiation from secondary hyperaldosteronism, in which an increase of plasma renin activity is obligatory). The main morphological diagnostic measures are contrast-enhanced CT with complementary aldosterone or cholesterol scintigraphy.

The therapy of choice for an andrenocortical tumor with hyperaldosteronismus is tumor excision. Aldosterone antagonists (spironolactone) can be used for conservative therapy. The use of aldosterone antagonists is also the therapy of choice in bilateral adrenocortical hyperplasia with hyperaldosteronism.

Hypoaldosteronism

A deficiency of aldosterone—a rare disease—can be caused by congenital enzyme defects, e.g., in 21-hydroxylase deficiency with sodium loss syndrome (see Congenital Adrenal Hyperplasia), by the various forms of adrenocortical insufficiency, iatrogenically (secondary to bilateral adrenalectomy), or medicinally (e.g., heparin).

Various causes of a secondary aldosterone deficiency (e.g., as a consequence of chronic nephropathy) must be differentiated from primary hypoaldosteronism. The diagnosis requires the demonstration of reduced aldosterone secretion and hypereninemia.

Hypercortisolism (Cushing Syndrome)

Hypercortisolism is an increase of serum glucocorticoids of any origin. The differential diagnosis must distinguish between Cushing disease (the ACTH-producing adenoma of the anterior pituitary), iatrogenic hypercortisolism (e.g., due to glucocorticoid medication), and primary autonomous (i.e., not pituitary-controlled) overproduction of glucocorticosteroids by the adrenal cortex. The possible main causes of primary hypercortisolism are, on the one hand, benign adenomas of the adrenal cortex and, on the other, rarely, carcinomas. The diagnosis always requires endocrinological demonstration of increased glucocorticosteroid secretion, e.g., by quantitative determination of glucocorticoid secretion in 24-hour urine or by functional diagnosis with dexamethasone. The most important parameter for differentiating between primary hypercortisolism and secondary or iatrogenic hypercortisolism is the determination of ACTH, which is suppressed in primary and iatrogenic, and increased in pituitary-dependent hypercortisolism. The symptomatology of Cushing syndrome, is very much the same as the of Cushing disease (see Chapter 2). In patients with adrenocortical adenomas and, particularly, carcinomas with hypercortisolism, however, the clinical symptoms can vary widely because of the underlying disease. In addition to endocrinological diagnosis, imaging procedures such as sonography, contrast-enhanced CT, and possibly also scintigraphic examination methods (cholesterol scintigraphy) are helpful in locating the lesion. The therapy of choice in primary hypercortisolism is tumor excision. Second-line therapy is the administration of drugs that inhibit corticosteroid secretion, e.g., mitotane, metyrapone, ketoconazole, aminoglutethimide, and others.

Hypocorticoidism (Hypoadrenocorticism)

Hypocorticoidism is defined as a reduced secretion of glucocorticosteroids by the adrenal cortex. Primary hypocorticoidism (Addison disease) is based on a disease of the adrenal cortices themselves, while secondary hypocorticoidism is caused by reduced glucocorticosteroid secretion due to reduced ACTH stimulation. The clinical symptomatology is independent of the cause of hypocorticoidism (see Table 5.2).

Increased cutaneous pigmentation (brown hand creases), particularly in areas exposed to light, is demonstrable only in primary hypocorticoidism (due to increased melanocyte-stimulating hormone [MSH] secretion) and not in the secondary form (so-called white Addison).

Primary hypocorticoidism is usually caused by autoimmune processes; previously, a frequent cause was tuberculosis. Numerous drugs, e.g., aminoglutethimide, ketoconazole, and others, can also inhibit glucocorticosteroid synthesis by way of various mechanisms. Other causes, e.g., meningococcal sep-

Table 5.2 Symptoms of adrenocortical insufficiency (hypocorticoidism)

General weakness and fatigue
Weight loss, anorexia
Hypotension, dizziness, tendency to collapse
Abdominal complaints
   pain, vomiting, nausea, diarrhea, constipation
Elektrolyte disturbances
   hyponatremia, hyperkalemia, salt graving
Muscle and joint pain
Reduced pubic and axillary hair
Vitiligo, hyperpigmentation (facultative)

sis (Waterhouse–Friderichsen syndrome), infiltrations of various causes, and others, are extremely rare. Secondary hypocorticoidism is almost always caused by anterior lobe insufficiency (e.g., mostly due to a pituitary adenoma or prolonged high-dosage glucocorticosteroid therapy).

The demonstration of reduced serum hydrocortisone secretion is essential to confirm the diagnosis. ACTH secretion is increased in primary hypocorticoidsm, but decreased in the secondary form. The therapy of choice is replacement with hydrocortisone.

Untreated adrenocortical insufficiency can lead to an Addison crisis, a life-threatening deterioration of this disease, frequently triggered by infections, with psychic and neurological complications as well as severe hypovolemia, circulatory shock, and renal failure.

Congenital Adrenal Hyperplasia (CAH)

CAH is caused by various congenital autosomally recessive hereditary enzyme defects of steroid biosynthesis by the adrenal cortex. The most common cause of CAH is 21-hydroxylase deficiency, which accounts for 95% of cases, followed by 11-β-hydroxylase deficiency (4%), and some very rare enzyme defects such as 3-β-hydroxysteroid dehydrogenase deficiency, 17-hydroxylase deficiency, 17,20-lyase deficiency, and others (see Fig. 5.4). Increased ACTH and androgen production is common to 21-hydroxylase deficiency and 11-β-hydroxylase deficiency in addition to reduced glucocorticosteroid secretion. About two-thirds of patients with 21-hydroxylase deficiency may also display reduced synthesis of mineralocorticosteroids, which leads to sodium-loss syndrome. The late onset type, a mild form of 21-hydroxylase deficiency, does not become clinically manifest until after puberty. This mild heterozygous enzyme defect, which is never associated with the sodium-loss syndrome, is one of the most common causes of increased androgen production, and 11-hydroxylase deficiency is similar. The main symptoms are, in girls, signs of virilization, particularly of the external genitals, and, in both sexes, rapid postnatal growth with premature closure of the epiphysial cartilages and resultant short stature. Sexual hair growth is increased. Hirsutism and ovarian insufficiency with amenorrhea develop in women, and men display all the symptoms of hypogonadotropic hypogonadism.

Hypotensive dehydration with hyponatremia and hyperkalemia predominates in patients with sodium-loss syndrome, whereas hypokalemic hypertension is characteristic for the 11-hydroxylase deficiency.

Where treatment is indicated at all, the therapy of all forms of CAH consists of the suppression of ACTH secretion by replacement with hydrocortisone and, in mineralocorticoid deficiency, by simultaneous replacement with fludrocortisone.

Steroid biosynthesis in the adrenal cortex

Mineralocorticoid — Glucocorticoid — Androgens

Cholesterol
↓ *Desmolase*
Δ^5-Pregnenolone —*17α-Hydroxylase*→ 17α-OH-pregnenolone —*17,20-Lyase*→ Dehydroepiandrosterone DHEA

3β-OH-Δ^5-steroid dehydrogenase; steroidisomerase | *3β-OH-Δ^5-steroid dehydrogenase; steroidisomerase* | *3β-OH-Δ^5-steroid dehydrogenase; steroidisomerase*

Progesterone —*17β-Hydroxylase*→ 17α-OH-progesterone —*17,20-Lyase*→ Δ^4-Androstenedione

↓ *21-Hydroxylase* | ↓ *21-Hydroxylase* | ↓ *17β-OH-steroid dehydrogenase*

11-Deoxycorticosterone (DOC) | 11-Deoxycortisol | Testosterone

↓ *11β-Hydroxylase* | ↓ *11β-Hydroxylase*

Corticosterone | Hydrocortisone

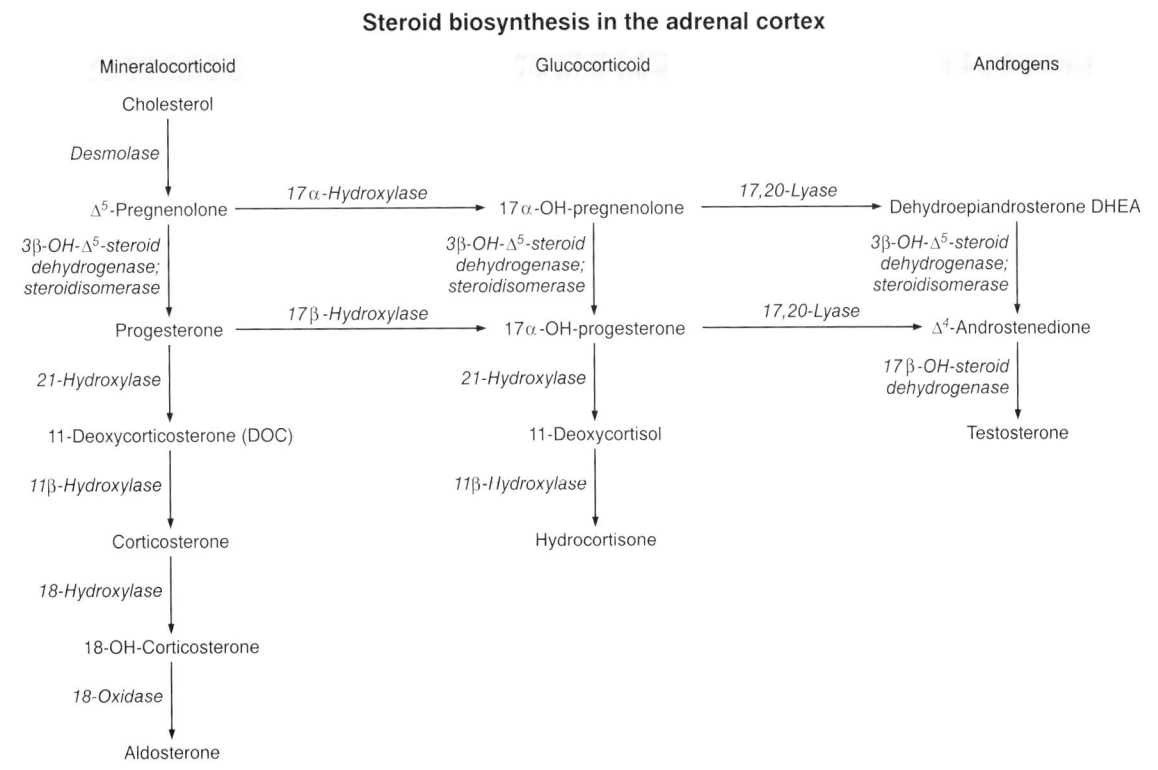

↓ *18-Hydroxylase*

18-OH-Corticosterone

↓ *18-Oxidase*

Aldosterone

Fig. 5.**4** Steroid biosynthesis in the adrenal cortex

Adrenocortical Tumors

The most common adrenocortical tumor is the "incidentaloma." These tumors are usually diagnosed by chance during abdominal sonography or CT. They are clinically asymptomatic, although usually slight endocrine activity is demonstrable in many cases during the diagnosis of endocrinological function. These benign adenomas, particularly those up to 3 cm in diameter, do not generally require treatment. Instead, sonographic follow-up is sufficient.

Hormonally active adenomas and carcinomas, and hormonally inactive carcinomas and metastases from other carcinomas must be distinguished in the differential diagnosis from the "incidentaloma." Where there is a reasonable clinical suggestion, the diagnosis must include increased endocrine activity due to an increased secretion of estrogens, androgens, glucocorticoids, mineralocorticoids, or catecholamine. Important aids in the further clarification of the nature of an andrenocortical tumor—particularly necessary for those that are more than 3 cm in diameter—are MRI, scintigraphy, angiography and computer-guided puncture with subsequent histological assessment of the tumor tissue.

With a yearly incidence of 1 per 1.5 million people, adrenocortical carcinoma is, overall, a very rare disease. It becomes clinically manifest only by virtue of its endocrine activity or its invasive growth. The main symptoms of the rare estrogen-producing adenomas and carcinomas in men are gynecomastia and testicular atrophy. The demonstration of increased estrogen production is often difficult in women. An increased common secretion of estrogen, androgen, and corticoids has also been demonstrated in a few cases. Far more frequent are glucocorticoid- and mineralocorticoid-producing adenomas and carcinomas, pheochromocytomas, and paragangliomas (see Adrenal medulla). The therapy of choice in hormonally active adenomas and in carcinomas of the adrenal cortex is tumor excision. It is of importance that a pheochromocytoma is ruled out preoperatively. The tumor region should always be irradiated after excision of large carcinomas in order to prevent local recurrence. Adrenolytic mitotane therapy is available for the medicinal therapy of glucocorticosteroid-producing adrenocortical carcinomas (e.g., in metastases or in tumor resection). Treatment with etoposide and cisplatin, doxorubicin, or with suramin can be attempted as an alternative in cases which do not respond to treatment with mitotane.

Hypertrichosis and Hirsutism

Hirsutism is defined as the occurrence of male-pattern hair in women. Hypertrichosis and virilization should be distinguished from this. Hypertrichosis is defined as increased hair growth over the whole body, usually as an idiovariation. While hypertrichosis constitutes an increase in the number of body hairs, hirsutism is characterized by the increased growth of terminal hair at typically male sites of predilection. The severity and extent of hirsutism are assessed using the classification proposed by Ferriman and Gallway, who used a scale of 0–4 for the severity of hirsutism. A total of nine hormone-dependent body areas is assessed: the upper lip, the chin region, the presternal region, the upper and lower abdominal region, the upper arms, the insides of the thighs, the thoracodorsal region and the lumbosacral region including the buttocks. The causes listed in Table 5.3 must be distinguished pathophysiologically.

The therapy of hirsutism depends entirely on the cause. Tumor excision is obviously required on demonstration of an adrenocortical or ovarian tumor with clinical symptoms. Hyperandrogenemia can be treated with, for example, antiandrogens, progestogen–estrogen combinations, or with corticosteroids.

Table 5.3 Causes of hirsutism

Adrenal causes
  Androgen-producing adenoma
  Androgen-producing carcinoma
  Adrenogenital syndrome
  Congenital adrenal hyperplasia
Ovarian causes
  Androgen-producing tumors
  Polycystic ovary syndrome (Stein–Levanthal syndrome
  Ovarian hyperthecosis
Acromegaly
Hyperprolactinemia
Hypercorticoidism
  (Cushing disease, Cushing syndrome)
Obesity
Menopause
Drugs

Adrenal Medulla

Pheochromocytoma

Pheochromocytoma is a benign (90%) or malignant (10%) neuroendocrine tumor (paraganglioma) of chromaffin cells in the adrenal medulla (90%), where it appears more often on the right side than on the left. It can also be a sympathetic paravertebral ganglioma, which appears in the region of the inferior mesenteric artery at the level of the aortic bifurcation, or Zuckerkandl bodies (10%). A distinction is made between sporadic (usually unilateral) and familial forms (frequently bilateral), which can occur in isolation or in association with MEN type IIa or III, or with the Hippel–Lindau syndrome (cerebellar hemangioblastoma with retinal angioma), and neurofibromatosis.

The incidence of pheochromocytoma is reported to be 1 per 1 million/year. It can occur at any age, but is seen more frequently in patients between the ages of 50 and 70.

Adrenal pheochromocytomas produce adrenaline and noradrenaline; the extraadrenal form usually produce only noradrenaline. The main clinical symptoms are palpitations, headache, tendency to perspire, weight loss, and episodic or manifest hypertension (incidence in hypertension about 0.1%). Specific diagnostic measures are required in the presence of the above-mentioned typical constellation of symptoms before surgery for a suprarenal tumor, in a suggested familial disposition, in hypertension recalcitrant to drug therapy, and in very young hypertensive patients. The determination of vanillylmandelic acid and metanephrine is inadequate on its own as a diagnostic tool; catecholamines in 24-hour urine should be measured also (repeatedly if necessary). MIBG scintigraphy should be performed in doubtful cases or in the event of pathologically elevated concentrations of catecholamines and their metabolites or both. Scintigraphy is preferable to MRI which, in turn, is superior to CT. Angiography is generally unnecessary.

Therapy, consists of surgical removal of the tumor. Pharmacotherapy should consist of α-blockers and, after adequate α-blockade, of β-blockers also. Before undergoing surgery for a pheochromocytoma, the patient must be treated with α-blockers for a sufficiently long period.

Ultrasound

L. Abet

Investigative Technique

The investigation and visualization of the adrenal glands through abdominal ultrasound is still a task that requires a great deal of skill and experience. Success is more dependent on the constitution of the patient, the quality of the equipment, and the skill of the investigator than for other organs. The patient should not eat before the investigation and should avoid foods or drinks that cause flatulence for three days before the investigation.

Sector or convex-array transducers with a frequency of 3–5 MHz are most suitable. Linear transducers are theoretically possible, but make access to the adrenal region more difficult. The patient is supine **and** positioned obliquely or laterally with a prop under the respective flank. Access to the right adrenal region is possible from a subcostal paramedian position as well as from a lateral intercostal position between the front and middle axillary line. The region of the left adrenal gland is accessible from a medial epigastric position as well as from a lateral intercostal position at the level of the posterior axillary line. When examining laterally from the right, the right lobe of the liver is used as an acoustic window; to see the left adrenal gland, the left lobe of the liver or the spleen serves as an acoustic window. In each of these four acoustic directions, transverse and longitudinal scans are acquired, inspiration and expiration are used to locate the optimal acoustic window.

Landmarks for finding the adrenal glands are the inferior vena cava, the upper kidney pole and the dorsal and caudal margin of the liver on the right, and, the aorta, the upper kidney pole, and the tail of the pancreas and the splenic vein or both on the left.

Normal Findings

Provided that high-resolution equipment and subtle examination technique is used, the normal adrenal glands can be identified with a reliability of between 70% and 97%. Because of the physiological hyperplasia, delineation of the adrenal glands is almost always possible in newborns. The hypoechoic cortex can be differentiated from the hyperechoic medulla (Fig. 5.**5**).

In adults, the definite visualization of normal adrenal glands as a poorly echogenic structure is considerably more difficult because of the lesser degree of impedance to the surrounding perirenal fat tissue. The right adrenal gland is easier to identify than the left. A differentiation of cortex and medulla is rarely possible.

Pathology

An adrenal gland tumor is always seen as a less echogenic mass in comparison to the retroperitoneal fat, irrespective of its malignancy or histological composition. The only exception is the rare myelolipoma (Fig. 5.**6**).

If the conditions of investigation (equipment technology, constitution of patient) are optimal, and the adrenal gland position is defined by the above-mentioned landmarks and no structure of reduced echogenicity to the surrounding structures can be delineated, an adrenal hyperplasia or an adrenal tumor of 2 cm or more in size can be excluded reliably.

On the other hand, an "empty" adrenal location does not justify the diagnosis of adrenal atrophy. **Adrenal atrophy,** including possible small speckled calcifications, may either be seen with difficulty in sonography or not at all. Therefore, Addison disease, hypopituitarism, autoimmune idiopathic adrenal atrophy, as well as chronic inflammation and corticoid therapy causing adrenal atrophy are not indications for sonography. On the other hand, to exclude hemorrhage or malignomas as the cause of hormonal defi-

136   5 Adrenal Gland

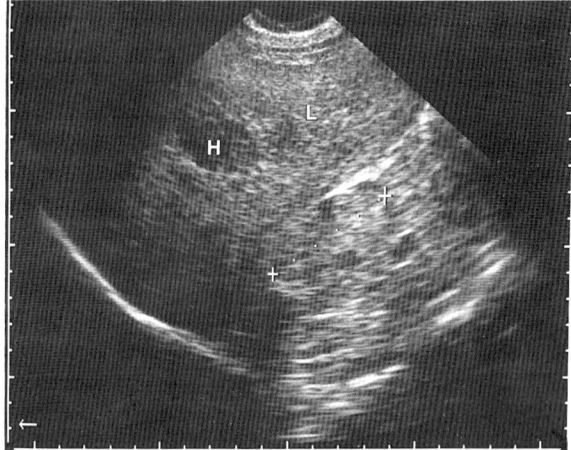

Fig. 5.6 Oblique section of an adenolipoma of the right adrenal gland (+...+) presenting as a hyperechoic tumor in a steatotic liver (L) with hypoechoic areas, smooth outer contour, 5.5 × 2.5 cm size. H = liver hemangioma

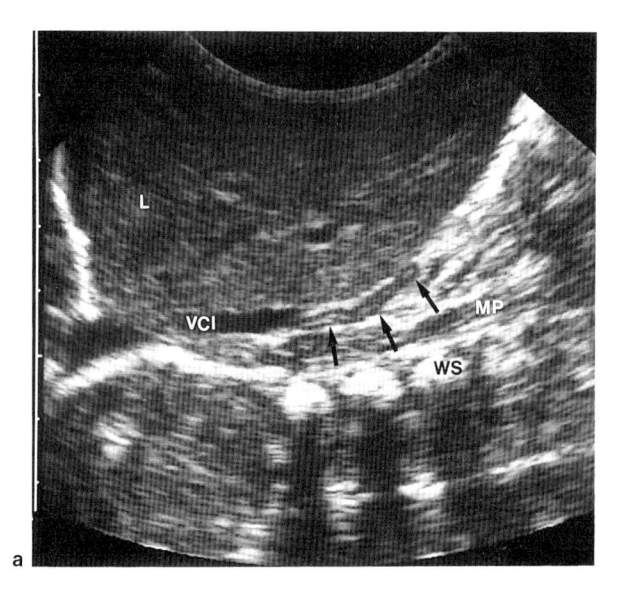

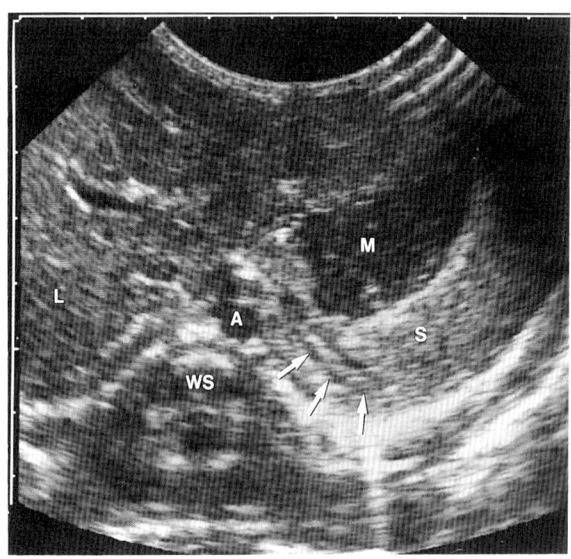

Fig. 5.5 Normal adrenal gland of a three-year-old newborn with echogenic marrow reflex and hypoechoic cortex. (**a**) Longitudinal section, (**b**) transverse section. L = liver, WS = vertebral bone, MP = psoas muscle, VCI = inferior vena cava, A = aorta, M = stomach

ciencies, sonography should be part of the basic diagnostic spectrum.

In **hyperplasia,** the adrenal glands retain their typical configuration in sonography, and a differentiation of cortex and medulla should be possible (Fig. 5.7). Findings generally appear bilaterally. If the medulla cannot be visualized as a central echogenic band, then it must be assumed that there is a mass that requires further investigation. Differentiation between homogeneous hyperplasia and the nodular, nonhomogeneous form is not always reliable in sonography.

Hemorrhages show varying echogenicity depending on age and size. In newborns especially, they are sometimes bilaterally seen as anechoic, inhomogeneous, or homogeneous masses. In the follow-up, the findings become smaller and echogenicity of the margins increases, sometimes combined with calicifications. Full recovery is also possible (Fig. 5.**8**).

In contrast to tumorous infiltration, the pyramid-shaped configuration of the organ is usually retained even with larger hemorrhages. Nevertheless, in the perinatal period the suggestion of adrenal hemorrhage must always bring to mind the differential diagnosis of neuroblastoma. Early bleeding and necrosis of the tumor may lead to a similar echogenicity as in hematoma.

Pseudocysts, resulting from hemorrhages or necrosis, parasitic and genuine **cysts,** and adenomas that have degenerated to cysts appear as round or oval, echofree structures with smooth margins and a relative enhancement of the posterior echo. They are usually less than 3 cm in size. From a differential diagnostic view, hemorrhage or liver, kidney, or pancreas cysts must be excluded. Greater mobility during breathing compared with the adjacent organs usually make it possible to accurately trace the structure to the organ of origin.

Hemangiomas (Fig. 5.**9**), lymphangiomas, and **granulamatous infections** such as **tuberculosis** or **histoplasmosis** are rare incidental findings, and established, sonomorphological criteria are not available. Only **myelolipomas** are hyperechoic tumors with homogeneous internal structure.

Adenomas appear as round or oval masses with smooth margins of decreased echogenicity. Their structure is mainly homogeneous and they are smoothly and well-demarcated against the adjacent structures. Ninety percent of all adenomas have diameters of less than 3 cm and they are predominantly

Ultrasound 137

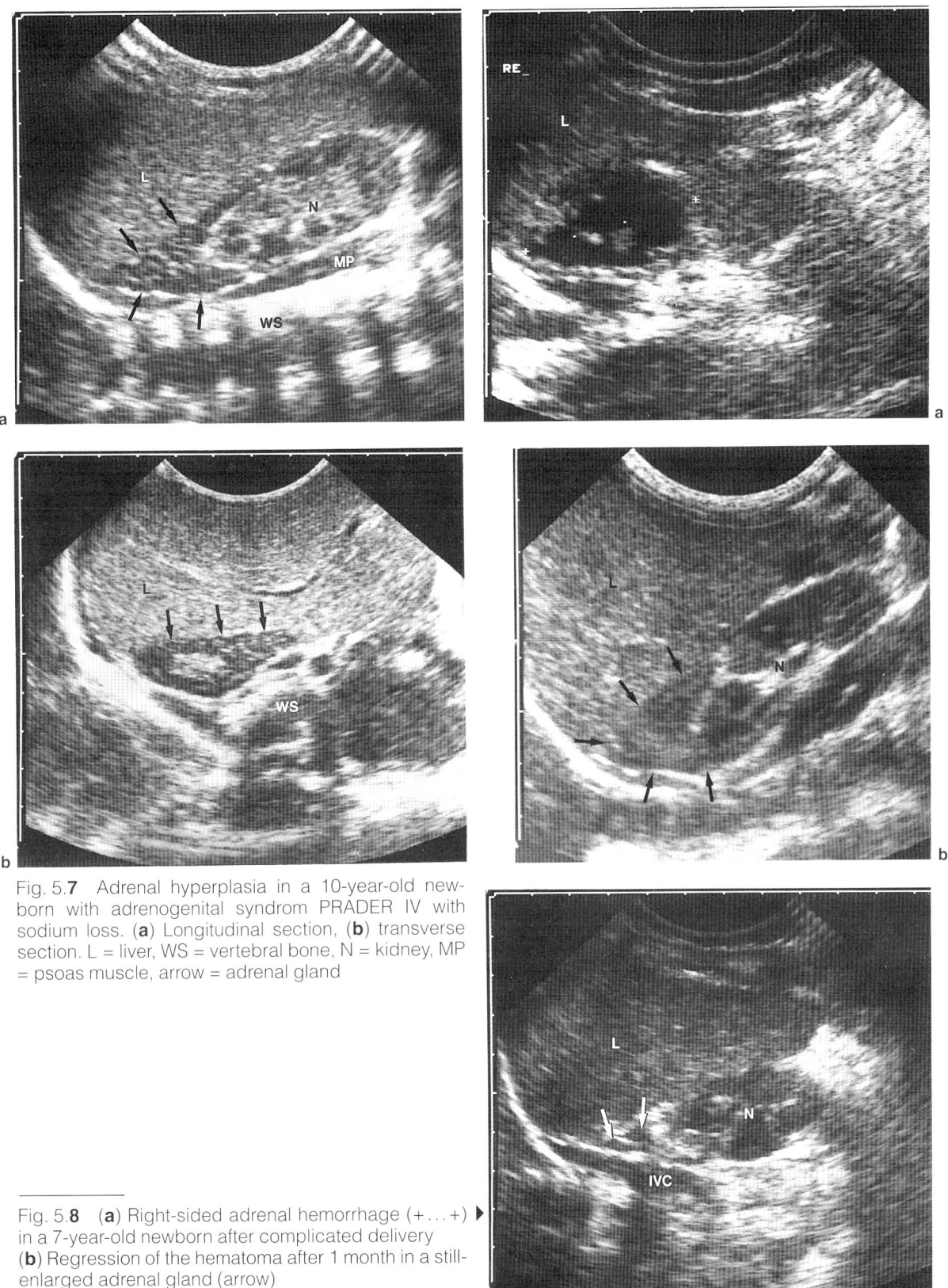

Fig. 5.7 Adrenal hyperplasia in a 10-year-old newborn with adrenogenital syndrom PRADER IV with sodium loss. (**a**) Longitudinal section, (**b**) transverse section. L = liver, WS = vertebral bone, N = kidney, MP = psoas muscle, arrow = adrenal gland

Fig. 5.8 (**a**) Right-sided adrenal hemorrhage (+...+) in a 7-year-old newborn after complicated delivery
(**b**) Regression of the hematoma after 1 month in a still-enlarged adrenal gland (arrow)
(**c**) Almost normal adrenal findings (arrow) after 3 months with differentiation between echogenic marrow and hypoechoic cortex. L = liver, N = kidney, IVC = inferior vena cava

5 Adrenal Gland

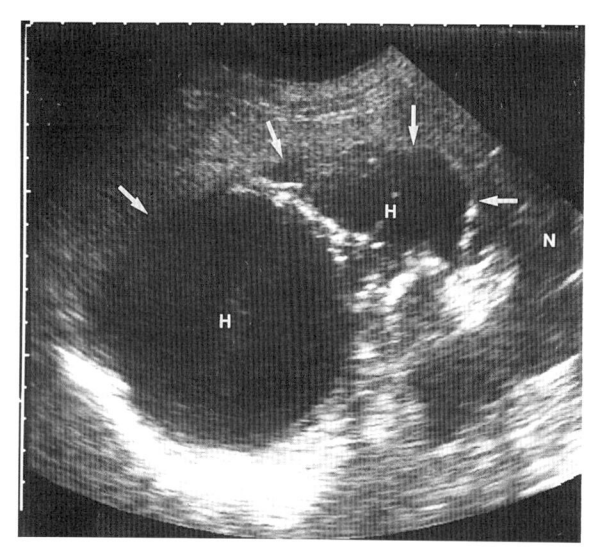

Fig. 5.**9** Oblique section of a right adrenal angioma with pseudocystic transformation (arrow) and posttraumatic bleeding, with a total size of 13 cm. H = hematoma, N = kidney, L = liver

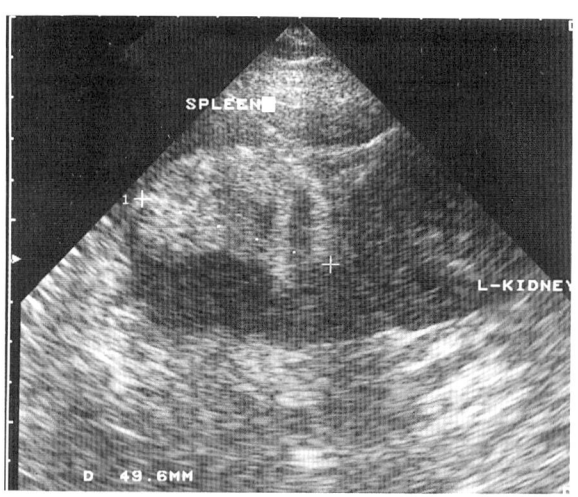

Fig. 5.**10** Longitudinal section of a left-sided 6.6 cm adrenal adenoma (+...+) in a patient with biopsy proven ovarian carcinoma. Inhomogeneous echo structure with hypoechoic and hyperechoic areas and shadowing by calcification after hemorrhage

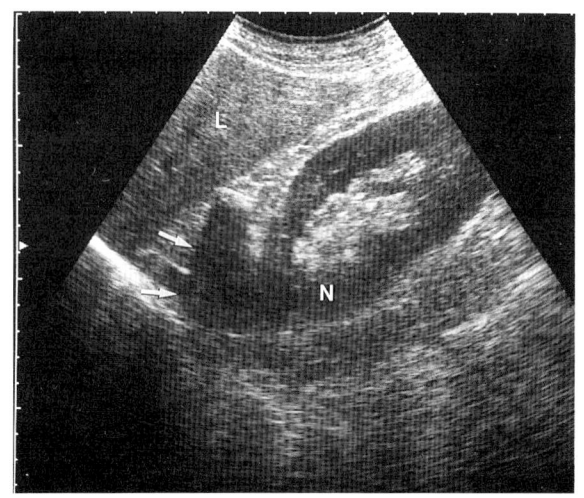

Fig. 5.**11** Longitudinal section of a right-sided 4.5 cm adrenal adenoma (+...+) as an incidental finding in a patient with esophageal carcinoma. Homogeneous structure, hypochoic to liver (L) and isoechoic to kidney (N)

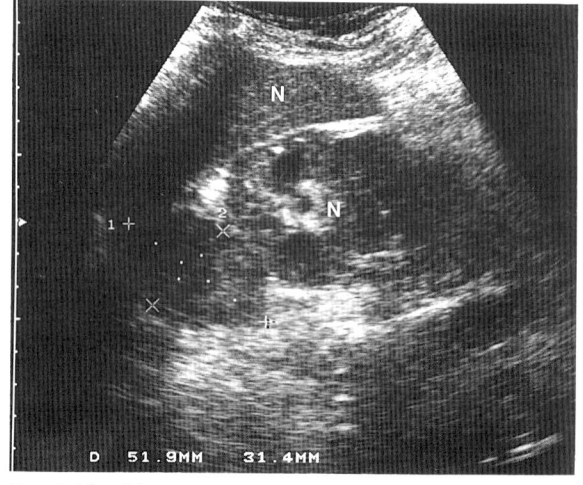

Fig. 5.**12** Pheochromocytoma of the left adrenal gland (+...+) with inhomogeneous echo structure, isoechoic to spleen (M) and kidney (N), smooth outer contour

found on the left. Differentiation from other benign or malignant masses is not possible (Fig. 5.**10** and 5.**11**).

Like adenomas, **pheochromocytomas** appear as well-demarcated, round or oval tumors with a marked propensity for the right adrenal gland. Early hemorrhages and regressive changes or necroses may lead to an inhomogeneous internal structure while the tumor is small in diameter. Because the clinical and paraclinical symptoms are already at hand, and have led to the correct diagnostic categorization, the main task of sonography is to locate the tumor. The presence of liver metastases indicates malignancy. Specific echo characteristics for pheocromocytomas do not exist making a differentiation from other benign or malignant tumors impossible (Fig. 5.**12** and 5.**13**).

Because of their often bland clinical symptoms and endocrinological findings, **primary malignomas** (carcinomas, sarcomas) remain often undetected until they have reached an advanced stage in which the margins of the organ have definitely been exceeded, the adjacent organs have been displaced and infiltrated, and lumbar lymph node metastases and vessel compression and infiltration have developed. The tumors then have irregular margins and an inhomogeneous

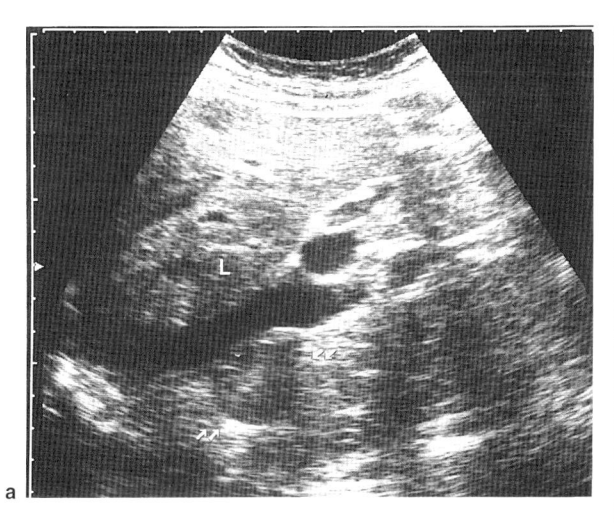

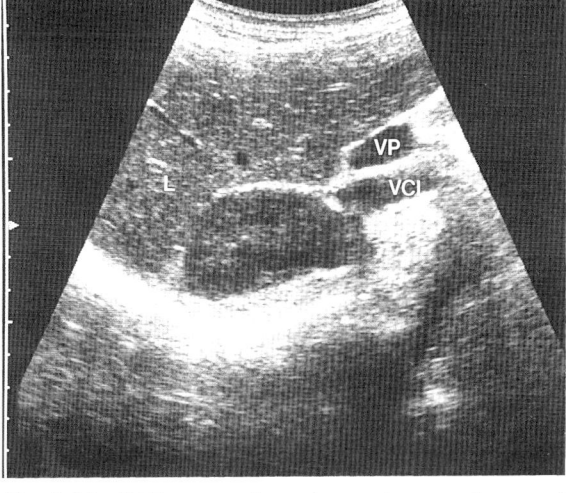

Fig. 5.14 Oblique section of an adenocarcinoma of the right adrenal gland, which is well demarcated from liver (L). VP = portal vein, IVC = inferior vena cava

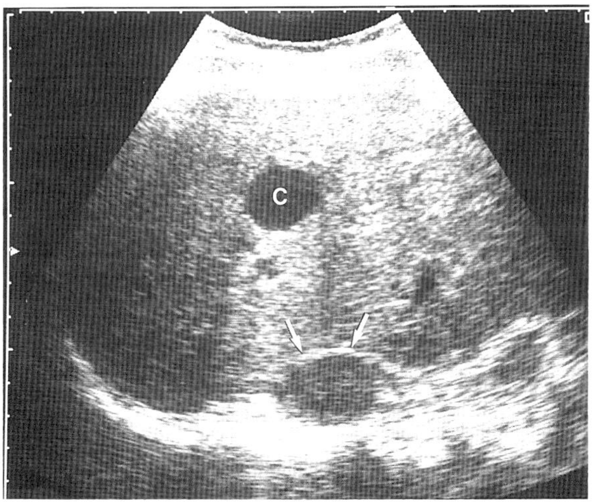

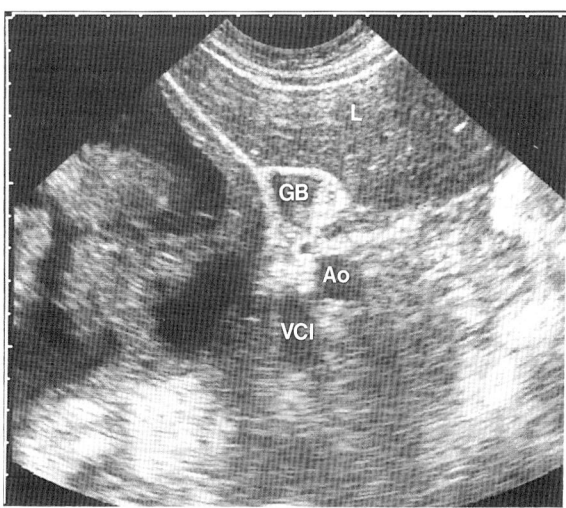

Fig. 5.13 Right-sided pheochromocytoma (+...+) 2.5 cm in size, isoechoic to liver (L), smooth contour. (**a**) Longitudinal and (**b**) oblique section. VCI = inferior vena cava, C = liver cyst

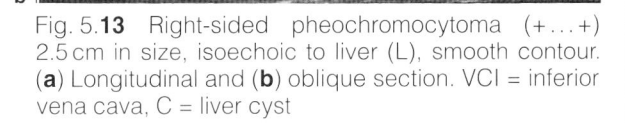

Fig. 5.15 Transverse section of a 13 cm right-sided adrenal carcinoma, well demarcated from liver (L). Inhomogeneous structure due to necrosis and hemorrhage. GB = gall bladder, VCI = inferior vena cava, A = aorta

echo pattern. It is then often difficult to clearly distinguish the adrenal gland as the organ of origin (Figs. 5.**14**, 5.**15** and 5.**16**).

Increasingly widespread use of routine prenatal and postnatal sonography have made it possible to detect **neuroblastomas** at a stage in which they have a more favorable prognosis, before the development of liver and lymph node metastases. At this stage, they are still well-demarcated, round tumors with relatively strong echogenicity (Fig. 5.**17**). The initially homogeneous echo structure can, however, soon become inhomogeneous because of hemorrhage and cystic necrotic decay.

Lymphomas appear as homogeneous adrenal gland enlargement and must be considered in the differential diagnosis of uncharacteristic tumors.

Metastases of the adrenal glands often occur bilaterally. Because there are no specific sonographic criteria, a unilateral affection makes differentiation from other benign or malignant findings impossible (Fig. 5.**18**).

Just as the normal adrenal gland is more difficult to delineate on the left, pathological findings are more difficult to visualize on the left. Para-aortic lymphomas, cysts of the pancreatic tail, accessory spleens, or parts of the stomach wall may simulate an affection of the adrenal gland. The splenic vein may help to trace a tumor to its origin in the tail of the pancreas or the adrenal gland because tumors of the pan-

5 Adrenal Gland

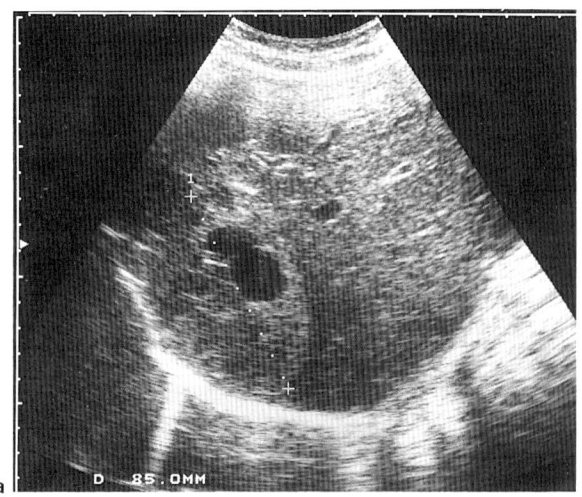

Fig. 5.**16** (**a**) Liver metastasis of an adrenal carcinoma with increased echogenicity and necroses.

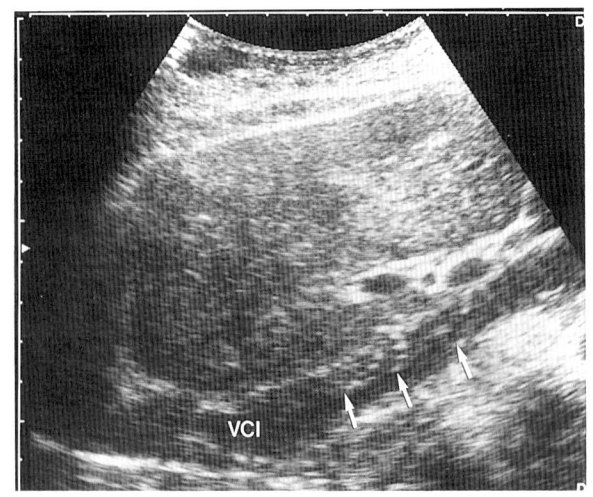

(**b**) Tumor-induced thrombosis (arrow) of the inferior vena cava (IVC) in the same patient

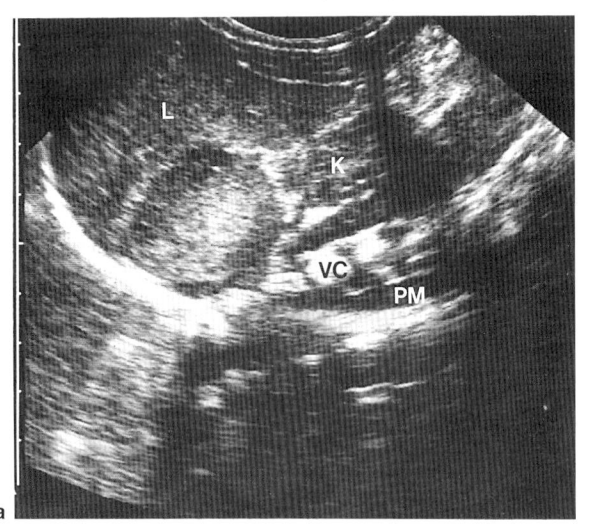

Fig. 5.**17** Right-sided fetal adrenal tumor, slowly growing since the 28th gestational week. Postpartum: 3 cm round tumor (+... +) with inhomogeneous echo structure and slightly undulated, sharp outer contour.

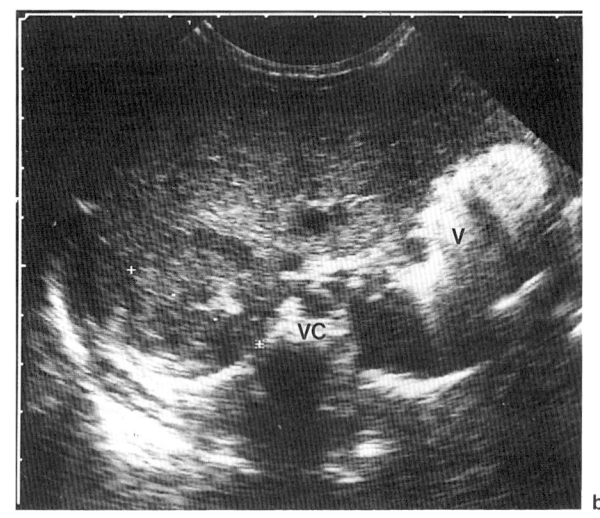

Surgical histology: neuroblastoma. (**a**) Longitudinal section, (**b**) transverse section. L = liver, WS = vertebral bone, MP = psoas muscle, N = kidney, M = stomach

creatic tail always lie ventrally; adrenal tumors lie dorsally to the vein.

Summary

Although the sonographic appearance of adrenal tumors is relatively unspecific, this does not distract from the value of sonography of the adrenal glands. In the hands of a skillful and experienced operator, sonography can provide valuable information that either makes more complex imaging techniques unneccessary or provides a basis for a more targeted approach. The variability of scanning planes and the use of breathing-dependent mobility of organs allows sonography to provide a more reliable evaluation of the relationship of an adrenal tumor to the adjacent organs (infiltration) than other imaging procedures. As part of a newborn screening procedure, indications for adrenogenital syndrome and neuroblastoma may be gained before clinical symptoms have appeared. Finally, the combination of sonography with immediate guided biopsy of an adrenal mass under certain clinical and paraclinical conditions may lead to a considerable reduction of the time needed for final diagnosis (Figs. 5.**19** and 5.**20**).

References

1 Bousvaros A, Kirks DR, Grossman H. Imaging of neuroblastoma: an overview. Pediatr Radiol 16:1986;89–196.
2 Hamper UM, Fishmann EK, Hartman DS. Primary adrenocortical carcinoma: sonographie evaluation with clinical and pathological correlation in 26 patients. AJR 1987;148:915.

Ultrasound 141

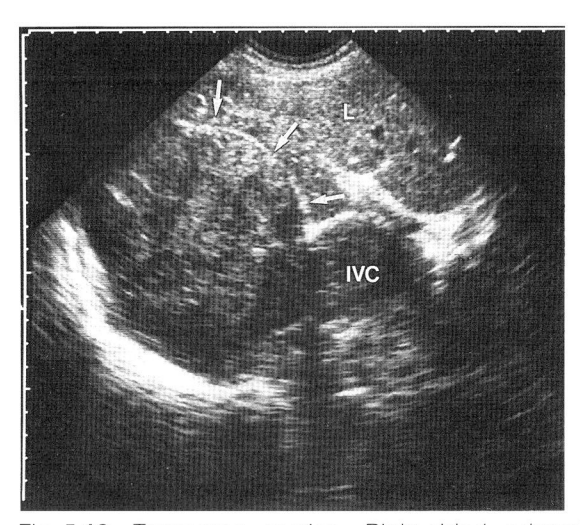

Fig. 5.**18** Transverse section. Right-sided adrenal metastasis (arrow) of a bronchial carcinoma, verified by sonographically guided biopsy. The tumor is isoechogenic to liver (L) and exhibits an inhomogeneous multinodular echo structure, smooth outer contour. Maximal diameter 12 cm. Thrombotic occlusion of the inferior vena cava (VCI)

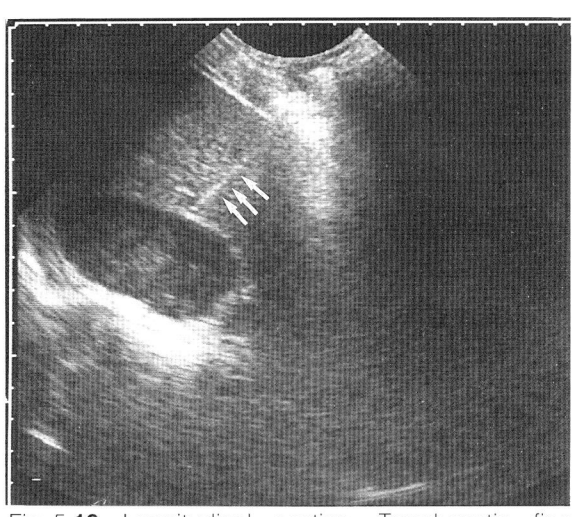

Fig. 5.**19** Longitudinal section. Transhepatic fine needle biopsy (arrow) of a right-sided adrenal tumor of 7 × 3 cm. Histology: poorly differentiated malignant tumor, probably carcinoma with extensive necroses. Largely reduced echogenicity compared to steatotic liver, smooth outer contour

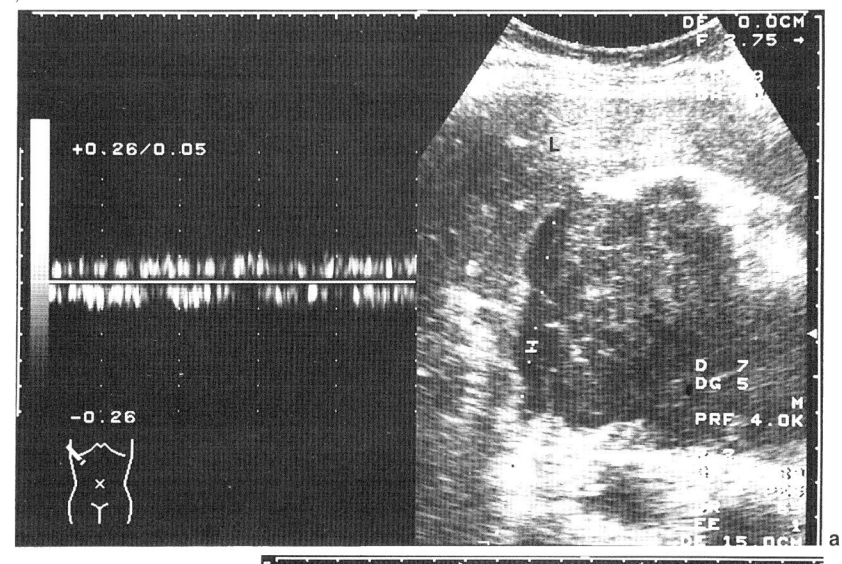

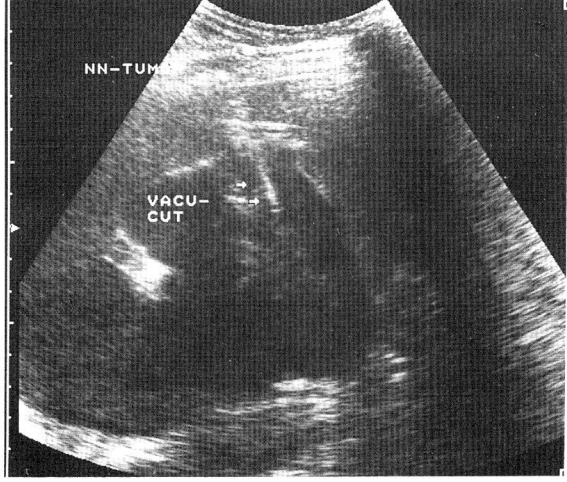

Fig. 5.**20** (**a**) Densely vascularized adrenal carcinoma on the right with reduced echogenicity, well demarcated from liver (L), inhomogeneous echo structure, polycyclic contour
(**b**) Transhepatic biopsy of the tumor using a Vacucut needle with a diameter of 1.2 mm

3 Hendry GMA. Cystic neuroblastoma of the adrenal gland – a potential source of error in ultrasonic diagnosis. Pediatr Radiol 1982;12:204–206.
4 Hirning T, van Kaick G, Gamroth A, Gambilohr R. Ultraschalldiagnostik raumfordernder Prozesse der Nebennieren mit Sektorscan-Technik. Ultraschall Klin Prax 1986;1:83–88.
5 Koischwitz D. Ultraschalldiagnostik bei Nebennieren-Erkrankungen. Ultraschall Klin Prax 1989;4:41–59.
6 Langer R, Kaufmann HJ, Stäblein W. Sonographische Befunde der postpartalen Nebennierenblutung. Monatschr Kinderheilk 1985;133:818–822.
7 Leidig E. Sonographie der Nebennieren-Erkrankungen des Neugeborenen. Ultraschall 1988;9:155–162.
8 Marchal G, Glin J, Verbeken E. High resolution realtime sonography of adrenal gland. J Ultrasonnal Med 1986;5:65.
9 Päivänsolo M, Merikanto J, Kallivinen M, Mc Aush G. Ultrasound in the detection of adrenal tumors. Eur J Radiol 1988;8:183.
10 Wernecke K, Galanski M. Perkutane Feinnadel-Biopsie der Nebennieren. Radiologe 1986;26:191.
11 Wilms G, Marchal G, Baert A, Adisoejoso B, Mangkuwerdojo S. CT and ultrasound features of post-traumatic adrenal hemorrhage. J Comput Assist Tomorgr 1987;11:112.
12 Winkler P, Abel T, Helmke K. Sonographische Darstellung der normalen Nebennieren bei normalen Nebennieren bei Kindern und Jugendlichen. Ultraschall 1987;8:271.
13 Yeh HC, Bhardwaj S, Gabrilove JL, Cuttner J. Imaging of diffused enlarged adrenal glands. Hospimedica 1991;9(9):37–42.

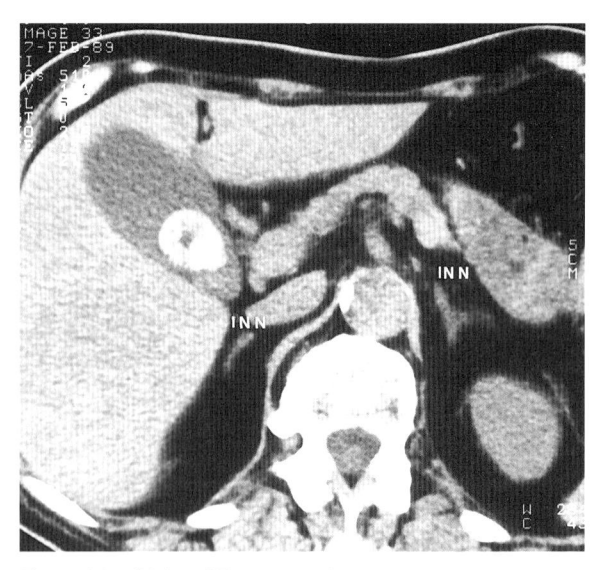

Fig. 5.**21** Plain CT scan of a normal linear right adrenal gland and an inverted Y-shaped left adrenal gland (1 NN). Secondary finding: cholecystolithiasis

Computed Tomography

C. Zwicker

From a developmental point of view, the adrenal cortex, which is derived from the coelomic mesoderm, must be distinguished from the adrenal medulla, which develops from the neural crest and the rudimentary forms of the sympathetic nervous system. This differentiation is, however, not possible in the imaging of the adrenals. Their small size and protected, retroperitoneal location limit the possibilities of sonographic imaging, whereas allows both organs to CT is be identified successfully in 95–100% of patients. In the cachectic patient without sufficient retroperitoneal fat, however, imaging may be difficult. According to Abrams a sensitivity of 84% and the specificity of 98% make CT the screening method of choice (1).

Technique

Targeted CT investigation of the adrenal glands should be carried out in slices using table increments of 4–5 mm in order to be able to detect subtle differences. If a mass is found, the analysis of contrast medium enhancement provides additional information. In this case, it is best to carry out a dynamic CT on the level of the main findings without table incrementation after the administration of a contrast medium bolus (e.g., 1 mL/kg body weight; flow: 4 mL/s) and to follow the development of enhancement with time–density curves.

Anatomy

The adrenal glands lie within the renal fascia in the adipose capsule, cephalad and medial to the upper kidney pole. The posterior part of the right adrenal gland is directly adjacent to the inferior vena cava. The right crus of diaphragm forms its medial border and the right liver lobe forms the lateral border. The left adrenal gland is often located more distally and may reach the left renal hilum. The ventral border is formed by the pancreatic cauda. Its cephalad–caudad length ranges from 20–40 mm (5). The median plain CT density comprises 25 H. The following variations in shape can be found:

Triangular
Linear
An inverted Y-shape
V-shaped
Delta-shaped

Pathology

Tumors of the Adrenal Cortex

Adenomas can be imaged if they are larger than 8 mm. Nonfunctioning tumors, "incidentalomas," are found by chance and are detected in 6% of all abdominal CT investigations. Depending on their lipid content, a wide variation of densities can be found, ranging from −15 H to 60 H. Because no information on steroid content can be gained from CT, hormonally active and inactive tumors cannot be distinguished. Due to their considerable increase in density in dynamic CT, Cushing adenomas can be differentiated from Conn adenomas and from nonenhancing kidney cysts with low contrast medium enhancement.

Carcinoma

Carcinomas can be distinguished from adenomas fairly reliably if they are 3 cm in size or larger. If the tumors are smaller, accurate differentiation is not possible. Additional criteria for malignancy are: irregular outer contours, infiltration into the vena cava and kidneys, lymph node enlargement, and liver metastases. If the tumors are large, they may show central necrosis. As opposed to vital tumor tissue, necrosis does not enhance with contrast medium (Fig. 5.**24**).

Adrenal Hyperplasia

Hyperplasia is usually the morphologic substrate of increased hormone production (e.g., Cushing syndrome with hormone-producing pituitary tumor) and can present with swelling and enlargement of both adrenal glands. Diagnosis, however, is difficult because of the great variation in shape, which limits the information provided.

Tumors of the Adrenal Medulla

Pheocromocytomas, Blastomas

The pheochromocytomas that are derived from the chromaffin cells of the adrenal medulla are difficult to evaluate for malignancy. The only definite indicator of malignancy is metastasis.

These tumors have smooth contours and are comparatively large. In dynamic CT they demonstrate a very intense contrast uptake because of their high arterial vascularization. Necrosis is not uncommon. In 10% of the patients, bilateral and extra-adrenal tumors occur along the sympathetic chain.

Neuroblastomas

Following nephroblastomas (Wilms tumor), neuroblastomas are the second most frequent malignancy in childhood. In 70% of all patients they arise from the adrenal medulla and less frequently from other loca-

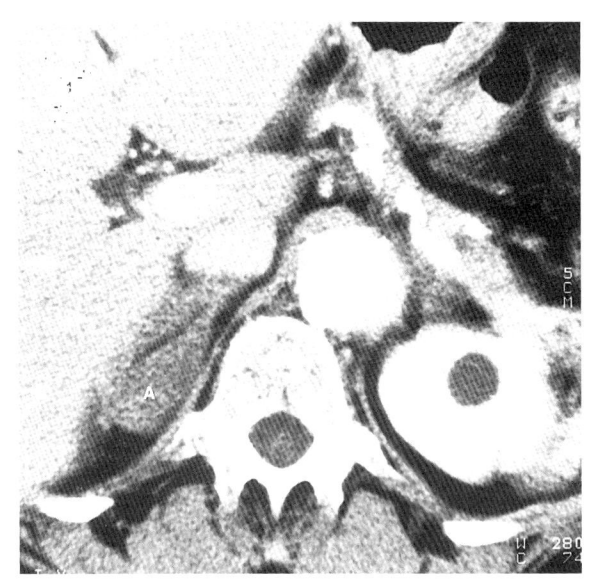

Fig. 5.**22** Extensive right-sided hormonally inactive adenoma without contrast enhancement in the dynamic CT (A). Secondary finding: renal cyst of the left kidney

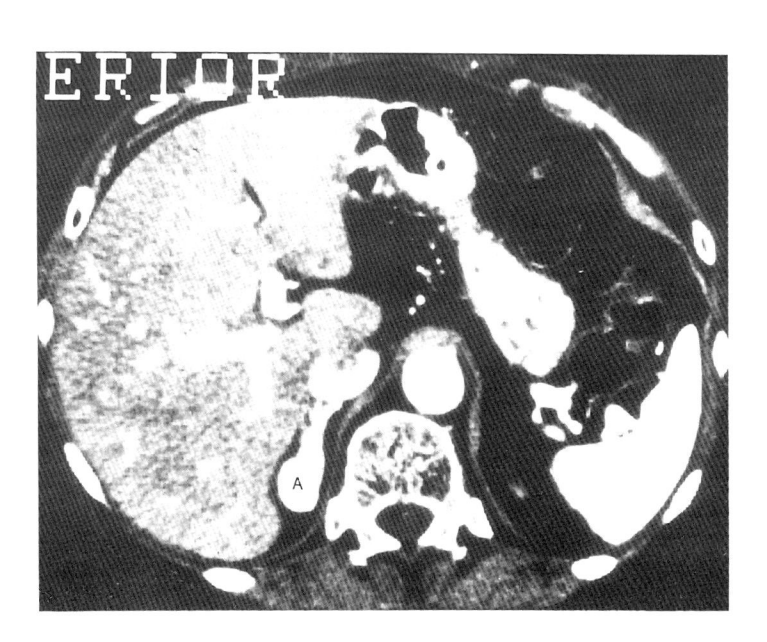

Fig. 5.**23** The dynamic CT series demonstrate an intense contrast-enhancing Cushing adenoma on the right (a)

144   5 Adrenal Gland

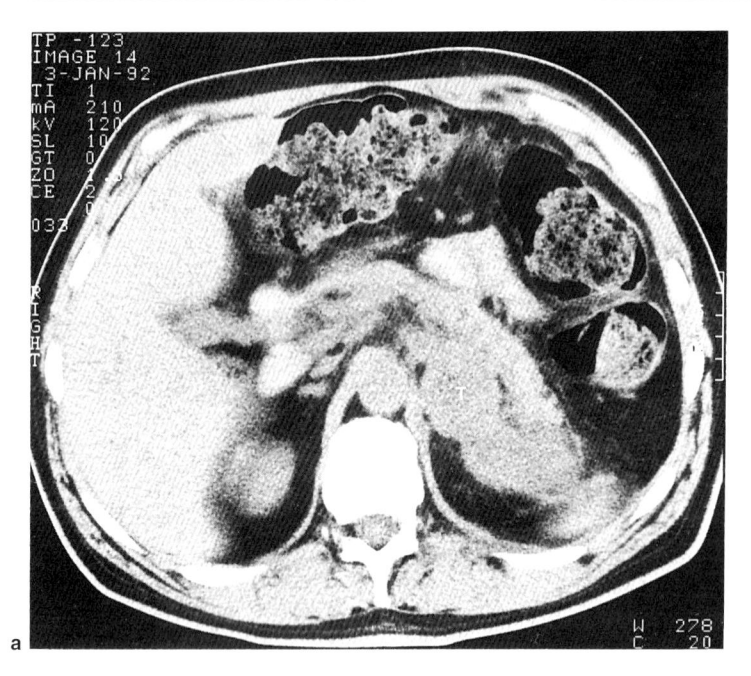

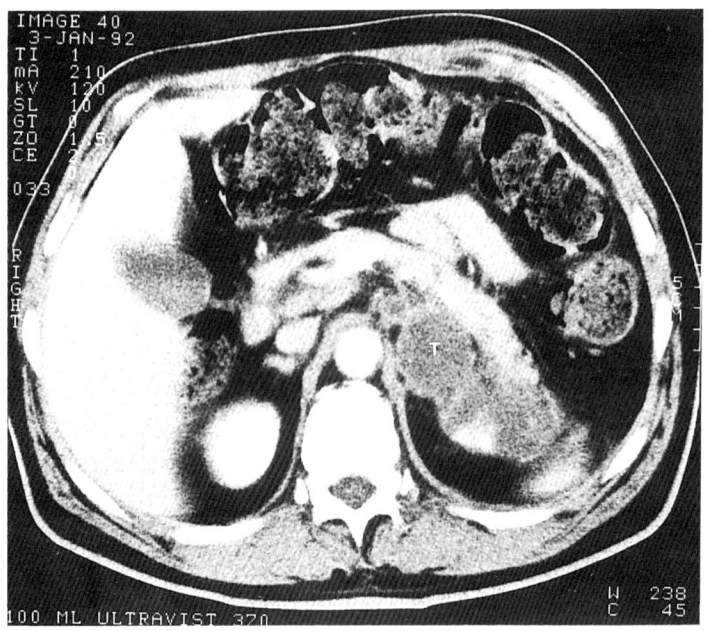

Fig. 5.**24** Large adrenal carcinoma (T) on the left with infiltration of pancreas and kidney. (**a**) Plain CT: mass of soft-tissue density in the left adrenal bed. (**b**) Dynamic contrast enhanced CT series: slightly enhancing mass infiltrating into adjacent organ structures

tions of sympathetic nervous tissue. CT scans show homogeneous, sometimes very large tumors of soft tissue density. According to Stark (8), calcifications can be found in 30% of all patients. Apart from the location, this can be indicative of neuroblastomas and may allow differentiation from Wilms tumor.

Other Tumors

Myelolipomas

On CT, nonfunctioning myelolipomas are incidental findings (7). Because of their lipid content, density is characteristically low at −50 to −80 H. Calcifications are seen in 25% of patients.

Adrenal Cysts

Adrenal cysts show water-equivalent density values and have smooth margins.

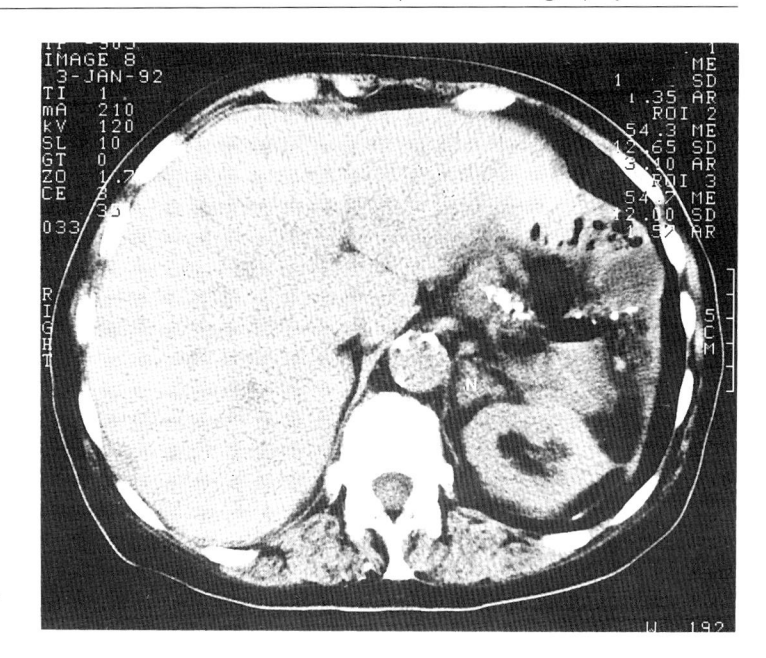

Fig. 5.**25** Hyperplastic enlargement of the left adrenal (N) by an endocrinologically active pituitary adenoma

Adrenal Metastases

Bronchial carcinoma is the most frequent primary tumor of unilateral or bilateral adrenal metastases, followed by breast and colorectal cancer (Fig. 5.**26**). Solid masses often show central necrosis that can be clearly delineated after contrast medium adminstration. Furthermore, the adrenals may be affected by Hodgkin and non-Hodgkin lymphomas.

Hemorrhages, Calcification

Bleeding of the adrenal glands occurs in about 2% of neonates and the initial high density values of around 60 H later drop to liquid values of around 10–15 H. Calcifications can be reliably visualized by CT and may either result from trauma or tuberculosis, or occur with tumors.

Summary

CT is a very accurate morphological procedure for the imaging of the adrenal glands because tumors can already be visualized at a size of 8–10 mm (2). Because of the great variation in shape, the differentiation of adrenal enlargement in hyperplasia is more difficult. If masses do not infiltrate or metastasize, or if they are not destructive, malignancy cannot be determined by CT. Thus, only 85% of the patients with malignant adrenal tumors can be correctly classified by CT (6).

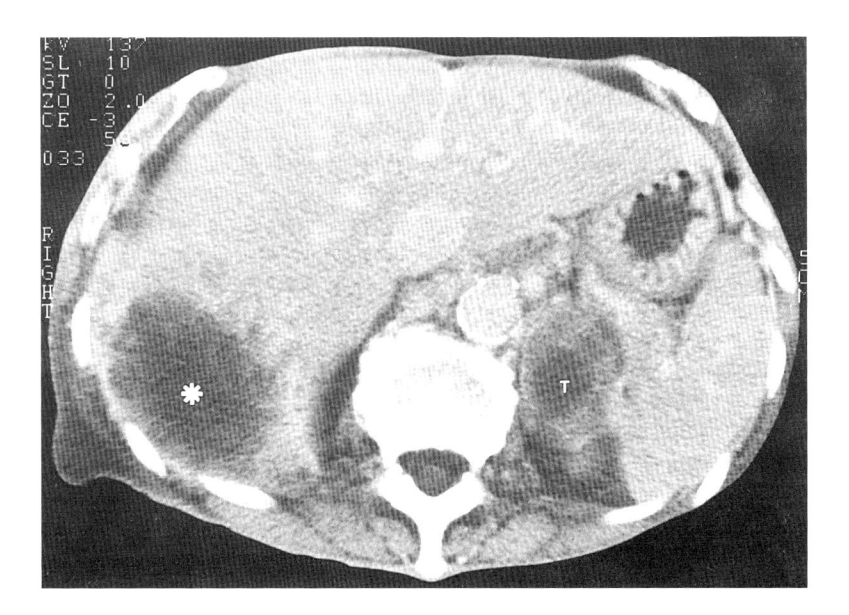

Fig. 5.**26** The dynamic contrast-enhanced CT series show a partially necrotic metastasis (T) of the left adrenal from a bronchial carcinoma. Secondary finding: extensive liver metastasis (*)

Perfusion characteristics in dynamic CT can be utilized to differentiate the arterially highly vascularized Cushing adenomas and pheochromocytomas from other masses.

References

1 Abrams HL, Siegelman SS, Adams DF, et al. Computed tomography versus ultrasound of the adrenal gland: a prospective study. Radiology. 1983;43:121–128.
2 Geisinger MA, Zelch MG, Bravo EL, Risius BF, Donovan PB, Borkowski GP. Primary hyperaldosteronism: Comparison of CT, adrenal venography and venous sampling. Am J Roentgenol. 1983;141:299–305.
3 Glazer HS, Weymann PJ, Sagel SS, Levitt RG, Mc Clennan BL. Nonfunctioning adrenal masses: incidental discovery on computed tomography. Am J Roentgenol. 1982;139:81–87.
4 Haertel M, Probst P, Bollmann J. Computertomographische Nebennierendiagnostik. Fortschr Röntgenstr. 1980;132:31–41.
5 Hübener KH, Grehn St, Schulze K. Indikationen zur computertomographischen Nebennierenuntersuchung; Leistungsfähigkeit, Stellenwert, Differentialdiagnostik. Fortschr Röntgenstr. 1980;132:37–46.
6 Katz RL, Patel S, Mackay B, Zornoza J. Fine needle aspiration cytology of the adrenal gland. Acta Cytol. 1984;28:269–282.
7 Leder LD, Richter HJ, Stambolis Ch. Pathology of renal and adrenal neoplasms. In: Löhr, E. Renal and Adrenal Tumors. Berlin: Springer; 1979.
8 Stark DD, Moss AA, Brasch RC. Neuroblastoma: diagnostic imaging and staging. Radiology 1983;148:101–108.

MR Imaging

I. R. Francis and A. M. Aisen

Introduction

The adrenal gland is well-suited for imaging by cross-sectional imaging techniques because it is surrounded by adequate retroperitoneal fat in most patients. Therefore, both CT and MR are equally adept at demonstrating the gland. The sensitivity for adrenal gland visualization by MR has ranged between 86% to 100% (1–4). Although CT and MR are capable of depicting most masses larger than 2 cm, CT is currently the preferred modality at most centers for evaluating the adrenal gland because of its superior spatial resolution. Using CT, a specific diagnosis can be made in only a limited number of conditions, such as most adrenal cysts and adrenal myelolipomas. However, the significant drawback of CT is its limited tissue specificity, including the inability to differentiate between adrenal tumors of different histologies (3, 5, 6). Though MR offers slightly poorer spatial resolution than CT, the superior contrast resolution more than compensates. In addition, MR has shown some promise in tissue characterization, particularly in distinguishing benign adenomas from malignant tumors of the adrenal cortex or medulla (7–16). MR is also capable of differentiating periadrenal vascular structures, including varices from the left adrenal gland, without the use of contrast enhancement (17).

Quantitative MRI is of some help in tissue characterization. Absolute measurements vary with scanner tuning, and do not reflect true tissue properties; thus, they are not useful. Instead, the ratios of the signal intensity of the adrenal lesions to other reference tissues such as liver, fat, muscle, and renal cortex or medulla have been employed, though these quantitative measurements also have limitations (1, 3, 4, 6). In practice, visually comparing the signal intensity of the lesion to the liver is as good an approach as any. The general rule is that adrenal adenomas are relatively darker than other lesions on T2-weighted images. Initial studies on adrenal tissue characterization performed on low and mid field units, showed that the accuracy for the diagnosis of adenomas was between 80% and 95%. A small number of adenomas were found to be brighter than usual, thus resembling malignant tumors (2, 9, 18). On the other hand, it was unusual for malignant neoplasms to appear as dark as adenomas (2, 7, 8, 10, 19). On high-field strength units (1.5 T), signal characteristics were less reliable than on lower field strength units. T2-relaxation times, however, were somewhat more useful in distinguishing adenomas from nonadenomas in two studies (10, 11).

More recently, chemical shift techniques using in-phase and out-of-phase imaging has been used with some success to make this distinction (20).

Techniques

In the past, spin-echo imaging with respiratory compensation has been most commonly used to evaluate the adrenals. A standard examination consists of T1- and T2-weighted images. The TRs have varied from 300–600 ms; TEs 15–40 ms for T1-weighted images and TRs from 1500–3000 ms; TEs 30–120 ms for T2-weighted images (4).

Other options that have been shown to improve image quality in upper abdominal imaging are respiratory-ordered phase encoding (ROPE), use of multiple acquisitions (NEX) for signal averaging, gradient moment nulling, spatial presaturation, the use of surface coils, fat-suppression techniques and breath-held imaging (21–31). However, some of these options have time penalties, thus increasing scan times; others have different imitations that restrict their potential for routine use. Recent studies have demonstrated the utility of contrast enhancement with intravenous contrast media based on Gd-DTPA (12). It is likely that contrast enhancement coupled with rapidly acquired gradient-echo imaging, which reliably demonstrates the phases of contrast enhancement, will prove useful in increasing the specificity of MRI. In the future, such a sequence may become part of the routine examination.

Spectroscopic imaging with separation of the water and fat tissue components has also shown some promise in tissue characterization (16). Recently, Mitchell and his colleagues have utilized chemical shift imaging successfully in distinguished between lipid-containing adenomas and lipid-poor malignant lesions.

Axial images are the most useful for evaluation of abnormalities of the adrenal gland. Coronal images can be used to determine the relationship of the adrenal mass to the upper pole of the kidneys and the liver, and sagittal images are useful to determine the relationship of adrenal masses to the inferior vena cava and the aorta.

At our institution, we begin the MR examination of the adrenal with T1-weighted coronal locator images. We then acquire respiratory compensated T1- and T2-weighted SE axial images. The technical parameters are TR of 300 ms and TE of 15 ms, 256 × 192 matrix, 4 NEX, using 5-mm-thick slices and an interslice gap of 1 mm for T1-weighted, and a TR of 2500 ms, TEs of 40 and 80 ms, 256 × 128 matrix, 2 NEX, using the same slice thickness and interslice gap. In addition, we are starting to use dynamic Gd-DTPA-enhanced imaging to determine the enhancement characteristics of adrenal masses. Presently this is done with fast, gradient-echo, multiplanar imaging, which provides rapid T1-weighted images at multiple tomographic planes. This allows both adrenal glands to be imaged in their entirety in a single breath-hold; the sequence is repeated serially to demonstrate the contrast dynamics. For T2-weighted imaging, we employ Fast Spin Echo techniques (FSE) with TRs between 2500–3000 ms and TEs of 17–40 ms for the first echo and 80–120 ms for the second echo. In addition, we now routinely use Gd-DTPA enhanced rapid dynamic imaging to determine the enhancement characteristics of adrenal masses. We also perform in-phase and out-of-phase gradient echo imaging to detect small amounts of fat, as suggested by Mitchell. We do not routinely use glucagon to suppress bowel motion or oral contrast medium to delineate the gastrointestinal tract for MR imaging of the adrenals.

In selected cases, angiographic sequences are helpful in identifying vascular structures or assessing vascular invasion of adrenal malignancies. Techniques based on "time of flight" (rapid T1-weighted gradient-echo sequences demonstrating the inflow of unsaturated spins in vessels as high signal) or phase contrast (which employ flow-sensitive magnetic field gradient pulses) are both useful. These sequences rarely work well in body imaging; thus, two-dimensional images acquired in single breath-holds are preferable.

Normal Glands

Anatomy

The normal glands have a varied appearance on CT and MR and are composed of a body and two limbs. The limbs usually have either have a vertical or horizontal orientation and appear V- or Y-shaped. The right adrenal gland is most often located posterior to the inferior vena cava, medial to the liver, anterolateral to the crus, and superior to the upper pole of the right kidney. The left gland is usually located posterior and medial to the splenic vasculature and the pancreas, anterior and lateral to the crus, lateral to the aorta, and anteromedial to the left kidney.

MR Appearance

The normal adrenal gland appears dark on both T1- and T2-weighted images in comparison with most other tissues. The gland is of similar or lower intensity (isointense or hypointense) when compared with liver and muscle on both T1- and T2-weighted images (Figs. 5.27 and 5.28). Generally the T1 images are used for anatomical definition, and the T2-weighted images are more often used for tissue characterization.

Nonfunctioning Tumors

Adrenal Cysts

Uncomplicated cysts are usually homogeneous, with a typical fluid appearance: they appear dark on T1-weighted images and markedly hyperintense on T2-weighted images (32). However, complicated cysts, either due to prior hemorrhage or calcification, appear heterogeneous and thus have a nonspecific appearance and can resemble other benign and malignant lesions.

Adrenal Myelolipomas

These uncommon tumors are benign and contain varying elements of fat and myeloid tissue (bone marrow elements). In fact, fat density demonstrated on CT in an adrenal mass is nearly pathognomonic for this entity. As with renal angiomyolipomas, the MR appearances of these lesions depends on the quantity of each component in the tumor. Thus, a variety of appearances have been reported. The masses can be homogenous with signal intensity similar to that of retroperitoneal fat, heterogeneous with areas of fat intensity, or may appear dissimilar to fat (33). The calcifications and ossifications sometimes seen in these tumors are usually difficult to detect by MR. It is important to note that in the small numbers of patients evaluated, MR was not helpful in making the diagnosis in patients with equivocal CT findings.

Hematomas

The MR appearance of hematomas depends upon the age of the hematoma as well as the field strength of the imager and the pulse sequence used (34, 35). In the acute phase they can appear hyperintense on the T1-weighted images, and in the subacute phase, they

148   5 Adrenal Gland

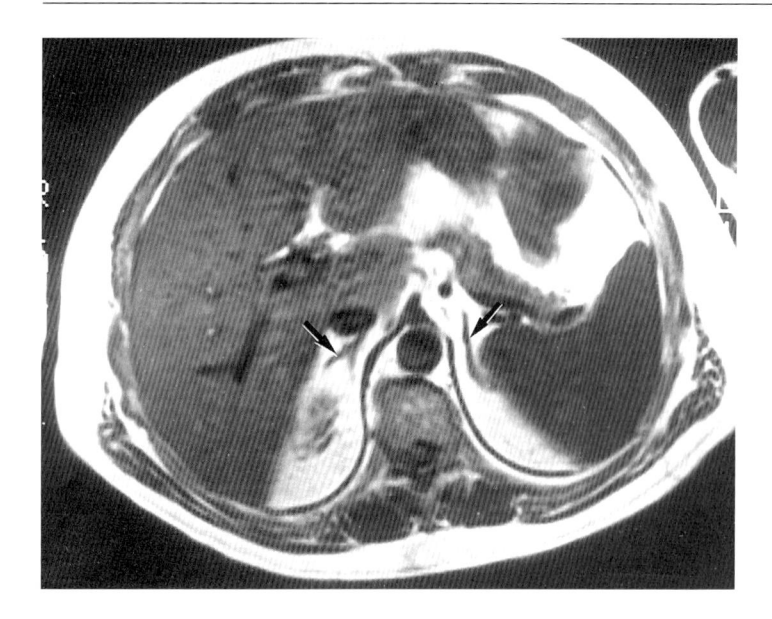

Fig. 5.**27** Normal adrenal glands (arrows) are either isointense or hypointense when compared to the liver on T1-weighted images

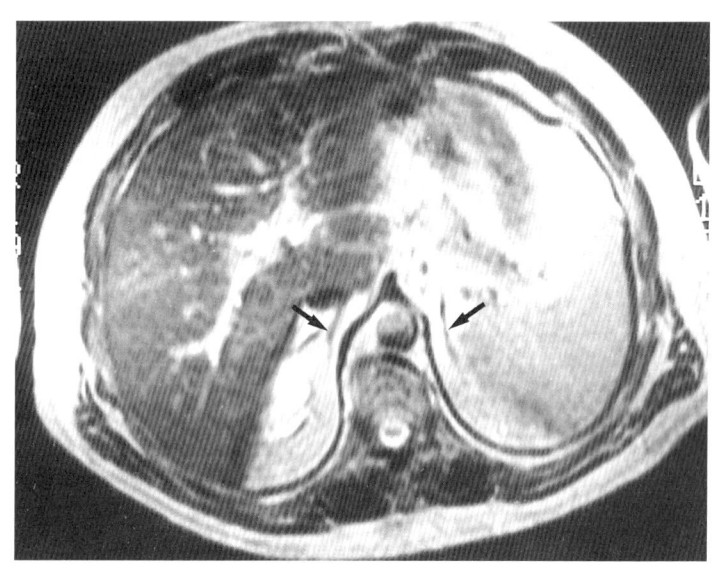

Fig. 5.**28** Normal adrenal glands (arrows) are either isointense or hypointense when compared to the liver on T2-weighted images

can develop a bright ring which progressively moves towards the center of the lesion. In the subacute and chronic phases, a thin dark rim of hemosiderin can be seen on both T1- and T2-weighted images.

Hyperfunctioning Adrenal Tumors

These can be divided into tumors of the adrenal cortex and medulla. We will discuss Cushing syndrome first, then hyperaldosteronism and finally, medullary tumors, specifically pheochromocytomas.

Adrenal Cortical Hyperfunction

Cushing Syndrome

Adrenal Adenoma
Adrenal adenomas account for 15–20% of patients with Cushing syndrome, with adrenal hyperplasia being the cause for the vast majority. As the average size of Cushing adenomas ranges from 2–2.5 cm (36), they can be readily localized by MR and CT. These tumors can have a variable appearance on spin-echo MR, being either hypointense to isointense with liver (Fig. 5.**29**), or even hyperintense on the T2-weighted images, thus resembling malignant tumors (37). Reimer et al. found that there was poor correlation of adrenal function with adrenal morphology and signal intensity ratios. In general, it appears that there is little difference in MR appearance between functioning and nonfunctioning adrenal adenomas (37).

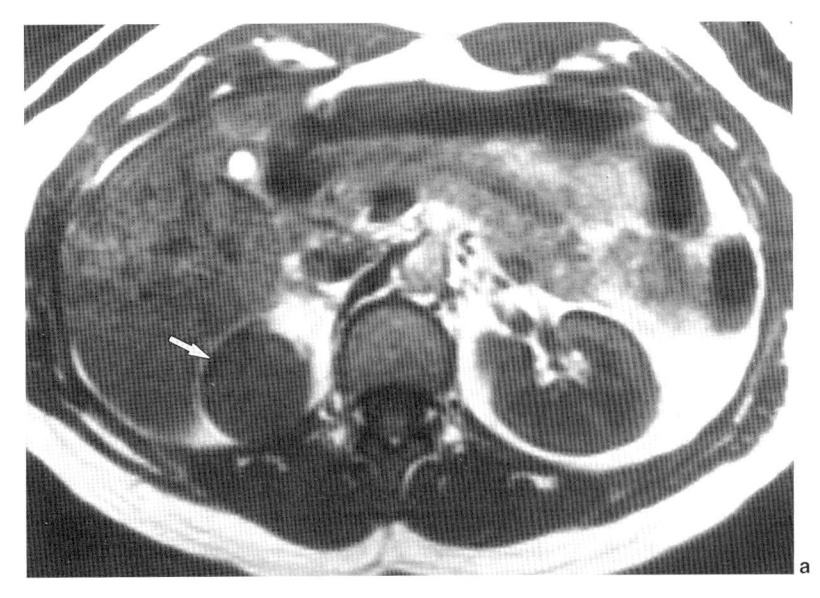

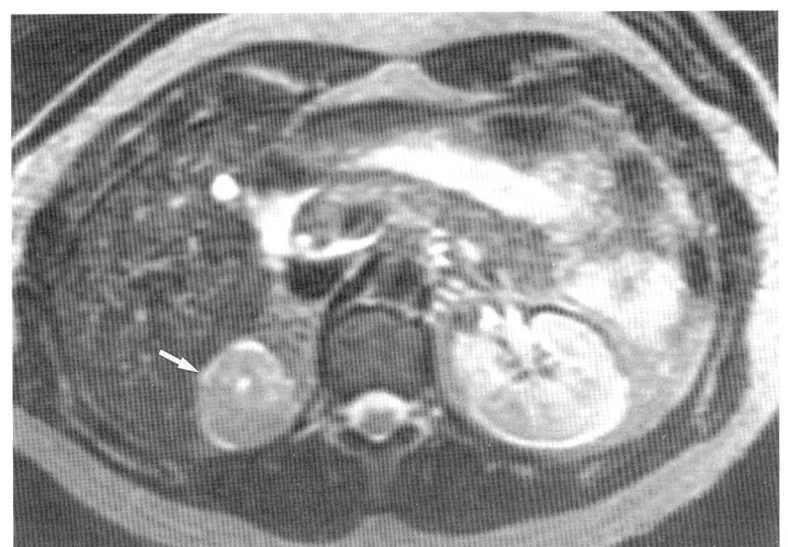

Fig. 5.**29** Cushing adenoma
a Right adrenal mass (arrow) in patient with Cushing syndrome
b Note that the lesion is hyperintense with the liver on the T2-weighted images on a 1.5 T imager (TR = 2000 ms, TE = 90 ms)

Adrenal Cortical Carcinoma

Adrenal cortical carcinomas account for 5–10% of patients with Cushing syndrome and roughly half of these tumors are functional (38–40). These tumors are usually large, heterogenous and are hyperintense on T2-weighted images (Fig. 5.**30**). Areas of calcification can be missed on MR, but MR has the advantage of being able to image in multiple planes. This feature is useful to evaluate the local extent of the tumor easily. Hepatic invasion and renal invasion can also be depicted more readily by coronal imaging (40, 41). Because these tumors can invade the inferior vena cava, caval involvement can be detected by MR using coronal or sagittal imaging without intravenous contrast enhancement as would be needed by CT. These findings can be easily seen using spin-echo, gradient-recalled imaging as well as on angiographic sequences.

Hyperaldosteronism (Conn Syndrome)

Aldosteronoma

In this syndrome, in contrast to Cushing syndrome, adenomas account for up to 80% of the patients. Bilateral adrenal hyperplasia accounts for the remaining 20%. In less than 1% of the cases, the cause for hyperaldosteronism is an adrenal cortical carcinoma.

The majority of the adenomas are small with a mean size of 1.6–1.8 cm (41). Thus, detection of these tumors even with current CT scanners using thin sections is about 80% (42). Ikeda et al. found that the smaller adenomas (less than 1 cm in size) went undetected by spin-echo MR using a 0.35 T imager, which

150   5 Adrenal Gland

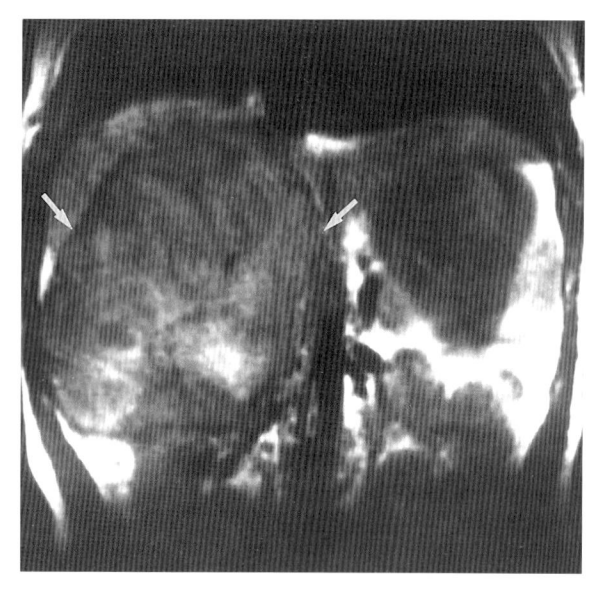

Fig. 5.**30** Large left adrenal cortical carcinoma (arrows)
a Coronal image. The mass is predominantly of low intensity (arrows)

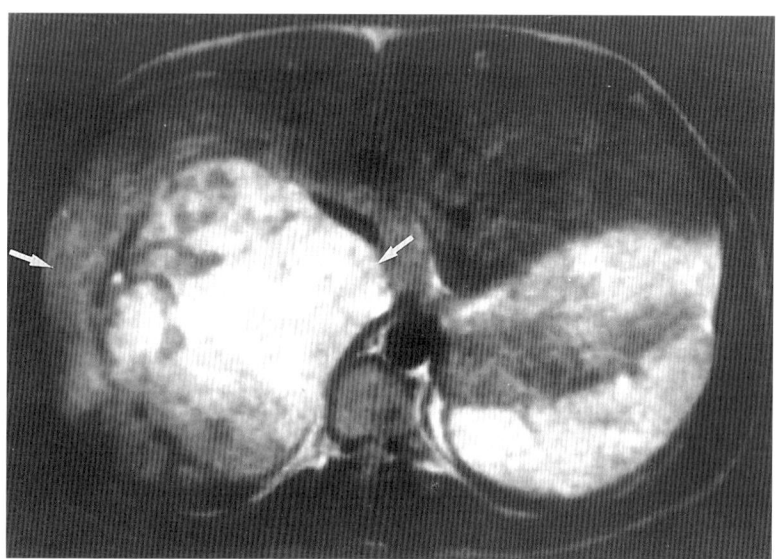

b Note areas of hyperintensity within the mass on the T2-weighted images (TR = 2000 ms TE = 60 ms, on a 0.35 T imager)

did not have many of the features available on the current generation scanners.

These functioning adenomas can resemble nonfunctioning adenomas and appear hypointense or isointense, or hyperintense with the liver on both T1- and T2-weighted images (Fig. 5.**31**) (37).

Role of MR in Adrenal Cortical Hyperfunction

Our early experience with a low field strength MR imager suggested that spin-echo MR imaging offers little additional information when compared to CT in the evaluation of hyperfunctioning adrenal cortical lesions (37). The increased spatial resolution of CT may offer an advantage in distinguishing bilateral hyperplasia from small unilateral adenomas. We are unaware of more recent studies with current generation scanners that have addressed this issue and could help determine the role of MR in adrenal cortical hyperfunction. At present, we feel that the routine use of MR in this setting is probably unnecessary. However, as stated above, MR may play a role in addressing specific issues such as caval involvement and hepatic or renal invasion in patients with functioning adrenal cortical carcinoma (42).

Adrenal Medullary Hyperfunction

Both pheochromocytomas and neuroblastomas fall into this category; Both tumors are briefly discussed.

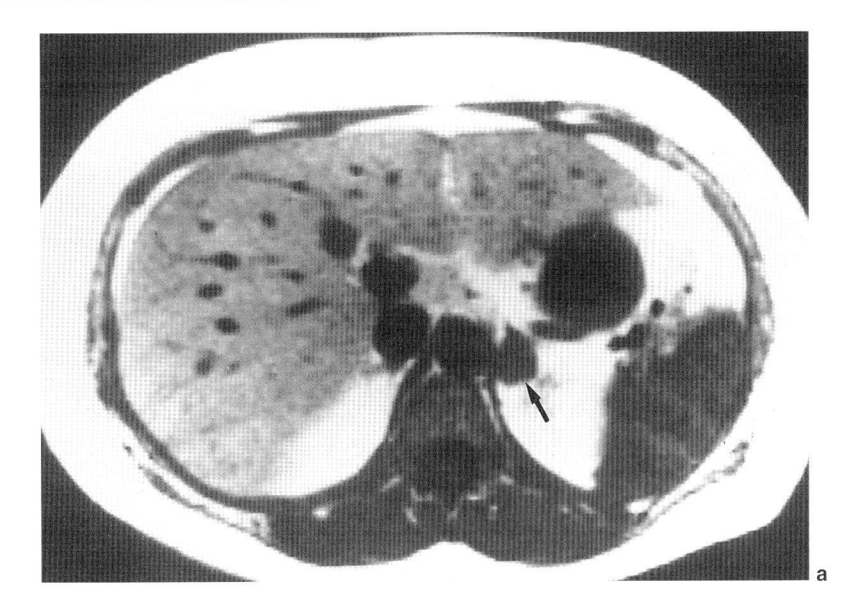

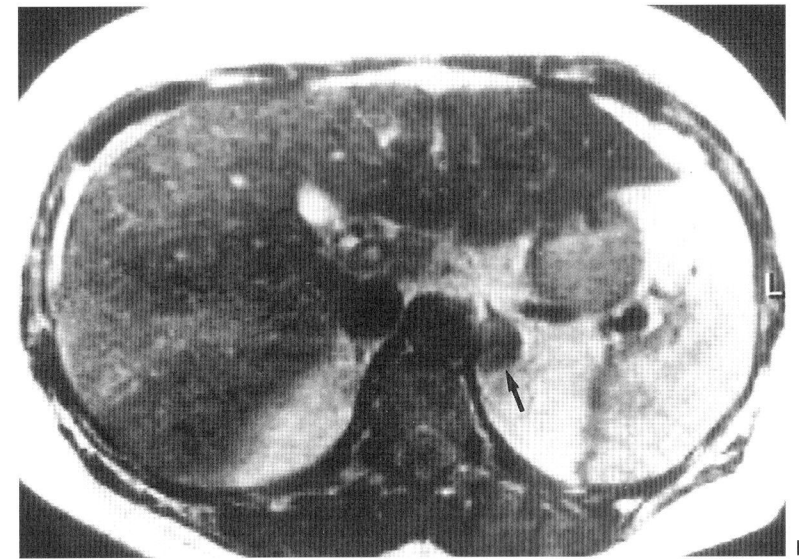

Fig. 5.**31** Aldosteronoma
a Small left adrenal aldosteronoma on T1-weighted image (arrow)
b Note that the lesion (arrow) resembles a nonfunctioning adenoma (TR = 2000 ms TE = 60 ms, on a 0.35 T imager)

Pheochromocytomas

Most pheochromocytomas (about 90%) are in the adrenal gland; the remaining 10% can be located anywhere along the sympathetic ganglia and chains. Even of the tumors located in extra-adrenal locations, most are located in the abdomen (46–48).

The tumors are usually sporadic but can be associated with certain specific syndromes. The common ones are the MEN type I, II syndromes, neurofibromatosis, and Hippel–Lindau disease. There is also a familial variety and in this condition as well as in the MEN syndromes, the tumors can be small and multicentric (48, 49).

Apart from the two exceptions described above, in general the tumors are usually large with a mean size of 3–5 cm and on CT can have a variety of appearances. The tumors can demonstrate areas of necrosis, fluid-fluid levels, and if intravenous contrast enhancement is used, they can show significant contrast enhancement (46, 48).

On low to mid field strength MR imagers, the tumors are very hyperintense on T2-weighted images in contrast to most typical adenomas (Fig. 5.**32**) (13–15). However, in one report, two low-intensity tumors have been reported mimicking adenomas. Our own limited experience on a high field strength imager has shown that at least some of these tumors are hyperintense on T2-weighted images. This hyperintense appearance has been attributed to the long relaxation times of these tumors (14).

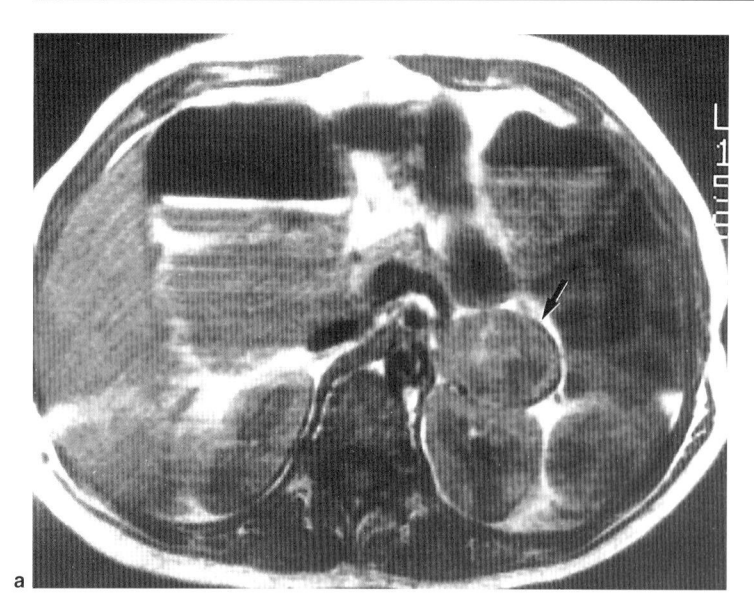

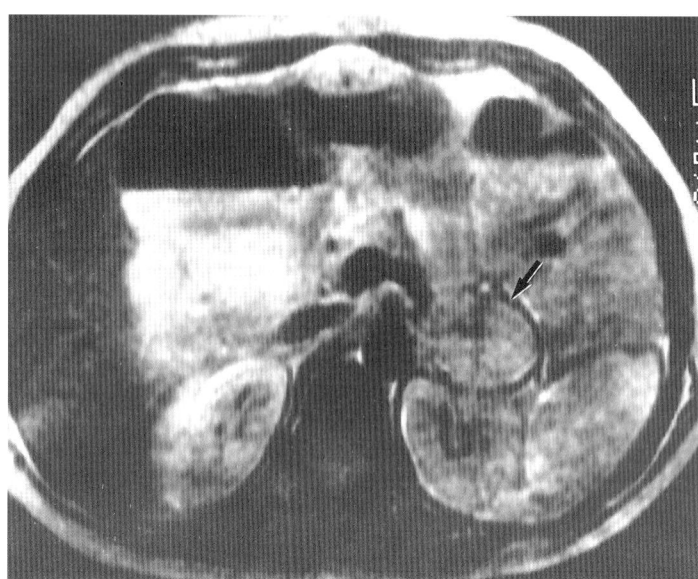

Fig. 5.**32** Pheochromocytoma
a Left adrenal pheochromocytoma on T1-weighted image (arrow)
b The mass (arrow) is hyperintense in comparison to the liver on the T2-weighted image (TR = 2000 ms TE = 60 ms, on a 0.35 T imager)

In a recent study Gd-DTPA has been used in an attempt to differentiate adenomas from nonadenomas, which included a small number of pheochromocytomas (12). The pheochromocytomas showed different contrast enhancement characteristics from adenomas. Adenomas showed early enhancement and quick washout in contrast to pheochromocytomas, which demonstrated strong persistent enhancement.

Neuroblastoma

Neuroblastoma is one of the most common solid tumors in childhood. Most of the tumors arise in the abdomen, and in 45% of children the presenting sign is the presence of an abdominal mass (50).

The tumors are generally large and appear hypointense on T1-weighted sequences and markedly hyperintense on the T2-weighted sequences. Imaging in the coronal plane is useful to determine the organ of origin of the abdominal mass i.e., distinguish a renal mass from an adrenal mass. Thus it can help differentiate a Wilms tumor and a hepatic neoplasm from a neuroblastoma (Fig. 5.**33**) (51–53).

Tumor staging is also an important aspect of tumor imaging and MR can depict the extent of the tumor because it is capable of depicting vascular anatomy and thus vascular encasement. Inferior vena caval involvement has been reported in these tumors (54), which can also be demonstrated on coronal or sagittal images using spin-echo, gradient-recalled, or MR angiographic techniques. Thus, resectable tumors can be differentiated from unresectable ones. Similarly, in patients with paraspinal tumors MR is capable of eval-

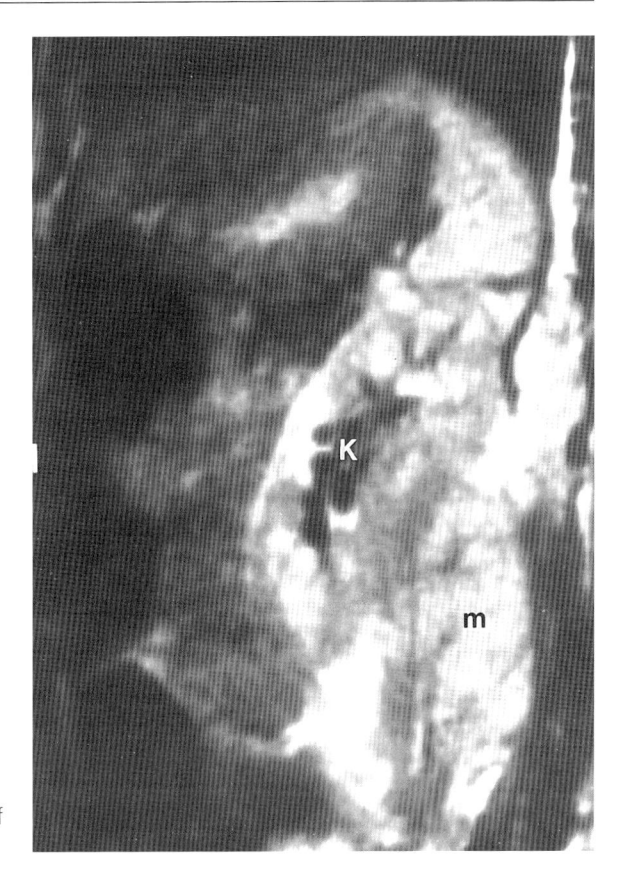

Fig. 5.**33** Neuroblastoma
a Sagittal T1-weighted image depicts separation of neuroblastoma (m) from kidney (k)

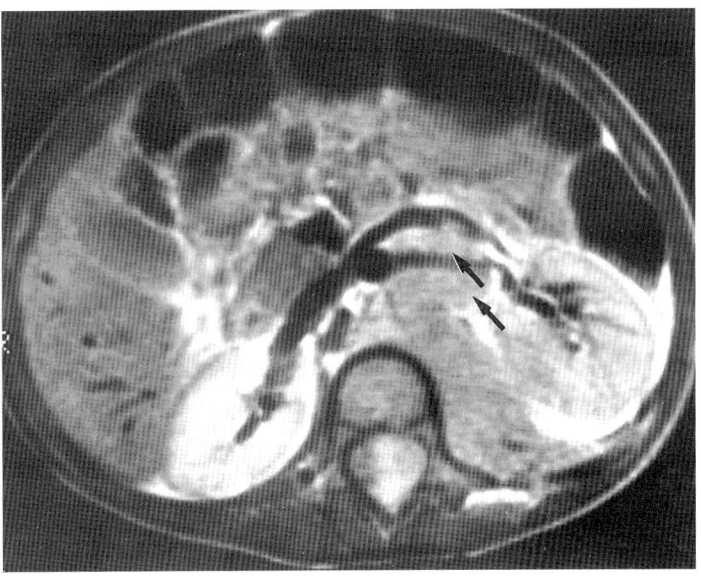

b Axial image in the same patient demonstrates that there is tumor encasement of left renal vascular pedicle (arrows)

uating the presence or absence of intraspinal extension of the tumor.

Skeletal and dural metastases are well demonstrated on T1-weighted images. The best imaging planes for demonstration of bone marrow involvement of the spine, which is common in this neoplasm, are either the coronal or sagittal planes (53).

Adenomas or Metastasis

Adrenal masses in patients with normal adrenal function must be evaluated in two clinical scenarios:

1. The incidental adrenal mass in the nononcologic patient

2. The adrenal mass in the patient with an underlying extra-adrenal primary malignancy

Adrenal Mass in the Nononcologic Patient

Most of these lesions are detected incidentally on CT examinations performed for other reasons and are often referred to as "incidentalomas." These tumors are generally under 5 cm and usually range in size from 1–3 cm. Lesions larger than 5 cm are generally considered more problematic, with a higher chance of occult malignancy, and are often removed regardless of imaging characteristics.

On CT, the incidentally discovered mass is homogeneous, well defined, low density lesions that do not show contrast enhancement (55–60). In equivocal cases, or in anxious patients, MR is of some use because a lesion that has low signal intensity on a T2-weighted sequence is much more likely to be benign. If the lesions have these features, they are, in most centers, assumed to be benign, nonfunctioning adenomas and are usually followed up with either CT or MR to confirm that there is no interval change in lesion morphology. At our medical center we use adrenal scintigraphy (using NP-59 [an iodocholesterol derivative]) as an additional tool to confirm the impression that the mass is indeed an adenoma (61, 62).

Adrenal Mass in the Oncology Patient

In this setting it becomes more crucial to distinguish an incidental nonfunctioning adenoma from a metastasis, as there are differences in clinical management.

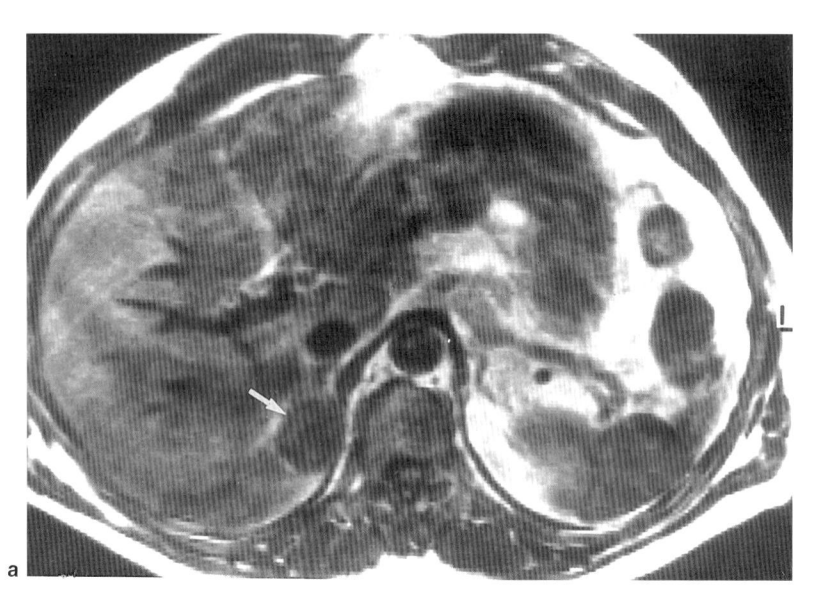

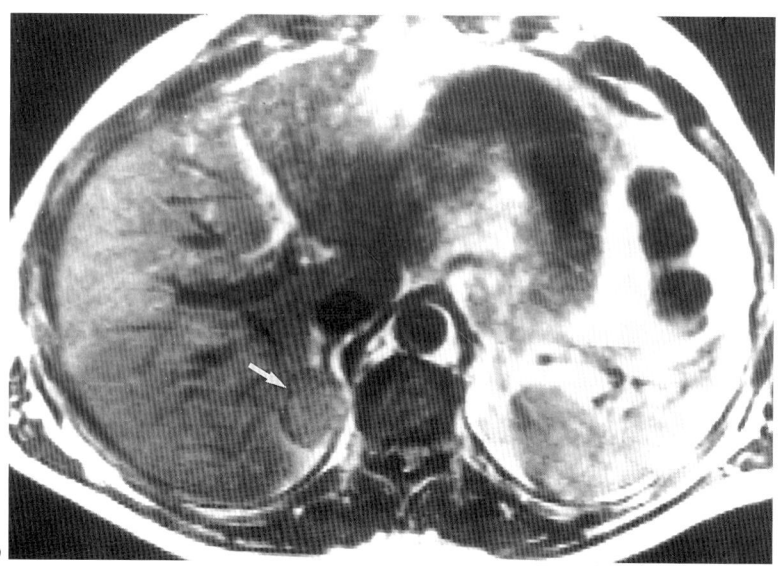

Fig. 5.**34** Nonfunctioning adenoma

a, b Typical, benign nonfunctioning adenoma (arrow) is hypo- or isointense with liver on T1- and T2-weighted images (TR = 2000 ms TE = 60 ms, on a 0.35 T imager)

Although several CT criteria have been used to attempt to make this distinction, it is not perfect because in about 20–30% of patients, there are no reliable CT criteria to make the distinction between adenomas and metastasis (58–60).

Several prior studies have addressed this issue using, low, mid and high field strength MR imagers (7–12). Using low to mid field strength imagers, most adenomas have been described as being hypointense to isointense to liver on both T1- and T2-weighted images (Fig. 5.**34**). Similarly most non-adenomas including metastases, have appeared hyperintense when compared to the liver on T2-weighted images (Fig. 5.**35**) (7–10). In studies by Glazer et al. and the other by Reinig, it was noted that there was a 20–30% crossover between adenomas an non-adenomas if signal intensity ratios were calculated.

Using high field strength imagers, it was noted that signal intensity ratios were not reliable and that adenomas could visually resemble malignant lesions (10, 11). In one study Kier and his colleagues concluded that on their 1.5-T high field strength imager, calculated T2 times were a more reliable indicator for determining whether a lesion was an adenoma or not. A cut-off of 60 ms seemed most appropriate with the least crossover between benign and malignant lesions. Lesions that had calculated T2 values less than 60 ms were most likely to be adenomas, and most with values greater than 60 ms were non-adenomas.

More recently, Krestin used contrast-enhanced breath-held gradient recalled MR imaging to differentiate between benign lesions such as adenomas from malignant adrenal tumors including metastases (12). In this study, the separation between benign and malignant lesions was nearly 90%. It showed that adenomas in general tended to show early enhancement but

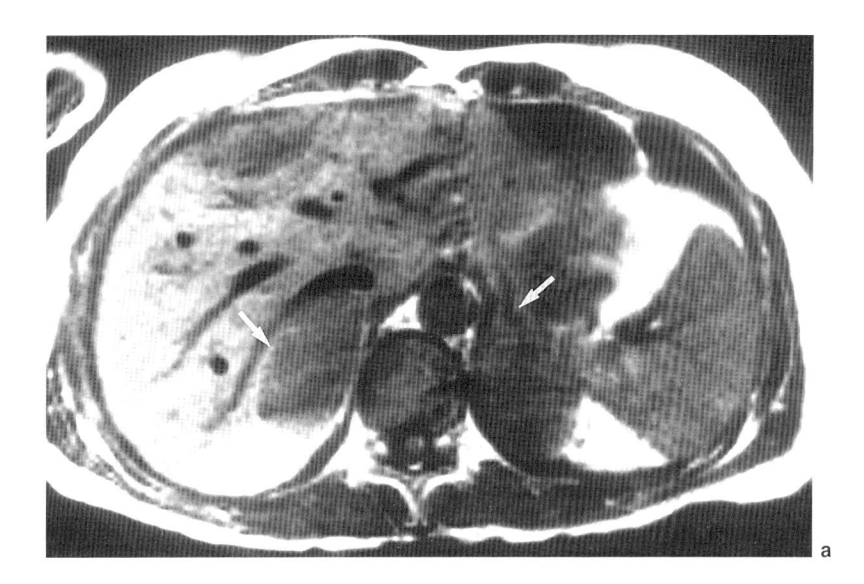

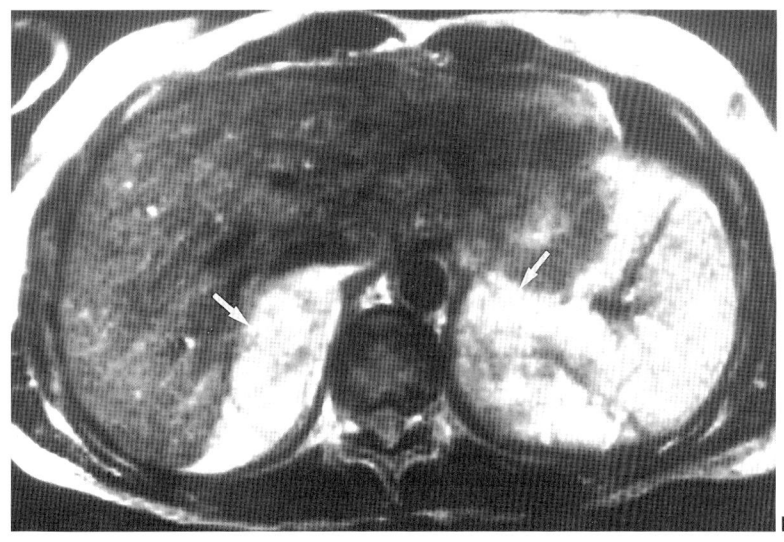

Fig. 5.**35** Bilateral adrenal lymphoma.
a The masses (arrows) are hypo- or isointense with liver on T1-weighted images
b On the T2-weighted images the masses (arrows) are hyperintense (TR = 2000 ms TE = 60 ms, on a 0.35 T imager)

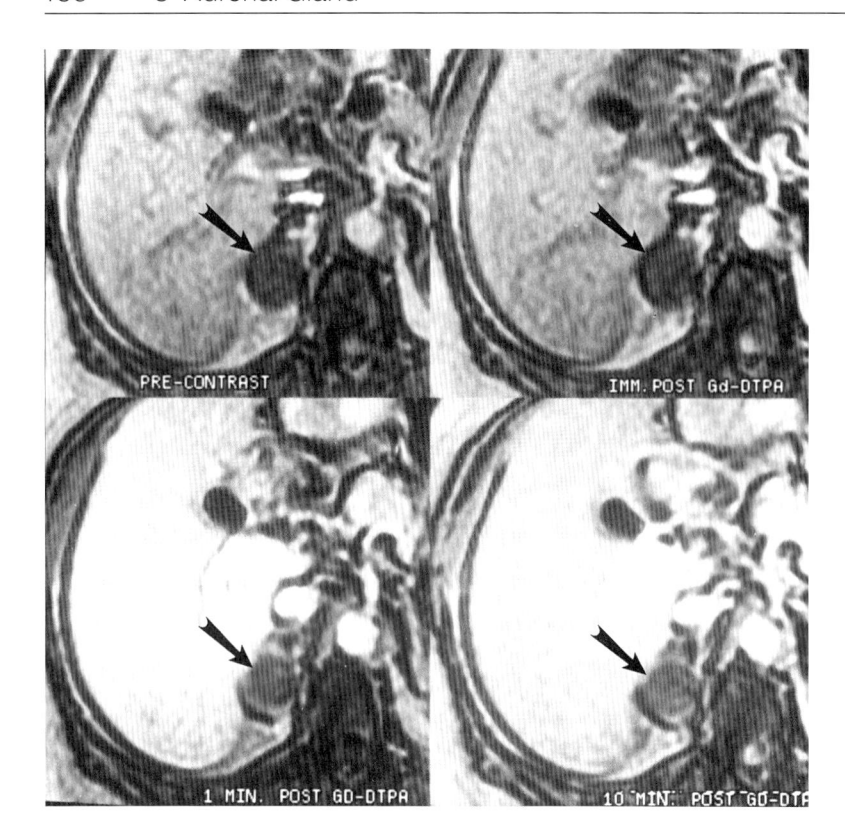

Fig. 5.**36** There is a right adrenal mass (black arrow) which shows relatively little contrast enhancement following enhancement with intravenous Gd-DTPA

quick washout, in contrast to malignant tumors, which showed slow, but persistent and greater enhancement. Our limited experience using Multiplanar Spoiled Gradient Recalled Imaging (Ultrafast SPGR) with contrast enhancement has shown similar results, as illustrated in Figs. 5.**36** and 5.**37**.

MR Spectroscopic Imaging

Leroy-Willig et al. have shown in initial work using spectroscopic imaging techniques that nonfunctioning adenomas can be separated from malignant tumors (adrenal cortical carcinomas) based on lipid content (16). The adenomas were shown in in vitro studies to contain more lipid than malignant tumors and thus could be separated from each other. However, one of the limitations of this technique is that the lesions have to be larger than 15 mm. Recently Mitchell and his colleagues reported their initial experience with gradient-echo imaging exploiting the chemical shift features of in and out of phase images (20). They successfully identified 25/26 adenomas in this study using these techniques. Using this technique, the lipid-rich adenomas lose signal and appear dark on the chemical shift out-of-phase images in contrast to their appearance ton the in-phase images. If this technique continues to reliably distinguish between lipid-containing adenomas and lipid poor non-adenomas, this will be an extremely useful test in the oncology patient.

Conclusion

MR is currently being used in some centers to evaluate incidentally discovered adrenal masses in patients with normal adrenal function, as an added method for confirming benignity of the lesion. However, we consider its role in the oncologic patient with an adrenal mass and normal adrenal function is at this time still investigational, although the study by Krestin et al. reported a high specificity for distinguishing between adenomas and metastases (12) using Gd-DTPA enhanced MR. Additional larger prospective studies to address this issue will be needed to determine if this technique will obviate the need for biopsy.

Spin-echo and gradient-recalled images as well MR angiography have been used to evaluate direct extension of large adrenal tumors into adjoining structures such as the kidney, liver, the renal vein, and the inferior vena cava without the need for intravenous contrast enhancement. Hence, these techniques are very valuable in patients with poor or borderline renal function.

MR Imaging 157

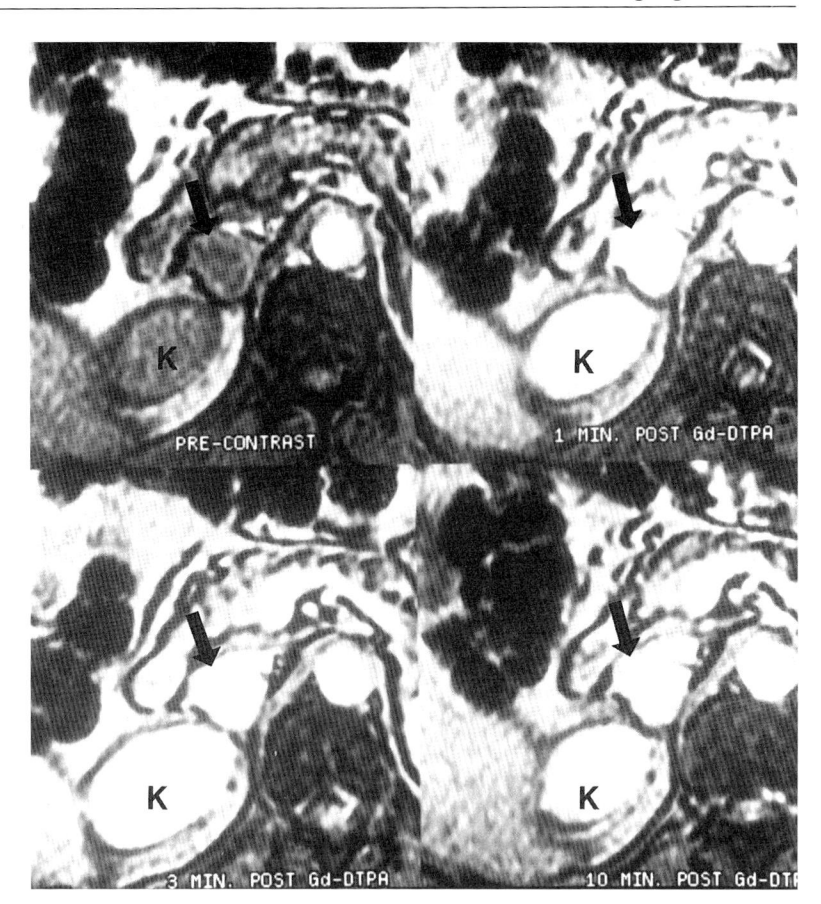

Fig. 5.**37** Mass (black arrow) anterior and medial to the right kidney (K) shows strong and persistent enhancement with Gd-DTPA. This proved to be a pheochromocytoma at surgery

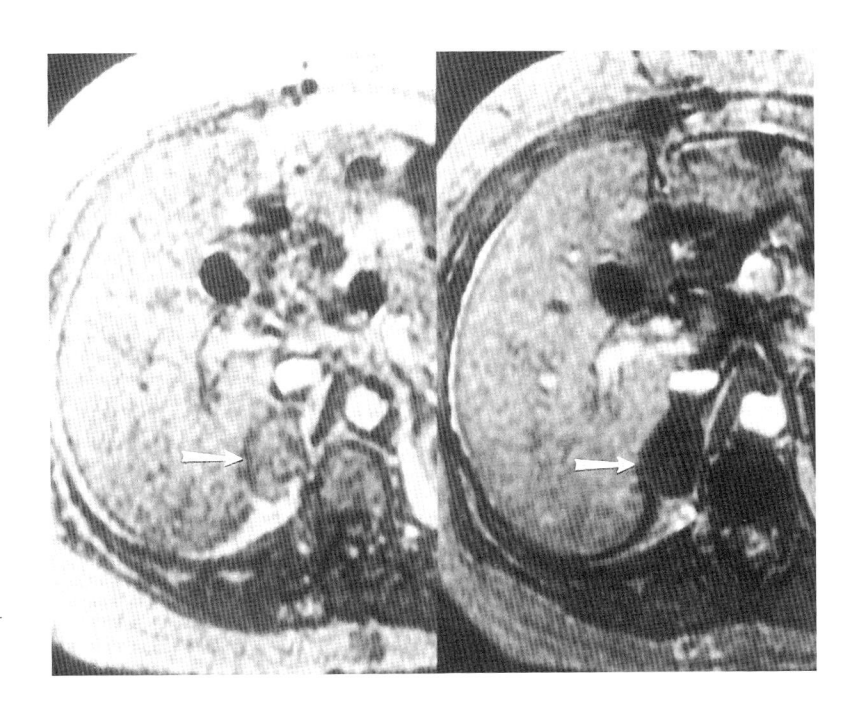

Fig. 5.**38** Right adrenal mass (white arrows) loses signal and appears dark on the out-of-phase image on the right in comparison to the in-phase image on the left

Currently MR is still used mainly as a problem-solving tool in the evaluation of adrenal disorders, and although new and fast methods are being used more commonly in the evaluation of the abdomen, it remains to be seen whether MR will replace CT as the primary imaging tool in the evaluation of adrenal disease.

References

1. Falke THM, Strake TE, Sandler MP, et al. Magnetic resonance imaging of the adrenal glands. Radiographics. 1987;7:343–370
2. Chang A, Glazer HS, Lee JKT, et al. Adrenal gland: MR imaging. Radiology. 1987;163:123–128.
3. Glazer GM, Francis IR, Quint LE. Imaging the adrenal glands. Invest Radiol. 1988;23:3–11.
4. Newhouse JH. MRI of the adrenal gland. Urol Radiol. 1990;12:1–6.
5. Korobkin MT. Overview of adrenal imaging: Adrenal CT. Urol Radiol. 1989;11:221–226.
6. Dunnick NR. Adrenal Imaging: Current status. AJR. 1990;154:927–936.
7. Reinig JW, Doppman JL, Dwyer AJ, Johnson AR and Knop RH. Distinction between adrenal adenomas and metastases using MR imaging. J Comput Assist Tomogr. 1985;9:898–901.
8. Glazer GM, Woolsey EJ, Borrello, J, et al. Adrenal characterization using MR imaging. Radiology. 1986;158:73–79.
9. Reinig JW, Doppman JL, Dwyer AJ, Johnson AR, Knop RH. Adrenal masses differentiated by MR. Radiology. 1986;158:81–84.
10. Baker ME, Blinder R, Spritzer C, Leight GS, Herfkens RJ, Dunnick NR. MR evaluation of adrenal masses at 1.5 T. AJR. 1989;153:307–312.
11. Kier R, McCarthy S. MR characterization of adrenal masses: Field strength and pulse sequence considerations. Radiology. 1989;171:671–674.
12. Krestin GP, Steinbrich W, Friedmann G. Adrenal masses: Evaluation with fast gradient-echo MR imaging and Gd-DTPA enhanced dynamic studies. Radiology. 1989;171:675–680.
13. Fink IJ, Reinig JW, Dwyer AL, et al. MR imaging of pheochromocytomas. J Comput Assist Tomogr. 1985;9:454–458.
14. Quint LE, Glazer GM, Francis IR, Shapiro B, Chenevert TL. Pheochromocytoma and Paraganglioma: comparison of MR imaging with CT and I-131 MIBG scintigraphy. Radiology. 1987;165:89–93.
15. van Gils APG, Falke THM, van Erkel AR, et al. MR imaging and MIBG scintigraphy of pheochromocytomas and extra adrenal functioning paragangliomas. Radiographics. 1991;11:37–57.
16. Leroy-Willig A, Bittoun J, Luton JP, et al. In vivo MR spectroscopic imaging of the adrenal glands: distinction between adenomas and carcinomas larger than 15 mm based on lipid content. AJR. 1989;153:771–773.
17. Glazer GM. MR imaging of the liver, kidneys and adrenal glands. Radiology. 1988;166:303–312.
18. Baker ME, Spritzer C, Blinder R, Herfkens RJ, Leight GS and Dunnick NR. Benign adrenal lesions mimicking malignancy on MR imaging: report of two cases. Radiology. 1987; 163:669–671.
19. Reinig JW, Doppman JL, Dwyer AJ and Frank J. MRI of indeterminate adrenal masses. AJR. 1986;147:493–496.
20. Mitchell DG, Crovollo M, Matteuci T, Petersen RO, Miettinen MM. Benign adrenocortical masses: Diagnosis with chemical shift MR imaging. Radiology 1992;185:345–351
21. Bailes DR, Gilderdale DJ, Bydder GM, et al. Respiratory ordered phase encoding (ROPE): a new method for reducing respiratory motion artifacts in MR imaging. J Comput Asst Tomogr. 1985;9:835–838.
22. Wood ML, Henkelman RM. Suppression of respiratory motion artifacts in magnetic resonance imaging. Med Phys. 1986;13:794–805.
23. Stark DD, Hendrick RE, Hahn PF, Ferrucci JT Jr. Motion artifact suppression with fast spin-echo imaging. Radiology. 1987;164:183–191.
24. Felmle JP, Ehman RL. Spatial presaturation: a method for suppressing flow artifacts and improving depiction of vascular anatomy in MR imaging. Radiology. 1987;164:559–564.
25. Edelman RR, Atkinson DJ, Silver MS, et al. FRODO pulse sequences: a new means of eliminating motion, flow, and wrap-around artifacts. Radiology. 1988;166:231–236.
26. Pattany PM, Phillips JJ, Chiu LC, et al. Motion artifact suppression technique (MAST) for MR imaging. J Comput Asst Tomogr. 1987;11:369–377.
27. Haacke EM, Lenz GW. Improving MR image quality in the presence of motion using rephasing gradients. AJR. 1987;148:1251–1258.
28. Mitchell DG, Vinitski S, Burk DL, et al. Motion artifact reduction in MR imaging of the abdomen: gradient moment nulling versus respiratory sorted phase encoding. Radiology. 1989;169:155–160.
29. Mitchell DG, Vinitski S, Saponaro S, et al. Liver and pancreas: improved spincho T1 contrast by shorter echo time and fat suppression at 1.5 T. Radiology. 191;178:67–71.
30. Semelka RC, Chew WM, Hricak H, et al. Fat-saturation MR imaging of the upper abdomen. AJR. 1990;155:1111–1116.
31. Edelman RR, Hahn PF, Buxton R, et al. Rapid MR imaging with suspended respiration: clinical application in the liver. Radiology. 1986;161:125–131.
32. Tung GA, Pfister RC, Papanicolaou N, et al. Adrenal cysts: Imaging and percutaneous aspiration. Radiology. 1989;173:107–110.
33. Musante F, Derchi LE, Bazzocchi M, et al. MR imaging of adrenal myelolipomas. J Comput Assist Tomogr. 1991; 15(1):111–114.
34. Falke THM, Strake TE, Shaff MI, et al. MR imaging of the adrenals: correlation with computed tomography. J Comput Assist Tomogr. 1986;10:242–253.
35. Itoh K, Yamashita K, Astoh Y, et al. MR imaging of bilateral adrenal hemorrhage. J Comput Assist Tomogr. 1988;12: 1054–1056.
36. Dunnick NR, Doppman JL, Gill JR Jr., et al. Localization of functional adrenal tumors by computed tomography and adrenal venous sampling. Radiology. 1982;142:429–433.
37. Remer EM, Weinfield RM, Glazer GM, et al. Hyperfunctioning and non hyperfunctioning benign adrenal cortical lesions: characterization and comparison with MR imaging. Radiology. 1989;171:257–260.
38. Hutter AM, Kayhoe DE. Adrenal cortical carcinoma. Am J Med. 1966;41:572–580.
39. Dunnick NR, Heaston D, Halvorsen R, et al. CT appearance of adrenal cortical carcinoma. J Comput Assist Tomogr. 1982;6:978–982.
40. Fishman EK, Deutch BM, Hartman DS, Goldman SM, Zerhouni EA, Siegelman SS. Primary adrenocortical carcinoma: CT evaluation with clinical correlation. AJR. 1987;148:531–535.
41. Dunnick NR, Doppman JL, Geelhoed GW. Intravenous extension of endocrine tumors. AJR. 1980;135:471–476.
42. Smith, Patel SK, Turner DA, Matalon DAS. Magnetic resonance imaging of adrenal cortical carcinoma. Urol Radiol. 1989;11:1–6.
43. Dunnick NR, Leight GS jr., Roubidoux MA, Leder RA, Paulson E, Kurylo I. CT in the diagnosis of primary aldoseronism in 29 patients AJR 1993;160:321–324
44. Geisinger MA, Zelch MG, Bravo EL, et al. Primary hyperaldosteronism: comparison of CT, adrenal venography and venous sampling. AJR. 1983;141:299–302.
45. Ikeda DM, Francis IR, Glazer GM, et al. The detection of adrenal tumors and hyperplasia in patients with primary hyperaldosteronism: comparison of scintigraphy, CT and MR imaging. AJR. 1989;153:301–306.
46. Welch TJ, Sheedy PF II, van Heerden JA, Sheps SG, Hattery RR, Stephens DH. Pheochromocytoma: value of computed tomography. Radiology. 1983;148:501–503.
47. Radin DR, Ralls PW, Boswell WD Jr, Colletti PM, Lapin SA, Halls JM. Pheochromocytoma: Detection by unenhanced CT. AJR. 1986;146:741–744.

48. Webb TA, Sheps SG, Carney JA. Differences between sporadic pheochromocytoma and pheochromocytoma in multiple endocrine neoplasia, type 2. Am J Surg Pathol. 1980;4:121–126.
49. Mathieu E, Despres E, Delepine N, Taieb A. MR imaging of the adrenal gland in Sipple disease. J Comput Assist Tomogr. 1987;11(5):790–794.
50. Donohue JP, Garrett RA, Baehner RL, et al. The multiple manifestations of neuroblastoma. J Urol. 1974;3:260–264.
51. Cohen MD, Weetman R, Provisor A, et al. Magnetic resonance of neuroblastoma with a 0.15T magnet. AJR. 1984;143:1241–1248.
52. Fletcher BD, Kopiwada SY, Strandjord SE, et al. Abdominal neuroblastoma: Magnetic resonance imaging and tissue characterization. Radiology. 1985;155:699–703.
53. Dietrich RB, Kangarloo H, Lenarsky C, et al. Neuroblastoma: The role of MR imaging. AJR. 1987;148:937–942.
54. Day DL, Johnson R, Cohen R, et al. Abdominal neuroblastoma with inferior vena caval tumor thrombus: report of three cases (one with right atrial extension). Pediatr Radiol. 1991;21:205.
55. Glazer HS, Weyman PJ, Sagel SS, Levitt RG, McClennan B. Non functioning adrenal masses: incidental discovery on computed tomography. AJR. 1982;139:81–85.
56. Mitnick JS, Bosniak MA, Megibow AJ, Naidich DP. Non functioning adrenal adenomas discovered incidentally on computed tomography. Radiology. 1983;148:495–499.
57. Oliver TW Jr., Bernardino ME, Miller JI, et al. Isolated adrenal masses in non small-cell bronchogenic carcinoma. Radiology. 1984;153:217–218.
58. Berland LL, Koslin DB, Kenney PJ, et al. Differentiation between small benign and malignant adrenal masses with dynamic incremented CT. AJR. 1988;151:95–101.
59. Hussain S, Belldegrun A, Seltzer SE, et al. Differentiation of malignant from benign adrenal masses: Predictive indices on computed tomography. AJR. 1985;144:61–65.
60. Lee MJ, Hahn PF, Papanicolaou N, et al. Benign and malignant adrenal masses: CT distinction with attenuation coefficients, size and observer analysis. Radiology. 1991;179:415–418.
61. Francis IR, Smid A, Gross MD, et al. Adrenal masses in oncologic patients. Functional and morphologic evaluation. Radiology. 1988;166:353–356.
62. Gross MD, Shapiro B, Bouffard AJ, et al. Distinguishing benign from malignant euadrenal masses. Ann Intern Med. 1988;109:613–618.

Angiography

Kyung J. Cho

The role of angiography and selective venous sampling in the evaluation of adrenal disease has diminished with the advent of the newer imaging modalities. Arteriography is used only in selected cases with adrenal lesions, when additional information about tumor resectability and vascular anatomy is needed following imaging studies. Selective venous sampling remains the most sensitive method for the localization of the source of primary aldosteronism and occult hypercorticism. This chapter reviews the current role of adrenal angiography and selective venous sampling in the diagnosis and localization of adrenal disease.

Vascular Anatomy

Successful performance and correct interpretation of adrenal angiography and selective venous sampling require a thorough understanding of the vascular anatomy. The adrenal glands are supplied by numerous branches of the superior, middle, and inferior adrenal arteries. The superior adrenal artery originates from the inferior phrenic arteries, which are branches of the aorta, celiac, or renal arteries. The middle adrenal artery usually arises from the aorta, whereas the inferior adrenal artery arises from the renal artery, the aorta, or occasionally from the superior polar or a capsular branch of the renal arteries.

A large central vein runs axially through the medulla and receives numerous venules from both the cortex and medulla. The left adrenal vein emerges from the adrenal hilum and is joined by the inferior phrenic vein before opeing into the superior aspect of the preaortic left renal vein (Fig. 5.**39**). When the left renal vein is retroaortic, crossing the aorta posteriorly, the left adrenal vein joins the cava separately, with a course similar to that of the preaortic left renal vein. When the left renal vein is circumaortic with both persistent ventral and dorsal limbs, the ventral (preaortic) limb is joined by the left adrenal vein. When the kidneys are ectopic or absent congenitally, the left adrenal vein drains into the small left renal vein. In contrast, the right adrenal vein almost always opens into the posterolateral aspect of the inferior vena cava between the right hepatic and renal veins. Small accessory hepatic veins arising from the same segment of the inferior vena cava may have a branching pattern similar to that of the right adrenal vein. These hepatic veins open into the anterolateral aspect of the cava, and an injection of contrast medium produces a dense accumulation of contrast medium with filling of other hepatic and portal veins (Fig. 5.**40**).

Technique

The angiographic technique used to evaluate adrenal disease has not been significantly modified over the past two decades except for use of digital subtraction technique. The arteriographic study begins with flush aortography and pelvic arteriography (for pheochromocytoma), and is followed by selective catheterization of the celiac, renal, lumbar, and inferior mesenteric arteries, depending on the abnormalities on the aortogram and prior imaging studies. An intra-arterial injection of epinephrine with a dose of 8–12 μg immediately before an injection of contrast medium into the renal and celiac arteries results in better filling of the adrenal branches. If the results of prior selective venous sampling suggest that the source of catecholamines is above the diaphragm, thoracic aortography, and subclavian and carotid arteriograms are obtained. Photographic subtraction of both the late arterial and capillary phases enhances tumor visualization. Inferior venacavography is performed via a femoral vein for evaluation of vena caval invasion.

5 Adrenal Gland

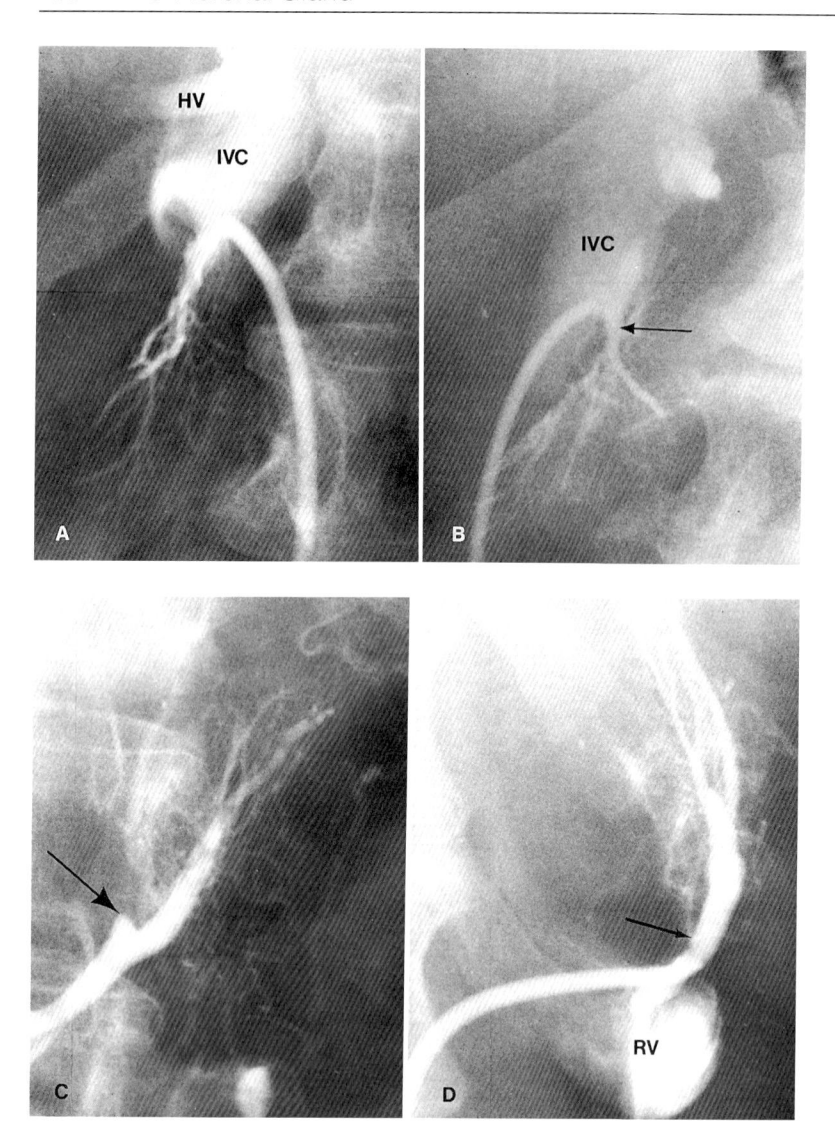

Fig. 5.**39** Normal adrenal venograms in a patient without biochemical evidence of adrenal disease. (**A**) Right adrenal venogram in the anteroposterior projection. The intraadrenal branches join a short main vein exiting at the superior part of the gland, which enters the right posterolateral aspect of the inferior vena cava. Right hepatic vein is filled from the inferior vena cava. (**B**) Right adrenal venogram in the right posterior oblique projection. The adrenal gland is projected posterior to the IVC. Note the short main vein (arrow). (**C**) Left adrenal venogram in the anteroposterior projection. The main adrenal vein receives the intra-adrenal branches while running along the axis of the adrenal gland and opens into the left renal vein after receiving the inferior phrenic vein (arrow). The renal capsular veins are filled from the surface of the gland. (**D**) Left adrenal venogram in the left posterior oblique projection. The adrenal vein (arrow) opens into the cranial aspect of the renal vein. HV = hepatic vein, IVC = inferior vena cava, RV = renal vein

Selective venous sampling is a safe procedure and provides useful diagnostic information. It is indicated in patients with suggested adrenal and extra-adrenal disorders in which diagnosis and localization are difficult. Since its description in 1967 (1), the technique of adrenal vein catheterization has been modified slightly. Both adrenal veins can be successfully catheterized in over 90% of cases. Because the procedure is safe and easy to perform, adrenal venous sampling can be performed on an outpatient basis. For the right adrenal vein, a 5 or 6.5 Fr cobra-shaped catheter is introduced into the inferior vena cava via a femoral vein, and the posterolateral aspect of the vena cava above the right renal vein is explored. Frequent injection of small amount of contrast medium facilitates catheterization. When the adrenal vein is entered and catheter position is confirmed by a test injection under fluoroscopy, blood sample is obtained. During sampling, the catheter is held in place and the patient is advised not to inhale deeply. For the left adrenal vein, a Simmonshaped catheter is introduced into the left renal vein and is slowly retracted while maintaining the tip directed cranially. When the left adrenal vein has not been entered after the tip has been retracted to near the vena cava, the catheter is advanced for a second exploration, or a straight soft-tipped guide wire is introduced to probe the orifice. When the tip of the catheter is near the adrenal vein, contrast medium is injected to identify the orifice. It is important that the tip is not placed in the inferior phrenic vein. Sampling is obtained from the adrenal vein either proximal or distal to the junction of the inferior phrenic vein. Simultaneous sampling using two catheters is helpful because hormone secretion may be episodic (Table 5.**4**).

For localization of pheochromocytoma, blood samples are obtained from various levels of the infe-

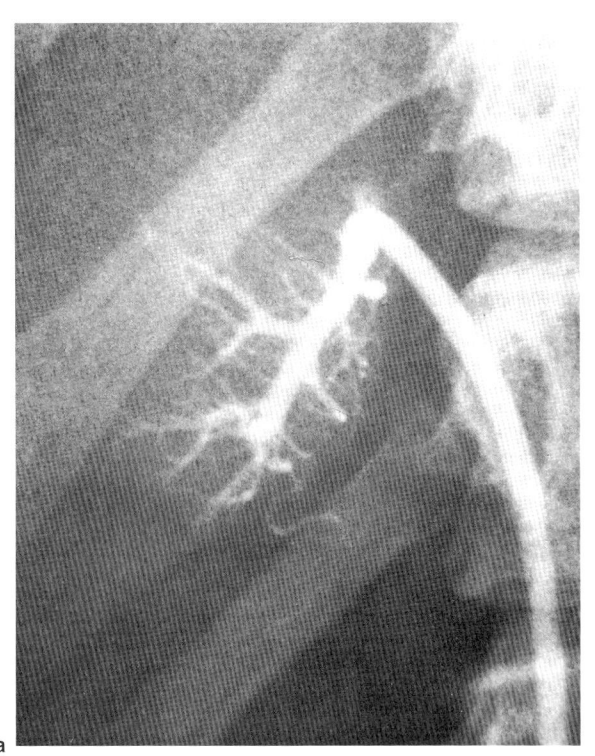

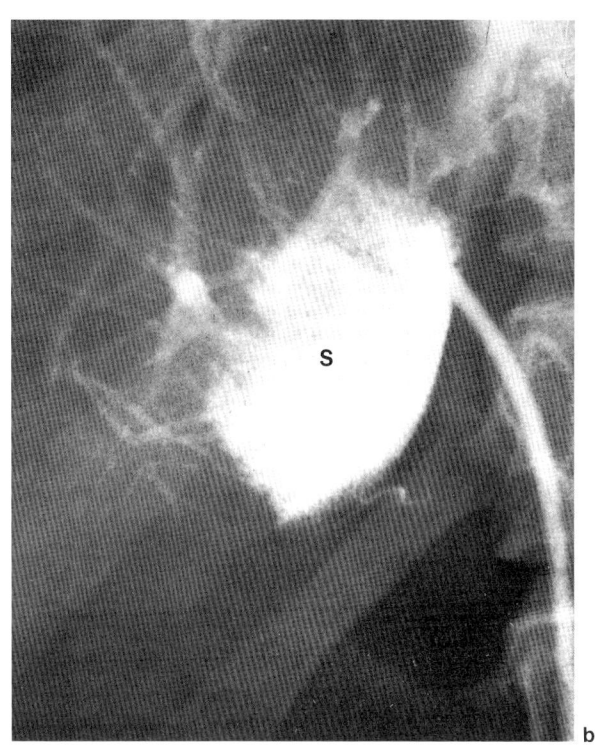

Fig. 5.40 An accessory hepatic venogram in the anteroposterior projection. (**a**) Early filling. The vein runs obliquely toward the right anterolateral aspect of the inferior vena cava. (**b**) Dense accumulation of contrast medium in the hepatic sinusoids (S) and filling of the hepatic and portal veins are typical of the accessory hepatic vein

rior vena cava, iliac, and jugular veins (2). Petrosal sinus sampling with ACTH assay is helpful in distinguishing pituitary from ectopic ACTH source (3, 4). In petrosal sinus sampling, catheters are percutaneously introduced via femoral veins and manipulated into the horizontal portions of both petrosal sinuses. Samples are also obtained from other veins including the jugular, thyroid, thymic, azygos, adrenal, and iliac veins, and superior and inferior vena cavas. Pulmonary veins are catheterized via the aorta for localization of pulmonary source of ACTH and the portal vein via the transhepatic approach for localization of the pancreatic source of ACTH.

Hypercorticism

Hypercorticism may be caused by autonomous function of an adrenal neoplasm, or excessive stimulation of the adrenal glands by a pituitary or ectopic ACTH-producing tumor. Successful treatment depends on accurate preoperative diagnosis and localization of the tumor. Both CT and adrenal scintigraphy are com-

Table 5.4 Episodic hormone secretion in a 38-year-old man with left aldosteronoma

	Aldosterone (ng/dL)			Hydrocortisone (µg/dL)			Norepinephrine (pg/mL)			Epinephrine (pm/L)			A/C Ratio		
	Right	Left	IVC	Right	Left	IVC	Right	Left	IVC	Right	Left	IVC	Right	Left	IVC
Initial	449	3004	38	714	22	16	2800	843	514	9785	2226	<20	0.6	136	2.3
Repeat	241	1167	21	401	18	11	1377	1632	484	4827	6708	<20	0.6	64	1.9

Note the significant changes in adrenal venous and caval hormone levels on repeat samples but the aldosterone ratios on both samples localize the tumor to the left adrenal gland. Hydrocortisone levels are higher in the adrenal vein without tumor. The A/C ratio in the normal side remains the same, whereas that in the adrenal vein with tumor decreased from 136 to 64.

IVC = Inferior Vena Cava

plementary methods and are capable of localizing most tumors. Venous sampling is a sensitive method but reserved for patients with inconclusive imaging studies. If inappropriate secretion of ACTH or a non-pituitary neoplasm producing ACTH is suggested, selective petrosal sinus sampling helps the surgeon plan the correct operation. If petrosal sinus sampling indicates an ectopic ACTH source, and imaging studies are normal, pulmonary venous sampling may be needed. Tumors that are known to produce ACTH are bronchial carcinoids, thymic carcinoids, pheochromocytomas, and islet-cell tumors.

Adrenal venography with hydrocortisone assay is useful in distinguishing neoplasm from hyperplasia. In a unilateral disease, hydrocortisone levels in the adrenal vein draining the tumor are significantly higher than those in the contralateral adrenal vein and the inferior vena cava. If catheterization is limited to either side, a hydrocortisone value in the adrenal vein similar to that of the inferior vena cava localizes a tumor to the opposite adrenal gland, whereas a hydrocortisone level significantly higher than that in the inferior vena cava with the venographic absence of a tumor and on CT or both, indicates bilateral adrenal hyperplasia. The venographic appearances of hydrocortisone producing adenoma are nonspecific and similar to those of other adrenal adenomas. The intraadrenal branches are displaced around the tumor and the contralateral adrenal gland may appear small with crowding of adrenal venous branches (Fig. 5.41). The venographic findings of bilateral adrenal hyperplasia include enlargement of the glands with spreading of adrenal venous branches. Arteriographically, adrenal adenomas exhibit tumor blush with subtle neovascularity.

Primary Aldosteronism

Primary aldosteronism is a rare clinical syndrome caused by autonomous secretion of aldosterone from a unilateral adrenocortical adenoma or bilateral adrenal hyperplasia. Since adrenalectomy is the treatment of choice in unilateral adrenal disease, preoperative diagnosis and differentiation between aldosteronoma and bilateral hyperplasia are important. CT and adrenal scintigraphy are complementary methods for

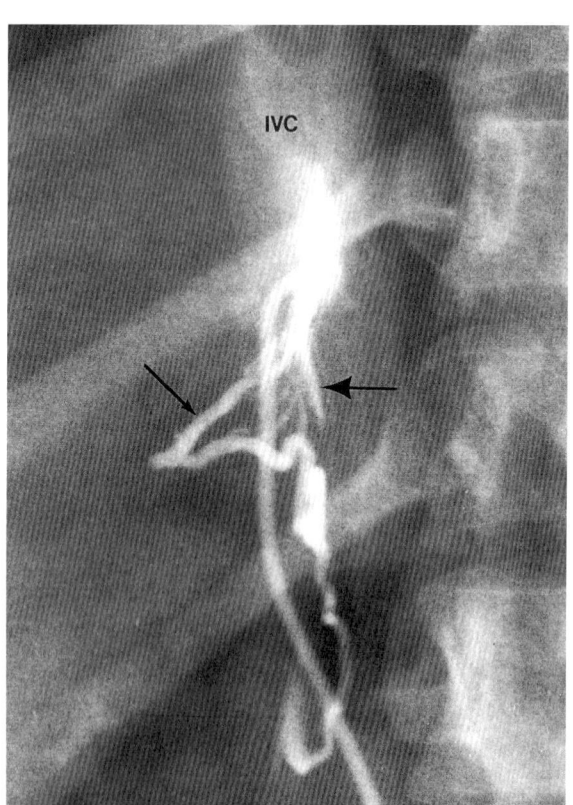

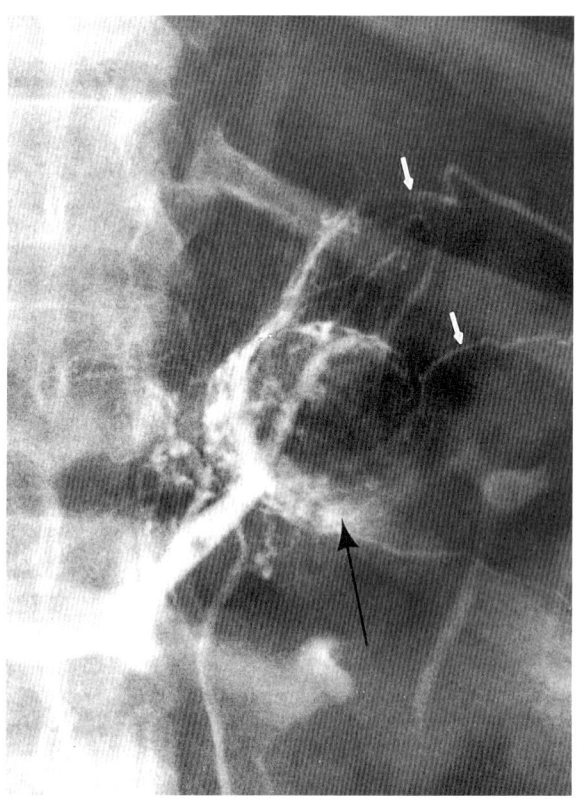

Fig. 5.41 Left adrenal adenoma in a 30-year-old woman with Cushing syndrome. (a) Right adrenal venogram. Right adrenal gland is atrophic with crowded intraadrenal branches (larger arrow). The adrenal capsular veins (smaller arrow) are dilated. (b) Left adrenal venogram. The intra-adrenal veins are distorted and displaced by the tumor (larger arrow), and the capsular veins are filled (smaller arrows). (From Cho KJ. Urologic Radiology 1982;3:249–255)

the diagnosis and localization of primary aldosteronism.

If prior imaging studies fail to localize an adenoma, or, if bilateral adrenal hyperplasia is suggested, selective adrenal venous sampling is indicated (5, 6). Determination of aldosterone and hydrocortisone levels in both adrenal venous effluent before and after ACTH stimulation can accurately localize the source of aldosterone excess and distinguish unilateral from bilateral adrenal disease. Adrenal venography may be used only for confirmation of catheter position. Although baseline sampling is highly accurate in diagnosis of aldosteronoma, a repeat sampling after ACTH stimulation may be required in selected cases. Measurement of hydrocortisone in each sample determines not only the accuracy of sampling, but also provides a means of compensating for differences in hormone concentration from catheter placement and dilution of the adrenal venous blood (6).

In unilateral aldosteronoma, aldosterone levels in the vein of the adrenal gland with tumor are significantly higher than those of the contralateral adrenal vein and inferior vena cava. In general, an aldosterone ratio of 3.0 or higher localizes an adenoma to the side with higher aldosterone levels and a ratio of less than 3.0 is evidence of bilateral hyperplasia (Table 5.5). The aldosteron elevel in the opposite adrenal gland in unilateral disease is slightly higher than or similar to those in the vena cava. Both aldosterone and A/C ratios may overlap between unilateral and bilateral adrenal disease, owing to episodic hormone secretion and to dilution of the adrenal venous blood. Difficulty of hormone analysis due to overlap can be resolved by a repeat selective sampling after ACTH stimulation. The aldosterone ratio may increase or decrease following ACTH stimulation but usually remains greater than 3.0 in unilateral adenoma, whereas a slight increase in the ratio but less than 3.0 is evidence of bilateral adrenal hyperplasia. The A/C ratios of 6.2 or higher localize unilateral disease, whereas an A/C ratio of 3.6 or lower indicates bilateral adrenal hyperplasia (6). In bilateral adrenal hyperplasia, both the aldosterone and A/C ratios in both adrenal veins are significantly higher than those in the vena cava (Table 5.6).

Arteriography has no diagnostic role in the evaluation of aldosteronoma. Arteriographically, aldosteronomas are vascular with moderate accumulation of a contrast medium with inconspicuous tumor vessels. The venographic appearance of aldosteronoma is similar to those of other small cortical adenomas. Venographically, bilateral adrenal hyperplasia shows nonspecific distortion of intra-adrenal veins (Fig. 5.42).

Adrenal Cortical Carcinoma

Adrenal cortical carcinoma is a rare tumor that may be biologically functional or nonfunctional. Approximately half of the tumors are functional and may present with Cushing syndrome, the adrenogenital syndrome, and hyperaldosteronism, depending on the type of hormone produced (7). No significant difference in survival has been found between functional and nonfunctional tumors (8). Early detection and radical surgery offer the best chances for long-term survival and the possibility of cure. Since the majority of adrenocortical carcinomas are greater than 5 cm in diameter, both CT and MRI can easily localize and stage the tumor, Angiographically, tumor vessels are demonstrated in over 90% of patients (8). Angiographic differentiation of an adrenal adenoma from a small carcinoma is difficult. Adrenal venography, selective adrenal and gonadal venous sampling are helpful for differentiating adrenal from extra-adrenal sources in feminizing tumors in males and virilizing tumors in females. Inferior vena cavography and renal venography are performed to evaluate venous involvement. Because it may be difficult to differentiate

Table 5.5 Results of adrenal venous sampling in a 45-year-old woman with right adrenal aldosteronoma

	Aldosterone (ng/dL)			Aldosterone Ratio	Hydrocortisone (µg/dL)			A/C Ratio			Ratio of A/C
	Right	Left	IVC		Right	Left	IVC	Right	Left	IVC	
Basal	3,872	38	30	102	11	24	2	352	1.5	15	235
				After ACTH							
5 min.	8,847	407	46	21.7	141	1,521	9	63	.27	5	225
10 min.	10,449	588	49	17.7	299	1,993	16	35	.3	3	117
20 min.	20,819	570	69	36.5	312	1,902	18	67	.3	3.8	223

Aldosterone levels in the right adrenal gland are higher than those of the left adrenal gland both before and after ACTH. The aldosterone level in the normal adrenal gland is similar to that of cava due to suppression. After ACTH stimulation, aldosterone levels in both adrenal veins increased but the aldosterone ratios decreased. Hydrocortisone response to ACTH is greater in the normal than the opposite gland.

Table 5.6 Adrenal venous sampling in a 53-year-old man with bilateral adrenal hyperplasia

	Aldosterone (ng/dL)			Aldosterone Ratio	Hydrocortisone (µg/dL)			A/C Ratio			Ratio of A/C
	Right	Left	IVC		Right	Left	IVC	Right	Left	IVC	
Basal	6409	3623	63	1.8	43	44	14	149	82	4.5	1.8
After ACTH											
10 min.	15,957	11,746	83	1.4	1,469	1,513	23	10.8	7.7	3.6	1.4
15 min.	17,628	12,845	104	1.4	1,488	1,631	25	11.8	7.8	4.2	1.5
25 min.	18,426	11,620	107	1.6	1,404	1,750	27	13.1	6.6	3.9	1.9

Aldosterone levels in both adrenal veins are higher than those in the inferior vena cava. The aldosterone (right/left) ratios are < 1.8 before and after ACTH. The ratios of A/C ratios are < 1.9.

adrenal from upper pole renal carcinoma with CT, angiography remains useful for this differentiation. The angiographic findings of adrenal carcinoma include fine, sparse neovascularity fed by the adrenal and capsular arteries and minimal puddling or shunting (9). In contrast, renal cell carcinomas usually demonstrate abundant coarse tumor vessels, fed by the renal and capsular arteries, with puddling and shunting.

Pheochromocytomas

Once the diagnosis of pheochromocytomas is established by the measurement of plasma and urinary catecholamines or their metabolites, CT, MRI, and ^{131}I-MIBG scintigraphy are performed to localize and stage the tumor. When imaging studies are inconclusive or localize a tumor adjacent to major vascular structures, arteriography and inferior vena cavogra-

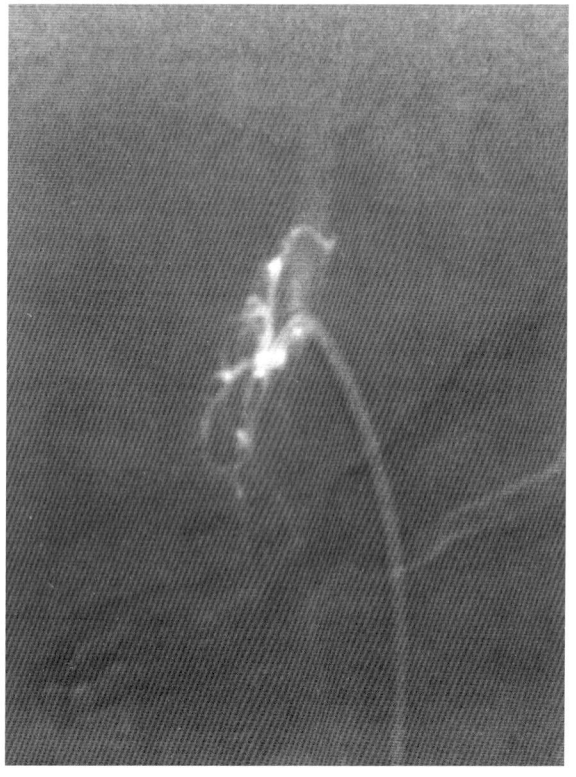

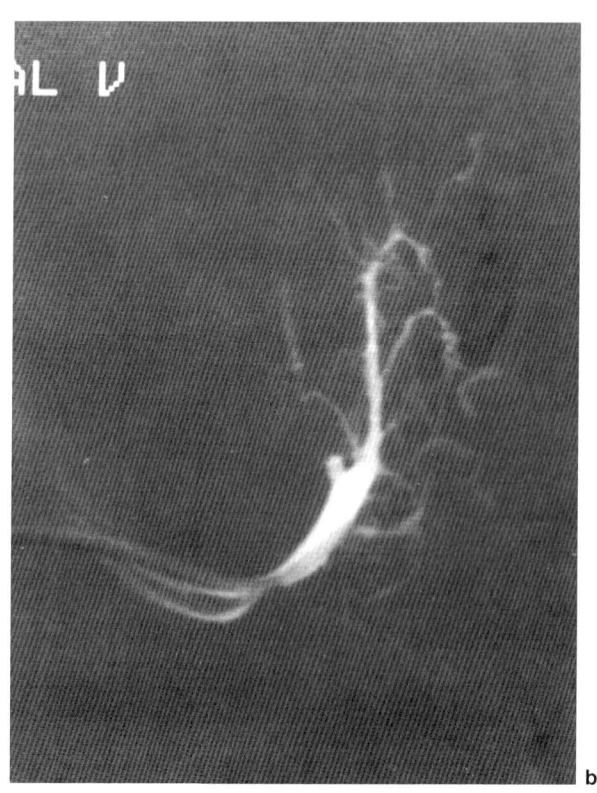

Fig. 5.42 Bilateral adrenal hyperplasia in a 53-year-old man with primary aldosteronism (same case in Table 3). (**a**) Right adrenal digital subtraction venogram showing arcuate displacement of the intra-adrenal veins. (**b**) Left adrenal venogram. The adrenal gland is enlarged and the intra-adrenal veins are distorted

Angiography 165

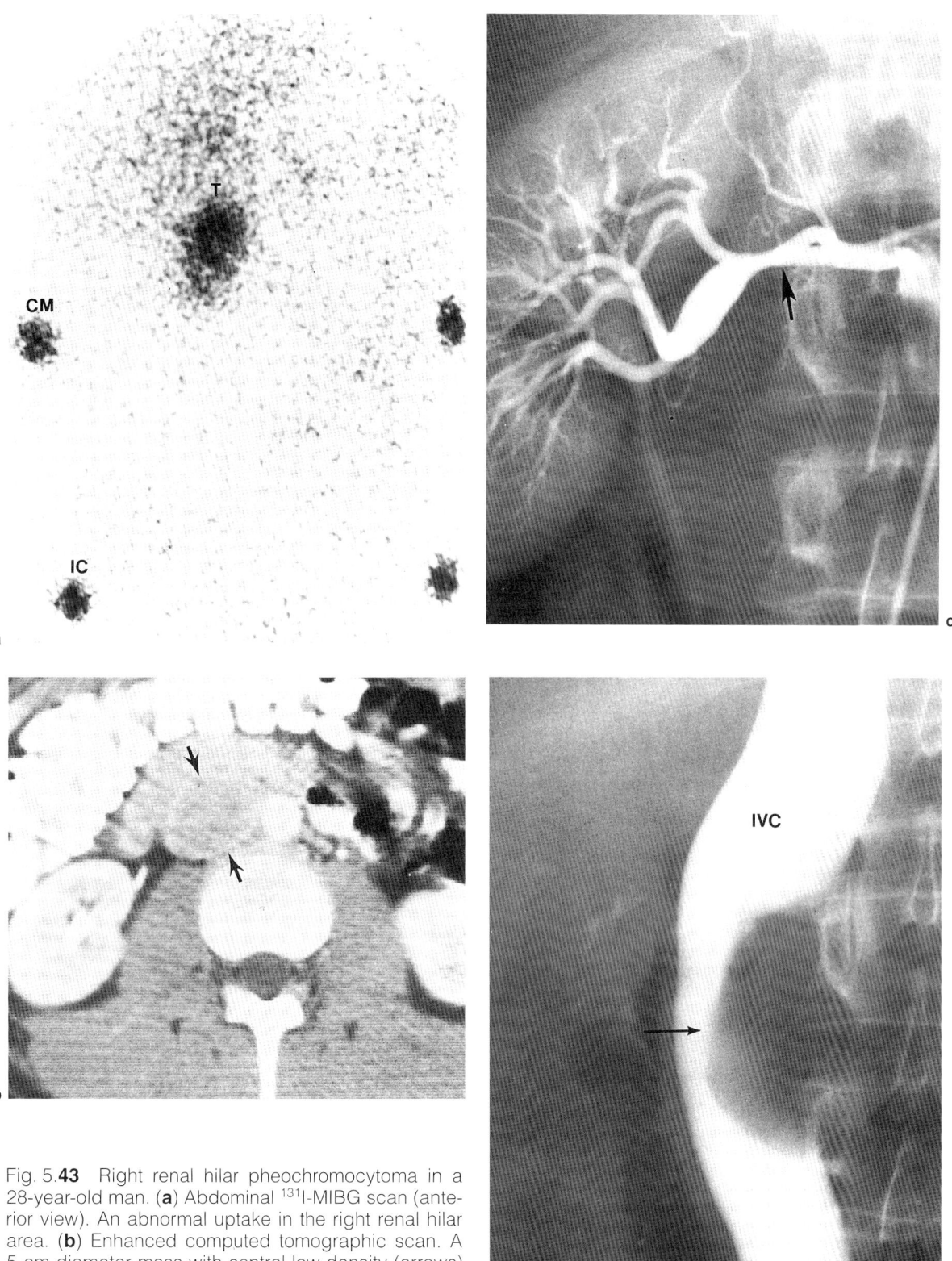

Fig. 5.**43** Right renal hilar pheochromocytoma in a 28-year-old man. (**a**) Abdominal ^{131}I-MIBG scan (anterior view). An abnormal uptake in the right renal hilar area. (**b**) Enhanced computed tomographic scan. A 5-cm diameter mass with central low density (arrows) in the region of the inferior vena cava. (**c**) Right renal arteriogram. The main renal artery is compressed by the mass (arrow). (**d**) Inferior vena cavogram. The inferior vena cava is displaced and compressed by the mass (arrow). T = tumor, CM = costal margin, IC = iliac crest, IVC = inferior vena cava

phy or both are performed to provide the necessary preoperative vascular information (Fig. 5.43).

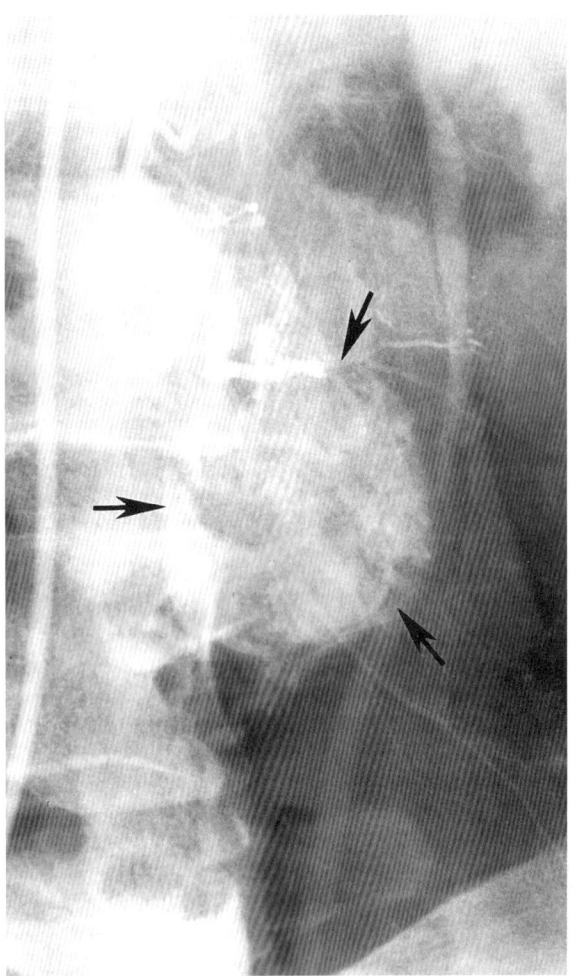

The patient in whom pheochromocytomas is suggested should be prepared with adrenergic blocking drugs to minimize the risk of hypertensive crisis and subsequent complications. Phenoxybenzamine hydrochloride (Dibenzyline), a long-acting adrenergic, α-adrenergic receptor blocking agent is administered orally before angiography. Phentolamine (Regitine), a short-acting agent, is administered intravenously if contrast injection induces significant hypertension. Propranolol hydrochloride (Inderal), a beta-adrenergic receptor blocking agent, is given orally to the patient with catecholamine-induced cardiac arrhythmias. During the arteriographic procedure, blood pressure should be checked before and after each injection of contrast medium and the ECG continuously monitored. Appropriate symphathetic blocking and stimulating agents should be at hand for immediate administration if necessary.

Angiographically, both adrenal and extra-adrenal pheochromocytomas are usually vascular with homogeneous accumulation of a contrast medium (Fig. 5.44). Small tumors have scanty neovascularity, with inconspicuous feeding arteries, whereas large tumors

Fig. 5.44 Pheochromocytoma arising from the organ of Zuckerkandl. Parenchymal phase of left third lumbar arteriogram showing homogeneous tumor blush (arrows). The left ureter is displaced laterally

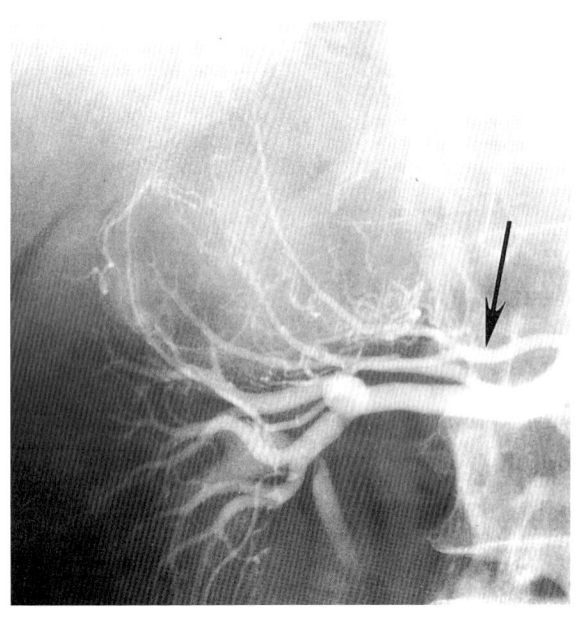

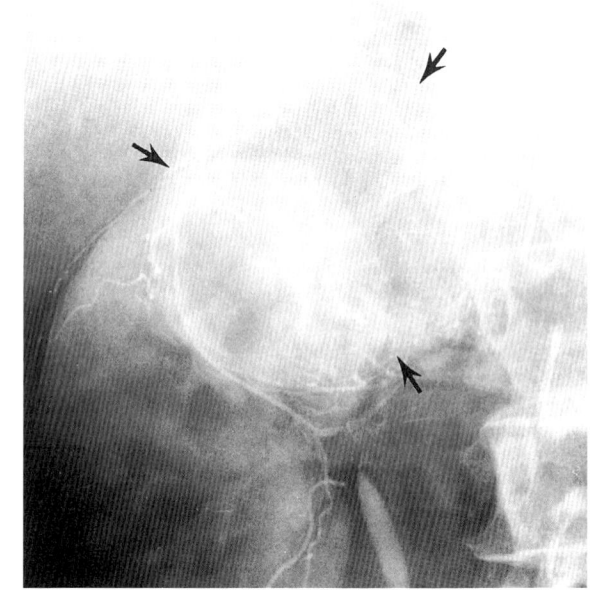

Fig. 5.45 Right adrenal cystic pheochromocytoma in a 57-year-old man with neurofibromatosis. (a) Right renal arteriogram showing dilated adrenal artery (arrow) and fine tumor vessels in periphery of the mass. (b) Parenchymal phase showing central lucency (arrows)

Angiography 167

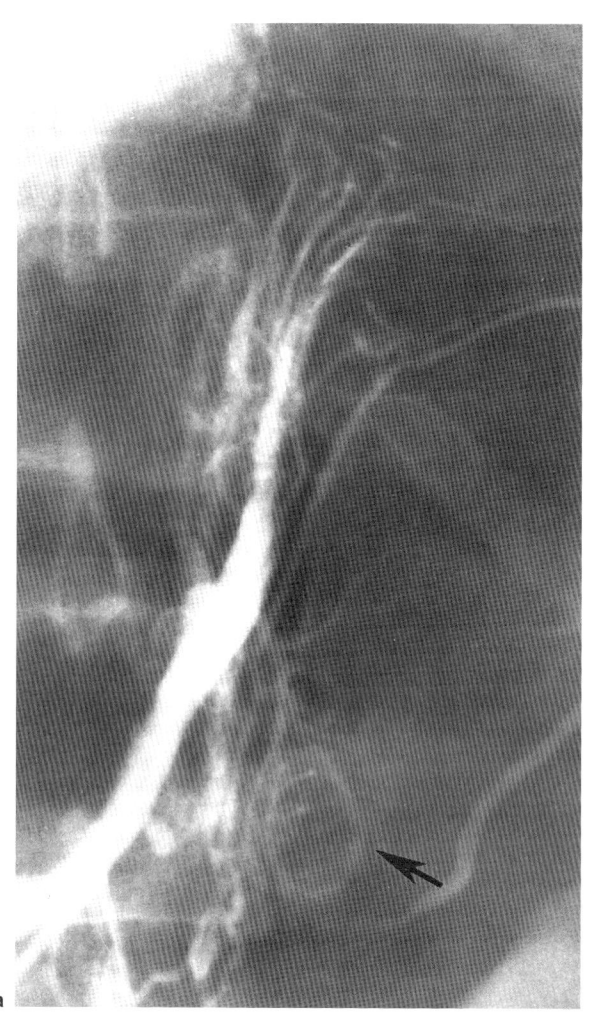

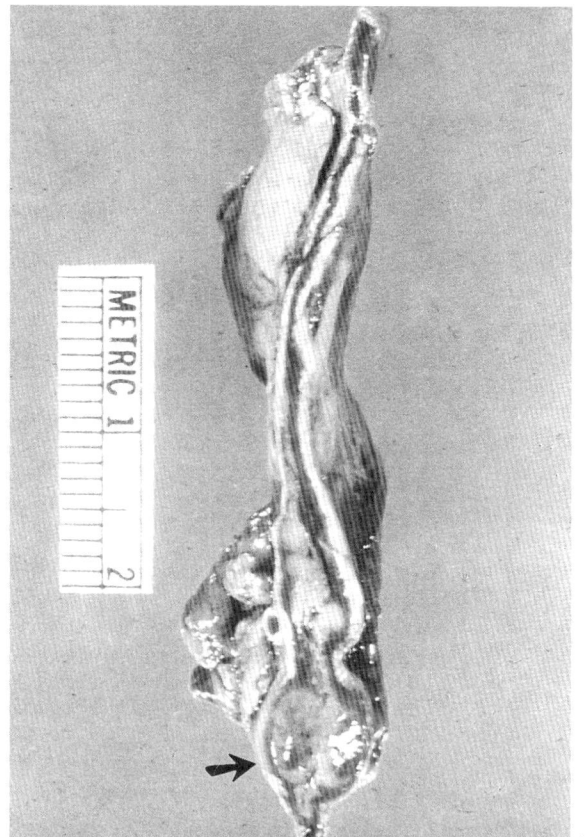

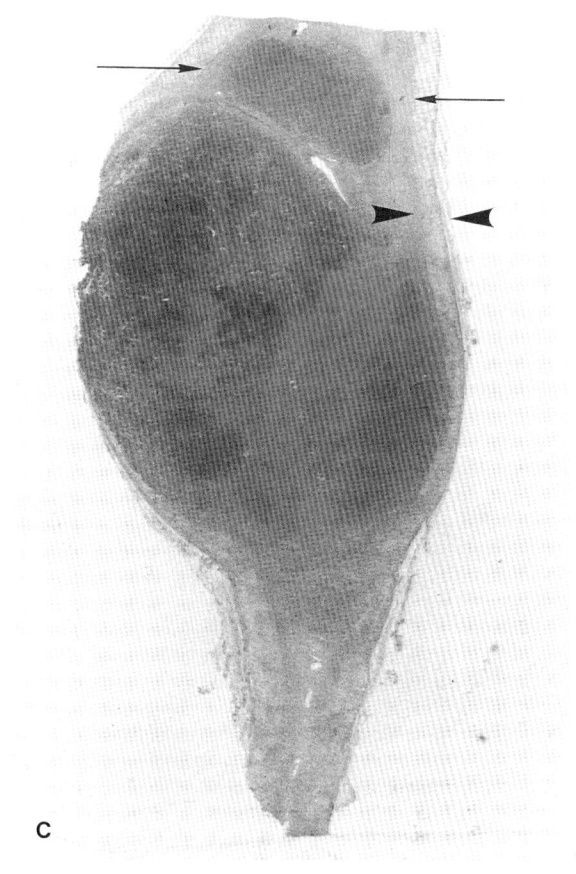

Fig. 5.**46** Bilateral adrenal medullary hyperplasia in a 24-year-old woman with MEN type II syndrome. (**a**) Left adrenal venogram showing an ovoid mass in the lower part of the adrenal gland (arrow). (**b**) Section of left adrenal gland showing nodular expansion of the medulla and a medullary nodule (1.2 cm in diam), pheochromocytoma (arrow). (**c**) Histological section of pheochromocytoma of left adrenal gland and adjacent nodular medullary hyperplasia. Expanded medulla (between arrows) and thin cortex (between arrowheads) (H and E × 4). (From Cho et al. AJR 1980; 134:23–29)

are more vascular with abundant tumor vessels and dilated feeding arteries. Tumor vessels may be coarse and arranged in a reticulated pattern, or converging toward the center in a spoke-wheel manner or distributed in the periphery of the mass. A combination of central lucency and peripheral tumor blush in the tumor with central necrosis gives the appearance of a "ring" (Fig. 5.**45**). About 10% of the tumors are hypovascular due to infarction and cystic changes, and may be missed at angiography. Intravenous extension of a pheochromocytoma into the inferior vena cava may demonstrate a linear vascular pattern parallel to the course of the vena cava. The origin of feeding arteries depends on the origin of the tumor. The adrenal tumor is supplied by the adrenal arteries, whereas the retroperitoneal pheochromocytomas receive their blood supply from the lumbar and inferior mesenteric arteries. The tumors of the pelvis and bladder receive blood from the internal iliac artery.

Renal artery stenosis may coexist with pheochromocytomas in the renal hilar region (Fig. 5.**43 c**). It may be secondary to compression of the artery by the tumor or to catecholamine released from the tumor. Surgical removal of the tumor may result in restoration of the artery. The arteriographic appearance and the results of renal vein renin sampling are helpful in determining whether the stenosis needs surgical correction. The relatively typical arteriographic appearance of the stenosis and its close proximity to the tumor allows differentiation from coexisting stenotic disease due to other causes such as fibromuscular dysplasia and arteriosclerosis. Angiography cannot be used to differentiate benign from malignant tumors unless metastases is present. Like primary tumors, both recurrent and metastatic tumors are usually vascular.

Adrenal venography and venous sampling are reserved for patients with inconclusive imaging studies. Venous sampling with determination of epinephrine and norepinephrine is useful in patients with suggested extra-adrenal pheochromocytomas (10). As with arteriography, the patient undergoing venography and venous sampling should be prepared with adrenergic blocking agents. Adrenal venography is sensitive in demonstrating small adrenal medullary nodules associated with MEN type II syndrome (11) (Fig. 5.**46**). Venographic findings of pheochromocytoma vary greatly depending on the tumor size. The adrenal venous branches are stretched arcuately similar to those caused by cortical adenomas. In larger tumors, the adrenal veins are dilated with prominent venous channels. When the tumor has central necrosis or cystic change, only a few dilated veins may be demonstrated. The venographic findings of adrenal medullary hyperplasia are similar to those of cortical hyperplasia. The adrenal gland may show enlargement with spreading of intra-adrenal venous branches. Nodular hyperplasia may produce minimal arcuate displacement of small adrenal venous branches.

Catheterization of the inferior vena cava with assay of plasma catecholamine is useful for the localization of tumors in patients in whom unusual sites of paraganglioma, malignant, or multiple tumors are suggested. Caval sampling is preferred to selective adrenal venous sampling because selective catheterization and injection of a contast medium may precipitate the release of a large amount of catecholamines. In caval sampling, a curve-tipped catheter with one or two side holes made near its tip is placed at the appropriate levels of the inferior vena cava to collect adrenal venous effluent and regional blood samples. Adrenal venous blood is collected from both sides of the inferior vena cava between the diaphragm and right adrenal vein, and from the left renal vein. Additional blood samples are obtained from both sides of the cava between the renal veins and caval bifurcation, the iliac, jugular, and innominate veins, and the superior vena cava.

Conclusion

Despite the availability of the newer imaging modalities, selective venous sampling continues to play an important diagnostic role in patients with hypercorticism and primary aldosteronism. Adrenal venous sampling is a safe procedure and can be performed on an outpatient basis. Arteriography is indicated only in selective patients in whom additional information is needed preoperatively. To date, percutaneous adrenal ablation through arterial and venous approaches has not been useful in the management of patients with adrenal disease (12–16).

References

1. Reuter SR, Blair AJ, Schteingart DE, Bookstein JJ. Adrenal venography. Radiology. 1967;89:805–814.
2. Harrison TS, Freier DT. Pitfalls in the technique and interpretation of regional venous sampling for localizing pheochromocytoma. Surg Clin North Am. 1974;54:339–347.
3. Doppman JL, Oldfield E, Krudy AG, Chrousos GP, Schulte HM, et al. Petrosal sinus sampling for Cushing's syndrome: Anatomical and technical considerations. Radiology. 1984;150:99–103.
4. Doppman JL, Nieman L, Miller DL, Pass HI, Chang R, et al. Ectopic adrenocorticotropic hormone syndrome: Localization sutdies in 28 patients. Radiology. 1989;172:115–124.
5. Yune HY, Klatte EC, Grim CE, Weinberger MH, Donohue JP, et al. Radiology in primary hyperaldosteronism. AJR. 1976;127:761–767.
6. Dunnick NR, Doppman JL, Mills SR, Gill JR, Jr. Preoperative diagnosis and localization of aldosteronomas by measurement of corticosteroids in adrenal venous blood. Radiology. 1979;133:331–333.
7. Richie JP, Gittes RF. Carcinoma of the adrenal cortex. Cancer. 1980;45:1957–1964.
8. Nader S, Hickey RC, Sellin RV, Samaan NA. Adrenal cortical carcinoma. A study of 77 cases. Cancer. 1983;52:707–711.
9. Fritzsche P, Andersen C, Cahill P. Vascular specificity in differentiating adrenal carcinoma from renal cell carcinoma. Radiology 1977;125:113–117.
10. Palubinskas AJ, Rizen MF, Conte FA. Localization of functioning pheochromocytomas by venous sampling and radioenzymatic analysis. Radiology. 1980;136:495–496.

11 Cho KJ, Freier DT, McCormick TL, Nishiyama RH, Forrest ME, et al. Adrenal medullary disease in multiple endocrine neoplasia type II. AJR. 1980;134:23–29.
12 Zimmerman CE, Kettyle WM, Eisenberg HR, Spark R, Rosoff CB, Cohen RB. Transvenous adrenalectomy. J Surg Res. 1972;12:124–127.
13 Zimmerman CE, Eisenberg HR, Spark R, Rosoff CB. Transvenous adrenal destruction: Clinical trials in patients with metastatic malignancy. Surgery. 1974;75(4):550–556.
14 Bunuan HD, Alltree M, Merendino RA. Gelfoam embolization of a functioning pheochromocytoma. Am J Surg. 1978;136:395–398.
15 Dunnick NR, Doppman JL, Gill JR Jr. Failure to ablate the adrenal gland by injection of contrast material. Radiology. 1982;142:67–69.
16 Horton JA, Hrabovsky E, Klingberg WG, Hostler JA, Jenkins JJ. Therapeutic embolization of a hyperfunctioning pheochromocytoma. AJR. 1983;140:987–988.

Nuclear Medicine
G. Barzen

In contrast to the radiological techniques used to image the adrenal gland, which are based on morphological appearance, scintigraphic imaging relies on the functional status of the adrenal gland.

This means that scintigraphic imaging is only possible and successful in case of hormone production of the adrenal gland (tracer, adosterol, and MIBG) or on the basis of available receptors (Somatostatin receptor imaging).

Differentation of the different diseases of the adrenal gland is not possible from the morphological appearance gained by scintigraphic studies. This is the domain of radiological methods (CT and MRI) because scintigraphic studies are insufficient here. The object of scintigraphy is to obtain further clues for interpretation (hormone production) of structures that are indistinguishable on CT and MRI and to search for the locations of excessive hormone production. Because different tracers have to be used to detect different adrenal pathologic lesions, the following questions should asked:

Is there any excessive hormone production in the adrenal cortex or medulla?
Which hormone or metabolites are elevated in the blood or urine?
What kind of disease is most probable?

Principles of Scintigraphic Imaging of the Adrenal Cortex

Scintigraphic imaging of the adrenal cortex is based on the ability of the adrenal tissue to produce steroid hormones. For imaging purposes, a labeled precursor of the steroidal hormones is given, which accumulates in the adrenal tissue depending on the rate of hormone production. The biosynthetic pathway for the production of the major mineralocorticoids (aldosterone), glucocorticoids (hydrocortisone) and androgens (testosterone) starts with cholesterol, derived from the diet and from endogenous synthesis through acetate.

For scintigraphic imaging, ^{131}I-labeled derivates of cholesterol have been investigated. Today only ^{131}iodomethyl-19-nor-cholest-5(10)-en-3β-ol (Adosterol), which has a greater affinity than the earlier used ^{131}I-19-iodocholesterol, is available for intravenous administration. A third tracer, ^{75}Se-6 β-selenomethyl-19-norcholesterol, which behaves nearly identically to ^{131}iodomethyl-19-nor-cholest-5(10)-en-3β-ol, is also used. ^{75}Se is a pure gamma emitter with a long physical half-life (119 days).

Because these tracers are like cholesterol precursors of minerolocorticoids, glucocorticoids, and androgens, differentation between these hormones is impossible, i.e., excessive production of minerolocorticoids (hyperoldosteronism) is not differentiable scintigraphically from excessive production of glucocorticoids (Cushing syndrome). Therefore, it is only demonstrable by scintigraphic means if there is a unilateral or bilateral excessive, reduced, lost, or normal steroid production. The causes and the affected hormones can not be demonstrated.

Technique

Administration

Before administration, thyroidal uptake of free radioiodine has to be blocked by administrating

Table 5.7 Dosimetry of ^{131}I-iodomethyl-19-norcholesterol (Adosterol), ^{75}Se-6β-selenomethyl-19-norcholesterol (SMC) and $^{123/131}$I-meta-iodobenzyl-guanidine

	Adosterol	SMC	^{123}I-MIBG	^{131}I-MIBG
Dose	37 MBq	9.25 MBq	370 MBq	37 MBq
Dosimetry (cGy/dose)				
Adrenals	28	6.1	8–30	100
Thyroid			22–35	36
ovaries	8.0	1.9	1.4	0.6–0.8
liver	2.4	2.4	1.0	0.4
whole body	1.2	1.4	0.2	0.1

Lugol's solution (strong iodine solution) potassium iodine, or perchlorate for 14 days; 0.25–0.5 MBq/kg body weight ^{131}iodomethyl-19-nor-cholest-5(10)-en-3β-ol (adosterol) minimal 20 MBq and maximal 74 MBq is slowly given intravenously. Specific activity is 37 MBq/mg. Rarely, allergic reactions are seen.

Acquisition

Images are acquired on a large FOV gamma camera with a parallel-hole, high-energy (^{131}I, 360 KeV) collimator. Planar dorsal and ventral projections are performed.

Studies are performed from 24 hours up to 7 days p.i., sometimes delayed images up to 12 days p.i. are recommended (M1.0). For suppression scintiscans (to demonstrate pathological hormone production), dexamethasone can be given orally in a dosage of either 2 mg daily (0.5 mg every 6 hours), starting 48 hours before tracer injection, or 4 mg daily (1 mg every 6 hours), starting 7 days before tracer injection, and continuing for the duration of the study.

Normal Distribution

Because ^{131}iodomethyl-19-nor-cholest-5(10)-en-3β-ol (Adosterol) and its metabolites are excreted by way of the kidney, liver, and biliary systems into the duodenum and bowel, the bladder, liver, and bowel are regularly visible (Fig. 5.**47**). Also, the normal adrenal cortex appears roughly symmetrical; the right adrenal gland may be a little bit more prominent in dorsal projections. The normal uptake per gland is between 0.07% and 0.3% of the injected dose.

Pathological Findings

Interpretation of missed or decreased tracer accumulation in scintigraphy is difficult because visualization of the adrenal cortex depends on dose, time after application, actual hormone production, drug interaction (oral contraceptives, spironolactone), and adrenal stimmulation by ACTH and angiotensin II or both. Therefore, it may be normal in most cases that the adrenal cortex is not, or only faintly visualized in patients after injection of small doses (20 MBq or less), whereas in high doses (40 MBq or more) the adrenal cortex should be seen in nearly all normal cases. Clearly, asymmetrical uptake (increased uptake) on one side (adenoma) or decreased (lost) uptake on the other side (anatomical destruction) is a pathological sign in most cases (see Table 5.**8**) because excessive hormone production on one side, which suppresses the ACTH serum level, is followed by suppression of the other adrenal gland. Nevertheless, hormone production is only partly dependent on ACTH.

In patients with Cushing syndrome, the uptake and size of the adrenal cortex reflect the underlying pathophysiology, but they appear normal in about 30–40% of patients (6, 14). In 60–70% there is an asymmetrically (adenoma) (Fig. 5.**48**) or symmetrically increased tracer uptake or an enlargement of the affected side (see also Table 5.**8**). In functioning adrenal carcinoma, the uptake of cholesterol on the affected side is low and therefore not visualized (13), whereas on the contralateral side, uptake is inhibited. In this case, adrenal carcinoma is suggested and unilateral adenoma excluded. Other causes of bilateral missed visualization such as hypercholesterolemia also have to be excluded.

In patients with aldosteronism caused by an adenoma (primary hyperaldosteronism [Conn Syndrome]) there is unilateral enlargement and increased uptake in most cases.

In secondary aldosteronism, there may be bilateral enlargement and increased uptake. Patients with virilism (androgenital syndrome) most often show a bilateral ACTH-induced increased uptake of the enlarged glands (Table 5.**8**).

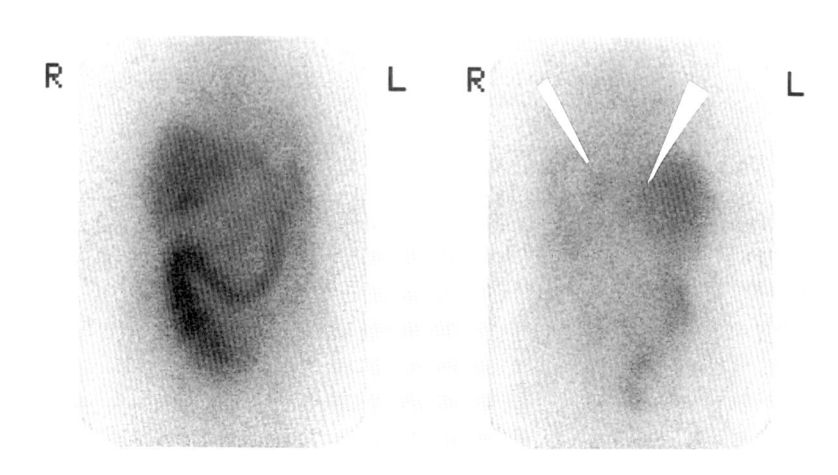

Fig. 5.**47** Normal distribution 48 hours after administration of ^{131}I-iodomethyl-19-norcholest-5(10)-en-3β-ol (Adosterol) the liver and the bowel are visible. The adrenals are seen in dorsal projection as faint accumulation

Table 5.**8** Scintigraphic Imaging of the Adrenal Cortex: findings with ^{131}iodomethyl-19-norcholest-5(10)-en-3β-ol (Adosterol^R)

Diagnosis	Findings	
	Size of the gland small/normal/enlarged	Intensity of accumulation reduced/normal/high
Cushing syndrome caused by		
Adrenal hyperplasia (secondary)	bilateral –/normal/enlarged	–/normal/high
Adrenal nodular hyperplasia	bilateral –/normal/enlarged	–/normal/high
Adrenal neoplasia		
Adenoma	unilateral of the affected site –/normal/enlarged	–/normal/high
Carcinoma	–/normal/enlarged	reduced/normal
echogenous	bilateral small/normal/–	reduced/–/–
Aldosteronism caused by		
primary (adenoma)	unilateral (affected side) –/normal/enlarged	–/normal/high
secondary	bilateral –/normal/enlarged	–/normal/high
Virilism Caused by		
Hyperplasia	bilateral –/normal/enlarged	–/normal/high
Adenoma/carcinoma	unilateral (affected side) –/normal/enlarged	–/normal/high
Adrenal insufficiency primary adrenal insufficiency		
anatomical destruction		
affected side:	uni-/bilateral in most cases not visible	reduced/–/–
unaffected side:	–/normal/–	–/normal/–
metabolic failure in hormone production	bilateral (glands in most cases not visible)	reduced/–/–
secondary adrenal insufficiency	bilateral (glands in most cases not visible, accumulation of tracer after application of ACTH demonstrable)	

Principles of Scintigraphic Imaging of the Adrenal Medulla

In the middle of the first trimester of fetal life, cells of the neural crest migrate from the thoracic region to form the sympathetic chain and other ganglia, and to invade the developing adrenal cortex, where they become the adrenal medulla (4). As a part of the neuroectodermal tissue (sympathetic system), the adrenal medulla, by way of biosynthesis, has the ability to produce Tyrosine—Dihydroxyphenylalanine—dopamine, norepinephrine (80%), and epinephrine (20%), which are released into the circulatory system on demand. For scintigraphic imaging of the adrenal medulla, ($^{123/131}$I-MIBG) is used. This physiological analog of norepinephrine and guanethidine was first synthesized by Wieland et al. (15). The uptake mechanism remains uncertain, but there is a passive diffusion process (5) and a sodium-dependent uptake, which could be inhibited by desipramine and cocaine, suggesting that uptake occurs by neuronally characterized uptake 1 system. Both mechanisms are re-

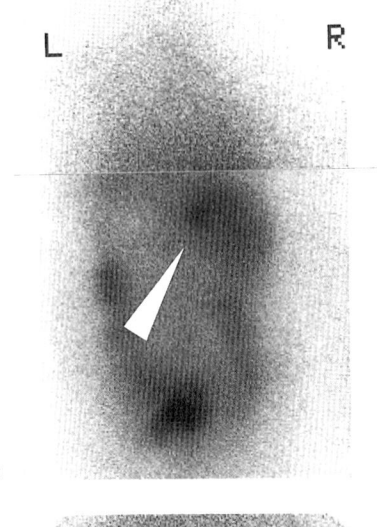

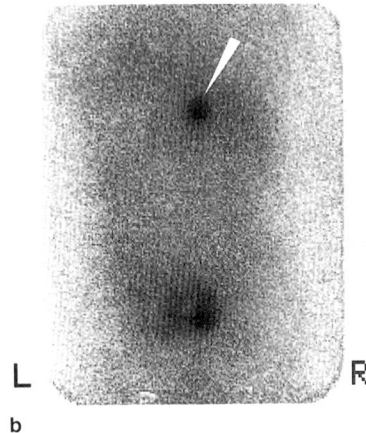

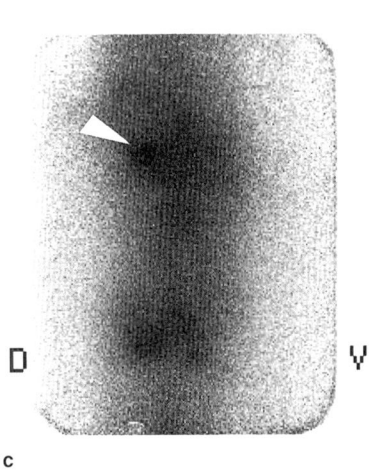

Fig. 5.48 Cushing syndrome In the dorsal projection ((**a**) 48 hours p. i. and (**b**) 144 hours p. i.), and in the lateral view ((**c**) 144 hours p. i.) in a patient with suggested Cushing syndrome, a unilateral accumulation in the region of the right adrenal gland is visible, whereas the left adrenal gland is not visible. High activity in the bowel and an adenoma of the right adrenal gland (histologically proven) are shown

sponsible for the uptake of $^{123/131}$I-MIBG in intracellular storage granules in the normal medulla, whereas the sodium-dependent uptake is seen in pheochromocytomas exclusively. In most cases, imaging is only successful if there is increased hormone production, which means that the level of epinehrine, norepinephrine or its metabolites in blood or urine shoud be elevated. A normal blood level, however, does not exclude successful imaging.

The adrenal medulla can be affected by three important diseases with increased uptake of MIBG: pheochromocytoma (paraganglioma), neuroblastoma, and ganglioneuroma (ganglioneurocytoma).

Technique

Administration

Before injection, thyroidal uptake of free radioiodine has to be blocked by administration of Lugol's solution (strong iodine solution), potassium iodine, or perchlorate. As a analog of norepinephrine, $^{123/131}$I-MIBG may theoretically displace it from the storage granules and precipitates a hypertensive crisis. Therefore, slow i.v. injection over 30 seconds is recommended.

^{123}I-MIBG and ^{131}I-MIBG are available for imaging studies. Twenty to 40 MBq, and sometimes up to 74 MBq ^{131}I-MIBG, is given, or 400 MBq ^{123}I-MIBG, which resembles a similar dosimetry of 20 MBq ^{131}I-MIBG and has superior imaging characteristics.

Acquisition

Images are acquired on a large FOV gamma camera with parallel-hole high-energy (^{131}I-MIBG, 360 KeV) or low-energy (^{123}I-MIBG, 159 KeV) collimator.

Imaging is always performed at 24 hours and 48 hours p.i., and additional images can be made up to 7 days p.i. if ^{131}I-MIBG is used. Dorsal and ventral planar projections are performed, and SPECT may be used 24 hours p.i. if 400–600 MBq ^{123}I-MIBG has been administered. Also, ^{99m}Tc-DMSA may be used to outline both kidneys to localize the MIBG accumulation exactly.

Normal Distribution

Using up to 40 MBq ^{131}I-MIBG, the adrenal medulla is normally not visualized, but with higher doses of up to 174 MBq, the normal medulla is visible as a faint area in the dorsal projections. This dose is, however, considerably higher than the dose that is now considered appropriate for routine imaging (3).

In normal cases ^{123}I-MIBG scintigraphy (400 MBq) routinely shows the normal medulla in dorsal projections. A number of drugs (cocaine, reserpine, tricyclic antidepressants, phenylpropanolamine, etc.) interfere with MIBG uptake and should be discontinued before imaging.

MIBG uptake is uniformly seen in the liver and spleen (Fig. 5.49) with a maximum of 24 hours p.i. and

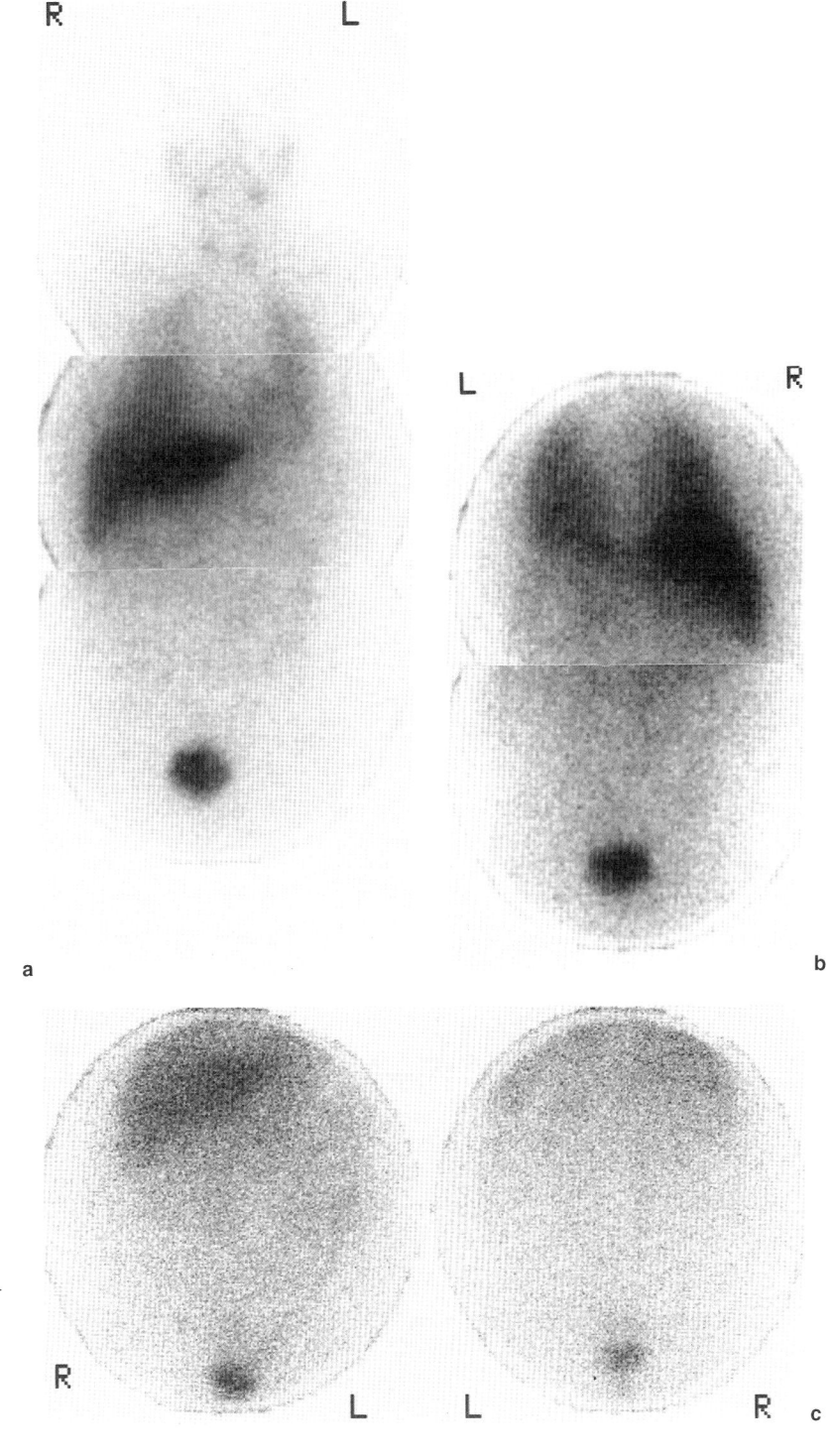

Fig. 5.49 Normal distribution 4 hours after application of 200 MBq ^{123}I-MIBG ((**a**) anterior projection and (**b**) posterior projection) the salivary glands, the thyroid, liver and bladder are visible. Visualization of the lungs is normal within the first 20 hours. Normal adrenal glands are not visible in the anterior and posterior projections 24 hours p.i. (**c**)

a rapid decrease up to 72 hours. Sixty percent of the injected dose is cleared within 24 hours by renal excretion, resulting in kidney and bladder activity that declines rapidly. However, for 48 and 72 hours p.i. (^{131}I-MIBG) there is still faint activity accumulation in the bladder and kidney region. In up to 30% of patients, especially within the first 24 hours p.i., there is tracer uptake in the bowel, especially in obstipated patients. Appropriate measures are recommended. Transitory uptake in the lungs within the first hours after injection has been reported, but is normally not visible 24 hours p.i. The salivary glands are normally visualized by neuronal uptake of $^{123/131}$I-MIBG and uptake of free iodine. Visualization of myocardium with $^{123/131}$I-MIBG is demonstrable in normal distribution, but is missed in cases of abnormally high uptake of MIBG in the adrenal medulla or MIBG-storing tumors (pheochromocytomas, neuroblastomas, ganglioneurocytomas, and MEN).

Pathological Findings

Decreased or missed visualization of the adrenal medulla may be normal (low-dose injection), and is caused by anatomical destruction of the adrenal medulla, reduced production of epinephrine and norepinephrine, or interfering medications. Because visualization is variable (60–100%) and depends also on dose and labeling (^{123}I/^{131}I), interpretation is often difficult and may give only hints for diagnosis (3, 11).

Increased uptake in the adrenal gland of MIBG is seen in the following:

Hyperplasia
Pheochromocytomas (benign, malignant, familial pheochromocytoma, MEN type II, neurofibromatosis, Hippel–Lindau disease)
Neuroblastoma
Gangliocytoma

Differentiation of these diseases is not possible using scintigraphy.

Pheochromocytoma

Pheochromocytoma is an uncommon tumor. The incidence in adults is between 0.01% and 0.001%, and in hypertensive patients, it is probably increased to 0.1% (6). Ten percent are malignant, 10% occur in children, 10% are extra-adrenal (6), and 10% are associated with one of the following autosomal dominant syndromes (especially if they are bilateral): MEN type IIa or IIb, neurofibromatosis (Recklinghausen disease), Hippel–Lindau disease, or familial pheochromocytomas.

Pheochromocytomas occur predominantly in the adrenal medulla (85–90% in adults and 70–80% in children); 10–20% are malignant, and if the location is extraadrenal, about 40% are malignant. Sensitivity of Scintigraphy with $^{123/131}$I-MIBG is 76–93% (2) for intra-adrenal and extra-adrenal locations, accuracy is 91–96% (Fig. 5.50).

Neuroblastoma

Neuroblastomas, like pheochromocytomas that arise from the neural crest, are the second most common solid malignancy in childhood. About 50% are lo-

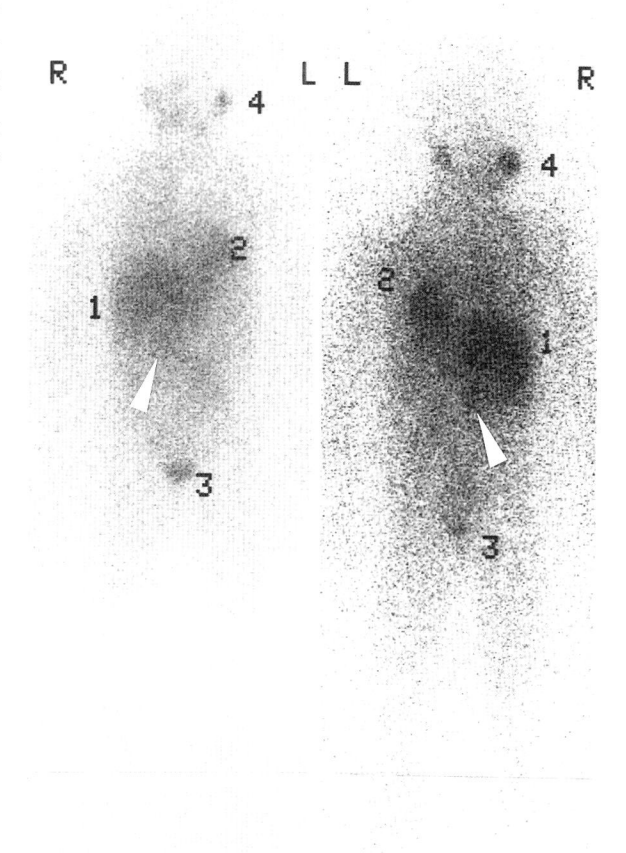

Fig. 5.50 Extra-adrenal pheochromocytoma Whole-body scan anterior (**a**) and posterior (**b**) projection of a 3-year-old girl with suggestion of a recurrent para-aortal extra-adrenal pheochromocytoma 24 hours after administration of 40 MBq ^{123}I-MIBG. In the dorsal projection, a faint para-aortal accumulation is visible, which is better seen in the high count single view image (**c**, T = recurrence) especially in the substraction image (**d**, *) after performance of a hepatobiliary study with delimination of liver and duodenum (**e**).
(1 = Liver, 2 = Heart, 3 = Bladder, 4 = salivary glands)

Fig. 5.50c-e

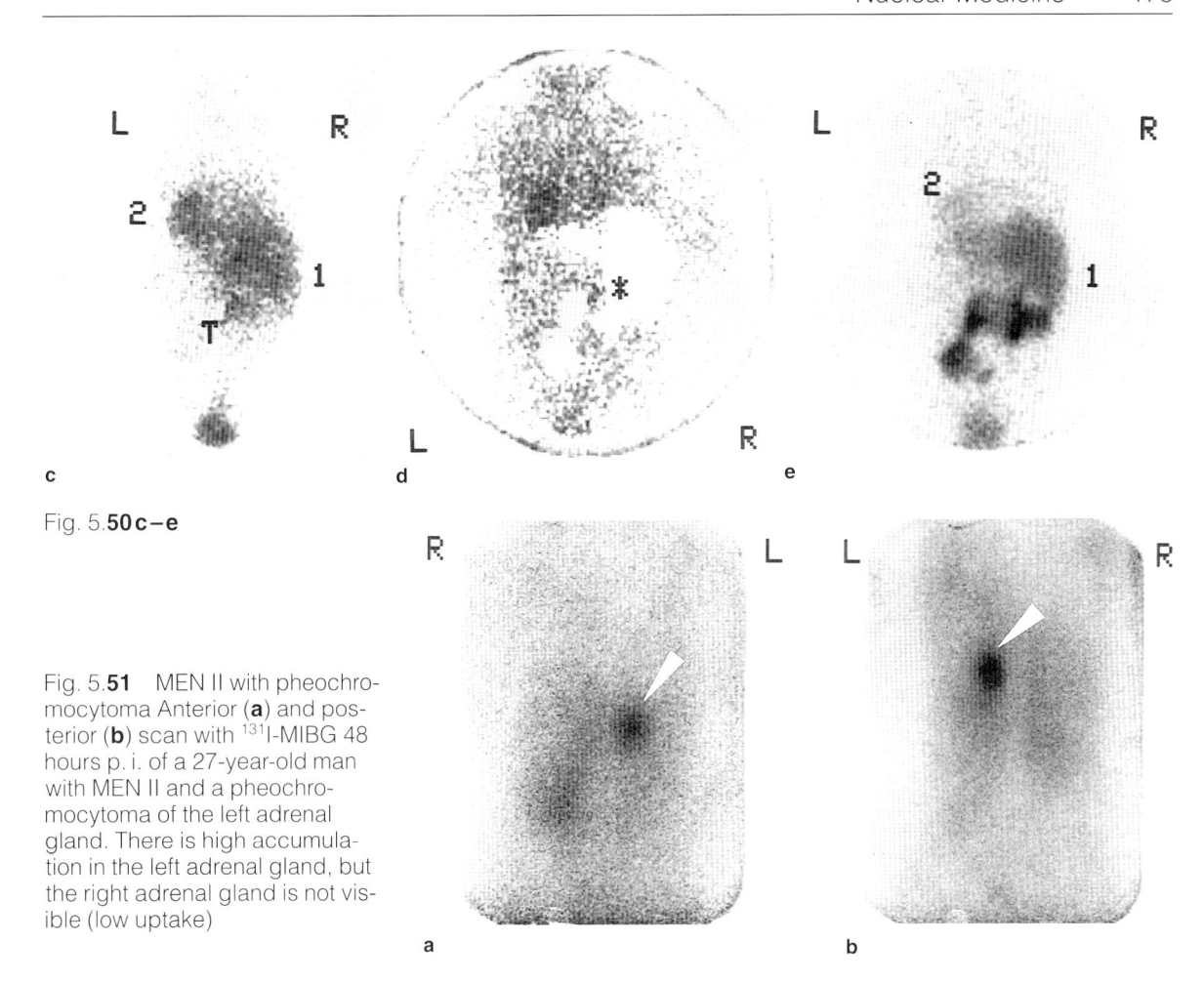

Fig. 5.51 MEN II with pheochromocytoma Anterior (**a**) and posterior (**b**) scan with ^{131}I-MIBG 48 hours p. i. of a 27-year-old man with MEN II and a pheochromocytoma of the left adrenal gland. There is high accumulation in the left adrenal gland, but the right adrenal gland is not visible (low uptake)

cated in the adrenal glands, 25% in the sympathetic ganglia, and 15% in the posterior mediastinum. Sensitivity for neuroblastomas by $^{123/131}$I-MIBG is (10) up to 95% (Fig. 5.52).

Typical Findings

The typical finding for pheochromocytomas and neuroblastomas arising from the adrenal medulla is a "hot spot" on the affected side in the typical region of the adrenal gland (Fig. 5.51). In dorsal projections, the tumors are often more prominent. The unaffected side may be suppressed and not visualized. Highly active endocrine lesions are often visible within 24 hours, but the best tumor-to-background contrast can be reached from 48–72 hours p.i. (if ^{131}iodine labeling is used). Hyperplasia of the adrenal medulla is difficult to differentiate from normal adrenal medulla. An enlarged medulla and or unusually good visualization of both glands raises the suggestion of hyperplasia or bilateral pheochromocytomas.

Principles of Receptor Imaging of the Adrenal Gland

In addition to scintigraphic imaging of the adrenal gland by precursors of the adrenal hormones, scintigraphic imaging with somatostatin receptors is possible. Somatostatin receptors have been demonstrated on normal tissue and on a variety of human tumors (8, 12) described by APUD characteristics (apudomas, pituitary tumors, endocrine pancreatic tumors, carcinoids, pheochromocytomas, neuroblastomas, paragangliomas, etc.). However, in a variety of different tumors without endocrine activity (meningioma, astrocytoma, Hodgkin and non-Hodgkin lymphomas, oat cell carcinoma, breast cancer, etc.), accumulation of Somatostatin and its analogs have been demonstrated by autoradiographic studies. Therefore, scintigraphy with somatostatin and its analogs is not specific for any adrenal disease or function, and only "hot spots" are pathological.

Two tracers (^{123}I-Tyr^3)-octreotide and (^{111}In-DTPA-D-Phe^1)-octreotide are currently available; but in general, ^{111}In-DTPA-D-Phe^1-octreotide is favored

176   5 Adrenal Gland

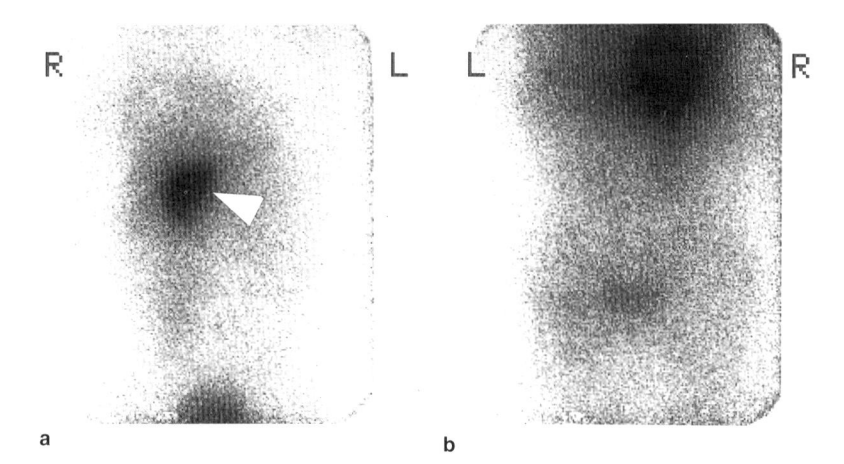

Fig. 5.52 Neuroblastoma Anterior (**a**) and posterior (**b**) scan of a 10-year-old girl, 72 hours after application of 37 MBq ^{131}I-MIBG with a high accumulation in the right adrenal region; surgically proven neuroblastoma

because of easier labeling and purification and the longer half-life of ^{111}In, which enables scintigraphy 24 hours p.i. Also, the profuse hepatobiliary excretion of (^{123}I-Tyr^3)-octreotide with variable fecal activity hampers the recognition of tumors located in the abdomen (7).

Technique

Administration

An i.v. injection of 111 MBq (i.e., 10 µg pentetreoide, for planar imaging 4 and 14 hours p.i.) or 222 MBq ^{111}In-DTPA-D-Phe^1-octreotide (for SPECT) is administered. To prevent artifacts due to radioactivity in the intestine, laxatives are given routinely starting on the day of administration.

Acquisition

Planar scanning and SPECT are performed 4 and 24 hours p.i. with a medium-energy parallel-hole collimator (^{111}In 171 keV and 245 keV), 24 and 48 hours p.i., 500 000 counts per frame should be collected. For the adrenal gland, anterior and posterior projections should be aquired. SPECT is possible 24 hours p.i. if 220 MBq ^{111}In-DTPA-D-Phe^1-octreotide has been given.

Normal Distribution

Normally, there is a faint visualization of the pituitary gland and thyroid, whereas the liver, spleen, and kidneys are clearly visualized. The small amount of the radiolabeled compound excreted by the biliary sys-

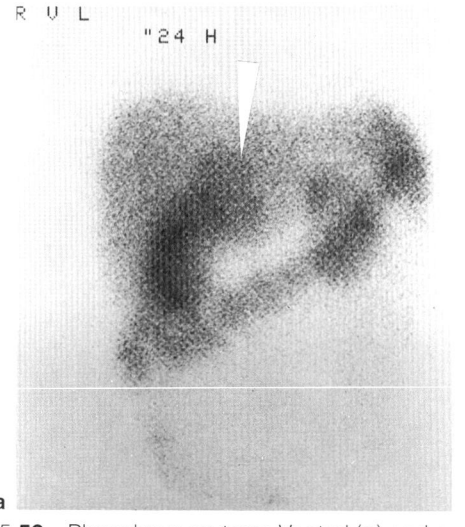

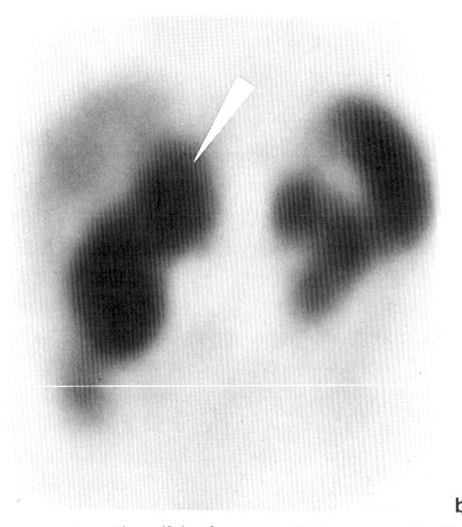

Fig. 5.53 Pheochromocytoma Ventral (**a**) and coronal SPECT reconstruction (**b**) of a scan 24 hours p. i. after application of 211 MBq ^{111}In-DTPA-D-Phe^1-octreotide in a 56-year-old man with a suggested pheochromocytoma. Accumulation cranial of the right adrenal gland, proven pheochromocytoma. Beneath the tumor, liver, spleen, kidney and intestine is visible (from Dr. M Bäder, Nuklearmedizin, Klinikum Berlin-Steglitz)

tem is already sufficient to visualize the large bowel on the 24-hour images if laxatives have not been used. The tumor-to-background ratio does not increase from the 24- to 48-hour images.

Pathological Findings

Pathological findings resemble a "hot spot" in the suspected region (Fig. 5.53). No further differentiation is possible. In case of pheochromocytoma, there is accumulation in the adrenal medulla.

Sensitivity of ^{111}In-DTPA-D-Phe^1-octreotide for pheochromocytomas, neuroblastomas, and neurogangliocytomas is suspected to be lower than that of MIBG. If there is any value of ^{111}In-DTPA-D-Phe^1-octreotide for detection of disease of the adrenal cortex had to be examined.

References

1. Beierwaltes WH, et al. Visualization of the human adrenal glands in vivo by scintilation scanning. JAMA. 1971;216:275–277.
2. Bomanji HE, Britton KE. Characterisation of meta-(I-123)-MIBG uptake by normal adrenal medulla in hypertensive patients. J Nucl Med. 1987;28:319–324.
3. Brown MJ, Fuller RW, Lavender JP. False positive diagnosis of bilateral pheochromocytoma by iodine-131-labelled meta-iodobenzylguanidine. Lancet. 1984;56.
4. Coupland RE. The natural history of the chromaffin cell. London: Longmans Green, 1965.
5. Jacques S, Tobes MC, Sisson JC, Baker JA. Mechanism of uptake of noerepinephrine and meta-iodobenzylganidine into cultured human pheochromocytoma calls. J Nucl Med. 1984;25:122.
6. Juni JE, Gross MD. Bilateral visualization on adrenal cortical sintigraphy. Semin Nucl Medicine. 1983;13(2):168–170.
7. Krenning EP, Backer WH, Kooij PPM, et al. Somatostatin receptor scintigraphy with Indium-111-DTPA-D-Phe-1-Octreotide in man: metabolism, dosimetry and comparison with iodine-123-Tyr-3-Octreotide. J Nucl Med. 1992;33:652–658.
8. Lamberts SWJ, Krenning EP, Reubi JC. The role of Somatostatin and its analogs in the diagnosis and treatment of tumors. Endocr Rev. 1991;12(4):450–482.
9. McEwan AJ, Shapiro B, Sisson JC, Beierwaltes WH, Ackery DM. Radio-iodobenzylguanidine for Scintigraphic Location and Therapy of Adrenergic Tumors. Semin Nucl Med. 1985;15(2):132–160.
10. Munkner T. 131I-meta-iodobenzylguanidine scintigraphy of Neuroblastomas. Semin Nucl Med. 1985;15(2):154–160.
11. Nakajo M, Shapiro B, Copp J, et al. The normal and abnormal distribution of the adrenomedullary imaging agent m-(I-131)iodobenzylguanidine (I-MIBG) in man: evaluation by scintigraphy. J Nucl Med. 1983;24:672–682.
12. Oel HY, Krenning EP, Lamberts SWJ. Somatostatin Rezeptor Imaging using OctresoScan(R) 111. Rotterdam, 1991.
13. Seabold JE, et al. Detection of metastatic adrenal carcinoma using 131I-6β-iodomethyl-19-norcholesterol total body scans. J Clin Endocrin Metabol. 1977;45:789–97.
14. Tragel KH, Czembirek H, Kletter K, Geyer G. Klinische Erfahrungen mit der szintigraphischen Nebennierendarstellung. Wiener Klin. Wochenschr. 1977;89:231–237.
15. Wieland DM, Swanson DP, Brown LE, Beierwaltes WM. Imaging the adrenal medulla with an I-131-labeled antiadrenergic agent. J Nucl Med. 1979;20:155–158.

A Radiologist's View

W. Auffermann

Imaging plays a crucial role in the differential diagnosis of endocrine disorders of the adrenal glands (2, 4, 6). MR imaging and CT are the main imaging tools for the evaluation of morphologic abnormalities (4), whereas scintigraphy and venous sampling may show functional abnormalities of the adrenals. Patients are referred for two main reasons: clinical symptoms and laboratory findings of endocrine dysfunction, or for the evaluation of an incidentally detected adrenal mass in abdominal sonography or CT performed for other disorders. In case of clinical suggestion of an adrenal tumor based on biochemical findings, sonography should be performed initially and followed by either CT or MR imaging.

Hyperplastic Glands

Because hyperplasia is not sufficiently demonstrated by sonography, CT is the first step in the ACTH-independent type of endocrine disorder (the ACTH-dependent type does not need further workup). However, small nodules (less than 1 cm) may not be visible. In case of bigger nodes, CT may not sufficiently differentiate hyperplasia from adenoma. Bilateral uptake in NP-59 scintigraphy confirms adrenal hyperplasia and may differentiate it from adenoma and carcinoma.

Adenoma

Sonography is not sufficiently sensitive for the detection of adenomas less than 2 cm in size. It may, however, be used as an initial approach for adenomas greater than 2 cm. In general, CT is the method of choice, since it has a wide field of view and can better define the shape of the abnormal gland. Para-aortic adenomas are characterized scintigraphically as a unilateral focus of ^{131}I NP-59 radioactivity (5). If adrenal scintigraphy is equivocal or not available and CT findings are inconclusive, one should proceed with adrenal venous sampling (4). Angiography is usually not required for the diagnosis of hyperplasia or adenoma.

Hemorrhage

Larger hematomas with the adrenal gland can be sufficiently diagnosed sonographically. However, smaller hemorrhages need to be evaluated properly by CT. Adrenal hemorrhage can be unilateral or bilateral. If bilateral hemorrhage is improperly treated, adrenal insufficiency and death can result (4).

Calcification

Extensive calcification may already be recognized in the abdominal radiograph. CT, however, is most sensitive for the recognition of subtle calcification.

Myelolipoma

Myelolipoma is an incidental finding seen on sonography or CT in patients studied for a variety of other suggested disorders and does not need further workup.

Cyst

Pathologically, four types of adrenal cysts are recognized: endothelial, epithelial, parasitic, and pseudocysts, which usually present as an incidental finding on sonography, CT, or MR imaging. Usually, they do not need further workup.

Carcinoma

Nonhyperfunctioning adenomas of more than 1 cm in size are detected incidentally in about 1% of abdominal CT studies and must be differentiated from carcinomas. CT criteria suggestive of malignancy are: a size of more than 5 cm, central necrosis, calcification, and signs of metastatic spread (1, 3, 8). MR criteria of malignancy are related to high-intensity on T_2-weighted images, whereas adenomas are mostly hypointense or isointense to liver tissue. The enhancement pattern after Gd-DTPA is also promising. However, the remaining overlap between benign and malignant lesions causes uncertainty in the differentiation between adenoma and carcinoma. Therefore, a biopsy should be taken if malignancy cannot clearly be ruled out. In histologically differentiated carcinomas, metastases are screened scintigraphically.

Metastasis

Adrenal metastasis can be unilateral or bilateral and is detected on CT with high sensivity. Scintigraphy or percutaneous biopsy may help in differentiating metastasis from adenoma. Dynamic gadopentetate-enhanced MR imaging has been promising in the distinction between benign and malignant adrenal masses (7).

Pheochromocytoma

Hyperfunctioning tumors of the adrenal medulla include pheochromocytomas and neuroblastomas. Ninety percent of pheochromocytomas originate from the adrenal medulla. The remaining extra-adrenal tumors originate from the paravertebral sympathetic ganglia, Zuckerkandl's organs, or the urinary bladder. In 10%, tumors occur bilaterally. Asymptomatic tumors are seen in about 50% of patients with MEN type II. Adrenal tumors are usually large enough for sonographic detection. In order to detect an extra-adrenal site or to exclude multiple occurence, preoperative CT or MR imaging is certainly indicated. Although CT, MR imaging, and MIBG scintigraphy all have equally high accuracy rates in the detection of adrenal pheochromocytomas, the first imaging test performed is whole-body MIBG scintigraphy covering chest, abdomen, and pelvis. CT or MR may be used to define the area of accumulation more precisely. If clinical suggestion remains strong despite a negative MIBG scan, or if MIBG is not available, whole-body CT or MR imaging may be necessary.

References

1 Dunnick NR, Doppman JL, Gill JR jr, et al. Localization of functional adrenal tumors by computed tomography and adrenal venous sampling. Radiology. 1982;142:429–433.
2 Dunnick NR. Adrenal imaging. Current status. AJR. 1990; 154:927–936.
3 Fishman EK, Deutsch BM, Hartman DS, Goldman SM, Zerhouni EA, Siegelman SS. Primary adrenocortical carcinoma. CT evaluation with clinical correlation. AJR. 1987;148:531–535.
4 Francis EK, Gross MD, Shapiro B, Korobkin M, Quint LE. Integrated imaging of adrenal disease. Radiology. 1992;184:1–13.
5 Gross MD, Shapiro B, Thrall JH, et al. The scintigraphic imaging of endocrine organs. Endocrin Rev. 1984;5:221–225.
6 Ikeda DM, Francis IR, Glazer GM, et al. The detection of adrenal tumors with primary hyperaldosteronism. Comparison of scintigraphy, CT, and MR imaging. AJR. 1989;153:301–306.
7 Krestin GP, Friedmann G, Fischbach R, Newlang KFR, Allolio B. Evaluation of adrenal masses in oncologic patients. Dynamic contrast-enhanced MR US CT. J Comput Assist Tomogr. 1991;15:104–110.
8 Lee MJ, Hahn PF, Papanicolaou N, et al. Benign and malignant adrenal masses. CT distinction with attenuation coefficients, size, and observer analysis. Radiology. 1991;179:415–418.

A Surgeon's View

H. D. Roeher

Localization and Diagnosis of Adrenal Tumors

The indication for surgical treatment and the decision of operative strategy definitely have to be preceded by a safe and reliable diagnosis of the underlying adrenal disease. On the basis of clinical presentation, this includes biochemical methods, adequate hormone assays of blood and urine, and if necessary, also provocation and stimulation tests. In general, adrenal tumors can be associated or unassociated with hyperfunction (excess hormone production). The need for a thorough diagnostic workup also applies to the "incidentoma."

The localization of adrenal lesions, whether they arise from the adrenal cortex or from the adrenal medulla, has to prove primarily unilateral, bilateral, or ectopic manifestation. Valuable information may be gained from localization studies in case of malignancy with regard to infiltration into the adjacent structures and organs (regional) and also with regard to possible metastatic spread. This information has a direct impact on the indication for treatment, particularly on the choice of surgical strategy and the access to the adrenal glands. The aim of this decision is directed toward the least operative burden on the patient, the best achievable exposition, and a reliable therapeutic result.

There are three major ways of exposing the adrenal gland: by a transabdominal approach suitable for bilateral lesions, larger tumors, malignant lesions including local infiltration or regional lymph node involvement, and in case of ectopic manifestation; by a lateral lumbar approach to the retroperitoneum in case of unilateral lesions of limited average size; by a dorsal paravertebral approach in case of small unilateral adenomas (i.e., Conn syndrome) or for bilateral procedures in case of hyperplastic disease (i.e., Cushing syndrome).

Ultrasound and CT are included in diagnostic routine for adrenal tumors. The sensitivity of both techniques lies between 80 and 100% (1, 2). For ultrasound identification, a tumor must have a diameter of approximately 2.0 cm. For smaller adenomas, for example in Conn syndrome or for androgen-producing tumors, this technique may be unsatisfactory. CT on the other hand allows the detection of smaller tumors down to a size of 0.5 cm in diameter (3, 4). In addition, it gives more reliable information about infiltrative growth to the region and of suggestive regional lymph node involvement. All tumors more than 5 cm in diameter have to be considered suggestive of malignancy. Additional CT-guided fine-needle aspiration biopsy does not provide any further valuable information. In fact, there is almost no support for its application because of a considerable danger for local cell implantation after damage to the tumor capsule.

An exception may apply only for pure cystic lesions with the simultaneous aim of therapeutic decompression. Furthermore, adrenal aspiration cytology almost never enables discrimination of benign and malignant lesions. MRI has no advantage over CT for the identification of adrenal tumors, but it provides information on tissue characterization regarding malignancy.

MIBG-scintigraphy for diagnostic proof and localization of pheochromocytoma is an excellent help in identifying unilateral, bilateral, or even ectopic and metastatic disease with a sensitivity of 80–90% and a specificity of 100%. Expected extra-adrenal localization is between 10 and 20% of all lesions. Lesions can be found in the neck next to the carotid artery, in the posterior mediastinum, in the para-aortal region (i.e., Zuckerkandl's organs), in the urinary bladder, and in the testicles. In case of familiar disease or MEN type II syndrome, MIBG-scintigraphy may even detect adrenal medullary hyperplasia in a screening examination of preclinical disease.

However, the use of adrenocortical scintigraphy by ^{131}I-norcholesterol is of less value and not applied routinely. It may perhaps be applied individually in case of a negative CT study.

In conclusion, a good reliable imaging technique for adrenocortical adenomas (Cushing syndrome, Conn adenoma) and for pheochromocytoma, the latter also MIBG-scintigraphy, is important in planning the operative strategy for succesful surgical treatment. Older invasive techniques, like selective catheter arteriography, are obsolete. In a continuous series of 100 operations in the past six years for various adrenal diseases, accepted localization methods have given way to a convincing success rate with only one doubtful unilateral finding in a borderline case with clinical manifestation of hirsutism and slight proof of excess androgen production.

References

1 Falke THM, Te Strake L, Shaff MI, et al. Mrlamging of the Adrenals: Correlation with Computed Tomography. J Computer Assist Tomogr. 1986;10:242–53.
2 Kenney PJ, Berlow ME, Ellis DA. Current Imaging of Adrenal Masses. Radiographics. 1984;4:743–83.
3 Schwarz RJ, Schmidt N. Efficient Management of Adrenal Tumors. Am J Surg. 1991;1961:576–9.
4 Reinig JW, Doppmann JL, Dwyer AJ, Johnson AR, Knopf RH. Distinction between Adrenal Adenomas and Metastases Using MR Imaging. J Computer Assist Tomogr. 1985;9:898–901.
5 Glazer GM, Woolsey EJ, Borrello J, et al. Adrenal Tissue Characterization using MR Imaging. Radiology. 1986;158:73–9.
6 Sisson JC, Shapiro B, Beierswaltes WH, Copp JE. Locating Pheochromocytomas by Scintigraphy Using 131-I-Metaiodobenzylguanidine. CA-A Cancer J Clinicians 1984;34:86–92.
7 Dupont J, Fleury-Goyon MC, Lahneche B, Mornex R. Localization of Pheochromocytomas by 131-I-MIBG scintigraphy. Ann Med Interne Paris. 1991;142:171–6.

6 Pancreas

Anatomy

J. Staudt

The pancreas develops from the gastrointestinal epithelium and moves ventrally and dorsally into the duodenal region. Already in the end of the second embryonal month after duodenal rotation, the ventral part lying on the left of the descending duodenal part merges with the dorsal part. Because of this rotational move, the tissue from the pancreatic head originates from both parts and contains the common pancreatic duct (Wirsung's duct). The accessory pancreatic duct flows into the main duct cranially to the Wirsung's duct (Fig. 6.1).

The pancreas weighs around 70 g to 90 g, measures between 13 cm and 18 cm in length, lies within the duodenal slope, and extends with its tail to the spleen. It projects onto the first and second lumbal vertebral body. The portal vein, which exits the venous confluens and runs from the left to the right, the inferior vena cava, and the abdominal aorta lie behind the pancreas (Fig. 6.2).

With its exocrine part, the pancreas is a purely serous gland that exhibits a lobular architecture. The islet cells (islets of Langerhans) are brighter in color and lie within the darker acinar lobuli (Fig. 6.3). Their number increases towards the pancreatic tail. The diameter of one round epithelial complex ranges from 100 to 500 μm. Four types of cells can be differentiated: A cells for glucagon, B cells for insulin (80–85%), D cells for somatostatin, and pp cells for the pancreatic polypeptides.

Endocrinology

R. A. Halvorsen Jr.

Endocrine tumors of the pancreas originate from cells of the islet of Langerhans. Islet cells are neuroectodermal in origin and share common cytochemical attributes of APUD. Depending upon the synthetic capability of an individual tumor, detectable hormonal production may or may not be present. There are at least five types of hormonally active tumors arising from

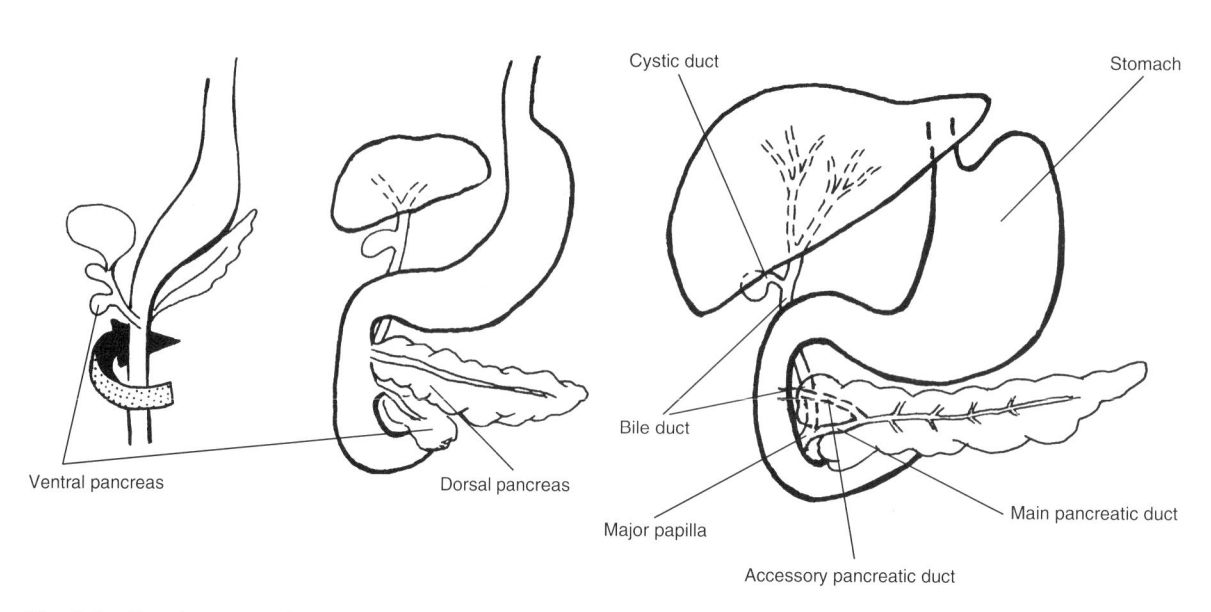

Fig. 6.1 Development of the pancreas

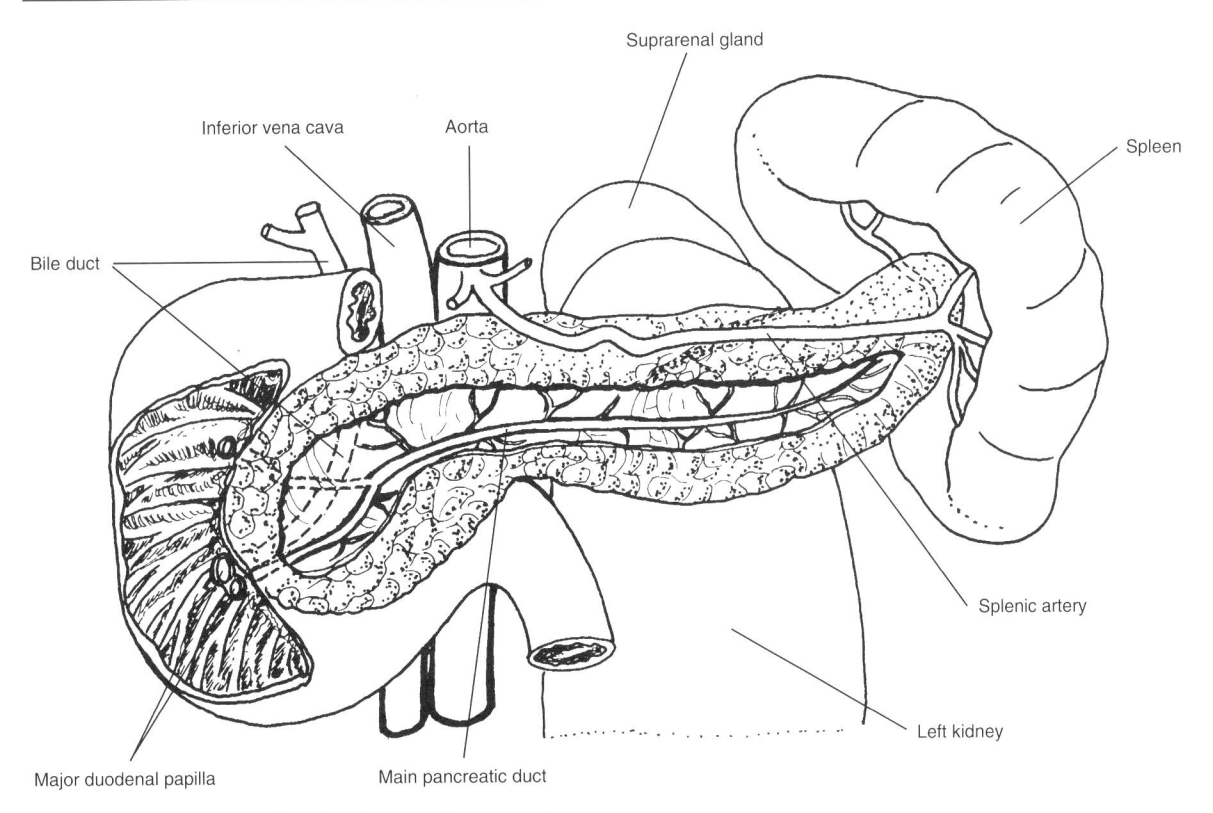

Fig. 6.2 A dissection showing the duodenum and pancreas

the endocrine pancreas. These include insulin-producing tumors (insulinoma), gastrinproducing tumors (gastrinoma), vasoactive intestinal-peptide-producing tumors (Vipoma), glucagon-producing tumors (glucagonoma), and somatostatin-producing tumors (somatostatinoma). These tumors demonstrate relative hypervascularity, detectable as enhancing lesions on imaging studies. Islet cell tumors also share histologic features; they are typically well differentiated with low mitotic activity, which makes distinguishing benign from malignant tumors difficult (1). Islet cell tumors are occasionally associated with MEN type I, also called Wermer syndrome. MEN type I syndrome includes tumors of the pituitary, pancreas, and parathyroid glands.

Islet cell tumors of the pancreas can be subdivided into three major categories: 1. nonfunctioning islet cell tumors, 2. insulinomas, and 3. all the remaining hormonally active tumors. Imaging of all islet cell tumors is important to stage the frequently malignant nonfunctioning tumors, localize insulinomas for curative resection, and determine which of the remaining tumors are surgically treatable.

Nonfunctioning islet cell tumors (non-hormone-producing) are usually large at diagnosis, often greater than 5 cm in diameter, frequently malignant, and often invasive of adjacent structures (2). The de-

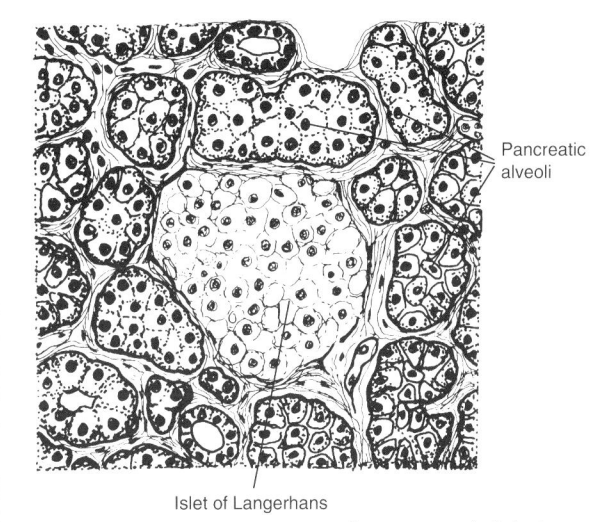

Fig. 6.3 Section of a portion of a pancreatic lobule

tection and staging of these relatively large tumors is straightforward with noninvasive imaging techniques, such as CT, transabdominal ultrasound, or MRI, and will not be discussed further.

Imaging of the functional or hormonally active tumors of the pancreas is useful in the localization, but not the diagnosis of these functional tumors. The diagnosis of tumors that produce active hormones is the

Table 6.1 Islet cell tumors, Tumor Characteristics

	Solitary	Multiple	Extrapancreatic	Malignant	MEN I
Insulinoma	80%	10%	rare	10%	10%
Gastrinoma	35%	20–40%	7–39%	61–90%	33%
Somatostatinoma	50%	6%	44%	91%	~50%
Vipoma	80%	20%	0	>68%	?
Glucagonoma	100%	0	rare	60–80%	?

Compiled from reference 3–8

province of the endocrinologist. Localization of the cause of the endocrine abnormality is the problem. Insulinomas are usually solitary, benign lesions that are potentially curable by surgery in the majority of patients.

The other functioning tumors of the pancreas are frequently malignant, diffuse, and often not amenable to surgical therapy (Table 6.2) (3–8). Other than insulinoma, which has a low incidence of malignancy usually estimated at 10%, most islet cell tumors, including vipomas, glucagonomas, somatostatinomas, as well as nonfunctioning tumors, will be dicovered to be malignant with diligent follow-up (3). For instance, gastrinomas are estimated to be malignant in 60–90% of cases. The reported numbers of the other types of islet cell tumors are small, but the majority of vipomas and glucagonomas are malignant. Despite the high frequency of malignancy, the noninsulin-secreting islet cell tumors are slow growing and indolent. Preoperative evaluation is important with these unusual tumors of identify those patients with limited disease, who are potentially curable with surgery.

References

1 Brenna MF, MacDonald JS. Cancer of the endocrine system. In: DeVita VT Jr., Hellman S, Rosenberg SA, eds. Cancer: Principles and Practice of Oncology. 2nd ed. Philadelphia: J.B. Lippincott; 1982:1206–1222.
2 Doppman JL, Shawker TH, Miller DL. Localization of islet cell tumors. Gastroenterol Clin North Am. 1989;18(4):793–804.
3 Norton JA, Doppman JL, Jensen RT. Cancer of the endocrine system. In: DeVita VT Jr., Hellman S, Rosenberg SA, eds. Cancer: Principles and Practice of Oncology. 3rd ed. Philadelphia: J.B. Lippincott; 1989:1314–1331.
4 Zollinger RM. Gastrinoma: the Zollinger-Ellison syndrome. Seminars in Oncol. 1987;14(3):247–252.
5 Parker CM, Hanke CW, Madura JA, Liss EC. Glucagonoma syndrome: case report and literature review. J Dermatol Surg Oncol. 1984;10;11:884–889.
6 Boden G. Insulinoma and glucagonoma. Seminars in Oncol. 1987;14(3):253–262.
7 Mekhjian HS, O'Dorision TM. VIPoma syndrome. Seminars in Oncol. 1987;14(3):282–291.
8 Vinik AI, Stroden WE, Eckhauser FE, et al. Somatostatinomas, PPomas, neurotensinomas. Seminars in Oncol. 1987; 14(3):263–281.

Computed Tomography

M. Bezzi, F. Orsi, P. Ricci, F. M. Salvatori, F. Maccioni, L. Broglia, P. Rossi

CT is a relatively noninvasive technique that is routinely used in the localization of functioning tumors of the pancreas. Modern scanners produce axial images of very high resolution, providing invaluable information to the surgeon concerning the location of the tumor and its relationships to the surrounding normal structures. Short scan times decrease problems due to respiratory and bowel motion artifacts and facilitate the performance of rapid scans following injection of contrast medium. Together with ultrasound, CT is the initial radiologic test of choice in the workup of a patient with a suggested apudoma of the pancreas because it is not invasive, it is not very expensive, and it provides high diagnostic accuracy in locating and staging the neoplasm.

Technique

The CT study should always be performed on a modern scanner in order to obtain images with high resolution in a short scan time. The stomach and small bowel loops are opacified with oral contrast medium; distension of the stomach is particularly helpful in examining the pancreatic tail. Baseline unenhanced scans are obtained from the level of the uncinate process to the dome of the liver with 5–8 mm thick slices at an 8–10 mm slice interval. Findings to look for on precontrast scans, other than obvious masses, are focal alterations of the pancreatic contour and calcifications (27, 40) (Figure 6.4). The unenhanced study of the liver is important to detect metastases, which are usually hypervascular (5).

The contrast-enhanced study is performed with overlapping 5–8 mm thick slices and a 4–6 mm interslice gap: the overlapping technique is used to reduce the effect of inconstant respiration, which may cause omission of some anatomic levels and leave small lesions undetected. Iodinated contrast medium is injected at a rate of 4–6 mL/s in an antecubital vein with an automatic injector in six or seven separate doses of 25–30 mL each, using contrast medium at a concen-

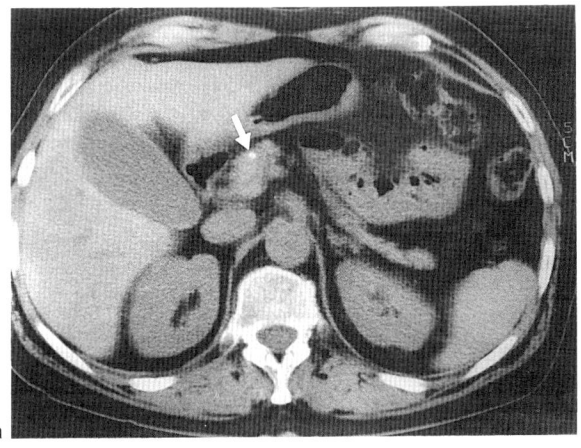

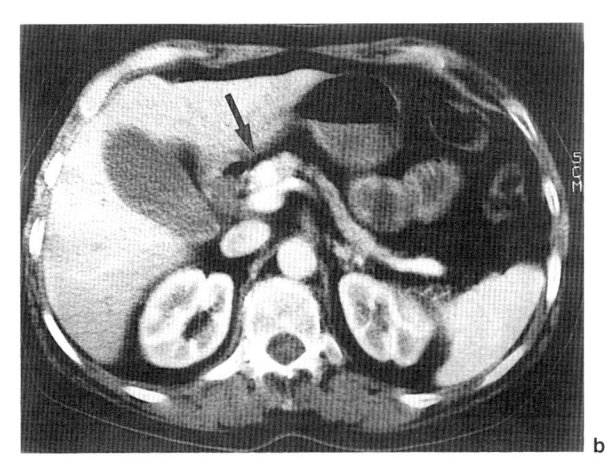

Fig. 6.4 Spiral CT in a case of insulinoma. (**a**) Unenhanced scan shows only small calcification at the level of the pancreatic isthmus (white arrow). (**b**) Postcontrast study demonstrates a focal area of parenchymal enhancement corresponding to a small endocrine tumor (arrow). (Courtesy of doctors Albert L. Baert and Guy Marchal)

tration of 300 mg Iodine/mL. The scans are obtained 14–20 seconds after each bolus, during the phase of peak arterial enhancement, and continued after the end of the bolus injections so that the whole gland is examined in a phase of maximal enhancement. An adequate amount of contrast medium is necessary to produce a detectable difference in enhancement between tumor and surrounding normal pancreatic tissue; some lesions are seen only after injection of more than 150 mL of iodinated contrast medium (300 mg I/mL) (29). If an abnormality or a lesion is seen on precontrast scans, contrast medium is injected at this level to study the region at the peak of both arterial and parenchymal enhancement, after this the rest of the gland is examined.

The intra-arterial injection of contrast medium through a catheter placed in the celiac or superior mesenteric artery has been suggested (1, 12) to obtain optimal pancreatic enhancement and possibly to decrease the total dose of iodine; artifacts produced by the catheter can, however, obscure small lesions and cause problems in image interpretation when the lesion is close to the catheter. It is conceivable that this technique may be able to localize, after a negative angiogram, the hypovascular endocrine pancreatic tumors that are occasionally reported, (12, 31) but experiences with the method are limited.

Spiral volumetric CT with the single breath-hold technique (10, 16) may ability of CT to detect small endocrine tumors; with spiral CT, all the data are obtained during one breath-hold, respiratory misregistration of scans is therefore not a problem. Once the volume of data is acquired, position, thickness, and number of planes can be arbitrarily selected for reconstructing images, so that the center of a lesion can always be depicted for size assessment and density measurements. Another potential advantage of the technique is that the whole pancreas can be examined in the phase of maximal enhancement, therefore increasing the differential blush between tumor and glandular tissue (10). Preliminary reports on the use of this technique in pancreatic disease (10) have demonstrated better opacification of vessels, improved visualization of anatomic details, and elimination of motion artifacts, as compared to conventional dynamic CT. An example of a small insulinoma detected with spiral CT is shown in Fig. 6.4.

Normal Findings

Thorough knowledge of the normal pancreatic anatomy and of the relationships between the gland and the surrounding structures is essential in the diagnosis of all pancreatic abnormalities. This is particularly true of endocrine neoplasms in which the abnormality may be very subtle, and a wrong diagnosis may be caused by misinterpretation of a normal anatomic structure.

Substantial variation exists in the size, shape, and location of the normal pancreas; the tail, particularly, may vary in location. In a patient with considerable retroperitoneal fat, the gland may be entirely straight, remaining in the same axial plane from the level of the neck to the end of the tail, thus allowing for a complete examination in a reduced number of scans. In other patients, the orientation of the tail may be oblique with the tip located high and lateral behind the gastric body. In these cases one should prolong the examination with the overlapping slice technique until the whole pancreas has been covered by the study.

The contour of the gland may be lobulated, and the lobules may appear even more prominent by the interdigitating peripancreatic fat; these focal, but normal, alterations of the contour usually show the same contrast enhancement of the rest of the gland and should not be interpreted as possible tumors (Fig. 6.5).

Interpretation of postcontrast scans may be difficult, and pitfalls include the erroneous diagnosis of a tumor when an area of increased attenuation is, in fact, an isolated segment of a tortuous vessel, or, conversely, the failure to detect a tumor that is assumed to be a vascular structure. The superior mesenteric artery and vein run straight and perpendicular to the pancreas, and do not present themselves as a problem in the differential diagnosis. The splenic vessels, on the contrary, may represent a diagnostic dilemma: the vein runs closely parallel to the posterior aspect of the gland from which it is often separated by a fat plane; the artery has a more tortuous course and sometimes enters deeper into the glandular tissue, without fat planes in between. Loops of these two vessels, more frequently the artery, cut by the axial scan plane may be interpreted has enhancing lesions (Fig. 6.6).

Finally, a pancreatic tumor may be simulated by loops of the proximal jejunum that, especially in thin patient, may lay directly against the pancreatic tail. Unopacified bowel loops may be misinterpreted as focal bulges of the glandular contours, particularly when, as it might happen, they enhance after injection of contrast medium. In these cases repeated scans after additional administration of oral contrast medium will be necessary to clarify the finding.

Pathological Findings

The characteristic CT features of islet cell tumors differ in relation to their clinical presentation, so that they can be divided in two groups: hormone-secreting neoplasms and nonfunctioning tumors.

The clinical presentation of a functioning islet cell tumor depends on the type of hormone secreted; usually the clinical signs and symptoms, together with the hormonal radioimmunoassays, allow for a correct categorization of the patient into one of the different endocrine syndromes. Once the presence of an islet cell tumor is suggested, the role of the radiologist is to localize it: Failure normally occurs because the tumor is too small to be detected by current imaging techniques, or the patient's symptoms are due to diffuse neuroendocrine cellular hyperplasia ("microadenosis") (21).

Insulinoma, together with gastrinoma, is the most common secretory tumor and is usually benign. The tumor is frequently small; 70% are less than 1.5 cm (24). In Stefanini's series (34), 5% were less than 0.5 cm, 34% were between 0.5 and 1 cm, and only 8% were larger than 5 cm. This explains why the CT study must be extremely accurate in order to detect such small nodules. The lesions are evenly distributed throughout the gland (26, 30, 34) (Fig. 6.7) and are multiple in 10% of cases. Fortunately, extrapancreatic insulinomas are very rare (1–4%) (24) and this, as opposed to what happens in patients with Zollinger–Ellison syndrome, permits the physician to focus the CT study on the gland only.

On unenhanced scans, insulinomas usually do not present differences in density with respect to the normal pancreatic tissue, but they can sometimes be suggested because of a focal distortion of the glandular contour; one case of an isodense insulinoma in a fatty replaced pancreas has been reported (7). Calcifications may be present, usually in clusters or clumps, and are more common in malignant than in benign neoplasms (40).

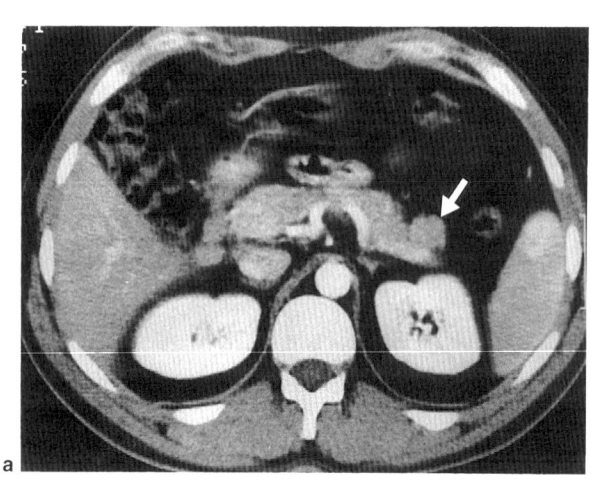

Fig. 6.5 Abnormal lobulation of pancreatic contour simulating an exofitic mass in a patient with suggested apudoma. (**a**) Precontrast study shows abnormality of pancreatic contour (arrow). (**b**) Postcontrast CT demonstrates that the suspected mass enhances to the same degree of the rest of the gland, therefore representing a lobule of pancreatic tissue

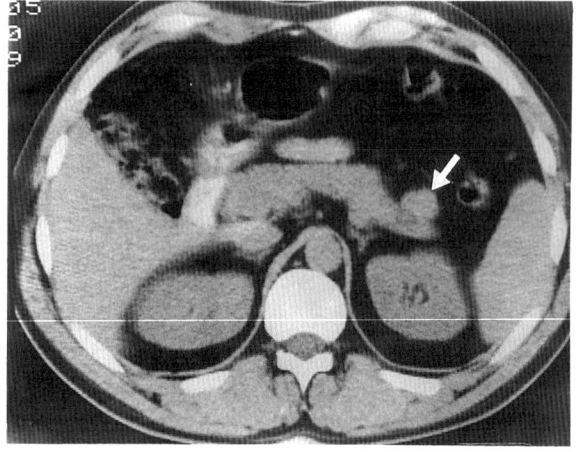

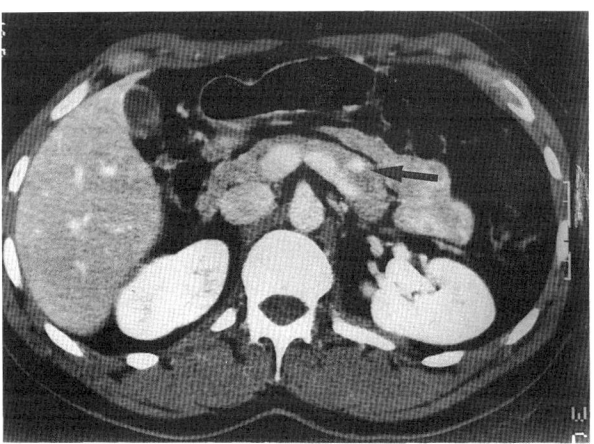

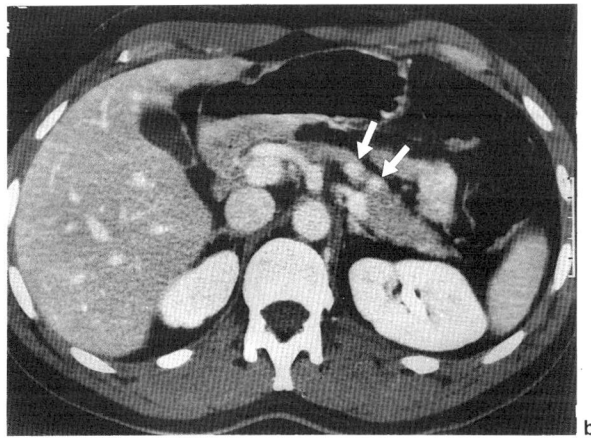

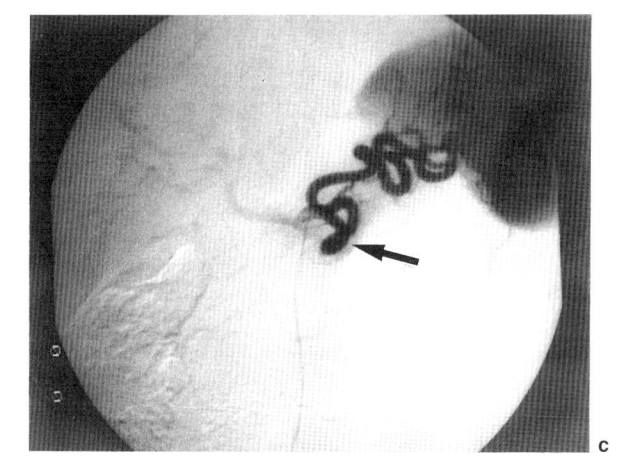

Fig. 6.**6** Possible diagnostic error in a patient with hyperinsulinism undergoing CT for tumor localization. (**a**) Contrast-enhanced CT of pancreas shows a focal, hyperdense area within the tail (arrow). (**b**) At a higher level it is apparent that the hyperdense areas (white arrows) represent a loop of the splenic artery cut along its short axis by the transverse plane of scan. (**c**) Splenic arteriogram demonstrates the vascular tortuosity responsible for the CT finding (arrow). Both CT and angiography were negative for insulinoma.

After contrast medium injection, most insulinomas, due to their rich vascularity, enhance and become hyperdense relative to the surrounding pancreatic tissue. This transient hyperdensity corresponds to the typical tumor "blush" seen on arteriography and is a characteristic CT feature of a functioning endocrine tumor (Figs. 6.**8**, 6.**9**, and 6.**10**). In small lesions, up to 4–5 cm in diameter, the enhancement is usually homogeneous; larger lesions may be inhomogeneous with a slightly hypodense center and tend to be more often malignant. Insulinomas, even when large, seldom undergo central necrosis because of their rich arterial network, which continues to develop as the tumor grows (35). Although the above-mentioned findings are seen in most patients, cases of hypodense or even cystic insulinomas have been reported (23, 31) (Fig. 6.**11**).

Gastrinomas originate within the pancreas only in 70–75% of cases, while the rest are mostly located in the duodenal wall, or in other sites such as the stomach, small bowel, omentum, or peripancreatic tissue (19, 41). Actually, 90% of all gastrinomas are found within an anatomic triangle that includes the head and neck of the pancreas, the duodenum, the hepato-

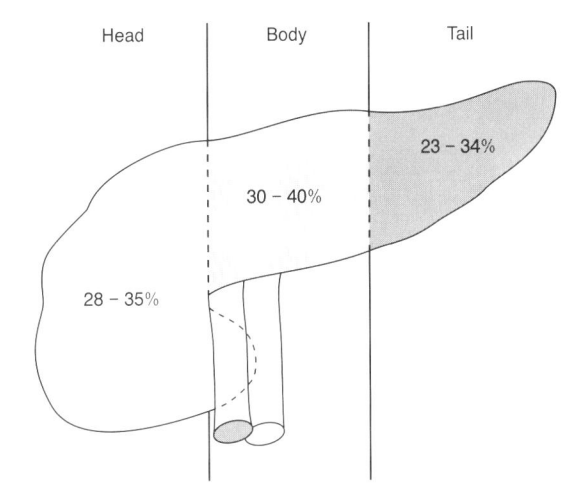

Fig. 6.**7** Pancreatic distribution of insulinoma (data from references 26, 30, 34)

duodenal ligament, and a portion of the stomach as shown in Fig. 6.**12** (32). Patients with Zollinger–Ellison syndrome tend to have multiple gastrinomas in

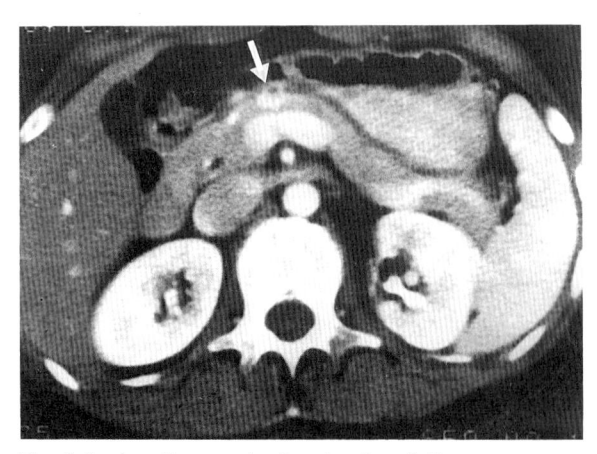

Fig. 6.**8** Insulinoma in the body of the pancreas. Highly vascular tumor, anterior to the confluence of the splenic vein into the portal vein (white arrow) (from reference 28, with permission)

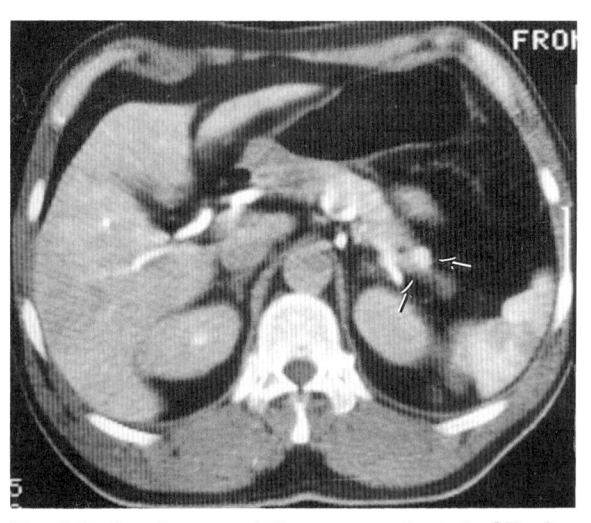

Fig. 6.**9** Insulinoma of the pancreatic tail. CT after intra-arterial injection of contrast medium shows marked enhancement of a small islet cell tumor (hatched arrows) (from reference 27, with permission)

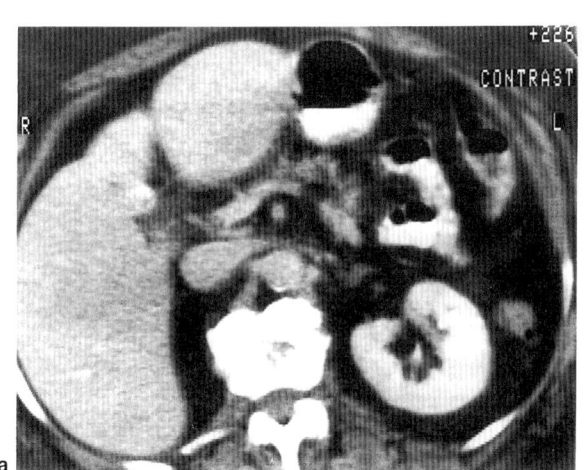

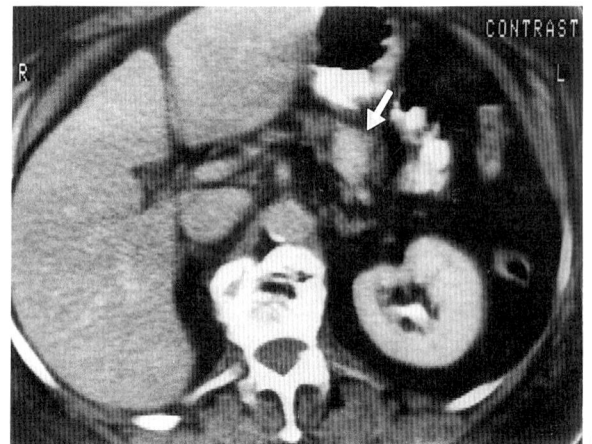

Fig. 6.**10** Insulinoma of the body in an atrophic pancreas. Contrast-enhanced CT: (**a**) The body of the pancreas is atrophic, with partial fatty replacement. (**b**) At a slightly higher level, a hyperdense lesion (arrow) is seen posterior to the stomach

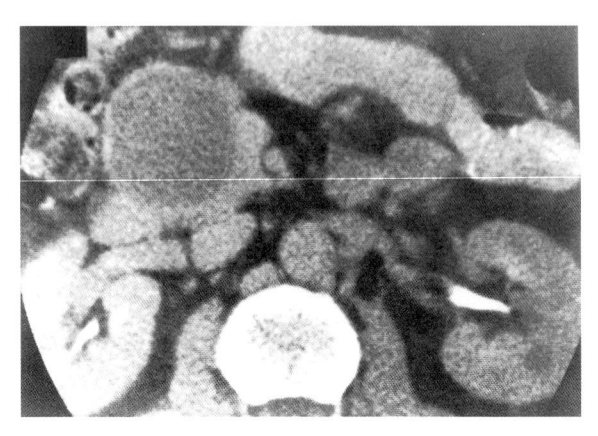

Fig. 6.**11** Cystic insulinoma. Hypodense, homogeneous mass in the pancreatic head, 6 cm in diameter. The CT features are similare to those of a pancreatic pseudocyst. (from reference 23, with permission)

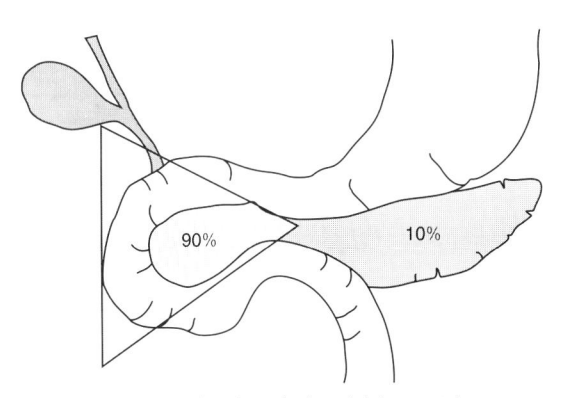

Fig. 6.12 Anatomic triangle in which gastrinomas are most often found (Adapted from reference 32)

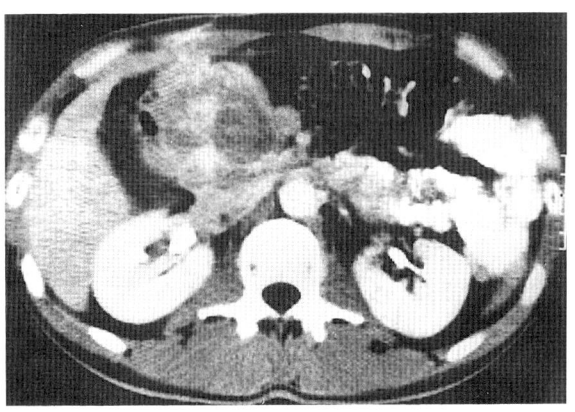

Fig. 6.13 Malignant apudoma of the pancreatic head, presenting with hyperincretion of more than one islet cell hormone. Contrast-enhanced CT: inhomogeneous mass in the head, adjacent to the duodenum, with no signs of bile duct obstruction

20–40% of cases (6). In addition, the tumors are often very small at the time of presentation (38% are less than 1 cm [38]). The small size and the frequent extrapancreatic location make CT localization of these tumors an extremely difficult task.

The CT pattern of gastrinomas is similar to that of insulinomas, and tumors usually present as hyperdense nodules after the injection of contrast medium; gastrinomas, however, tend to be less homogeneous. Extrapancreatic gastrinomas, although difficult to localize, present similar CT features.

Because a high percentage (approximately 60% [8,42]) of gastrinomas are malignant, metastases may be already present at the time of diagnosis. If this is the case, therapy is directed toward amelioration of symptoms rather than radical surgical cure. In this case, primary and metastatic lesions are studied for different purposes. The primary lesion is evaluated in those patients with large lesions and advanced disease who may benefit from tumor debulking if their endocrine symptoms are not controllable by drug therapy (2). Evaluation of metastatic foci is done to stage the disease, to assess resectability, which is possible in a small number of cases (20), and, eventually, to judge the response to chemotherapy.

Secondary liver lesions from either insulinoma or gastrinoma are usually hypervascular. This type of metastases is visualized as areas of high attenuation in the first 20–40 seconds after contrast medium injection, during the peak of arterial enhancement, and may then become rapidly isodense to the liver. Because it is impossible to study the whole liver during the peak arterial enhancement, in approximately one-third of patients these lesions remain undetected (5). Precontrast scans are often helpful in showing lesions not seen on postcontrast scans. Moreover, in these cases, MRI, due to its superior intrinsic liver lesion contrast, may be used to detect small secondary foci and stage the disease better than CT (37).

The other functioning tumors of the pancreas (glucagonoma, vipoma, somatostatinoma, PP-oma) are much rarer than insulinoma and gastrinoma; they tend to reach larger sizes and the majority have metastasized by the time of clinical presentation. From a radiological point of view they do not represent a diagnostic problem since localization, due to their dimensions, is not difficult (4, 15, 36) (Fig. 6.13). The CT study is mainly aimed at correctly staging the tumor when chemotherapy or debulking surgery are planned.

Nonfunctioning endocrine tumors are clinically silent until they cause late symptoms due to their size or to the presence of liver metastases. Therefore, at the time of diagnosis they are much larger than hormonally active lesions, ranging from 4 cm to more than 10 cm in size (Fig. 6.14). It is crucial to discriminate between these tumors and pancreatic adenocarcinomas, because the prognosis is more favorable and specific chemotherapy can be started. The most distinctive features are calcifications, which are seen in 20–30% of malignant apudomas, but are rare in adenocarcinomas. In addition, these tumors usually tend to encase the superior mesenteric and the portal veins rather than the celiac or superior mesenteric arteries (3, 11). Whenever a nonfunctioning apudoma is suggested on CT and needs to be confirmed in order to decide the treatment, a CT-guided biopsy of the lesion, with immunohistochemical stains, will help in the differential diagnosis from other pancreatic neoplasms.

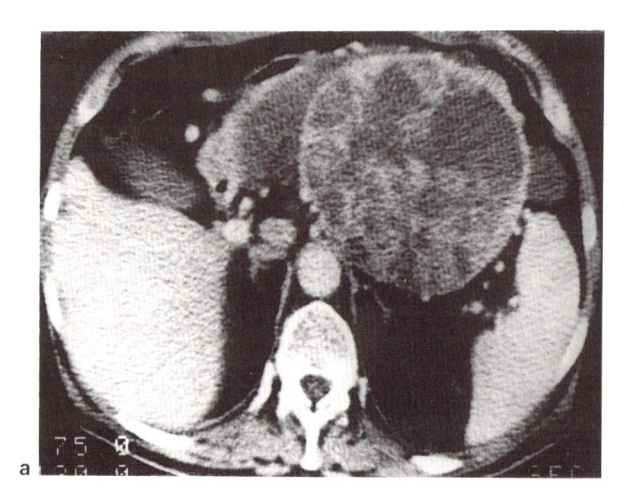

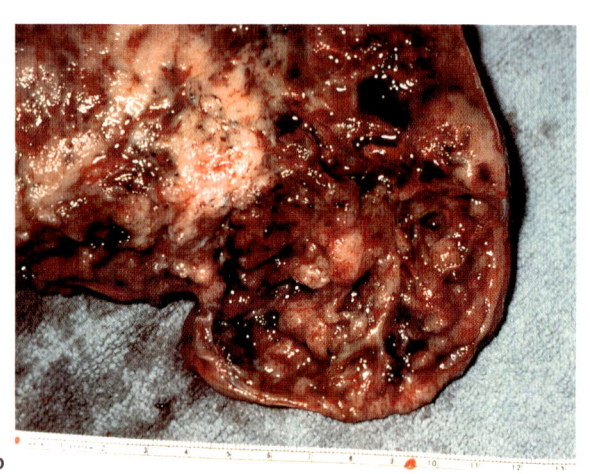

Fig. 6.**14** Large, nonfunctioning apudoma located in the pancreatic tail (**a**), with internal cystic degeneration. (**b**) Operative specimen: sarcomatous changes were present within the tumor. (Courtesy of Dr. Albert L. Baert)

Diagnostic Accuracy

Many articles report on the ability of CT in the localization of the islet cell tumors, but most of them tend to consider all the tumors together and do not give specific results for the different histologic types. From all papers, however, emerges that diagnostic accuracy correlates to tumor size: in fact, the highest detection rates are observed in lesions larger than 2–3 cm (13, 28). We refer here to the results of the most significant works on the two most frequent clinical syndromes.

Insulinoma

CT is fairly sensitive in the localization of insulinoma with sensitivity values ranging from 47% to 74% (9, 22, 27, 28, 33). The specificity is 67–100% (27, 28, 33). Values close to 100%, however, reflect a bias in the selection of the "gold standard" used to confirm the diagnosis, as explained later in this chapter. When adequately performed, CT is sufficiently accurate in localizing and staging the disease in the majority of patients. The false-positive results with CT are very rare, but a negative CT study, in the presence of the clinical evidence of the syndrome, should be followed by other noninvasive tests, such as MRI, and perhaps by angiography.

Gastrinoma

The diagnostic accuracy of CT should be considered separately for the primary lesion and for the hepatic metastases. Extrahepatic gastrinoma (i.e., the primary tumor) can be detected with a sensitivity of 45–59%, with a high specificity (95–100%), but with a low negative predictive value (15–54%) (13, 18, 38). This indicates that a positive CT result is a reliable indicator of the location of the lesion. However, because of low negative predictive values, a negative CT result should not be used as a basis to exclude surgical exploration.

Liver metastases are identified with a sensitivity of 71–72%, high specificity (98–100%), and high negative predictive value (90%) (13, 18, 38). These results show that CT is an excellent method for tumor staging, only slightly inferior to angiography. Therefore, if the CT study is positive for liver secondary lesions, no further studies should be undertaken unless metastases resection is planned.

Interpreting the International Literature on the Localization of Endocrine Pancreatic Tumors

One must pay extreme attention when analyzing the world literature on islet cell tumor localization, because the wide range of success rates quoted for the different techniques and for the same techniques from different centers is somewhat confusing.

There are several reasons for these differences. First, the relative rarity of these neoplasms encourages many radiologists to publish series involving small numbers of patients, which carries an intrinsic statistical bias. Second, the most important articles on the subject come from a few specialized centers, each with its own area of particular diagnostic expertise. Therefore, the statistics are difficult to compare because of the differences in equipment, operator experience, and procedural methods. In addition, some series are accumulated over a period of 5–10 years (22), and therefore include patients studied with different equipment, introducing another potential source of statistical error.

Third, the parameters used in each paper to evaluate success and failure in the radiological localization of islet cell tumors are very important. Usually, the radiologist, when analyzing the results of his investigation, wishes to establish the number of both true- and false-positive radiological diagnoses and true- and false-negative diagnoses. This is not always so easy. The true- and false-positives are usually obtained by analyzing patients who have undergone operations, but the data is not completely accurate because the surgeon may not find some small tumors correctly identified by the radiologist. Only a careful follow-up may reveal this error. A complete analysis of true- and false-negative values should include all the unoperated patients in whom radiological results were negative. Again, the data may not be valid, as the real incidence of missed tumors in unoperated patients can never be known.

Finally, the attitude of the surgeons may introduce a further bias. If a surgeon places great reliance on his or her radiologist and does not operate on patients in whom radiological results are negative, but elects to treat the patients by medical means (for example H_2receptor antagonists in case of Zollinger–Ellison syndrome), then the number of patients undergoing surgery with a radiologically negative diagnosis in that institution will be very small and the published results will show highly accurate "positive" data, and little in the way of "negative" data. In fact, the patients that never come to surgery cannot appear in any series based on "surgically confirmed" cases. To find out the true-negative and false-negative rates in such a group would require years of follow-up so that the final outcome of all referred patients could eventually be established. In a series in which radiological success and failure is based only on "surgically proven cases," rather than careful follow-up, the real number of true-negative results can never be assessed with certainty. Such a series should not include specificity values (as specificity is defined by the ratio: true negative ÷ [true negative + false positive]).

For the radiologist publishing in this field, it is almost impossible to overcome these difficulties in a way that allows his or her material to be presented in a form that is accurate and coherent without being misleading. It is therefore important that anyone reviewing the literature on this subject be aware of the foregoing caveats.

References

1. Ahlstrom H, Magnusson A, Grama D, et al. Preoperative localization of endocrine pancreatic tumors by intra-arterial dynamic computed tomography. Acta Radiol. 1990;31:171.
2. Andersen DK. Current diagnosis and management of Zollinger-Ellison syndrome. Ann Surg. 1989;210:685.
3. Bok EJ, Cho KJ, Williams DM, Brady TM, Weiss CA, Forrest MA. Venous involvment in islet cell tumors of the pancreas. AJR. 1984;142:319.
4. Breatnach ES, Han SY, Rahatzad MT, Stanley RJ. CT evaluation of glucagonomas. J Comput Assist Tomogr. 1985;9:25.
5. Bressler EL, Alpern MB, Glazer GM, Franzis IR, Ensminger WD. Hypervascular hepatic metastases: CT evaluation. Radiology 1987;162:49.
6. Bonfils S, Bernades P. Zollinger-Ellison syndrome: natural history and diagnosis. Clin Gastroenterol. 1974;3:539.
7. Cohen DJ, Fagelman D. Pancreas islet cell carcinoma with complete fatty replacement: CT characteristics. J Comput Assist Tomogr. 1986;10:1050.
8. Creutzfeldt W, Arnold R, Creutzfeldt C et al. Pathomorphologic, biochemical and diagnostic aspects of gastrinomas (Zollinger-Ellison syndrome). Hum Pathol 1975;6:47.
9. Dunnick NR, Long JA Jr, Krudy A, Shawker TH, Doppman JL. Localizing insulinomas with combined radiographic methods. AJR. 1980;135:747.
10. Dupuy DE, Costello P, Ecker CP. Spiral CT of the pancreas. Radiology. 1992;183:815.
11. Eelkema EA, Stephens DH, Ward EM, Sheedy PF II. CT features of nonfunctioning islet cell carcinoma. AJR. 1984;143:943.
12. Fink IJ, Krudy AG, Shawker TH, et al. Demonstration of angiographically hypovascular insulinoma with intraarterial dynamic CT. AJR. 1985;144:555.
13. Frucht H, Doppman L, Norton JA, et al. Gastrinomas: comparison of MR imaging with CT, angiography, and US. Radiology. 1989;171:713.
14. Gunther RW, Klose KJ, Ruckert K, et al. Localization of small islet-cell tumors. Preoperative and intraoperative ultrasound, computed tomography, arteriography, digital subtraction angiography, and pancreatic venous sampling. Gastrointest Radiol. 1985;10:145.
15. Hercot O, Legmann P, Humbert M, et al. Diagnostic du glucagonome. Interet du scanner, de l'echographie et de l'arteriographie. A propos de deux observations et revue de la litterature. J Radiol. 1989;70:309.
16. Kalender WA, Seissler W, Klotz E, Vock P. Spiral volumetric CT with single-breath-hold technique, continuous transport, and continuous scanner rotation. Radiology. 1990;176:181.
17. Krudy AG, Doppman JL, Jensen RT, et al. Localization of islet cell tumors by dynamic CT: comparison with plain CT, arteriography, sonography, and venous sampling. AJR. 1984;143:585.
18. Maton PN, Miller DL, Doppman JL, et al. Role of selective angiography in the management of patients with Zollinger-Ellison Syndrome. Gastroenterology 1987;92:913.
19. McCarthy D, Jensen R. Zollinger-Ellison syndrome-current issues. In: Cohen S, Soloway R, eds. Hormone-Producing Tumors of the Gastrointestinal Tract. New York: Churchill Livingstone; 1985:25–55.
20. Norton JA, Sugarbaker PH, Doppman JL, et al. Aggressive resection of metastatic disease in selected patients with malignant gastrinoma. Ann Surg. 1986;203:352.
21. Norton JA, Shawker TH, Doppman JL, et al. Localization and surgical treatment of occult insulinomas. Ann Surg. 1990;212:615.
22. Paivansalo M, Makarainen H, Siniluoto T, Jalovaara P. Ultrasound compared with computed tomography and pancreatic arteriography in the detection of endocrine tumors of the pancreas. Europ J Radiol. 1989;9:173.
23. Pogany AC, Kerlan RK Jr, Karam JH, Le Quesne LP, Ring EJ. Cystic insulinoma. AJR. 1984;142:951.
24. Proye C. Surgical strategy in insulinoma: clinical review. Acta Chir Scand. 1987;153:481.
25. Proye C, Boissel P. Preoperative immaging versus intraoperative localization of tumors in adult surgical patients with hyperinsulinemia: a multicenter study of 338 patients. World J Surgery. 1988;12:685.
26. Rasbach D, Van Heerden J, Telander R, et al. Surgical management of hyperinsulinism in the multiple endocrine neoplasia type 1 syndrome. Arch Surg. 1985;120:584.
27. Rossi P, Allison DJ, Bezzi M, et al. Endocrine tumors of the pancreas. Radiol Clin North Am. 1989;27:129.
28. Rossi P, Baert A, Passariello R, et al. CT of functioning tumors of the pancreas. AJR. 1985;144:57.
29. Rossi P, Baert A, Marchal W, et al. Multiple bolus technique vs. single bolus infusion of contrast medium to obtain prolonged contrast enhancement of the pancreas. Radiology. 1982;144:929.
30. Service F, Van Heedern J, Sheedy P. Insulinoma. In: Service F, ed. Hypoglycemic disorders – Pathogenesis and treatment. Boston: GK Hall Medical Publishers; 1983;111.

31 Smith TR, Koenigsberg M. Low density insulinoma on dynamic CT. AJR. 1990;155:995.
32 Stabile B, Morrow D, Passaro E. The gastrinoma triangle: Operative indications. Am J Surg. 1984;147:25.
33 Stark DD, Moss AA, Goldberg HI, Deveney CW. CT of pancreatic islet cell tumors. Radiology. 1984;150:491.
34 Stefanini P, Carboni M, Patrassi N, Basoli A. Beta-islet cell tumors of the pancreas: results of a study on 1067 cases. Surgery. 1974;75:597.
35 Thompson NW, Eckhauser FE, Vinik AI, Lloyd RV, Fiddian-Green RG, Strodel WE. Cystic neuroendocrine neoplasm of the pancreas and liver. Ann Surg. 1984;199:158.
36 Tjon A Tham Rto, Jansen JBMJ, Falke THM, et al. MR, CT, and ultrasound findings of metastatic vipoma in pancreas. J Comput Assist Tomogr. 1989;13:142.
37 Tjon A Tham Rto, Falke THM, Jansen JBMJ, Lamers CBHW. CT and Mr imaging of advanced Zollinger-Ellison Syndrome. J Comput Assist Tomogr. 1989;13:821.
38 Wank SA, Doppman JL, Miller DL, et al. Prospective study of the ability of computed axial tomography to localize gastrinomas in patients with Zollinger-Ellison syndrome. Gastroenterology. 1987;92:905.
39 Wise SR, Johnson J, Sparks J, et al. Gastrinoma: the predictive value of preoperative localization. Surgery. 1989;106:1087.
40 Wolf EL, Sprayregen S, Frager D, Rifkin H, Gliedman ML. Calcification in an insulinoma of the pancreas. Am J gastroenterol. 1984;79:559.
41 Wolfe M, Alexander R, McGuigan J. Extrapancreatic, extraintestinal gastrinoma: effective treatment of surgery. N Engl J Med. 1982;306:1533.
42 Zollinger R. Gastrinoma: factors affecting prognosis. Surgery. 185;97:49.

MR Imaging

P. Pavone, M. Di Girolamo, G. P. Cardone,
C. Catalano, G. Albertini Petroni,
and R. Passariello

A certain diagnosis of a pancreatic islet cell tumor is based on the presence of characteristic clinical symptomatology, on the evaluation of hormonal values, and on positive stimulation tests. In case of pancreatic apudomas, the primary role of diagnostic imaging is the correct localization of the tumor within the glandular parenchyma, and in case of malignant apudomas, such as gastrinomas, the identification of liver metastases. A presurgical, correct localization of the tumor is of utmost importance in making successful intervention and reducing surgical repetition 1. One has to consider that the surgical removal of islet cell tumors is curative in benign cases, which are the most frequent.

Surgical exploration may have negative results when the tumor is small, deeply rooted in the pancreas, or has a consistency similar to that of surrounding parenchyma at palpation 2. Therefore, a correct preoperative localization of pancreatic islet cell tumors remains one of the most challenging tasks of diagnostic radiology 3. In fact, 90% of pancreatic islet cell tumors are less than 2 cm in size at clinical diagnosis 4.

For presurgical detection and localization of pancreatic islet cell tumors, preoperative ultrasound examinations have a sensitivity of 60% in the best series, according to the literature 5.

With CT, the alteration of pancreatic border is evident in 60% of cases, and bulging of pancreatic contour is not a reliable finding. CT reliability has been improved by performing a dynamic injection of contrast medium, leading to a sensitivity of 40% to 77% (6); its specificity, however, still remains low. A careful injection technique of large doses of contrast medium is needed to detect the hyperdensity of the islet cell tumors.

Over the last 20 years, invasive diagnostic procedures like angiography and portal venous sampling have been the most reliable modalities for detecting functioning tumors of the pancreas. Therefore, these procedures are routinely performed to detect such lesions, with a sensitivity of 54–90% with angiography (5), and a sensitivity of 83% with portal venous sampling (7).

MRI has not provided satisfactory results until recently. In one reported series, in fact, only two lesions larger than 3 cm were detected using this technique (8); more recently, a 20% sensitivity was reported in the detection rate of pancreatic gastrinomas (9).

The recent improvements in motion artifact reduction technique, optimization of intrinsic contrast of MRI pulse sequences, and an accurate preparation of the upper gastrointestinal tract, have allowed to obtain good image quality of the pancreas in most clinical cases and to propose MRI in the preoperative detection of islet cell tumors of the pancreas.

In this chapter we evaluate the results obtained with MRI in the preoperative detection of pancreatic insulinomas (beta cell tumors) in a clinically selected series. The same patients were examined using to CT, performed with i. v. injection of multiple boli of contrast media, and selective angiography. MRI findings were subsequently compared to CT and angiography results.

MRI of the Pancreas: Method of Study

The partial suppression of breathing artifacts was obtained by reducing the echo time and repetition time of spin-echo T_1 sequences, and by increasing the NEX. This technique for studying the abdomen was proposed by Stark in 1987 (10). We employed T_1-weighted sequences with a TR of 260–320 ms and TE of 16 ms, the lowest time allowed by the available software. Eight is a more appropriate number of excitations for improving image quality and maintaining low acquisition times. The highest spatial resolution was provided by a 256 × 256 matrix.

T_2-weighted and proton density sequences were characterized by a TR of 2000 ms and TEs of 30 and 70 ms, a NEX of two and a matrix of 128 × 256.

The images were acquired on axial plane, with a slice thickness of 10 mm, and adopting an interslice gap of 3 mm, as opposed to 5 mm employed by Stark. With these two sequences it is possible to examine the pancreas in about 20 minutes.

For a better evaluation of the pancreatic parenchyma, it is very important to correctly prepare the upper gastrointestinal tract. Tap water (250 mL) was given as an oral contrast medium immediately before the study. In order to avoid peristaltic movement, i.m. scopolamine was administered 15–20 minutes before the examination. Using this method, a good definition of the duodenum and gastric lumen was always obtained.

The use of specific oral contrast media may also be proposed to improve the delineation of the pancreas by MRI. Actually, oral contrast media for the opacification of the alimentary tract are undergoing clinical tests. They include positive compounds, such as oral Gd-DTPA (11), which shows high signal intensity within the lumen, and negative compounds, such as viscous compounds of particles containing iron oxide (12), which show low signal intensity within the lumen.

Normal Findings

On T_1- and T_2-weighted sequences, the pancreas shows the same signal intensity of liver parenchyma.

The head of the pancreas is surrounded by some anatomical structures such as the inferior vena cava posteriorly, the superior mesenteric vein and artery anteriorly, and the second portion of the duodenum, laterally. In the posterior portion of the head of the pancreas, it is possible to distinguish the distal choledochus, which, in normal conditions, has a caliber smaller than 8 mm and presents low signal intensity on T_1-weighted images and high signal intensity on T_2-weighted images (Fig. 6.**15**).

The isthmus is localized between the head and the body region of the pancreas. Behind the isthmus, the superior mesenteric vein merges into the splenic vein to form the portal vein. On spin-echo sequences, the portal system shows the characteristic signal void, which is typical of vessels with flow. In the inferior isthmal portion, posteriorly to the splenomesenteric confluence, is the uncinate process.

Because of oblique position of the pancreas, the body and the tail region are localized in more cranial planes than the pancreatic head. Superiorly or posteriorly to the pancreatic body and tail region, or within the pancreas, the splenic vein is evidenced with its linear course and characteristic signal void.

Due to its low spatial resolution, MR imaging is not able to evaluate the intrapancreatic Wirsung's duct under normal conditions.

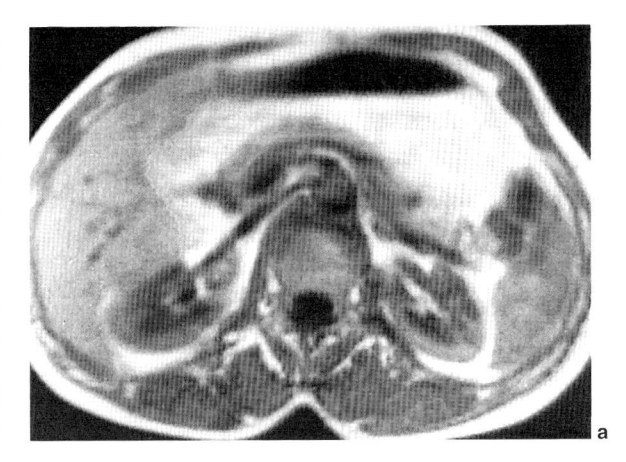

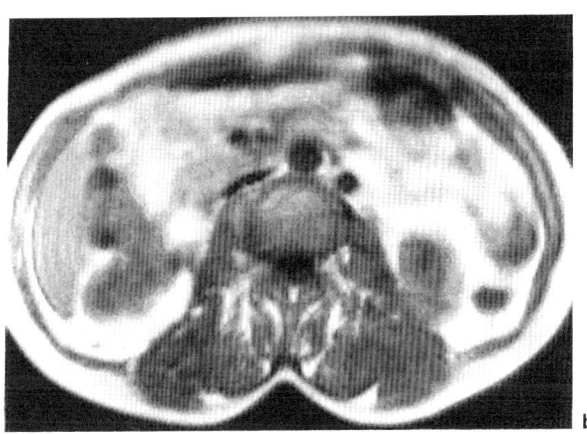

Fig. 6.**15** Normal anatomy of the pancreas. The upper gastrointestinal tract has been opacified with Gd-DTPA. In the first axial image (**a**) the body–tail region of the pancreas is evidenced with the splenoportal junction and the origin of celiac trunk. In a more caudal axial image (**b**) the head of the pancreas surrounded posteriorly by the inferior vena cava, the mesenteric vein and artery antero-medially and the second portion of duodenum laterally is depicted

Pathological Findings

In the eleven patients included in our study, the diagnosis of pancreatic insulinoma was based on positive hormonal tests, and all the patients underwent surgery. All patients had previously undergone selective angiography and CT.

The clinical diagnosis was made on the basis of the fasting plasma glucose/insulin ratio (less than two strongly suggests the presence of insulinoma), prolonged fasting tests, and dynamic studies of insulin secretion: insulin-induced hypoglycemia (IIH, 0.1 U/kg i.v. in 60 minutes) with plasma C-peptide assessment, diazoxide (DZX, 600 mg i.v. in 1 hour), and somatostatin (SRIF, 25–50–100 µg i.v. during first, second and third hour, respectively) tests to evaluate the suppressibility of beta cell secretory function (13, 14). In our experience, both IIH and DZX are very important for the diagnosis, whereas the SRIF test provides more information on the degree of differentiation of the tumor cells.

In ten patients, a beta cell tumor of the pancreas was surgically removed, and in all of them, MRI identified the lesions. In one patient, previously referred to surgery for removal of an insulinoma, multiple micrometastases of the liver were found during surgery with no lesion of the pancreas.

The appearance of islet cell tumors on MRI was that of a nodular lesion of variable diameter and different signal intensity. Hypointensity on T_1-weighted sequences was predominant and the lesion was isointense to normal pancreas in one case only. On T_2-weighted images the lesions were hyperintense in eight cases; in two cases they were not detected, due to isointensity in one case and to the presence of significant motion artifacts in the other. The lesion size was smaller than 1 cm in three patients, between 1 and 2 cm in five patients, and between 2 and 3 cm in two patients. The tumors were located in the body-tail region of the pancreas in four patients (Fig. 6.16), in the head in four patients (Fig. 6.17), and in the isthmus in two patients (Fig. 6.18).

In our series, MRI studies were performed after CT, from which the results were already known. CT scans were acquired with rapid i. v. injection of contrast medium, and third generation equipment was used. Contiguous slices of 10 mm thickness were acquired during the dynamic phase of the contrast enhancement. When detected with CT, the lesions showed a characteristic nodular hyperdense appearance after administration of contrast media. In one case only, alteration of pancreatic contours was evident. In seven cases, lesions were not seen with CT, including that of hepatic micrometastases. The sensitivity of CT in our series was therefore low, with only four detected lesions out of 11. False-positive results are a frequent occurrence with CT when focal areas of hyperdensity are detected. This is due to the presence of intraparenchymal vessels, which, in contrast, are easily depicted using MRI.

The evaluation of angiographic studies permits diagnosis of beta cell tumors of the pancreas in 54–90% of patients. In our study, angiography results were negative in three patients, also considering the patient with multiple hepatic micrometastases, and in one patient, repeated angiography after initial MRI led to detection of the lesion, with careful study technique

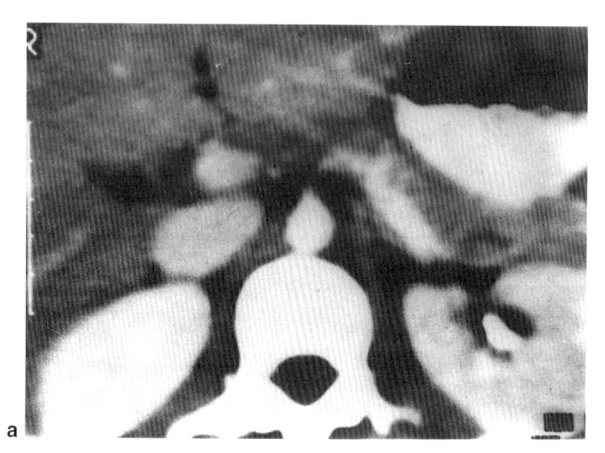

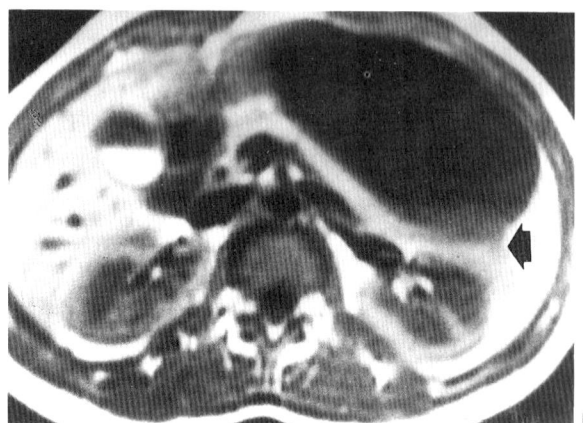

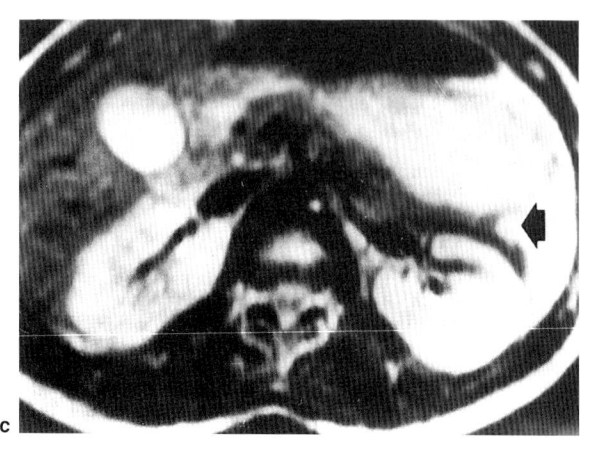

Fig. 6.**16** Insulinoma of the tail of the pancreas. The enhanced CT (**a**) does not show relevant hyperdensity in the pancreas. Retrospectively, a minor bulging of the tail could be identified. MRI shows a slightly hypointense area in the T1-weighted image (**b**, arrow), with marked hyperintensity in the T2-weighted image (**c**, arrow). The comparison of the two images helped to identify the lesion, with indentation of the normal pancreas. A 0.8 cm insulinoma was removed at surgery

MR Imaging 193

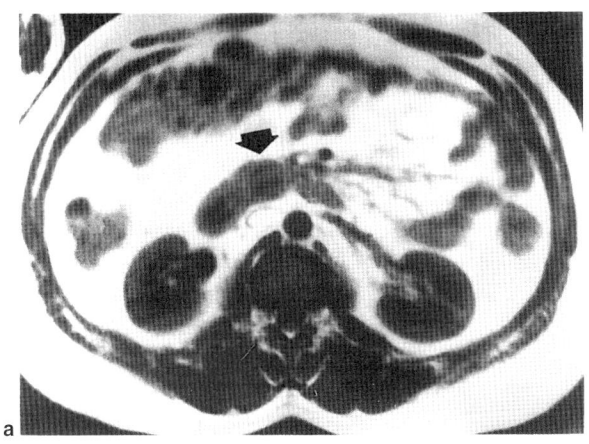

Fig. 6.**17** Insulinoma of the head of the pancreas. Although the lesion measured more than 2 cm at surgery, it did not cause any bulging of the pancreatic contour, justifying two previous negative CT studies.

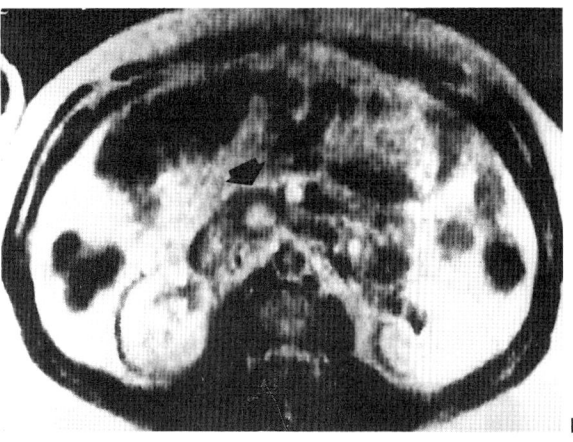

At MRI the pancreatic head insulinoma is evident with slight hypointensity in the T1-weighted image (**a**, arrow) and marked hyperintensity in the T2-weighted image (**b**, arrow)

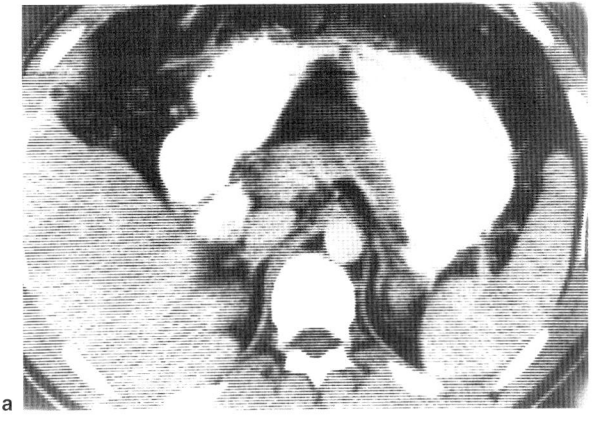

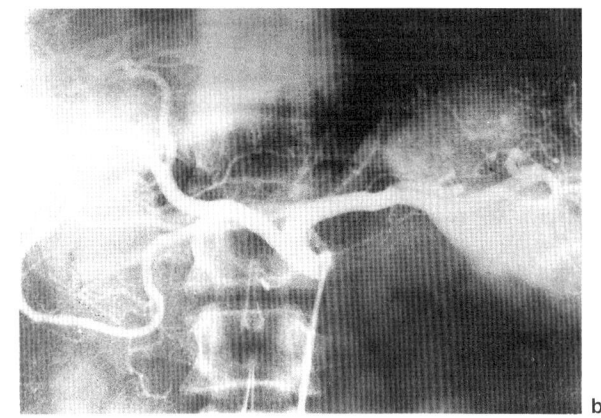

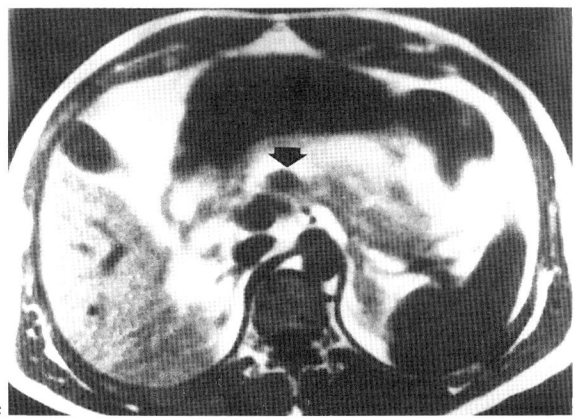

Fig. 6.**18** Insulinoma of the pancreatic isthmus. The CT scan (**a**) and the Angiography (**b**) of this patient did not show a relevant hypervascular lesion and were considered negative. MRI performed afterwards showed a 2-cm, hypointense lesion at the pancreatic isthmus on the T1-weighted image (**c**, arrow). The lesion was isointense or slightly hyperintense on the T2-weighted image (**d**, arrow)

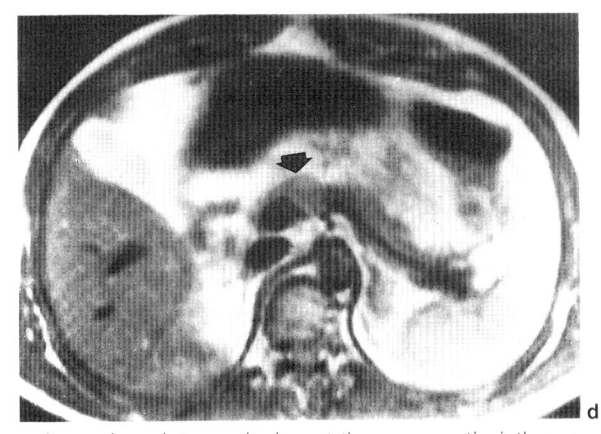

and gas filling of the stomach. The angiography was performed using a selective catheterization of the celiac trunk and superior mesenteric artery. In four patients superselective catheterization of the dorsal pancreatic and gastroduodenal arteries was done. Angiography, however, is an invasive procedure and does not show the anatomical relationship of the lesion to the intrapancreatic structures, the bile duct, or the peripancreatic vessels.

Conclusions

Based on our experience, MRI seems to be a promising technique for the localization of islet cell tumors.

The resolution of motion artifacts obtained at medium field strength, in fact, allows for good image quality in abdominal MRI in most cases, with excellent intrinsic contrast. A careful technique is of utmost importance in evaluating the pancreas with MRI and can explain the good results of our series, contrary to previously reported series.

The positive MRI findings in this series suggest a definite role for this technique in the preoperative evaluation of islet cell tumors. In presence of positive clinical and biochemical findings, MRI could be substituted for CT in the detection of these lesions, following preoperative ultrasound. The use of invasive preoperative procedures, such as angiography, when MRI findings are positive, could be avoided. MRI can also detect the presence of liver metastases in case of pancreatic apudomas, like gastrinomas, with malignant biological behaviour.

Although promise exists in the use of MRI to detect pancreatic islet cell tumors, its real clinical role needs to be established after larger series are acquired.

References

1. van Heerden JA, Edis AJ, Service FJ. The surgical aspects of insulinomas. Ann Surg. 1979;189:677–682.
2. Stefanini P, Carboni M, Patrassi N, Basoli I. Beta-islet cell tumors of pancreas: results of a study on 1067 cases. Surgery. 1974;75:579–609.
3. Gunther RW, Klose KJ, Ruckert K, Beyer J, Kuhn FP, Klotter HJ. Localization of small islet-cell tumors: preoperative and intraoperative ultrasound, computed tomography, arteriography, digital subtraction angiography, and pancreatic venous sampling. Gastrointest Radiol. 1985;10:145–152.
4. Friesen SR. Tumors of endocrine pancreas. N Engl J Med. 1982;306:580–590.
5. Galiber AK, Reading CC, Charbonneau JW, et al. Localization of pancreatic insulinoma: comparison of pre- and intraoperative US with CT and angiography. Radiology. 1988;166:405–408.
6. Rossi P, Baert A, Passariello R, Simonetti G, Pavone P, Tempesta P. CT of functioning tumors of the pancreas. AJR. 1985;144:57–60.
7. Passariello R, Feltrin GP, Miotto D, Pedrazzoli S, Rossi P, Simoneti G. Transhepatic portal catheterization with pancreatic venous sampling versus angiography in the localization of pancreatic functioning tumors. Front Radiol. 1982;1:51–69.
8. Tscholakoff D, Hriack H, Thoeny R, Winkler ML, Margulis AR. MR imaging in the diagnosis of pancreatic disease. AJR. 1987;148:703–709.
9. Frucht H, Doppman JL, Norton JA, et al. Gastrinomas: comparison of MR imaging with CT, angiography, and US. Radiology. 1989;713–717.
10. Stark DD, Hendrick RE, Hahn PF, Ferrucci JT Jr. Motion artifact reduction with fast spin-echo imaging. Radiology. 1987;164:183–191.
11. Laniado M, Kornmesser W, Hamm B, Clauss W, Weinmann MJ, Felix R. MR imaging of the gastrointestinal tract: value of Gd-DTPA. AJR. 1988;150:817–821.
12. Rink PA, Smevik O, Nielsen G, et al. Oral magnetic particles in MR imaging of the abdomen and pelvis. Radiology. 1991;178:755–780.
13. Tamburrano G, Lala A, Mauceri M, Leonetti F, Andreani D. Diazoxide infusion test in patient with single benign insulinoma. Horm Res. 1983;17:141–146.
14. Tamburrano G, Leonetti F, Mauceri M, Lala A, Falluca F. Effect of low doses of somatostatin on plasma insulin levels in patients with insulinoma. Serono Symposia Review. 1984;3:202–206.

Angiography

M. Bezzi, F. M. Salvatori, F. Orsi, M. Rossi, G. Natali, and P. Rossi

Arteriography was the first imaging modality employed in the localization of endocrine pancreatic tumors (27), and for many years before the introduction of cross sectional imaging, has been the only tool available to radiologists and surgeons to obtain preoperative informations on the number, site, and dimensions of these rare neoplasms. When properly applied, the accuracy of arteriography can come close to 80–85% (1, 11, 33); however, in modern diagnostic imaging, the role of angiography is complementary to CT and MR, which are the primary methods of evaluation. Other angiographic techniques used for localization of pancreatic apudomas include transhepatic portal venous sampling and intra-arterial stimulation with hepatic venous sampling, which are briefly discussed in this chapter.

Technique

The high rates of islet cell tumor localization by arteriography found in the literature (1, 11, 14, 33) can be achieved only when excellent radiography is combined with meticulous arteriographic technique. Actually, there are very few other areas of angiography in which the difference between a technically mediocre study and an optimal study is so critical in terms of diagnostic accuracy.

The first step of the procedure is an anteroposterior plain abdominal film that may reveal some small calcifications: This is not a specific finding for an apudoma but it may serve to draw the angiographer's attention to that area (21). Moreover, prior to angiography, it is advisable to obtain the distention of the stomach and duodenum with gas and induce bowel paralysis, in order to eliminate the confusing images caused by gastroduodenal mucosal folds (Fig. 6.**19**) and to give a "clear" view, particularly of the pancreatic

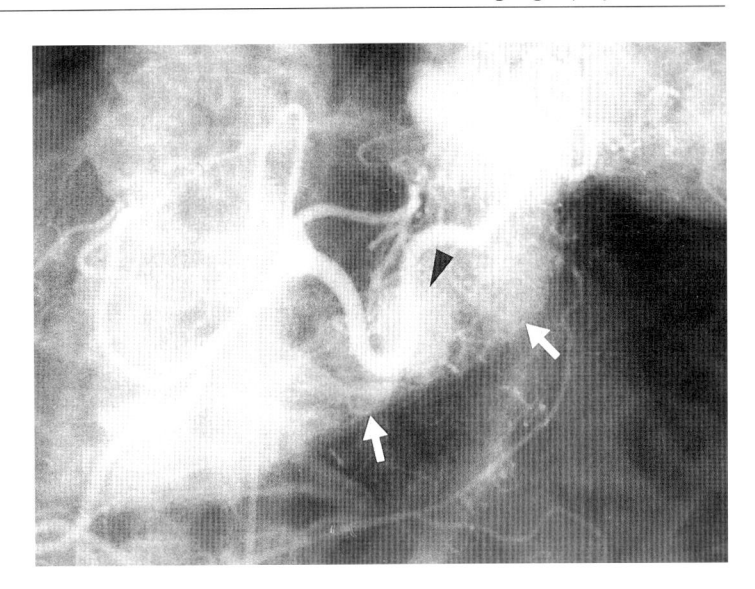

Fig. 6.**19** Gastric blush in a case of insulinoma located between the body and the tail of the pancreas. The celiac axis injection determines a strong opacification of the walls of the undistended stomach (white arrows), thus almost obscuring the nodular blush (arrowhead)

body and tail during splenic artery injection (Fig. 6.**20**). With a correct use of this technique it is also possible to achieve a finer superselective gastroduodenal arteriogram without the superimposed dense blush of the duodenal mucosa.

Selective abdominal angiography is commonly performed via a femoral approach with small Cobra or Simmons I type catheters (5 or 6 Fr), inserted through an introducer sheath that allows for easier catheter exchange. The celiac trunk, the splenic, superior mesenteric (SMA), gastroduodenal (GDA), dorsal pancreatic, and pancreaticoduodenal arteries should be selectively catheterized and injected whenever technically feasible; this technique requires experience and time, but the diagnostic accuracy will be greatly increased if the pancreas can be examined by more selective angiograms (Fig. 6.**21**). The superselective injections increase the relative amount of contrast medium delivered to the pancreas, minimizing the opacification of superimposed organs. The modalities of injection are reported in Table 6.**2**; however, one should remember that in order to obtain better results, it is advisable to conform the injection rate to the arterial flow, as judged under fluoroscopy; the administration of high doses of contrast medium is justified by the presence of several anastomoses within the arterial network of the gland.

The quality of the final arteriogram also depends on the radiographic technique that should conform to some simple but important rules: small focal spot, correct radiographic centering, right exposure factors (some authors suggest the use of a low voltage technique, within the 70 to 75 Kilovolt [peak] range, to demonstrate the smallest pancreatic vessels [5]), close film collimation, and photographic subtraction technique if necessary. The use of high-quality digital subtraction angiography is recommended, whenever available.

Radiographs are usually obtained in the anteroposterior view, but oblique views may be extremely helpful in doubtful cases. During injection of the splenic artery, particularly useful is a 15–20° right posterior oblique projection, which is used to separate the pancreatic tail from the spleen (Fig. 6.**20**).

Normal and Pathological Findings

The panoramic study of the celiac trunk is an important first step in pancreatic angiography because it demonstrates the vascular anatomy of the liver and pancreas, it may reveal the presence of hepatic metastases, and it shows the venous return with opacification of the splenic and portal veins. In case the tumor is directly shown by the celiac trunk injection (Fig. 6.**22**), superselective studies are still suggested in order to demonstrate multiple tumors.

During superselective injections, the angiographic pattern of the normal gland is characterized by the filling of a fine arterial network, followed by the parenchymal blush. Sometimes an excessive volume of contrast medium, superselectively delivered in one of the pancreatic arteries, may induce an intense glandular blush that may simulate a hypervascular nodule. This may be a cause of false-positive arteriographic diagnosis (27). It is beyond the purposes of this chapter to discuss the angiographic anatomy of the pancreas, which can be found elsewhere (36); however, a thorough knowledge of the normal and usual variations of the pancreatic vascular anatomy is necessary in order to understand small changes in course and distribution of vessels, which are often the basis for either negative or positive film interpretation.

The arteriographic pattern of the different islet cell tumors is similar, due to a basically similar type of vascularity, and does not permit a differential diagnosis of the various histologic types. Differences can be

196   6 Pancreas

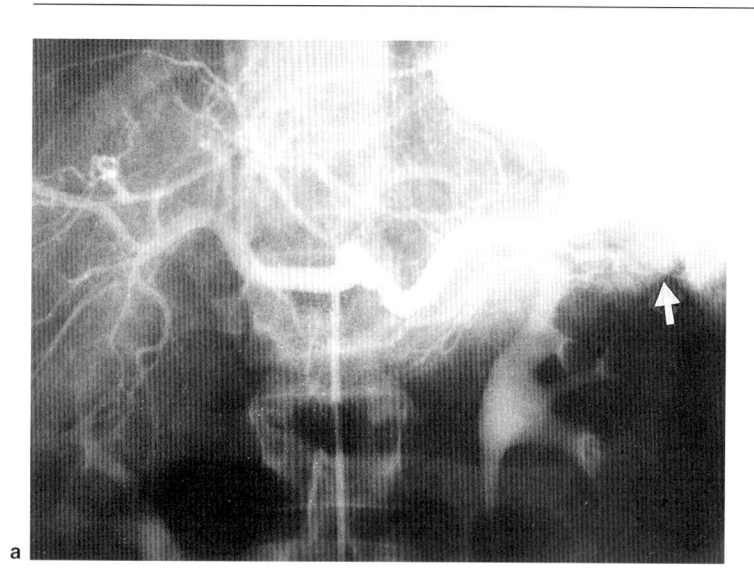

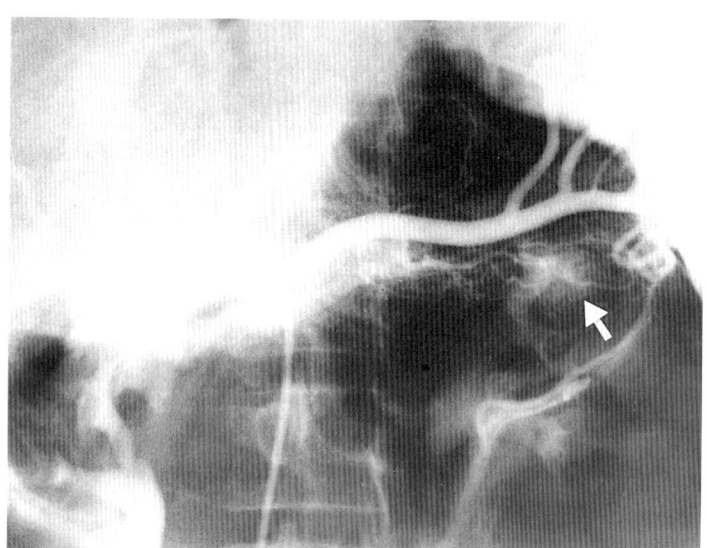

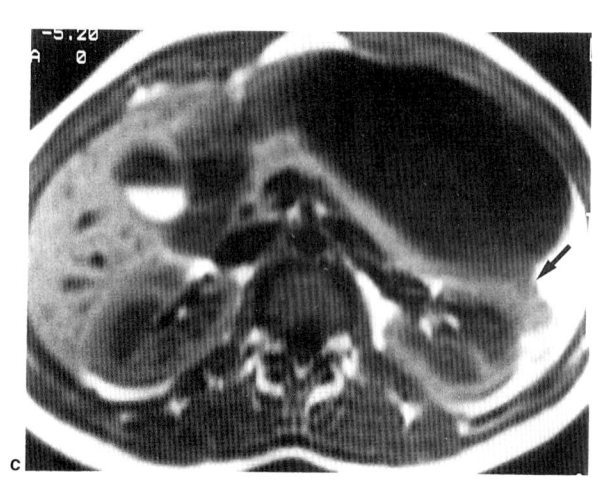

Fig. 6.**20**   Insulinoma of the tail. Sequence illustrating value of stomach distention and oblique projections. Parenchymal phase of a celiac arteriogram performed in AP projection: an area of focal pancreatic blush (arrow) is suspected but almost completely obscured by the spleen. (**b**) Splenic injection in the RPO projection after gastric distension: the tumor is now clearly apparent (arrow). (**c**) T_1-weighted MR axial scan shows small hypointense tumor in the tail (arrow) (MR scan courtesy of Dr. P. Pavone)

Angiography 197

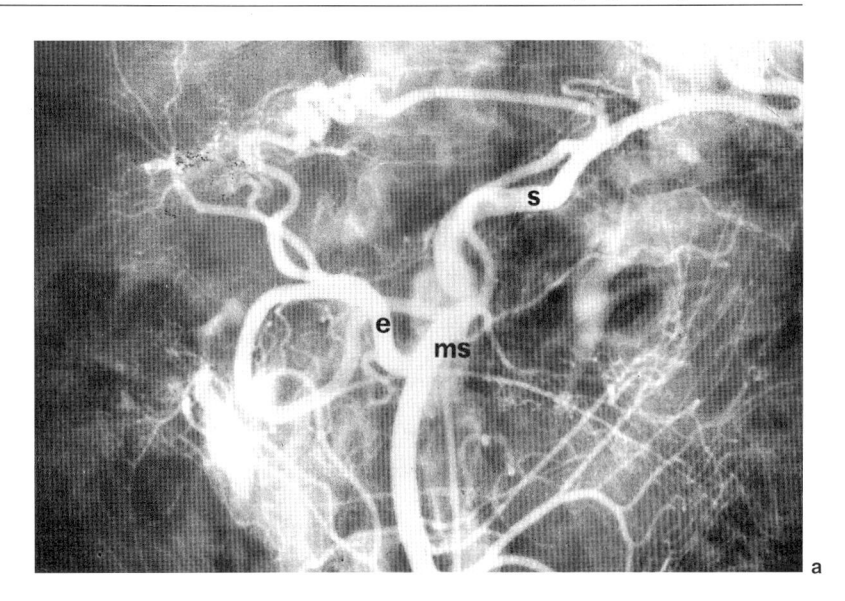

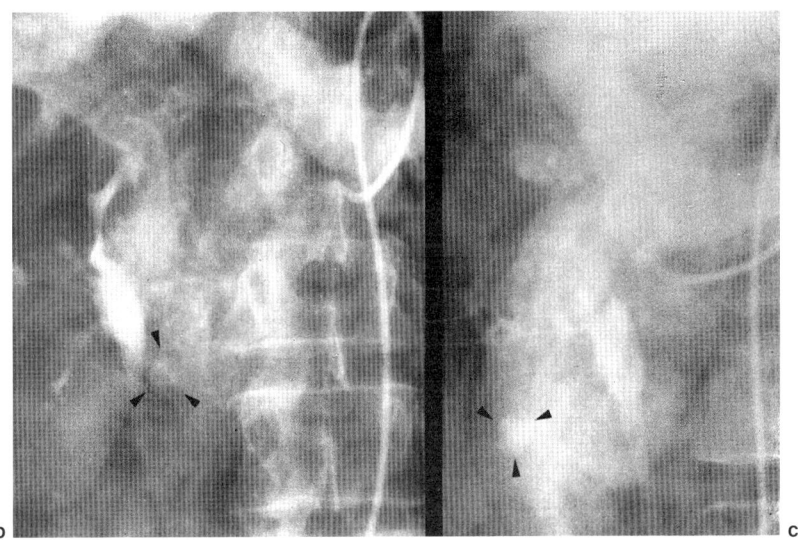

Fig. 6.**21** Gastrinoma of the head, value of selective studies. (**a**) Nonselective arteriogram is not diagnostic. Note anomalous origin of the common hepatic artery from the SMA (e = hepatic artery; s = splenic artery; ms = SMA). (**b**) A small round area of contrast blush within the head is demonstrated in the late phase of a selective GDA injection (Arrowheads). (**c**) An RPO projection after GDA injection helps define the tumor

Table 6.**2** Volumes of contrast medium and injection rates for conventional selective pancreatic angiography. (The amount of contrast medium is considerably reduced with the use of DSA)

Injection site	Total volume	Flow rate
Celiac trunk	50–70 mL	6–8 mL/s
Superior mesenteric artery	50–60 mL	6–8 mL/s
Splenic artery	35–45 mL	5–8 mL/s
Gastroduodenal artery	12–15 mL	3–4 mL/s
Dorsal pancreatic artery	9–12 mL	2–3 mL/s
Inferior pancreaticoduodenal artery	12–15 mL	3–4 mL/s

seen in relation to tumor functional conditions, size or malignancy, but they are not specific.

An area of dense, circumscribed, and homogeneous capillary blush is the most characteristic appearance of these lesions (Figs. 6.**21**, 6.**22**, and 6.**23**). This area of increased vascularity, which is supplied by one or more hypertrophic pancreatic arteries, is usually round or oval. The filling of a fine reticular network of normal arteries may precede the angiographic parenchymal phase (Fig. 6.**24**). The tumor blush usually appears in the late arterial–capillary phase, reaches its maximum approximately 4–7 seconds after injection, and may persist for 12–16 seconds after injection. Typically, small apudomas are round and relatively well defined.

Irregular and dilated feeding vessels are more likely to be seen in larger tumors. Often in these cases, there is also a characteristic displacement and bowing

198   6 Pancreas

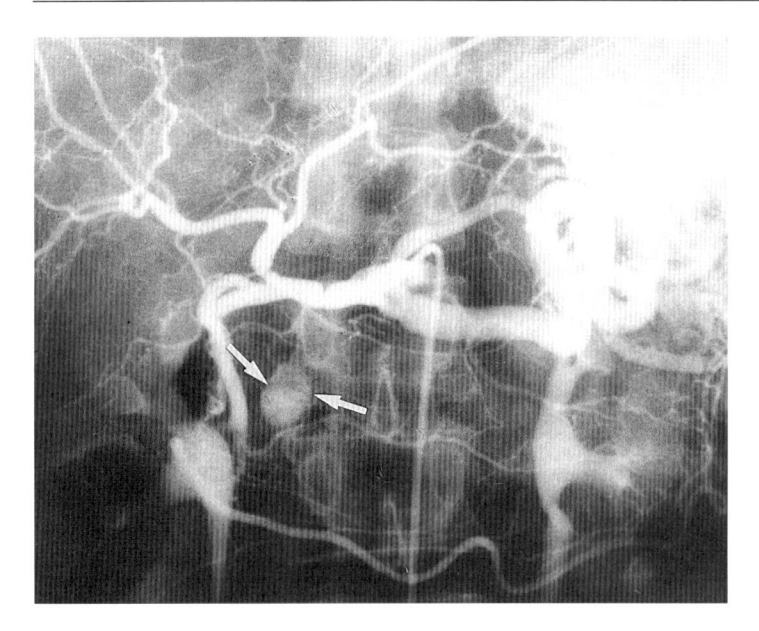

Fig. 6.**22** Insulinoma of pancreatic head. A hypervascular lesion is well demonstrated (arrows) on the celiac arteriogram. The need for selective injections is always justified by the possible presence of multiple tumors

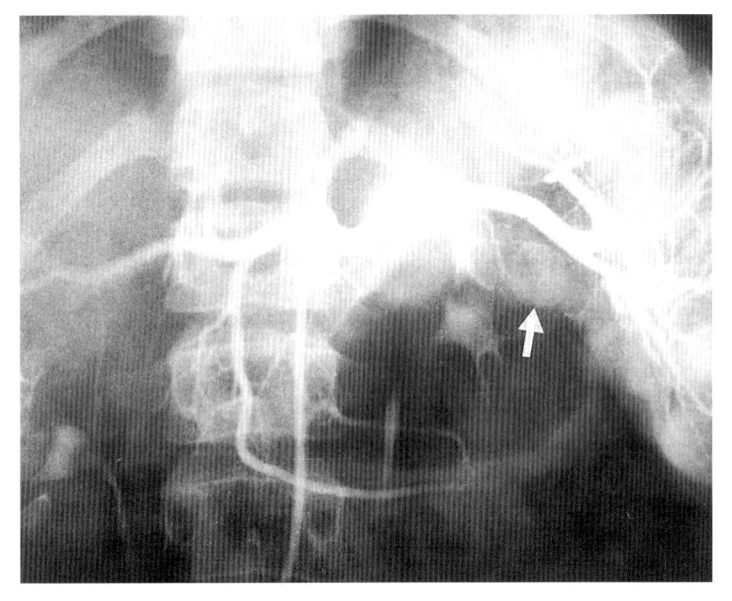

Fig. 6.**23** Insulinoma of the tail. Note clear, well-defined, tumor blush, nicely demarcated from the spleen (arrow). In this case the RPO projection was determined unnecessary

of slightly enlarged pancreatic arteries around the lesion (Fig. 6. **25**). In addition, the tumor stain in large lesions may be irregular and inhomogeneous, as compared to small ones.

The venous phase does not have a characteristic appearance. Nevertheless, superselective injections are followed by early visualization of pancreatic venous outflow, and enlarged veins draining from a tumor may be observed occasionally.

Hypovascular lesions are less frequent than hypervascular ones. They may be demonstrated as negative defects on the parenchymal phase (30), but, if large enough, are more often suggested on the basis of vascular displacement and arterial bowing (Fig. 6.**25**).

Features suggestive of a malignant lesion include irregular tumor outline with blurred borders and inhomogeneous opacification, marked irregularity of the feeding arteries with vascular encasement and obstruction or both. However, the only unequivocal radiological sign of malignancy is the demonstration of metastatic lesions in the liver or in the lymph nodes (Fig. 6.**26**). Hepatic angiography is particularly indicated in patients with Zollinger–Ellison syndrome because it is highly sensitive in detecting secondary lesions from gastrinoma (15, 24).

Angiography 199

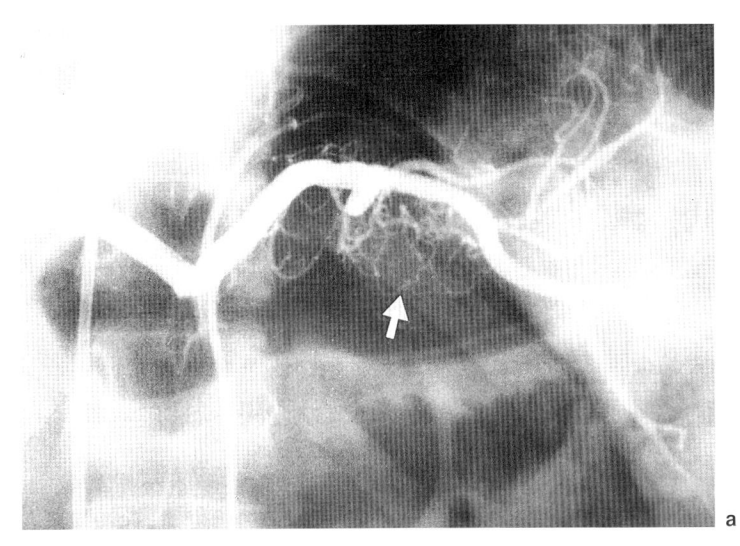

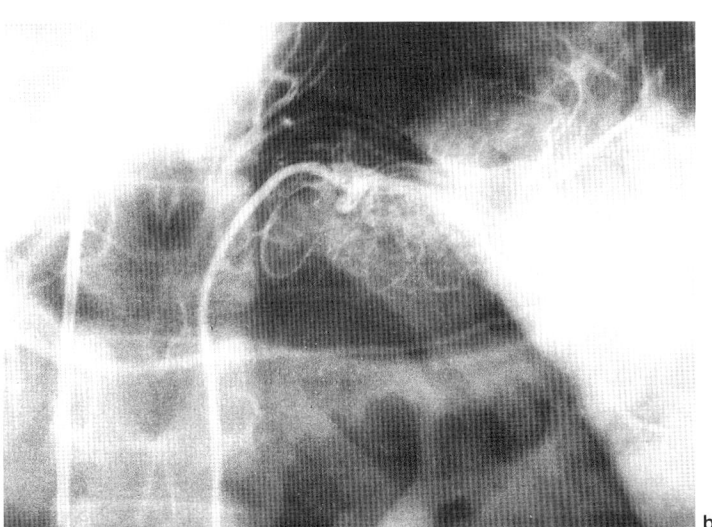

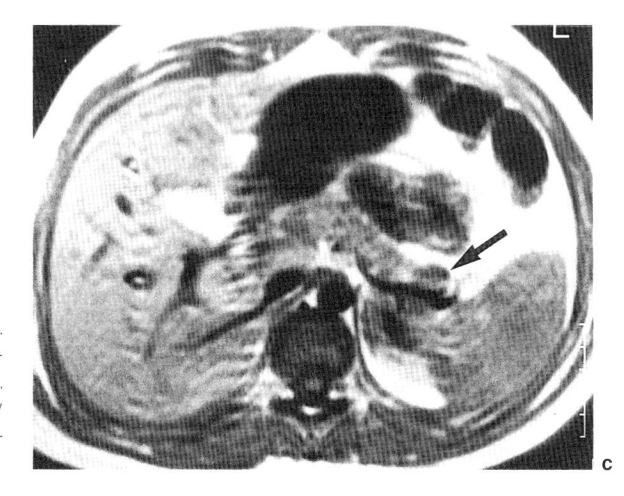

Fig. 6.**24** Insulinoma of the tail of the pancreas. (**a**) Selective splenic arteriogram after gastric distention shows initial filling of a fine arterial network (arrow). (**b**) Later phase of same injection: initial capillary blush. (**c**) T1-weighted MR axial scan shows hypointense nodule of pancreatic tail (arrow)

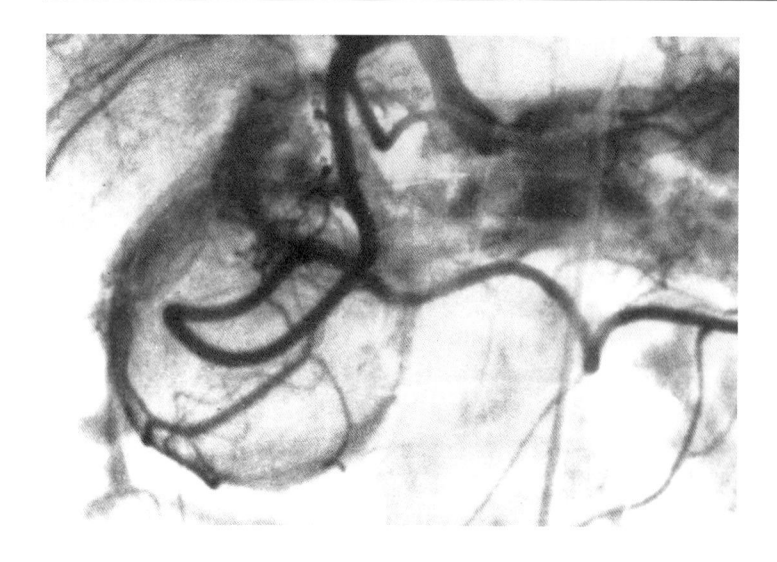

Fig. 6.25 Cystic insulinoma of the pancreatic head. Common hepatic arteriogram: large, centrally avascular mass with a hypervascular rim; note displacement and bowing of arteries at the perifery of the lesion (from Reference 30)

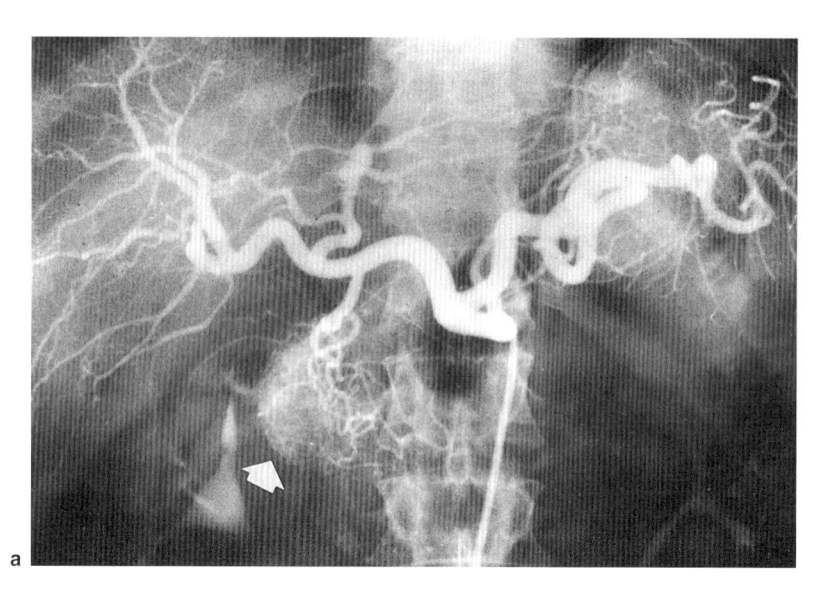

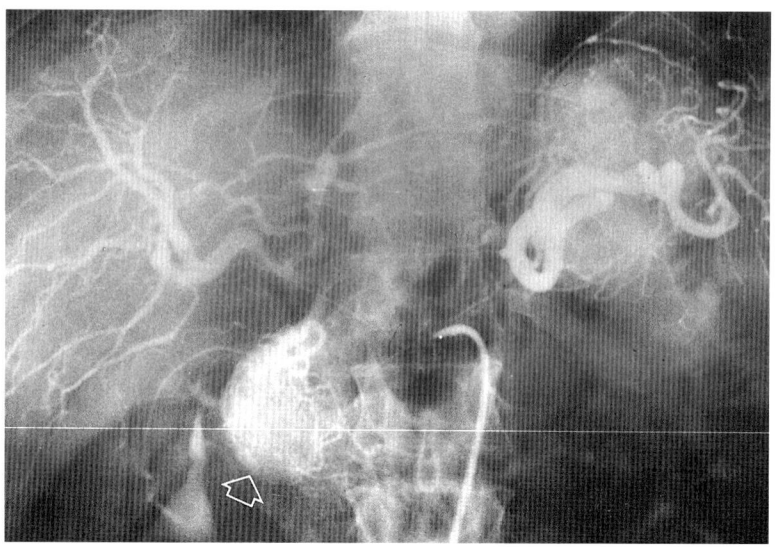

Fig. 6.26 Gastrinoma metastatic to peripancreatic nodes. (a) Early phase of celiac arteriogram shows a mass with a rich neovascularity that originates from the GDA (arrow); (b) in a later phase there is an intense well-defined blush (open arrow). Surgery revealed that the mass consisted of metastatic lymph nodes anterior to the pancreatic head; the primary gastrinoma was not found

The factors influencing the diagnostic results of arteriography in islet cell tumors are:

1. *Vascularity* of the lesion: most tumors are highly vascular and are easily detected, even when small. Tumors with poor arterial supply, even when relatively large, tend to escape localization because they do not determine a perceptible contrast blush (13, 37). However, even a highly vascular tumor may sometimes remain undetected if the volume or the injection rate of contrast medium is inadequate to obtain optimal tumor opacification. Another hypothesis that might account for unsuccessful localization of hypervascular tumors is that the lesion may not always present the same degree of endocrine activity. This may explain why a negative angiogram, in the same patient, is sometimes followed a few weeks apart by a positive study, often performed with the same technique (personal observation).

2. *Site and dimension:* small tumors localized within the pancreatic head may be difficult to demonstrate because of the superimposed contrast blush of the duodenal or gastric wall. Apudomas of the pancreatic tail more easily escape detection because they are masked by the opacification of the spleen at the hilum (Fig. 6.**22**), while a pancreatic body lesion may project over the spine. However, the angiographic examination may permit a confident diagnosis of hypervascular lesions 8–10 mm in size if principles of accurate radiographic technique, particularly oblique views and gastric distension, are carefully respected (Fig. 6.**23**).

There are a number of conditions that may cause errors in film interpretation, causing both overdiagnosis or underdiagnosis of pancreatic apudoma. False-negative diagnosis may occur because the lesion is too small or is not hypervascular; in other instances it is the mediocre quality of the exam that does not permit tumor identification. False-positive diagnoses may be caused by many factors: misinterpretation of vascular blushes due to normal duodenum, stomach, or splenic lobulations. Other common sources of error include accessory spleens, hyperplastic lymph nodes (22), or the abundant superselective opacification of portions of normal pancreas (1). More rarely, a false-positive angiogram may be due to peptic ulcer, chronic pancreatitis, pseudocysts (22), or hypervascular lesions of the liver that project onto the pancreatic area.

In addition to its role in tumor detection, angiography may also play a role in the therapy of malignant apudomas, by embolizing liver metastases with specific intra-arterial cytotoxic drugs mixed with Gelfoam powder, or even by embolizing the primary tumor in the occasional appropriate case (33).

Diagnostic Accuracy

Insulinoma

Although the published rates for successful localization of insulinomas vary widely from 29% to 89% (1, 11, 12, 14, 16, 31, 32, 33, 34), it is the experience of most specialized centers that when meticulous angiographic technique is observed, accurate localization can be achieved in 75% to 85% of patients (11, 14, 33). For these reasons selective arteriography has been for many years the single most accurate modality to detect beta cell pancreatic tumors. However, recent works from two tertiary care centers, the Mayo Clinic, Rochester, Minn. and the NIH, reported a large number of occult insulinomas, with angiographic detection rates between 50% and 60% (10, 16, 26), clearly inferior to the detection rates published by the same groups in previous years (11, 14). This decrease in sensitivity probably reflects two aspects. The development of highly sensitive assays for insulin has resulted in an earlier diagnosis of insulinoma. Therefore, the radiologist is increasingly called to localize lesions that are less than 1.5 cm in size (16). A second aspect, probably common to all tertiary care centers in the world, reflects a change in patient referral pattern, wherein only patients with negative CT and angiographic results at their local hospital, are referred for tumor localization, therefore causing a real bias in patient selection and increasing the number of "occult" tumors in the series of specialized centers (6).

Gastrinoma

Modern studies (15, 24) tend to consider the ability of angiography to identify the primary tumor and the secondary liver lesions separately. The rationale for this separation is that spread of gastrinoma is the major determinant of long-term survival in patients with Zollinger-Ellison syndrome (38), therefore, staging and assessment of hepatic metastases resectability is as important as localization of primary tumor.

Angiographic localization of extrahepatic gastrinoma (i.e., pancreatic or peripancreatic primary) can achieve a sensitivity of 68% to 80% (15, 24) with a high specificity (94–100%) but with a low negative predictive value (33–53%).

Hepatic secondary lesions are detected with a sensitivity of 71% to 86% (15, 24), high specificity, and with a high negative predictive value (89–94%), which makes angiography a reliable method in tumor staging. These results are superior to previous studies that did not separate the hepatic from extrahepatic disease and had an overall sensitivity of 15–54% (25, 32, 35, 38) and a specificity of 61% to 84% (25, 32, 35, 38). It is preferable not to consider the results from other series with small number of cases, due to their inherent low statistical significance.

In any case it must be underlined that the problems in interpreting the medical literature on the angiographical localization of islet cell tumors (33) are identical to those stated for CT.

The other endocrine tumors are usually large and are commonly diagnosed by CT or MR; the indications for angiography in these cases is to stage the disease and provide vascular anatomy if surgery is undertaken.

Transhepatic Portal Venous Sampling (PVS)

This technique is used to detect a localized peak in hormonal concentration within the tributaries of the portal system and therefore identify the site of a tumor regardless of its size and vascularity. The method is employed almost only to detect insulinomas and gastrinomas.

Essentially, the right portal vein is entered transhepatically, and serial samples are taken at 1–1.5 cm intervals along the splenoportal trunk and superior mesenteric vein. The technique, however, is certainly more accurate when numerous samples are selectively taken from the smaller veins draining the different pancreatic regions (32), because the extensive intrapancreatic venous network means that analysis of samples taken only from the larger veins may be misleading (28, 32). This superselective catheterization requires greater technical experience together with a thorough knowledge of venous anatomy and increases the time required for the procedure. The site of each sample is noted on a "map" drawn from the splenoportogram. Peripheral venous blood samples are taken to monitor both glucose and insulin levels.

For the interpretation of the data it is necessary to determine how much of a hormonal gradient is necessary for accurate tumor localization, and many different criteria have been proposed (4, 7, 19, 28, 32). An analysis of the different criteria has been made by Pedrazzoli et al. (29), who suggested calculating the mean and the standard deviation of all portal values and considering diagnostic a level greater than two standard deviations above the mean.

Although the diagnostic criteria differ among various authors, the results reported in the literature show a high diagnostic accuracy for this modality. In patients with insulinoma the sensitivity can be as high as 95% (32), but diagnostic accuracy usually ranges between 83% and 87% (18, 28, 29); these values are comparable to those of the largest arteriographic series. In case of gastrinoma the sensitivity in one series was found to be 94% (32), whereas in other series, the range of sensitivity was reported to be between 63% and 88% (3, 28), which compares favorably to the results obtained by arteriography.

The procedure is invasive and not without risk. Major complications, although rare, include pneumothorax, hemothorax, puncture of the inferior vena cava, biliary tree (4, 32) or gastrointestinal tract, intraperitoneal bleeding (17, 28), and mesenteric vein thrombosis (23). The risk of bleeding can be minimized by embolizing the catheter track through which sampling is performed with gelatin sponge. Modern angiographic materials and increased skills in performing transhepatic puncture, however, have greatly reduced the complications of this procedure. Therefore, considering the risk/benefit ratio of PVS in an era of modern diagnostic imaging, the use of this technique should be restricted to those cases in which all other localizing tests, including the intra-arterial stimulation test (see below) have failed.

Intra-arterial Stimulation Test (IAS)

This test is based on the stimulation of hormone release by selective intra-arterial injection of a secretagogue substance. This technique was introduced by Imamura et al., (20) who used secretin to localize gastrinomas, and then applied by Doppman et al. (8, 9) on larger groups of patients with suggested gastrinomas or insulinomas. The rationale for this localizing technique is to detect a peak of hormone secretion in the venous effluent to the liver after injection of specific substances into the different arteries feeding the pancreas, and thereby to localize the tumor in the pancreatic region supplied by the artery whose injection determined the hormonal peak.

The test follows standard diagnostic pancreatic angiography and actually adds only a few minutes to this procedure. Before angiography, a catheter is placed in the right hepatic vein to allow for venous sampling (initially both left and right hepatic veins were catheterized, but no differences in hormonal gradients were encountered (6), and therefore left hepatic vein sampling is no longer performed). The substances commonly used to stimulate hormone secretion are secretin in patients with Zollinger–Ellison syndrome and calcium gluconate for insulin-producing tumors (2, 39). Secretin is administered in doses of 30 IU each, while the amount of calcium gluconate in each single dose is 0.025 mEq Ca^{++}/kg; both substances are diluted in saline to a 5 mL bolus. The technique of injection and sampling is the same for both types of tumors.

Selective injections are made into the GDA, SMA (Fig. 6.**27**), proximal splenic, and hepatic artery. The dorsal pancreatic artery is not injected because localization would be imprecise; a variable portion of pancreatic head, neck, and body are supplied by this vessel (36). In addition, a concentrated solution of Ca^{++} injected into a small artery may induce focal pancreatitis. The secretagogue substances are rapidly inoculated in 5 mL boluses through the catheter positioned in the proximal portion of each artery; 5 mL samples of blood are taken from the hepatic vein

Angiography 203

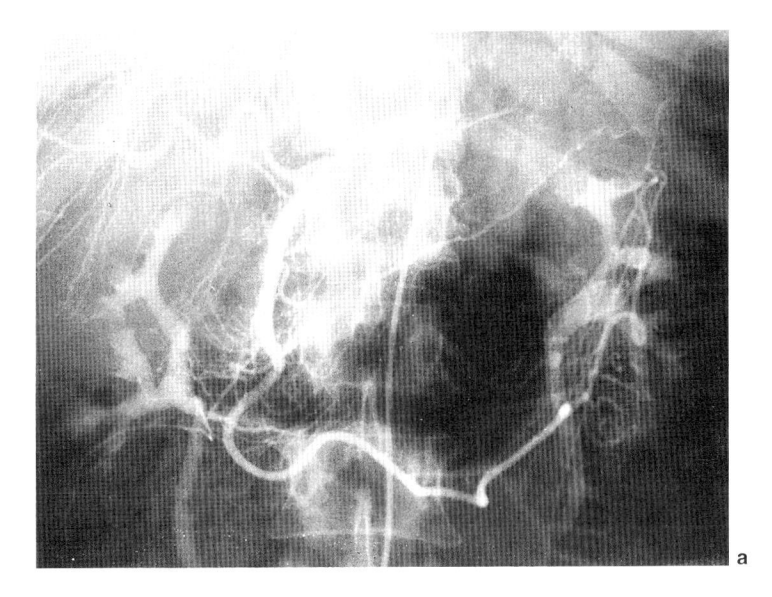

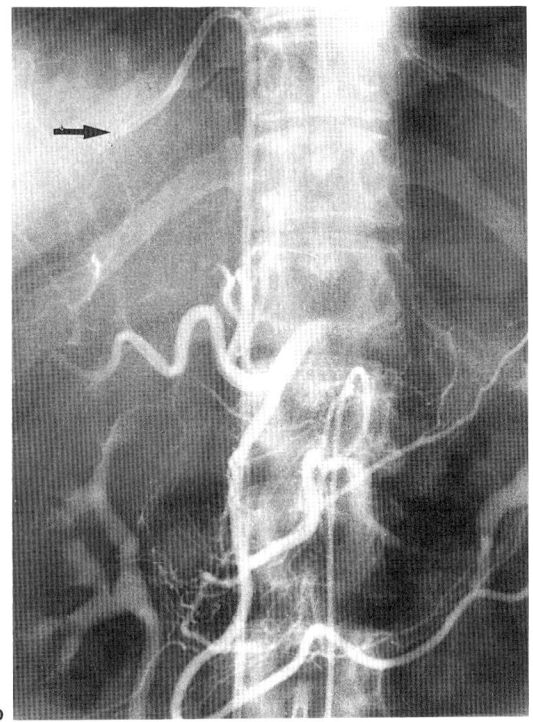

Fig. 6.**27** Positive IAS test in pancreatic head insulinoma. (**a**) Selective injections of GDA and (**b**) of inferior pancreatico-duodenal artery during SMA arteriogram show no evidence of tumor (note catheter in right hepatic vein for venous sampling (arrow). (**c**) IAS test shows rise in insulin levels on the 30-, 60-, and 90-second samples after SMA injection of calcium, therefore localizing the lesion in the inferior portion of the pancreatic head. There is no rise in the other samples after GDA, splenic, or hepatic artery injection. (**d**) Enucleation of the pancreatic head insulinoma at surgery

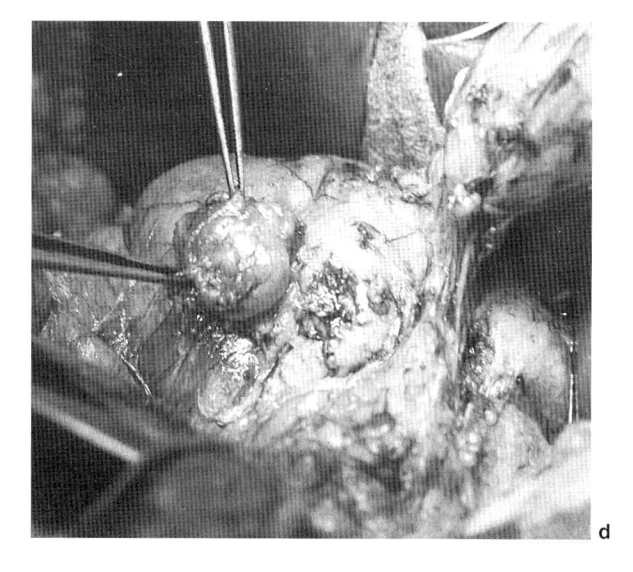

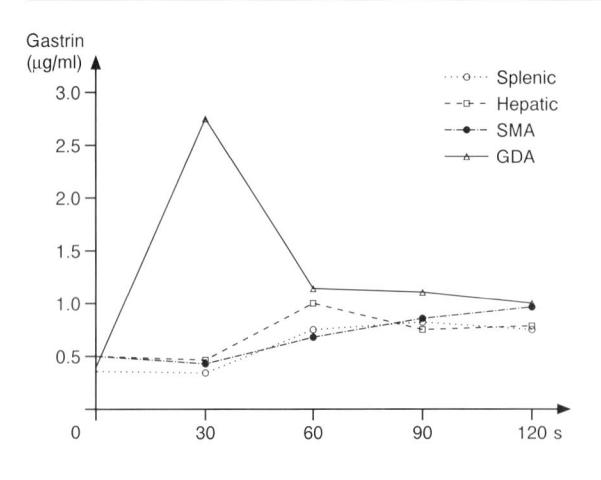

Fig. 6.**28** Results of IAS test for gastrinoma localization (adapted from Reference 8). Characteristic positive response on the 30-second venous sample after selective secretin injection in the GDA; a 5-mm tumor was found at surgery in the wall of the second portion of duodenum

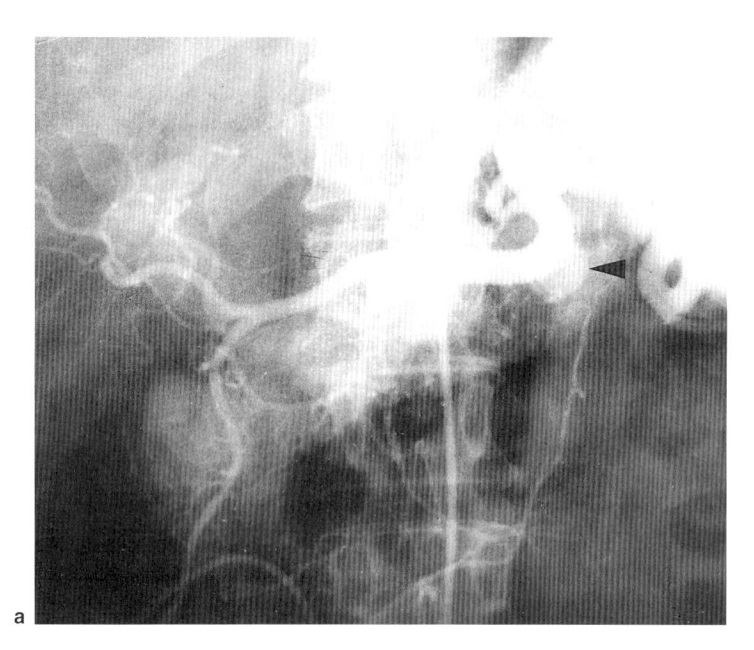

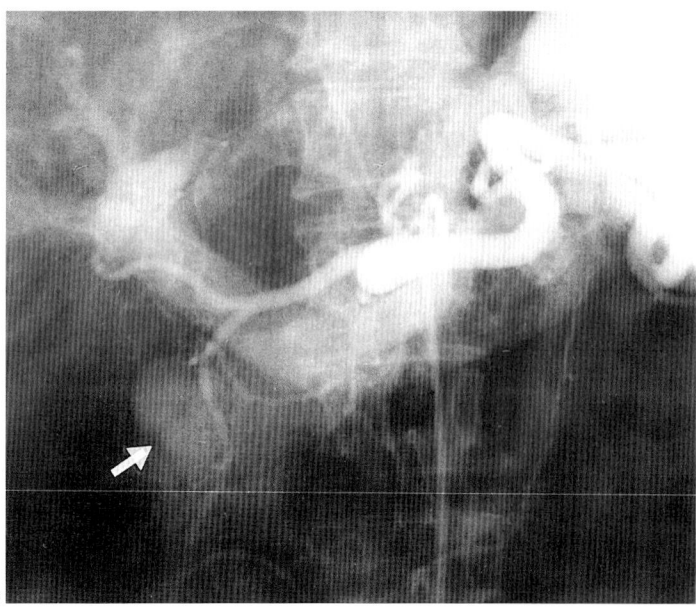

Fig. 6.**29** Multiple insulinomas. Celiac axis arteriogram (**a**) in an initial phase the lesion of the tail (arrowhead) is more apparent, whereas in a later phase, (**b**) the tumor located in the head becomes more evident (arrow)

before injection and 30, 60, 90, and 120 minutes after the bolus.

A positive test result is indicated by an elevation of hormone levels in the 30 and 60 second samples (Fig. 6.27 and 6.28) (8, 9), while a gradual elevation in the delayed samples is related to systemic recirculation of the stimulating substance and is not considered a localizing response. The regions in which the rise in hormone levels permits localization of the apudoma after each arterial injection are as follows:

- GDA →superior portion of pancreatic head (or duodenal wall in case of gastrinoma)
- SMA →inferior portion of head and uncinate process (Fig. 6.27) (or duodenal wall in case of gastrinoma)
- Splenic artery →pancreatic body and tail
- Hepatic artery →metastasis in the right lobe of liver

The potential advantage of the IAS test is to combine in the same procedure a morphologic angiographic study with a sampling test conceptually similar to PVS, therefore achieving with a single examination a higher diagnostic accuracy. In addition, the IAS study is technically easier to perform than PVS, does not involve additional costs, and is not associated with the morbidity that may be seen after transhepatic portal catheterization.

This technique has been introduced in clinical practice only in recent years and the number of patients studied is still limited. Therefore, the results reported in the literature, although interesting and encouraging, must be considered preliminary. Doppman et al., (8) in a series of 13 patients with suggested gastrinoma, reported that the IAS test was positive in 54% of patients (7, 13), while selective angiography was positive in 38% of patients (5, 13). As a combined study, however, angiography and the IAS test were positive in 77% of cases, which represented a detection rate higher than any single localizing study in that series. In the same small group of patients, PVS was positive only in 46% of patients. In another study from the same group (6), nine patients with suggested insulinoma were studied with the IAS test and angiography; calcium stimulation predicted the correct site of the tumor in all patients (100% detection rate), while angiography was positive in 66% of patients.

The method is still under development, and studies are being carried out with regard to the site and strength of injection as well as to the site of venous sample (right or left hepatic vein). However, if preliminary results are confirmed, it seems that the combination of angiography and the IAS test may approach a localization rate of 80% in case of gastrinoma and 100% in case of insulinoma, therefore replacing PVS in the localization of small "occult" tumors.

References

1. Boijsen E, Samuelsson L. Angiographic diagnosis of tumours arising from the pancreatic islets. Acta Radiologica Diagnosis. 1970;10(fasc3):161.
2. Brunt LM, Veldhuis JD, Dilley WG, et al. Stimulation of insulin secretion by a rapid intravenous calcium infusion in patients with beta-cell neoplasms of the pancreas. J Clin Endocrinol Metab. 1986;62:210.
3. Cherner JA, Doppman JL, Norton JA, et al. Selective venous sampling for gastrin to localize gastrinomas: a prospective assessment. Ann Intern Med. 1986;105:841.
4. Cho KJ, Vinik AI, Thompson NW, et al. Localization of the source of hyperinsulinism: Percutaneous transhepatic portal and pancreatic vein catheterization with hormone assay. AJR. 1982;139:237.
5. Clouse ME, Costello P, Legg M, et al. Subselective angiography in localizing insulinomas of the pancreas. AJR. 1977;128:741.
6. Doppman JL. An intrarterial stimulation test and intraoperative ultrasound for detection of insulinomas. Proceedings of G.R.A.D.O.4: Giornate di Radiologia Diagnostica Oncologica. Bologna:Monduzzi editore;1991:25.
7. Doppman JL, Brennan MF, Dunnick NR, et al. The role of pancreatic venous sampling in the localization of occult insulinomas. Radiology. 1981;138:557.
8. Doppman JL, Miller DL, Chang R, et al. Gastrinomas: localization by means of selective intrarterial injection of Secretin. Radiology. 1990;174:25.
9. Doppman JL, Miller DL, Chang R, Shwaker TH, Gorden P, Norton JA. Insulinomas: localization with selective intrarterial injection of Calcium. Radiology. 1991;178:237.
10. Doppman JL, Shwaker TH, Miller DL. Localization of islet-cell tumors. Gastrointest Clin North Am. 1989;18:793.
11. Dunnick NR, Long JA Jr, Krudy A, Shawker TH, Doppman JL. Localizing insulinomas with combined radiographic methods. AJR. 1980;135:747.
12. Epstein HY, Abrams RM, Berambaum FR, et al. Angiographic localization of insulinomas: High reported success rate and two additional cases. Ann Surg. 1969;169:349.
13. Fink IJ, Krudy AG, Shawker TH, Norton JA, Gorden P, Doppman JL. Demonstration of an angiographically hypovascular insulinoma with intrarterial dynamic CT. AJR. 1985;144:555.
14. Fulton RE, Sheedy PF II, McIllarath DC, Ferris DO. Preoperative angiography localization of insulin-producing tumors of the pancreas. AJR. 1975;123:367.
15. Frucht H, Doppman JL, Norton JA, et al. Gastrinomas: comparison of MR imaging with CT, Angiography, and US. Radiology. 1989;171:713.
16. Galiber AK, Reading CC, Charbonneau JW, et al. localization of pancreatic insulinomas: comparison of pre and intraoperative ultrasound with CT and angiography. Radiology. 1988;166:405.
17. Gothlin J, Lunderquist A, Tylen U: Selective phlebography of the pancreas. Acta Radiol Diagn. 1974;15:474.
18. Gunther RW, Klose JK, Ruckert K, Beyer J, Kuhn FP, Klotter HJ. Localization of small islet-cell tumors. Preoperative and intraoperative ultrasound, computer tomography, arteriography, digital subtraction angiography, and pancreatic venous sampling. Gastrointest Radiol. 1985;10:145.
19. Hsien-Chiu H, Chong-Zheng Y, Sou-Xian Z. Percutaneous transhepatic portal vein catheterization for localization of insulinoma. World J Surg. 1984;8:575.
20. Imamura M, Takahasha K, Adacha H, et al. Usefulness of selective arterial secretin injection test for localization of gastrinoma in Zollinger-Ellison syndrome. Ann Surg. 1987;205:230.
21. Imhof H, Frank P. Pancreatic calcification in malignant islet-cell tumors. Radiology. 1977;122:333.
22. Korobkin MT, Palubinskas Aj, Glickman MG. Pitfalls in angiography of islet-cell tumors of the pancreas. Radiology. 1971;100:319.
23. Luska G, Langer HE, Le Blanc S. Mesenterialvenenthrombose nach perkutantranshepatischer Pfortadersondierung (PTP) bei der Lokalisationsdiagnostik eines Insulinomas. Fortschr Rontgenstr. 1984;141:68.
24. Maton PN, Miller DL, Doppman JL, et al. Role of selective angiography in the management of patients with Zollinger-Ellison syndrome. Gastroenterology. 1987;92:913.

25. Mills S, Doppman JL, Dunnick NR, McCarthy DM. Evaluation of angiography in Zollinger-Ellison syndrome. Radiology. 1979;131:317.
26. Norton JA, Shawker TH, Doppman JL, et al. Localization and surgical treatment of occult insulinomas. Ann Surg. [In press].
27. Olsson O. Angiographic diagnosis of an islet cell tumor of the pancreas. Acta Chir Scand. 1963;126:346.
28. Passariello R, Feltrin GP, Miotto D. Transhepatic portal catheterization with pancreatic venous sampling versus angiography in the localization of pancreatic functioning tumors. Front Eur Radiol. 1982;1:51.
29. Pedrazzoli S, Pasquali C, Miotto D. Transhepatic portal sampling for preoperative localization of insulinomas. Surg. Gynecol Obstet. 1987;165:101.
30. Pogany AC, Kerlan RK Jr, Karam JH, Le Quesne LP, Ring EJ. Cystic insulinoma. AJR. 1984;142:951.
31. Proye C, Boissel P. Preoperative imaging versus intraoperative localization of tumors in adult surgical patients with hyperinsulinemia: a multicenter study of 338 patients. World J Surg. 1988;12:685.
32. Roche P, Raissonier A, Gillon-Savouret MC. Pancreatic venous sampling and arteriography in localizing insulinomas and gastrinomas: procedure and results in 55 cases. Radiology. 1982;145:621.
33. Rossi P, Allison DJ. Endocrine tumors of the pancreas. Radiol Clin North Am. 1989;27:129.
34. Rossi P, Baert A, Passariello R, Simonetti G, Pavone P, Tempesta P. CT of functioning tumors of the pancreas. AJR. 1985;144:57.
35. Ruszniewski PN, Mignon M, Rene E, Bonfils S. Localization of tumoral process in Zollinger-Ellison syndrome (ZES): a retrospective study in 79 patients (abstr.). Gastroenterology. 1986;90:1610.
36. Ruzicka F Jr, Rossi P. Normal vascular anatomy of the abdominal viscera. Radiol Clin North Am. 1970;8:3.
37. Smith TR, Koenigsberg M. Low-density insulinoma on CT. AJR. 1990;155:995.
38. Thompson JC, Beverly JR, Lewis MD, et al. The role of surgery in Zollinger-Ellison syndrome. Ann Surg. 1983;197:594.
39. Wollheim CB, Sharp GWG. Regulation of insulin release by calcium. Physiol Rev. 1981;61:914.

A Radiologist's View
R. A. Halvorsen Jr.

Imaging Techniques

A wide spectrum of noninvasive and invasive preoperative and intraoperative techniques are available for the localization of pancreatic masses. These include ultrasonography, CT, MRI, arteriography, and transhepatic percutaneous venous sampling. The role of these imaging modalities depends on the specific tumor type, lesion size, and to a certain extent, the experience of the radiologist.

Sonography

Abdominal sonographic examination of the pancreas is the least invasive of the imaging tests available. Sensitivity for the detection of these tumors has been reported to range from 15–64%, with more recent studies suggesting a sensitivity of approximately 60% (9–13). In the past, ultrasound has often been used as the first, and if positive, only preoperative imaging procedure due to the noninvasive nature of this relatively inexpensive test. In many institutions, CT has replaced sonography as the first imaging test because of its higher sensitivity rate.

Computed Tomography

CT has a reported sensitivity ranging from 17–80% in the detection of insulinomas (13–14). A limitation of many older studies reporting a low sensitivity with CT was that they were performed with slow scanners, thick sections and following, rather than during, a bolus of intravenous contrast media. A meticulous technique is required to detect small lesions. Currently, most authors recommend thinly collimated images of 3–5 mm through the pancreas during the administration of a bolus of contrast media. A recent study using state-of-the-art CT equipment reported a sensitivity of 100% for insulinomas larger than 1.5 cm, and a sensitivity of 71% for lesions 1 cm in diameter (15).

Magnetic Resonance Imaging

The role of MRI of pancreatic neoplasms has yet to be determined. Early reports were not promising. In a study of patients with insulinomas studied with MRI, Doherty et al. reported that only two of eight (25%) patients had true positive MRI studies (14). Using a newly developed MRI technique that includes fat saturation and gradient-echo images with injection of Gd-DTPA, Thoeni et al. reported much improved results (16). In this prospective study of nine patients with insulinomas, they found the T_1-weighted spin-echo images with fat saturation to be the pulse sequence that produced the best images and identified eight of nine tumors (89%).

Arteriography

Celiac angiography has a moderate reported success rate in the localization of insulinomas, with many studies reporting sensitivities in the 60–70% range (13). Doppman et al., at the NIH, reported a sensitivity of less than 50% for insulinomas but recommended the technique for the workup of all patients with insulinomas because arteriography remains the most sensitive study for the detection of liver metastases (greater than 90%) (2).

Transhepatic Percutaneous Portal Venous Sampling

In patients in whom less invasive tests have not localized endocrine-secreting tumors of the pancreas, PVS is another possibility. PVS requires a liver puncture, generally in the mid-axillary line, with an 18- or 20-gauge needle (17). A catheter is placed through this needle into the portal venous system, and multiple samples are obtained from the splenic, superior mesenteric, inferior mesenteric, and portal veins, as well as in pancreatic collaterals. Though technically difficult and expensive, PVS has a low morbidity and a high sensitivity for the detection of insulinomas and is the only test capable of detecting diffuse abnormalities of the pancreas that produce hyperinsulinism. PVS is less useful in patients with solitary gastrinomas (18) and appears to be of no utility in patients with diffuse gastrinomas (usually associated with MEN type I syndrome) (19–20).

Intraoperative Ultrasound

In addition to preoperative imaging, intraoperative examination of the pancreas and liver is now possible with ultrasound due to recent improvements in transducer technology. The use of high-resolution transducers (7.5 and 10 MHz) allows for detection of many pancreatic tumors. The ultrasound transducer is covered with a sterile sheath and placed intraoperatively into a peritoneal cavity that is filled with sterile saline. The transducer is held approximately 1 cm anterior to the pancreatic surface. Using anatomical landmarks such as superior mesenteric artery and vein, splenic vein, and duodenum, the pancreas can be identified (21). Intraoperative ultrasound can detect some focal lesions that are not palpable. Sensitivity for the detection of masses with intraoperative sonography ranges from 75–90% (12, 13, 15, 21). Most authors now feel that intraoperative ultrasound combined with surgical palpation is the single best technique for the detection of focal lesions of the pancreas. The question that arises is: If the patient is going to undergo surgical palpation and intraoperative ultrasound, are any preoperative imaging tests justified?

Insulinoma

Insulinomas are the most common islet cell tumors and are small in size, which poses a problem in localization. Insulinomas are generally treated surgically as there is no effective medical treatment for this disorder. Surgical localization is often simple when the tumors are easily palpable but may be difficult when the tumors are small or deep within the pancreatic parenchyma. Insulinomas in general are relatively small, ranging from 1–2 cm in diameter, but are occasionally less than 0.5 cm (22). Nonpalpable tumors are reported in 5–25% of operations (15). Some cases of hyperinsulinism are due not to a solitary tumor, but rather to diffuse pancreatic abnormalities. Approximately 20–25% of patients with insulin-producing islet cell abnormalities have diffuse disease (13). Diffuse disease is caused by three disease processes: adenomatosis, nesidioblastosis, and diffuse hyperplasia. Adenomatosis, which consists of either multiple macroadenomas or microadenomatosis interspersed between normal islets combined with one or more macroadenomas, occurs in approximately 5–18% of patients with hyperinsulinism. Nesidioblastosis, a diffuse and disseminated neoproliferation of insulin-producing cells from pancreatic ductules, is a frequent cause of hyperinsulinism in newborns and infants, but also occurs in adults and represents approximately 5% of all patients with hyperinsulinism. Nesidioblastosis may be diffuse or limited to one portion of the pancreas, such as the head of the pancreas (13). Diffuse hyperplasia of the islet cells has been reported in adults. In one study of 1137 cases of hyperinsulinism, 94% were caused by insulinomas, and 6% by diffuse islet cell disease (13, 23). In a study of 82 patients with hyperinsulinism, 76% had solitary adenomas, while 6% had carcinoma, and the remainder (18%) had diffuse pancreatic abnormalities (13). In general, diffuse abnormalities, such as adenomatosis, hyperplasia, and nesidioblastosis, are not detectable by the surgeon during surgery, and detectable by imaging only with PVS.

Intraoperative ultrasound is a relatively new technique that appears to increase the detectability of focal pancreatic masses in patients with endocrine-secreting tumors. Some authors have suggested that preoperative imaging tests are no longer necessary because a combination of surgical palpation with intraoperative ultrasound produces an acceptable detection rate for focal lesions. However, because of the frequent occurrence of diffuse hyperinsulinism resulting from microadenomas, hyperplasia, and nesidioblastosis, others think that it is premature to depend on intraoperative sonography and palpation alone (13). In addition, accurate preoperative localization provides other benefits (13). First, small tumors that are located preoperatively may be difficult to localize at operation. Preoperative localization avoids the higher risk of lengthy, extensive operations. Second, preoperative localization obviates the need for blind partial pancreatectomies. Third, in reoperations when postoperative fibrosis makes palpation difficult, preoperative localization is essential.

Gastrinoma

The workup of patients with gastrinoma is different from that of patients with hyperinsulinism. Both insulinomas and gastrinomas are derived from the same cell line, but differ in site of origin, potential for malignancy, association with multiple endocrine syndromes, and responsiveness to medical therapy (2). Insulinomas are uniformly distributed throughout the parenchyma of the pancreas, while gastrinomas are usually found in the pancreas but also occur in the duodenum (6–23%) and other peripancreatic tissue (1–16%) (22). Gastrinomas are frequently malignant (80%), while insulinomas are malignant in approximately 10% of cases. Gastrinoma is also more frequently involved with multiple endocrine syndromes (40%), whereas only 5 percent of insulinomas are associated with multiple endocrine syndromes.

In general, the localization of gastrinomas is more difficult than that of insulinomas because of the more common extrapancreatic location, more frequent multiplicity, and often, the smaller size of gastrinomas. In a review of the experience of the NIH in the detection of gastrinoma, Doppman et al. found that CT and ultrasound were positive in less than 30% of cases (2). In their hands, MRI was less successful than CT. Selective arteriography is useful in the detection of hepatic metastases and extrahepatic gastrinomas, whether in the pancreas, bowel wall, or other locations. Maton et al. reported in a series of 70 consecutive patients with Zollinger–Ellison syndrome that arteriography had a specificity of 100% and sensitivity of 86% for liver metastases and specificity of 94% and sensitivity of 68% for extrahepatic gastrinomas (24). They recommended an abdominal CT scan as the initial technique of tumor localization. If the CT suggests unresectable liver tumor, the patient can be spared an unnecessary laparotomy. A selective angiogram is recommended if the CT suggests resectable metastases or no metastatic disease, to confirm the extent of tumor in the liver and to possibly localize extrahepatic gastrinoma. PVS for gastrin appears to be incapable of reliably localizing gastrinomas (18). Intraoperative sonography is effective in detecting some gastrinomas, but compared to insulinomas, its overall performance is less, due to the difficulty in detecting tumors in the bowel wall (2).

Summary

The wide variety of preoperative and intraoperative imaging tests provides a list of options that at first appears confusing. A reasonable approach in the workup of patients with biochemically proven functioning islet cell tumors is to use imaging tests in a step-by-step fashion (Fig. 6.**30**). After biochemical tests indicate a hormonally active islet cell tumor and exclude the MEN type 1 syndrome, the first imaging test should be CT. The preoperative CT scan can detect not only focal lesions in the pancreas, but also liver metastases. If the CT result is positive for a focal lesion, then no other preoperative study is warranted. However, if the CT results are negative, the second step is arteriography, both in the search for the primary tumor and liver metastases. If arteriography fails to detect either a focal lesion or a metastasis, then an exploratory laparotomy with careful palpation of the pancreas, supplemented by intraoperative ultrasound, is warranted. This step-by-step approach will detect the large majority of resectable tumors, as well as metastatic disease in the majority of patients.

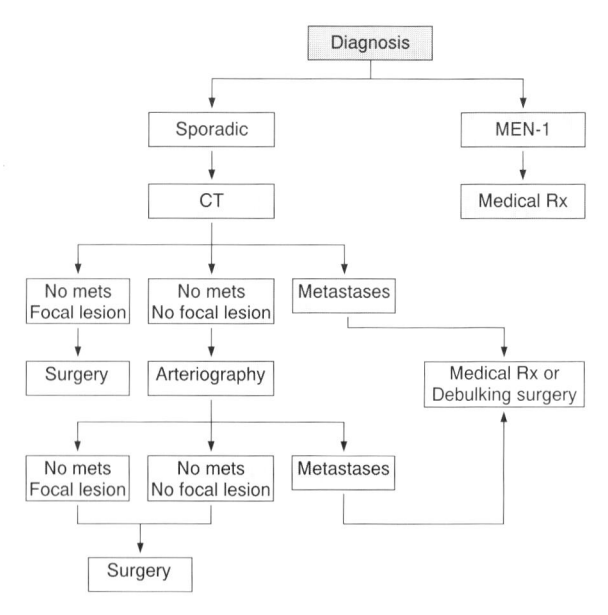

Fig. 6.**30**

This stepwise approach is unsuccessful in diagnosing the unusual patient with diffuse pancreatic lesions and no metastases. PVS is not efficacious in the detection of diffuse gastrinomas, and its role in vipomas, somatostatinomas, and glucagonomas is unclear. PVS has proven utility only in those patients with hyperinsulinism due to diffuse pancreatic disease. Therefore, PVS is restricted to those patients with insulinoma and no detectable focal lesion.

In the operating room, the role of intraoperative ultrasound is also controversial. Some authors recommend intraoperative ultrasound on all patients, even if a palpable lesion is present, either to help determine the location of the pancreatic ducts, or in the search for other nonpalpable nodules. Other authors recommend intraoperative ultrasound only if the surgeon cannot palpate a lesion. One obvious inference from currently available information is that because intraoperative ultrasound is such an important technique in the localization of masses, it is mandatory that radiologists become skilled in the technique of intraoperative ultrasound in hospitals where pancreatic surgery is performed.

References

1 Brenna MF, MacDonald JS. Cancer of the endocrine system. In: DeVita VT Jr., Hellman S, Rosenberg SA, eds. Cancer: Principles and Practice of Oncology. 2nd ed. Philadelphia: J.B. Lippincott; 1982:1206–1222.
2 Doppman JL, Shawker TH, Miller DL. Localization of islet cell tumors. Gastroenterol Clin North Am. 1989;18(4):793–804.
3 Norton JA, Doppman JL, Jensen RT. Cancer of the endocrine system. In: DeVita VT Jr., Hellman S, Rosenberg SA, eds. Cancer: Principles and Practice of Oncology. 3rd ed. Philadelphia: J.B. Lippincott; 1989:1314–1331.
4 Zollinger RM. Gastrinoma: the Zollinger-Ellison syndrome. Seminars in Oncol. 1987;14(3):247–252.

5. Parker CM, Hanke CW, Madura JA, Liss EC. Glucagonoma syndrome: case report and literature review. J Dermatol Surg Oncol. 1984;10;11:884–889.
6. Boden G. Insulinoma and glucagonoma. Seminars in Oncol. 1987;14(3):253–262.
7. Mekhjian HS, O'Dorision TM. VIPoma syndrome. Seminars in Oncol. 1987;14(3):282–291.
8. Vinik AI, Stroden WE, Eckhauser FE, et al. Somatostatinomas, PPomas, neurotensinomas. Seminars in Oncol. 1987;14(3):263–281.
9. Angelini L, Bezzi M, Tucci G, et al. The ultrasonic detection of insulinomas during surgical exploration of the pancreas. World J Surg. 1987;11:642–647.
10. Gorman B, Charboneau JW, James EM, et al. Benign pancreatic insulinoma: preoperative and intraoperative sonographic localization. AJR. 1986;147(5):929–934.
11. Klotter HJ, Rückert K, Kümmerle F, et al. The use on intraoperative sonography in endocrine tumors of the pancreas. World J Surg. 1987;11:635–641.
12. Galiber AK, Reading CC, Charboneau JW, et al. Pancreatic insulinoma: localization with intraoperative US. Radiology. 1988;166:405–408.
13. Fajans SS, Vinik AI. Insulin-producing islet cell tumors. Endocrinol Metab Clin North Am. 1989;18:45–74.
14. Doherty GM, Doppman JL, Shawker TH, et al. Results of a prospective strategy to diagnose, localize, and resect insulinomas. Surgery. 1991;110:989–97.
15. Böttger TC, Weber W, Beyer J, Junginger T. Value of tumor localization in patients with insulinoma. World J Surg. 1990;14:107–114.
16. Thoeni RF, Do NK, Shyn P. Islet cell tumor of the pancreas: a role for MRI? Proceedings: Society of Gastrointest Radiol. 1992;87.
17. Brunelle F, Negre V, Barth MO, et al. Pancreatic venous sampling in infants and children with primary hyperinsulinism. Pediatr Radiol. 1989;19:100–103.
18. Cherner JA, Doppman JL, Norton JA, et al. Selective venous sampling for gastrin to localize gastrinomas. Ann Intern Med. 1986;105(6):841–847.
19. Glowniak JV, Shapiro B, Vinik AI, et al. Percutaneous transhepatic venous sampling of gastrin: value in sporadic and familial islet-cell tumors and G-cell hyperfunction. New Engl J Med. 1982;307(5):293–297.
20. Roche A, Raisonnier A, Gillon-Savouret M-C. Pancreatic venous sampling and arteriography in localizing insulinomas and gastrinomas: procedure and results in 55 cases. Radiology. 1982;145:621–627.
21. Grand CS, van Heerden J, Charboneau JW, James EM, Reading CC. Insulinoma: the value of intraoperative ultrasonography. Arch Surg. 1988;123:843–848.
22. Fraker DL, Norton JA. Localization and resection of insulinomas and gastrinomas. JAMA. 1988;259(24):3601–3605.
23. Stefanini P, Carboni M, Patrassi N, et al. Beta-islet cell tumors of the pancreas: results of a study on 1067 cases. Surgery. 1974;75:597–609.
24. Maton PN, Miller DL, Doppman JL, et al. Role of selective angiography in the management of patients with Zollinger-Ellison syndrome. Gastroenterology 1987;92:913–918.

A Surgeon's View

H. D. Roeher

The most frequent endocrine tumors with or without hormonal activity of the gastroenteropancreatic system (GEP) are insulinomas, gastrinomas, and carcinoids. Some significantly less common tumors are glucagonoma, vipoma, somatostatinoma, PP-oma, etc. The diagnosis of the underlying disease should be supported by evident biochemical and hormone analytical proof including positive stimulation or provocation tests. Surgical removal of endocrine tumors is the only definitive means of treatment and relief from hyperfunctional status. With powerful drugs like omeprazole and octreotide, most clinical symptoms can be controlled for a certain period of time, thus allowing surgical removal of a gastrin-producing adenoma at a later stage, when it is expected to be larger and easier to localize. This is of even greater importance for gastrointestinal hormone-producing tumors within MEN type I syndrome, in which tumor multiplicity is a routine finding.

Successful surgical treatment of all endocrine tumors of the GEP system largely depends on the correct localization of single or multiple lesions and their complete removal. Unfortunately, all preoperative localization studies with presently available imaging techniques including ultrasound, CT, MRI, selective catheter angiography, endosonography, and receptor scintigraphy have been rather limited. Many gastrinomas and insulinomas of 1 cm to 2 cm in diameter or larger have been correctly localized by various techniques. However, the underlying lesions are often significantly smaller and are missed in some preoperative studies. Selective subtraction angiography has shown a higher sensitivity for insulinomas only. The majority, in fact, is big enough to be palpated or even visualized in a superficial location by an experienced surgeon, anyway. It is well-known that tumors that are not visible and not palpable and are in occult locations and also are more likely not to be detected by imaging techniques. Nevertheless, CT should be performed often mainly to identify larger tumors with infiltrative growth and suggestion of malignancy or to detect and to exclude distant metastases, mostly in the liver. The use of MRI for localization studies of hormonally active endocrine tumors of the GEP system has been quite disappointing.

Three techniques have to be discussed as valuable tools for tumor localization: (a) selective transhepatic portal venous catheterization; (b) somatostatin receptor scintigraphy; and (c) intraoperative ultrasound. For most endocrine tumors of the GEP system, of somatostatin receptor scintigraphy should be considered for two reasons: first, to identify the tumor in its location and to facilitate the surgical removal; second, to discriminate the functional receptor activity to support senseful application of medical control with the synthetic analog in case of surgical failure or incurable malignant disease.

Selective venous catheterization is effective only in expert hands and thus has limited availability. On the other hand it is invasive and not as successful as sometimes advertised. Furthermore, it cannot be accepted as a highly specific localization technique but as a "regionalization test" with respect to the complex venous drainage in this particular anatomic area. Therefore, it may have a place only in selected cases after a previously unsuccessful operation by an experienced surgeon and an urgent need for reintervention. Intraoperative ultrasound has turned out to be a very useful and effective tool to improve surgery and is strongly recommended for any operation. As can be gathered from recent literature it is the best aid in locating occult adenoma and thus minimizing operative failure. The question must even be raised whether patients should only be treated surgically under such preconditions.

All imaging methods for the localization of hormone-producing tumors of the GEP system have to compete with the "palpating finger" of the surgeon, provided he or she has enough experience. Among the most common tumors, insulinomas have a surgical success rate well above 95%, whereas the surgical success rate for gastrinomas is only about 70% to 90%. Imaging techniques all together do not have success rates above 50% to 70%. It must be decided when and when not to use these techniques. Positive results are achieved in comparatively larger, and therefore mostly visible and palpable adenomas, whereas tumors less than 5 mm in diameter frequently remain undetected.

CT has become a routine method for preoperative localization studies. Even with a 50% success rate, it may be accepted because at the same time it primarily excludes or detects expanded or metastatic growth (liver). Endosonography may be a promising method, however it has yet to prove its real value. There is almost no place and justification for invasive catheter techniques as a primary choice. Selective portal venous catheterization may have a certain value in planning reoperative surgery after previous failure. Somatostatin receptor scintigraphy may find support for wider application than localization, but only to support long-term treatment with the synthetic analog. The problem seems to be not to search for an appropriate localization technique but to know the address of an expert surgeon!

References

1 Cherner JA, Doppman JL, Norton JA, et al. Selective Venous Sampling for Gastrin to Localize Gastrinomas. Ann Int Med. 1986;105:841–7.
2 Kaplan EL, Horvath K, Udekwu A, et al. Gastrinomas: A 42-Year Experience. World J Surg. 1990;14:365–76.
3 Norton JA, Cromack DT, Shawker TH, et al. Intraoperative Ultrasonographic Localization of Islet Cell Tumors. Ann Surg. 1988;207(2):160–8.
4 Rothmund M et al. Surgery for Benign Insulinoma: An International Review. World J Surg. 1990;14:393–9.
5 Starke AAR, Frilling A, Becker H, Röher HD, Berger M. Are cat-scans necessary for preoperative localization of insulinomas? EJM. 1992;1(7):411–3.
6 Thompson NW, Bondeson AG, Bondeson L, Vinik A. The surgical treatment of gastrinoma in MEN I syndrome patients. Surgery 1989;106(6):1081–6.
7 Wolfe MM, Jensen RT: Zollinger-Ellison Syndrome. N Engl J Med. 1987;317(19):1200–09.

7 Carcinoid

Anatomy
J. Staudt

Carcinoid syndrome is generally related to the degeneration of enterochromaffin cells. This degeneration is associated with an increased serotonin excretion. The syndrome can also be simulated by other vasoactive substances, which cause the leading symptoms of the carcinoid syndrome. The carcinoid syndrome, with its low malignancy grade, has similar features to the apudoma. Primary manifestations sites of the carcinoid syndrome are the ileum, the appendix, and other parts of the gastrointestinal tract, and less often the pancreas and the bronchial tree. Occasionally, ectopic manifestation is due to teratogen scattering. It usually grows very slowly, but then infiltrates and metastazises into the liver. The prognosis is relatively good. An increased, sex-independent incidence is observed in the fifth decade of life.

Endocrinology
H. E. Bechtel

Carcinoid Tumors

Carcinoid tumors and islet cell carcinomas account for less than 1% of all malignancies, but they are the most common gastrointestinal endocrine tumors, accounting for approximately 55% of such neoplasms (1, 2, 3, 4, 5). These tumors differ from others in their ability to synthesize a variety of peptide hormones and in their indolent clinical course (5).

About 85% of carcinoid tumors arise in the gastrointestinal tract—foregut, midgut, hindgut—in the three parts of the original primitive bowel, 10% in lung and bronchus, and 5% in the larynx, thymus, kidneys, ovaries, prostate and skin. Most carcinoid tumors are located in the appendix and ileum (47).

Carcinoid tumors, which arise from enterochromaffin cells are usually found in the appendix, ileum, bronchus (6, 7, 24), and rectum (40). Biliary duct carcinoids are exceedingly rare (12, 13, 14, 15). Thymic carcinoids may be associated with hyperparathyroidism or Cushing syndrome (1, 8, 9). Other neuroendocrine neoplasms located in the mediastinum like the **thymic carcinoid** are small cell carcinomas, parathyroid tumors, and aortopulmonary or paravertebral paragangliomas (10). **Gastric carcinoids** are related to atrophic, antrum-sparing type A gastritis. The prevalence of gastric carcinoid in patients with pernicious anemia and achlorhydria is 2–9%. The incidence of gastric carcinoids may also be increased in patients with Hashimoto thyroiditis. Also, purely intramucosal carcinoids are described. A precursor lesion is probably the hyperplasia of endocrine cells in the atrophic fundic mucosa (11, 16). **Carcinoids of the brochus** and small intestine may occur in association with MEN I syndrome (6, 7, 24). Small bowel and bronchial carcinoids have a more malignant course. Symptoms from hormone secretion and early metastasis are more common (4, 17, 18, 19). A rare localization is the **carcinoid of Meckel's diverticula** (20, 21). **Appendiceal and colorectal carcinoids,** which may also be the sources of entopic or ectopic hormogenesis, have a relatively benign course and are usually more asymptomatic (4, 14, 22, 23, 25). The appendiceal carcinoid tumor is one of four main types of appendiceal neoplasms. The others are mucinous cystadenocarcinomas, colonic adenocarcinomas, and adenocarcinoid tumors (goblet cell carcinoid (26)). The adenocarcinoid tumors have a dual cell origin, a predilection for developing ovarian metastasis, and a malignant potential between carcinoid tumors and colonic adenocarcinomas (22).

Another rare manifestation of carcinoid tumors is found in gastrointestinal involvement in **Recklinghausen disease.** It is a distinct glandular, somatostatin-rich carcinoid of the periampullary region of the duodenum that contains psammoma bodies and may be associated with pheochromocytoma (27). Serotonin-producing carcinoids are found in a specialized type of **mature teratomas** (30). **Carcinoid tumors of the larynx** are rare tumors. Atypical and typical carcinoids of the larynx have been described. Typical carcinoid neoplasms are extremely rare. The total number of known and documented cases is likely no more than 13, whereas Woodruff analyzed 127 published cases of atypical laryngeal carcinoid. Typical laryngeal carcinoids are less aggressive than their atypical counterparts, but late, distant metastatis and death may occur (31, 32, 33).

The neuroendocrine tumors of the pancreas are discussed later in the chapter. They may become apparent by the symptoms caused by the hypersecretion of hormones such as VIP, glucagon, gastrin, or the secretory products of carcinoid tumors, e.g., 5-Hydroxytryptamine and tachykinin (25, 28, 29).

The initial diagnosis of carcinoid tumors is often delayed and difficult, because patients present a conglomeration of clinical symptoms that are often considered nonspecific and treated symptomatically. When diagnosed, the greater proportion of functioning endocrine tumors have already metastasized. As a result, complete surgical removal of the growth is possible in only a small number of patients. This gives considerable importance to palliative treatment (5, 34).

In a late state, carcinoid tumors may present with

 gastrointestinal bleeding
 abdominal pain
 obstruction from tumor growth
 tumor-induced mesenteric fibrosis causing intestinal kinking, obstruction, and vascular compromise.

Carcinoid Syndrome (1, 35, 36, 37, 39)

Enterochromaffin cells secrete a variety of hormones and are embryologically related to thyroid C cells, adrenal medullary cells, and melanocytes. Distinctive and debilitating effects are caused long before local growth or metastatic spread is apparent.

The carcinoid syndrome include the triad of

 cutaneous flushing,
 diarrhea (commonly secretory and hypermotility induced),
 valvular heart disease by endocardial fibrosis

and less commonly

 teleangiectasis,
 wheezing,
 paroxysmal hypotension (systolic blood pressure falls 20 to 30 mm HG.

Early in the course of the disease, symptoms are usually episodic and may be provoked by stress, catecholamines, and ingestion of food and alcohol. Approximately 5 of all patients with carcinoid tumors experience one or more symptoms of the carcinoid syndrome.

Small bowel carcinoids, especially, are associated with systemic manifestations in 30 to 60%, lung carcinoids 3,5%, appendix carcinoids 1%, and rectal carcinoids virtually never. In patients with intestinal carcinoids, the humoral symptoms only develop in the setting of metastatic disease to the liver. Extraintestinal carcinoids, whose hormone products are not immediately cleared by the liver, may produce the syndrome in the absence of metastasis. Patients with foregut carcinoid syndrome more often have dramatic cutaneous flushing involving the whole body than those with tumors of midgut or hindgut organs. In bronchial carcinoids, the flush may be prolonged for hours to days. Excessive lacrimation, salivation, facial edema, and significant hypotension are to be noticed. Gastric carcinoids are often associated with cutaneous manifestations, which last only minutes, are well circumscribed, and are characterized by pruritus and high levels of histamine secretion. In midgut carcinoid syndrome the flushing is less severe, and the facial teleangiectasis appears late in the course, whereas cardiac manifestations and peritoneal fibrosis are more frequently associated.

Pathophysiological and Biochemical Aspects of Carcinoid Syndrome

Serotonin (5-hydroxytryptamine, 5-HT) is the most common secretory product of carcinoid tumors. It is synthesized by the tumor by enzymatic modification of circulating tryptophan (Figs. 7.**1** and 7.**2**).

Up to 50% of the dietary intake of tryptophan can be converted to serotonin by these cells, which may leave inadequate substrate for the incorporation into proteins and conversion to niacin copying symptoms of protein malnutrition.

 Serotonin induces intestinal secretion, inhibits intestinal absorption, and stimulates intestinal motility causing diarrhea in most cases of carcinoid syndrome
 Serotonin stimulates fibroblast growth
 Serotonin secretion alone does not account for cutaneous flushing. The vasomotor changes are caused by multiple monamine and peptide factors

Monamine and Peptide Hormones

Histamine	Catecholamine
Somatostatin	Bradykinin
Tachykinin	Neurotensin
Enkephalin	Endorphin
Substance P	Vasopressin
Gastrin	Neurokinin A
Motilin	Prostaglandin
Adrenocorticotrophin	

The relative constrictions of each to the carcinoid syndrome remain to be identified.

Diagnosis

Serotonin is metabolized in the blood to 5-hydroxyindoleacetic acid (5-HIAA), which is cleared by the kidneys. Plasma and platelet serotonin and urinary 5-HIAA levels are usually elevated in the setting of carcinoid syndrome. Measurement of urinary

Fig. 7.**1** Biosynthesis and degradation of Serotonin

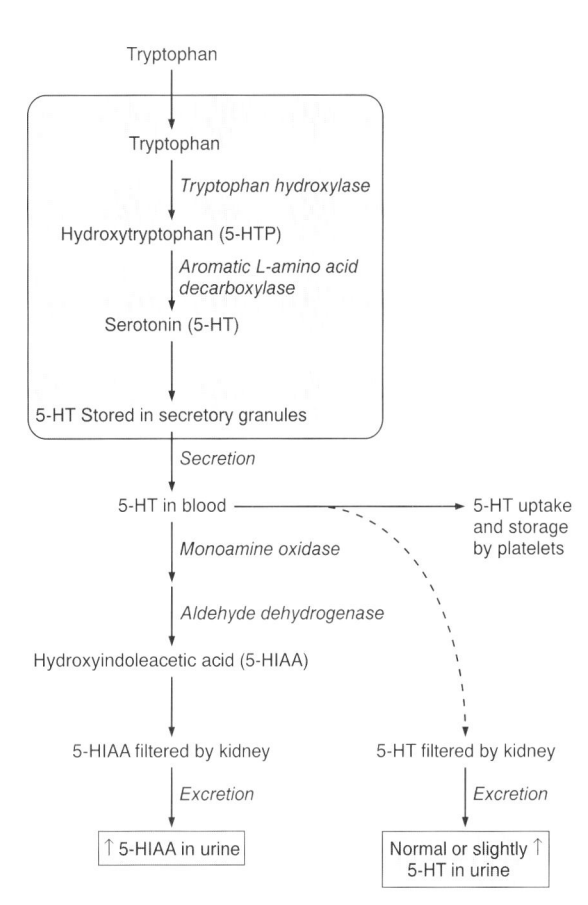

Fig. 7.**2** Metabolic pathway of serotonin in carcinoid syndrome

5-HIAA excretions is the most useful and practicable diagnostic test, and approximately 75% of patients excrete more than 80 mol/d (15 mg/d). Specificity of this test approaches 100% after exclusion of ingested substances known to elevate 5-HIAA-levels. These include bananas, pineapples, plantains, pecans, kiwifruits, walnuts, plums, and avocados. Aspirin and levodopa can cause a falsely depressed 5-HIAA level. But it has to be kept in mind, that in typical gastrointestinal carcinoid tumors usually no serotonin elevation and no carcinoid syndrome is found, because the serotonin of the portal vein is inactivated in the liver, or because many gastric carcinoid tumors lack the aromatic L-amino acid decarboxylase and convert 5-hydroxytryptophan (5-HTP) serotonin with low efficiency. Since 5-HTP is not metabolized to 5-HIAA, urinary studies may be misleading (1, 35, 36, 41).

Foregut carcinoid tumors (bronchus, stomach, duodenum, pancreas) synthesize only little serotonin, sometimes 5-hydroxytryptophan (5-HTP), ACTH, and bone metastasis may be found. Usually, typical carcinoid symptoms are only found in cases of liver metastasis.

Midgut carcinoid of tumors (jejunum, ileum, colon ascendens) synthesize a lot of serotonin, seldom secrete 5-HTP; ACTH and bone metastasis are seldom found.

Hindgut carcinoid tumors (colon transversum, colon decendens, rectum) seldom contain serotonin and also rarely secrete 5-HTP and ACTH. Bone metastases are found.

In regard to this pathophysiological specialty, in addition to urinary 5-HIAA excretion measurement, serum serotonin and 5-HTP concentration determination is necessary to confirm the diagnosis.

Another diagnostic tool is the provocation of cutaneous flushing by ethanol, pentagastrin, or small quantities of epinephrine (1, 24, 35, 36, 39, 41).

References

1 Feldman, JM. Carcinoid tumors and syndrome. Semin Oncol. 1989;14:237.
2 Nordheim I, et al. Malignant carcinoid tumors: An analysis of 103 patients with regard to tumor localisation, hormone production, and survival. Ann Surg. 1987;206:115.
3 Godwin JD. Carcinoid tumors: An analysis of 2837 cases. Cancer. 1975;36:560.

4. Wilander E, Lundquist M, Oberg K. Gastrointestinal carcinoid tumors. Histogenetic, histochemical, immunohistochemical, clinical and therapeutic aspects. Prog Histochem Cytochem. 1989;119(2):1–84.
5. Ajani JA, Carrasco OH, Samaan NA, Wallace S. Therapeutic options for patients with advanced islet cell- and carcinoid tumors. Reg Cancer Treat. 1991;3(5):235–242.
6. Elhassani NB. Bronchial carcinoid tumors. Ann Saudi Med. 1988;8(1):35–39.
7. Martensson H, et al. Bronchial carcinoids: Ananalysis of 91 cases. World J Surg. 1987;11:356.
8. Wollensak G. et al. Primary thymic carcinoid with Cushings' syndrome. Virchows Arch (A). 1992;420(2):191–195.
9. Division of Cardiac and Thoracic Surgery, Henry Ford Hospital, Detroit, Michigan. Carcinoid tumors of the thymus. Ann Thorac Surg. 1990;50(1):58–61.
10. Wick MR, Rosai J. Neuroendocrine neoplasms of the mediastinum. Sem Diagn Pathol. 1991;8(1):35–51.
11. Borch K. Atrophic gastritis and gastric carcinoid tumors. Ann Med. 1989;21(4):291–297.
12. Bumin C, et al. Carcinoid tumor of the biliary duct. Int. Surg. 1990;75(4):262–264.
13. Vinik AJ, Mc Leod MK, et al. Clinical features, diagnosis and localisation of carcinoid tumors and their management. Gastroenterol Clin North Am. 1989;18(4):865–896.
14. Wynick D, Bloom SR. Clinical Review 23: The use of the long acting somatostatin analog octreotide in the treatment of gut neuroendocrine tumors. J Clin Endocrinol Metab 1991;73(1):1–3.
15. Brown WM, et al. Carcinoid tumor of the bile duct. A case report and literature. Ann. Surg. 1990;56(6):343–6.
16. Wormsley KG. Therapeutic achlorhydria and risk of gastric cancer. Gastroenterologia Jpn. 1989;24(5):585–596.
17. Muller NL, Miller RR. Neuroendocrine carcinoma of the lung. Semin Roentgenol. 1990;25(1):96–104.
18. Thorson A, et al. Malignant carcinoid of the small intestine with metastasis into the liver. A clinical and pathologic syndrome. Am Heart J. 1954;47:795.
19. Zucker KA, et al. Malignant diathesis from jejunal-ileal carcinoma. Am J Gastroenterol. 1989;84(2):182–186.
20. Dixon A, Mc Anaw M, et al. Dual carcinoid tumors of Meckel's diverticula presenting as metastasis in an inguinal hernia sac. Case report with literature review. Am J Gastroenterol. 1988;83(11):1283–88.
21. Weber JD. Mc Fadden DW. Carcinoid tumors in Meckel's diverticula. J Clin Gastroenterol. 1989;11(6):682–686.
22. Rutledge RH, Alexander JW. Primary appendiceal malignancies. Rare but important. Surgery. 1992;111(3):244–250.
23. Moertel CG, et al. Carcinoid tumor of the appendix: Treatment and prognosis. N Engl J Med. 1987;317:1699.
24. Dieckmann ME, et al. Das Bronchialkarzinoid. Med Welt. 1987;38:732.
25. Hall JT, et al. Gastrointestinal and pancreatic endocrine tumours. Bailliere's Clinical Endocrinology and Metabolism 1992/1 (121–152)
26. Luedtke-Handjery A. et al. Goblet cell carcinoid of the vermiform appendix. Leber Magen Darm. 1991;21(5):226, 229–230.
27. Fuller CE, Williams GT. Gastrointestinal manifestations of type 1 neurofibromatosis (von Recklinghausens' disease). Histopathology. 1991;19(1):1–110.
28. Wiedemann B, Rath U. Neuroendocrine tumors of the gastroenteropancreatic system. Diagnosis and therapy. Inn Med. 1989;16(1):19–23.
29. Hoering E, von Gaisberg U. Neuroendokrine Tumoren des Pankreas und Gastrointestinaltraktes. Dtsch Med Wochenschr. 1991;11631–32:1197–1202.
30. Morgan LS. Hormonally active gynecologic tumors. Sem Surg Oncol. 1990;6(2)83–90.
31. Woodruff JM, Senie RT. Atypical carcinoid tumor of the larynx. A critical review of the literature. ORL. 1991;53(4):194–209.
32. El Naggar AK, Batsakis JG. Carcinoid tumor of the larynx. A critical review of the literature. ORL. 1991;53(4):188–193.
33. Larsen LG, Jacobsen GKP. Carcinoid tumor of the larynx. APMIS. 1989;97(8):748–753.
34. Muller MK, Niederle N, et al. Endocrine tumors of the gastrointestinal tract—part 1 and 2. Modern therapeutic concepts. Fortschr Med. 1992;110(4):37–45.
35. Oates JA. The carcinoid syndrome. N Engl J Med. 1986;315:702.
36. Sleisenger MH, Fordtran JS, eds. Gastrointestinal Disease. Pathophysiology, Diagnosis, Management. 4th ed. Philadelphia: Saunders; 1989:1560–70.
37. Saini A, Waxman J. Management of carcinoid syndrome. Postgrad Med. 1991;67(788):506–508.
38. Biosynthese und Abbau des Serotonins. In: Buddecke E. Grundriss der Biochemie. Berlin: de Gruyter; 1989.
39. Kaplan LM. Endocrine Tumors of the gastrointestinal tract and pancreas. In: Brunswald E, et al., eds. New York: McGraw; 1987.
40. Tomoda H, et al. A rectal carcinoid tumor of less than 1 cm in diameter with lymph node metastasis: A case report and a review of the literature. Jpn J Surg. 1990;20(4):468–472.
41. Feldman JM. Urinary serotonin in the diagnosis of carcinoid tumors. Clin Chem. 1986;32:840.
42. Brown NJ. Octreotide, a long acting somatostatin analog. Am J Med Sci. 1990;300(4):267–273.
43. Parmer H, Bogden A, et al. Somatostatin and somatostatin analogues in oncology. Cancer Treat Rev. 1989;16(2):95–115.
44. Kvols LK, et al. Therapeutic considerations for the malignant carcinoid syndrome. Acta Oncol. 1989;28(3):433–438.
45. Akerstrom G. Surgical treatment of carcinoids and endocrine pancreatic tumors. Acta Oncol. 1989;28(3):409–414.
46. Akerstroem G, et al. Abdominal surgery in patients with midgut carcinoid tumors. Acta Oncol. 1991;30(4):547–553.
47. Creutzfeldt W, Stöckmann F. Carcinoids and carcinoid syndrome. Am J Med. 1987;82(5B):4–15.

Computed Tomography

L.-E. Lörelius and E. Sugimoto

The primary carcinoid tumor is located in the bowel mucosa and is, in the majority of cases, reported to be less than 1 cm in diameter (7). Therefore, CT is a poor method for detection of the primary tumor (9). The tumor spreads first to the mesenteric lymph nodes. Further spread occurs either via the mesenteric root to the retroperitoneal lymph nodes, or via the portal vein to the liver.

Mesenterial metastases are very common and are found in 80% of the patients at diagnosis (7, 8). With increasing size, they may form a usually noncalcified mass in the mesentery, which is detectable by CT (1, 5, 9, 11). This mass may be seen either close to the bowel wall where it indicates the location of the primary tumor (Fig. 7.**3**), or more centrally, close to the mesenteric root (Fig. 7.**4**). The metastases induce fibrosis and shrinkage in the mesentery, which leads to retraction and kinking of bowel loops (3, 9, 11), sometimes seen with CT as a tornado-like configuration of the bowel loops (Fig. 7.**5**). This finding is often combined with abdominal pain and diarrhea as symptoms of intermittent bowel obstruction. Branches from arteries, veins, and lymph vessels may become encased and occluded either by the fibrosis or by vascular elastosis (4, 10). The concommitantly impaired vascular drainage from the bowel is frequently seen as stellate densities in the mesentery peripheral to a mesenteric mass (Fig. 7.**6**). Rarely, this finding is combined with a thickened bowel wall (Fig. 7.**7**) indicating an edema corresponding to the so-called blue ischemia of the bowel. Even more rare is the finding of ascites, which

Computed Tomography 215

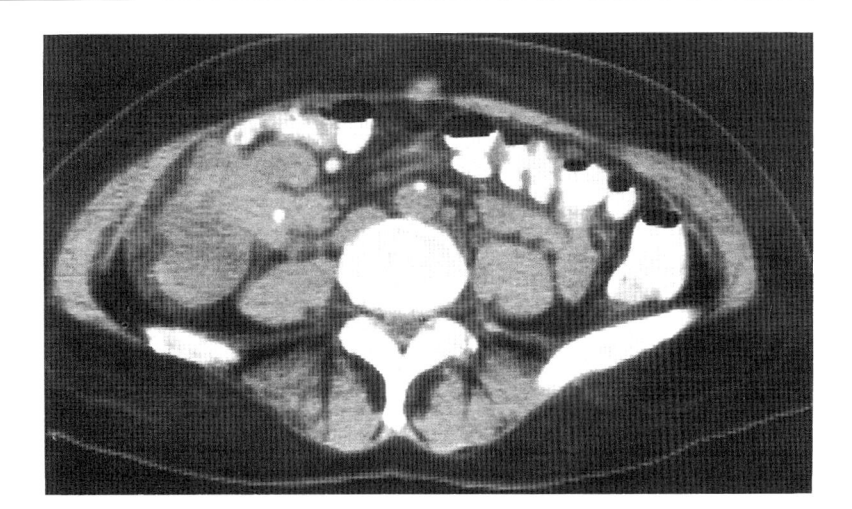

Fig. 7.**3** Partly calcified mesenterial mass in right hypocondrium surrounded by not contrastfilled bowel loops in a 62-year-old woman with diarrhea and flush

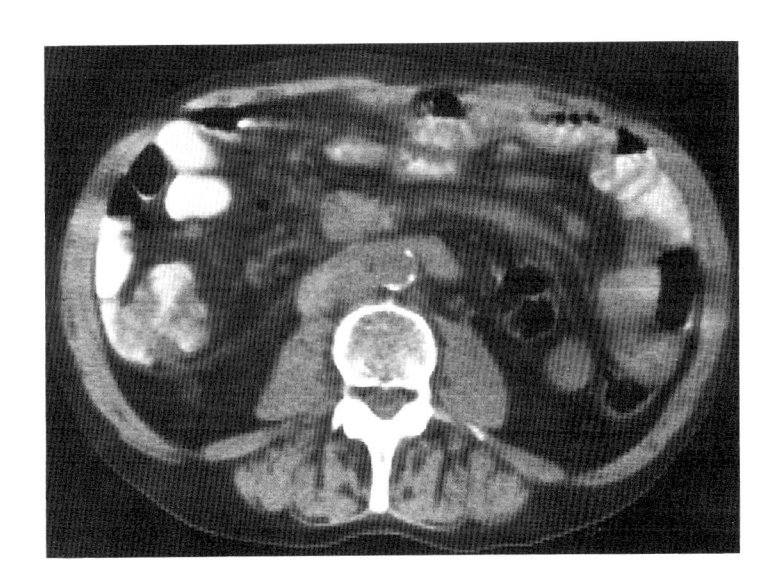

Fig. 7.**4** Centrally located mesenteric mass with stellate densities in the mesenteric fat and enlarged retroperitoneal lymph nodes around the aorta in a 71-year-old man with flush and elevated 5-HIAA

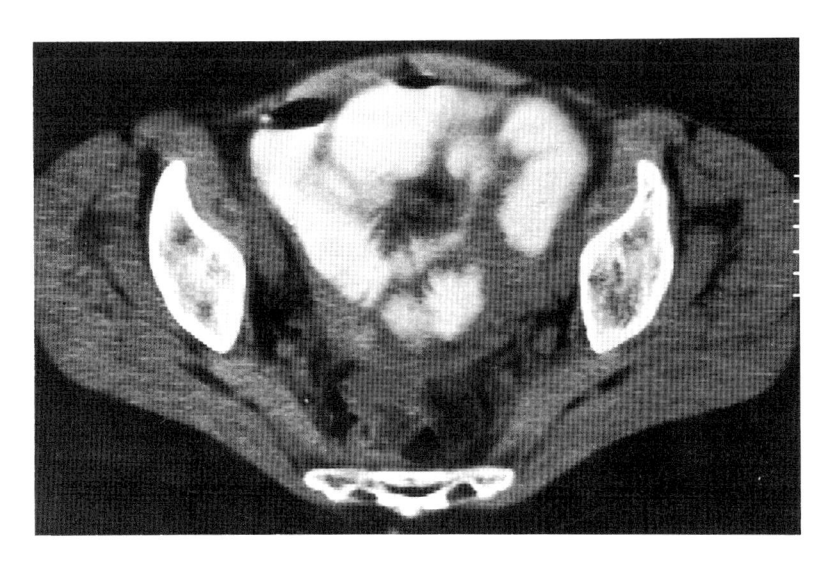

Fig. 7.**5** Moderately dilated loops of small bowel twisted around a small hypodense mesenteric mass in a 66-year-old woman with relapsing attacks of abdominal pain

216   7 Carcinoid

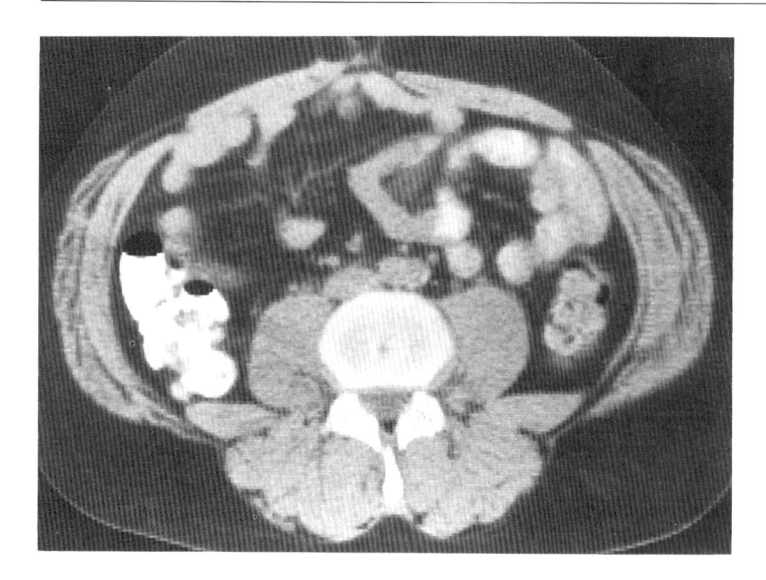

Fig. 7.**6** Thickened vascular densities radiating toward a relatively small mesenteric mass in a 46-year-old man with carcinoid syndrome but no abdominal symptoms

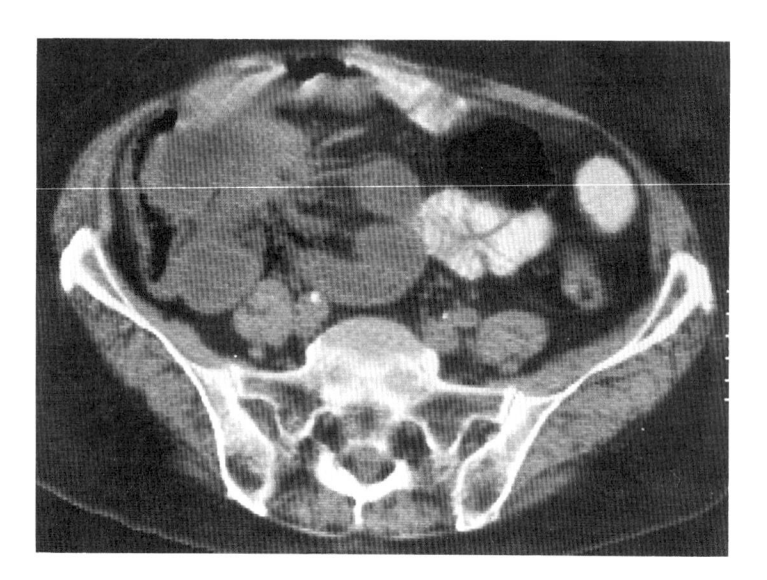

Fig. 7.**7** Loops of small bowel with thickening of the bowel wall around a mesenteric mass in a 73-year-old woman with carcinoid syndrome and diarrhea

may occur with or without liver metastases, but is usually combined with a mesenteric mass (Fig. 7.**8**).

Retroperitoneal metastases may be found both in patients with and without liver metastases. The metastases are located adjacent to the aorta and inferior vena cava (Fig. 7.**9**); they may also be found behind the crus of the diaphragm (9).

Liver metastases are the most frequent type of metastases found in CT of patients with carcinoid tumors, and are supposed to be a prerequisite for the development of carcinoid syndrome. They are often multiple and spread to both liver lobes (7, 9) (Fig. 7.**10**). Their attenuation may be similar to liver parenchyma and a small camera window is therefore recommended during the examination. It is often necessary to investigate with plain and with contrast-enhanced scans (Fig. 7.**11**). A special problem may occur during follow-up of patients treated with interferon because the normal liver sometimes changes attenuation due to fatty infiltration induced by interferon (1, 2, 14) (Fig. 7.**12**). When the metastases are identified, the radiologist should always have possible surgery in mind, because these patient's symptoms come from the hormone release more than from the tumor burden. It is therefore possible that the patient may even benefit from palliative tumor resection (Fig. 7.**12**). Totally atypical tumor resections have also been reported (7). If surgery is still recommended as the primary choice of treatment (13), medical treatment with interferon and somatostatin analog may definitely change the outcome of disease for a large group of the patients (6, 14). In these cases, remarkable regression of tumor size as well as reduction of hormone release may be seen (Fig. 7.**13**).

Differential diagnosis: Mesenteric masses also occur in ovarian carcinoma, non-Hodgkin lymphoma,

Computed Tomography 217

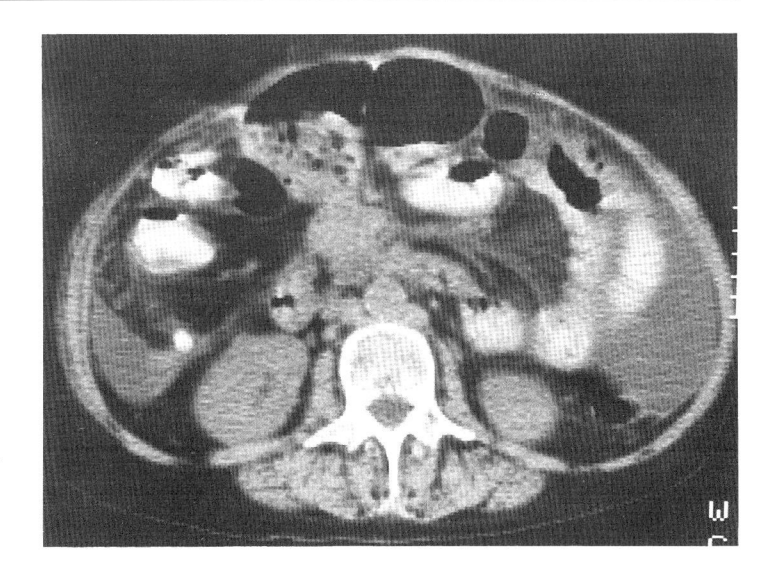

Fig. 7.**8** Mesenteric mass with stellate densities in the mesenteric fat, retroperitoneal lymph nodes, and ascites in a 56-year-old woman with carcinoid syndrome abdominal pain and diarrhea

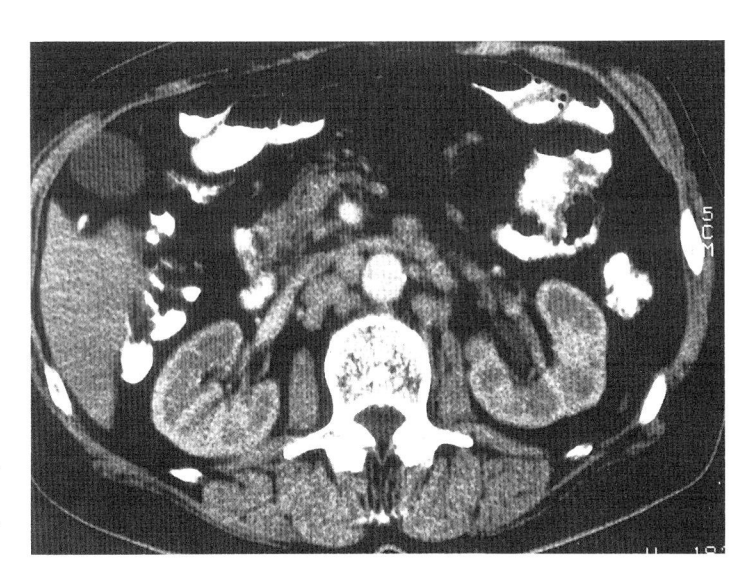

Fig. 7.**9** Enlarged retroperitoneal lymphnodes around the aorta and inferior vena cava in a patient with carcinoid syndrome, diarrhea, and abdominal pain

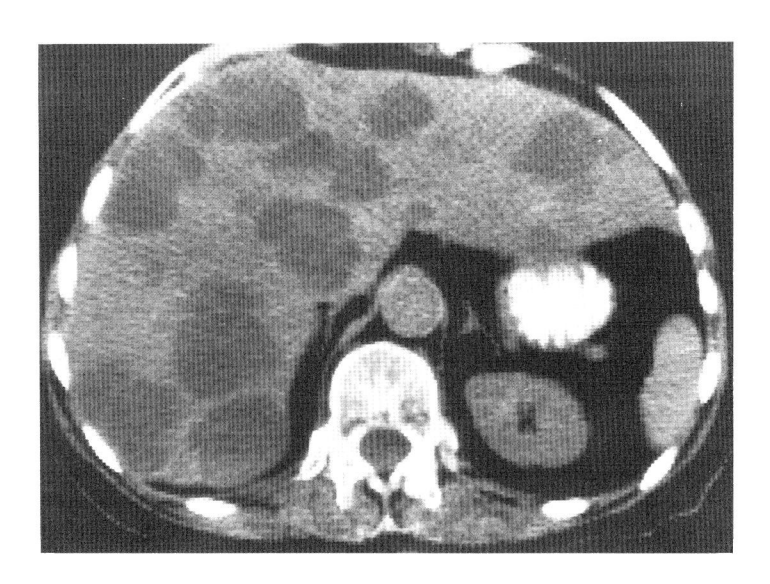

Fig. 7.**10** Multiple liver metastases from carcinoid tumor seen without contrast enhancement in a 72-year-old woman with carcinoid syndrome

218   7 Carcinoid

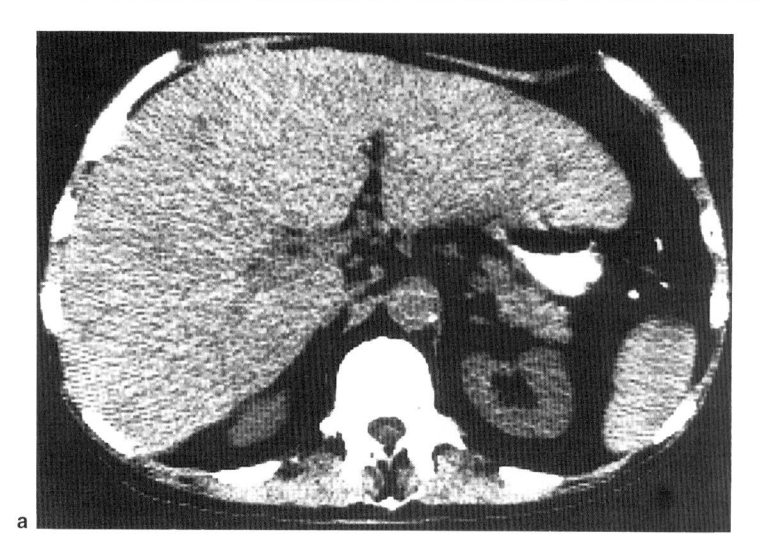

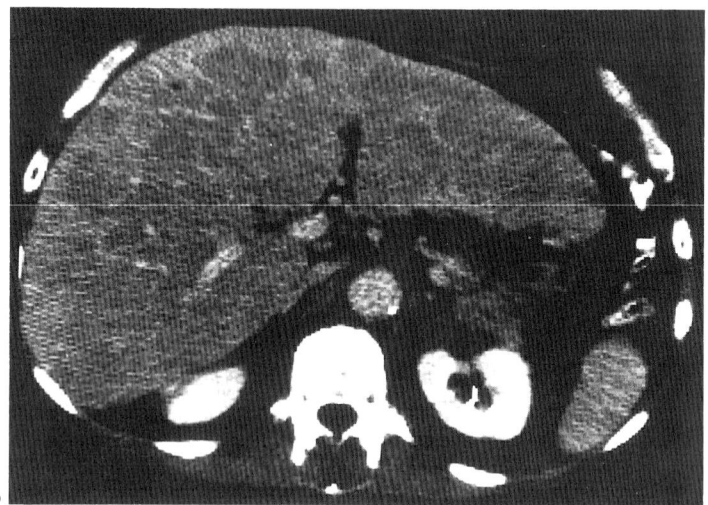

Fig. 7.**11** Liver metastases from carcinoid tumor isodense with the liver (**a**) before and (**b**) after contrast enhancement in a 79-year-old man with carcinoid syndrome and diarrhea

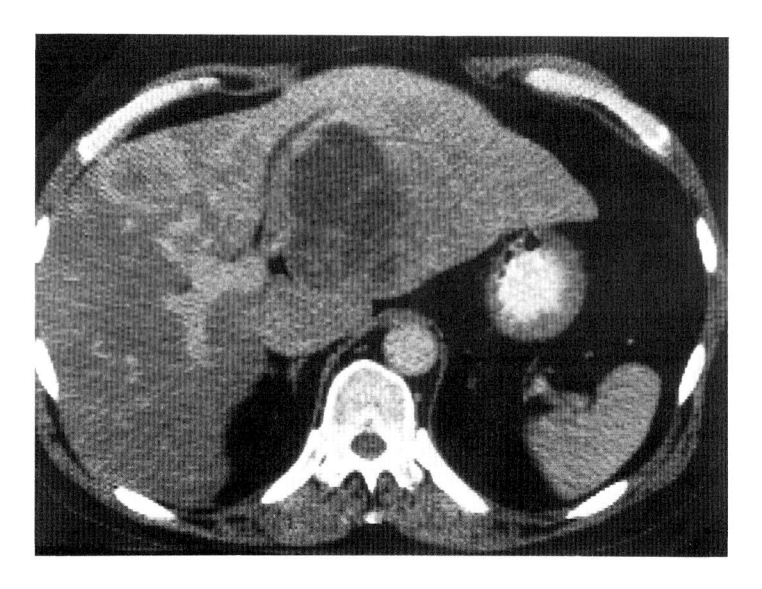

Fig. 7.**12** Liver metastases predominantly in the left liver lobe in a 50-year-old man with severe flushing, free from symptoms after surgical resection of the left lobe. Note the low density in the right lobe due to fatty infiltration caused by interferon

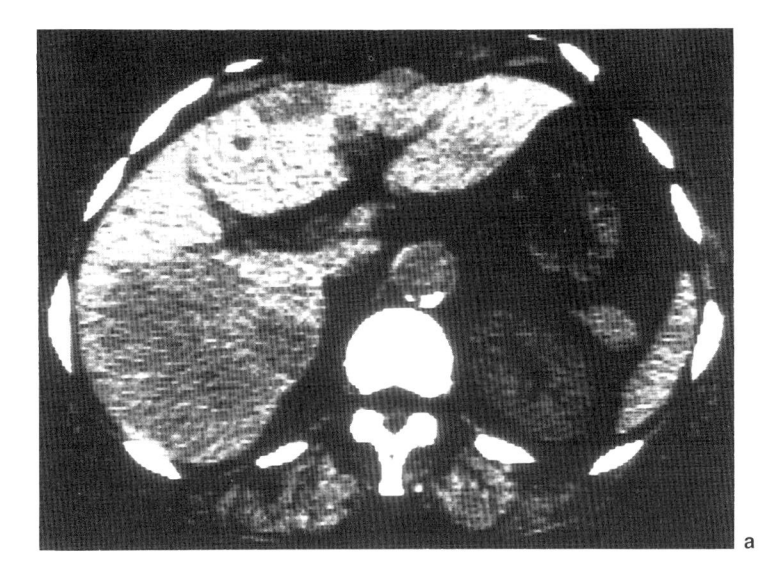

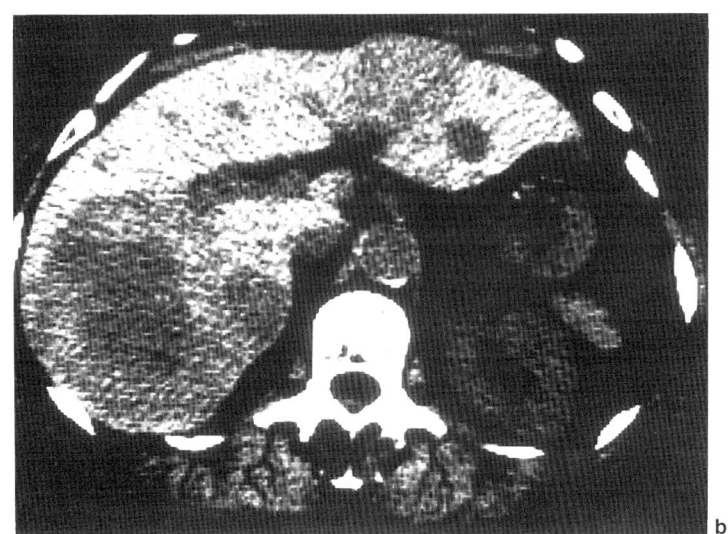

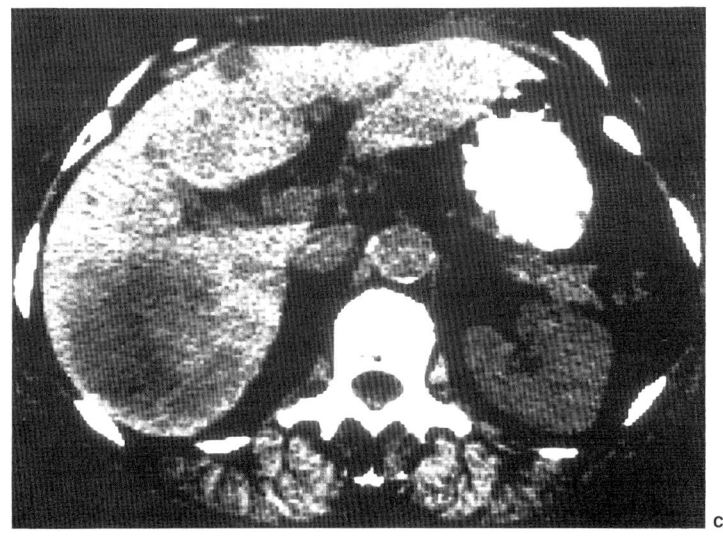

Fig. 7.**13** Liver metastases in both lobes in a 55-year-old woman with carcinoid syndrome and diarrhea (**a**) at referal (**b**) progress in size of metastases one year after treatment with Streptozotocin (S) and 5 Fluoro uracil (5FU) (**c**) Regression of metastases one year, (**d**) 3 years, (**e**) 6 years, (**f**) 9 years after beginning of treatment with interferon. (**g**) The levels of 5 HIAA in urine during 9 years of treatment in the same patient. MU = Million Units, INF = interferon. Note the morphological delay in response compared to the hormonal levels

Continued p. 220 ▶

220   7 Carcinoid

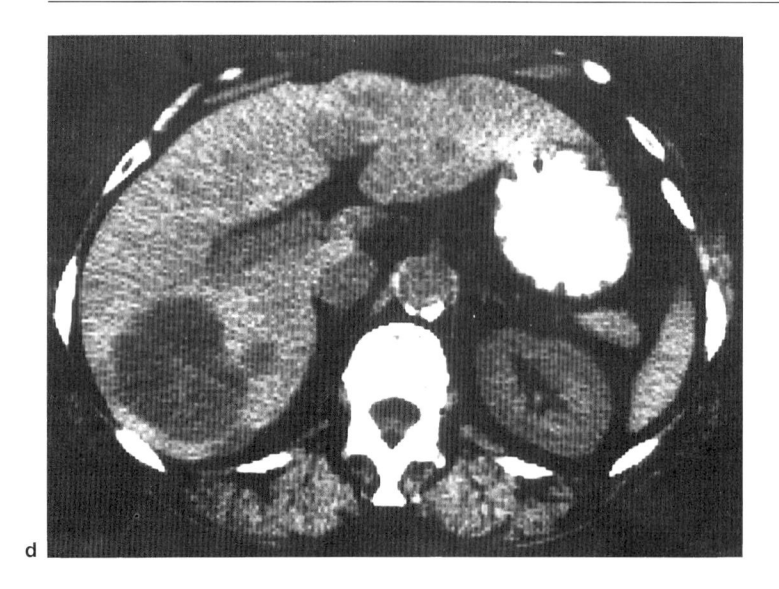

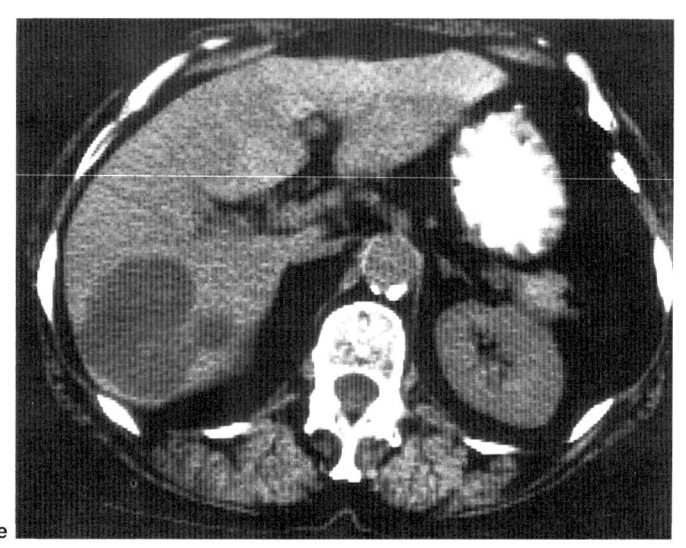

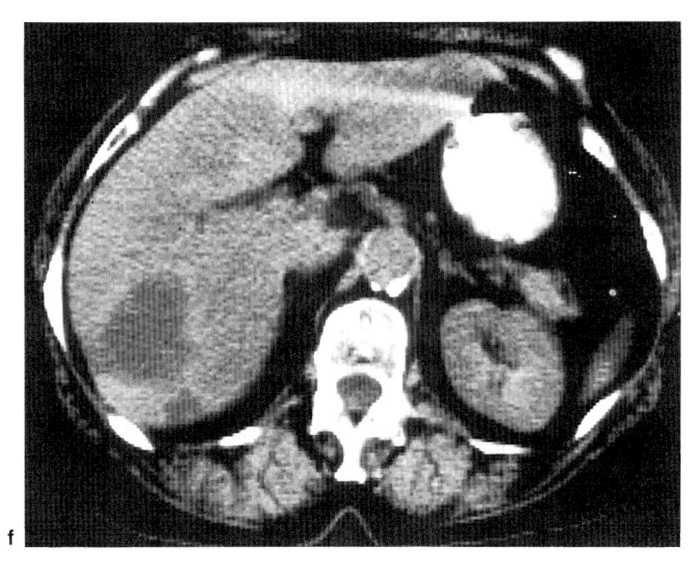

Fig. 7.**13e–f**

U-5HIAA
μmol/24 h

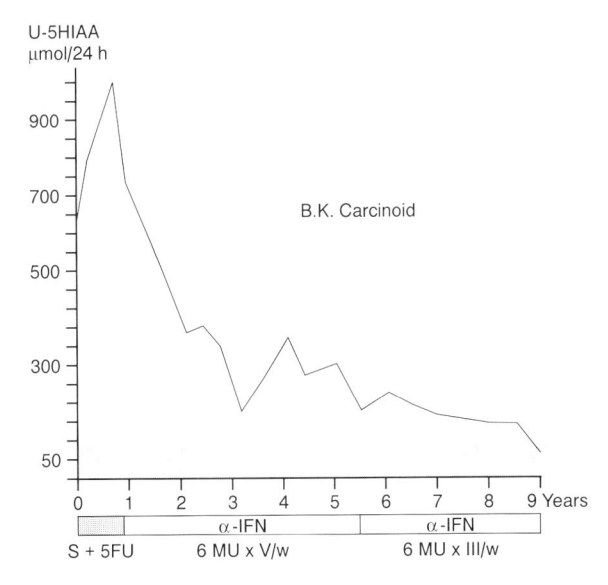

B.K. Carcinoid

S + 5FU | α-IFN 6 MU x V/w | α-IFN 6 MU x III/w

Fig. 7.**13g**

leukemia, cancer of the colon and pancreas, peritoneal mesothelioma, mammary cancer, and retractile mesenteritis (11, 12). The retroperitoneal metastases are similar to those found in lymphomas, and testicular and ovarian carcinomas.

It is not possible to separate these liver metastases radiologically from any other type of liver metastases, but when they occur, the patients usually have the clinical picture of carcinoid syndrome.

References

1. Andersson T, Wilander E, Eriksson B, Lindgren PG, Öberg K. Effects of interferon on tissue content in liver metastases of human carcinoid tumors. Cancer Res. 1990;50:3413–3415.
2. Andersson T, Eriksson B, Lindgren PG, Wilander E, Öberg K. Percutaneous ultrasonography-guided cutting biopsy from liver metastases of endocrine gastrointestinal tumors. Ann Surg. 1987;206:728.
3. Bernardino M, Jing BS, Wallace S. Computed tomography diagnosis of mesenteric masses. AJR. 1979;132:33–36.
4. Eckerhauser FE, Argenta LC, Strodel WE, et al. Mesenteric angiopathy, intestinal gangrene, and midgut carcinoids. Surgery. 1981;90:719–728.
5. Gould, M, Johnsson, RJ, Computed tomography of abdominal carcinoid tumour. Brit J Radiol. 1986;59:881–885.
6. Kvols LK, Moertel CG, O'Connell MJ, Schutt AJ, Rubin J, Hahn RG. Treatment of the malignant carcinoid syndrome. Evaluation of a long-acting somatostatin analogue. N Engl J Med. 1986;315:663.
7. Makridis C, Öberg K, Juhlin C, et al. Surgical treatment of midgut carcinoid tumors. World J Surg. 1990;14:377–385.
8. Moertel CG, Sauer WG, Dockerty MB, Baggenstoss AH. Life history of the carcinoid tumor of the small intestine. Cancer. 1961;14:901–912.
9. Picus D, Glazer HS, Levitt RG, Husband JE. Computed tomography of abdominal carcinoid tumors. AJR. 1984;143:581–584.
10. Qizilbash AH. Carcinoid tumours, vascular elastosis, and ischemic disease of the small intestine. Dis Colon Rectum. 1977;20:554–560.
11. Seigel RS, Kuhns LR, Borlaza GS, McCormick TL, Simmons JL. Computed tomography and angiography in ileal carcinoid tumor and retractile mesenteritis. Radiology. 1980;134:437–440.
12. Whitley NO, Bohlman M-E, Baker LP. CT patterns of mesenteric disease. J Comput Assist Tomogr. 1982;6(3),490–496.
13. Åkerström G, Makridis C, Johansson H. Abdominal Surgery in patients with midgut carcinoid tumors. Acta Oncol. 1991;30:547–553.
14. Öberg K, Norheim I, Lind E, et al. Treatment of malignant carcinoid tumors with human leukocyte interferon: Long term results. Cancer Treat Rep. 1986;70:1297–1304.

Angiography and Interventional Radiology

L.-E. Lörelius

Normal Vascular Anatomy

In order to interpret findings using angiography or to plan interventional procedures in patients with gastrointestinal tumors, a thorough knowledge of the normal vascular anatomy and its variations is necessary (16, 22). Some aspects of the anatomy should be emphasized especially when dealing with patients with carcinoid tumor disease. The superior mesenteric artery runs from the anterior aspect of the aorta behind the pancreas caudally in the retroperitoneal space and enters the mesentery at the border of the pancreatic neck and the horizontal part of the duodenum. Distal to this point, it runs inside the duplication of the visceral peritoneum known as the mesentery, where it shares space with concomitant veins, nerves, lymph vessels, lymph nodes, connective tissue, and fat. The main branches of the superior mesenteric artery to the duodenum, pancreas, jejunum, ileum, and the ascending and transverse colon all have side branches that communicate with each other. The arcades of communication formed in this way often exist in several levels with the most peripheral one at the mesenteric border of the bowel. This terminal arcade gives off the anterior and the posterior vasa recta to the bowel wall, and consequently, the bowel has its arterial and nervous supply as well as its venous and lymphatic drainage through a thin opening in the mesentery.

Carcinoid Tumors

These tumors can be divided according to their embryological origin into foregut (lung, thymus, gastric mucosa, and duodenum), midgut (jejunum ileum and the ascending and transverse colon), and hindgut (distal colon and rectum) tumors. This also has implications for a variable production of amines and peptides (25). Foregut carcinoid tumors frequently produce gastrin, somatostatin, and histamine, and are often polypoid, and angiography is rarely needed for diagnosis. The midgut "classic" carcinoids mainly produce serotonin and various tachykinins. When liver metastases occur, a "carcinoid syndrome" is often present implying flush, diarrhea, bronchoconstriction, and right-sided heart failure.

Midgut carcinoid tumors have a tendency to induce changes in the connective tissue both in the neighboring mesentery, as well as in mesenteric arteries and veins close to and remote from the tumor and farther away, for example in the pulmonary artery and the tricuspid heart valve. The changes within the right side of the heart generally consist of subintimal fibrosis, whereas the arterial and venous changes seem to consist mainly of adventitial deposits of elastin. These vascular changes, named vascular elastosis (3, 10, 19), are found in high frequency in arteries and veins in connection to the mesenteric metastases from midgut, but have not been described in association with foregut or hindgut carcinoid tumors. As trigger mechanisms for the development of this elastosis, different tumor-related chemical agents have been suggested including bradykinin, prostaglandin, and platelet-derived growth factor (PDGF), but so far a responsible agent has not been identified.

Carcinoid Anatomy

The primary carcinoid tumor is in itself almost always too small to be visualized by angiography. Multiple intestinal cardinoid tumors seem to occur in at least 25% of patients. The carcinoid spreads through the connective tissue and lymphatic pathways into the mesentery through the thin space at the mesenteric border of the gut and metastases in the regional lymph glands, which may be detected by radiological methods including angiography (6). The mesenteric lymph gland metastases from midgut carcinoid tumors tend to induce fibrosis, which fairly often retracts the bowel to sharp loops. The tumor also often invades the perivascular space and may encase or occlude both arterial and venous branches; it is then often combined with more or less pronounced vascular elastosis (3, 10, 19).

The normal anatomy of the mesenteric vessels, with multiple levels of arterial and venous arcades, usually allows rather extensive arterial occlusions until intestinal ischemia supervenes. Veins, together with lymph paths, that drain the gut also tend to be occluded. In particular, impairment of venous drainage may result in venous gangrene in these patients.

Angiographic Findings

The findings at angiography may frequently be diagnostic of a midgut carcinoid tumour. These findings were first described by Reuter and Boijsen in 1966 (20) and have been related to a retraction of the mesentery at the site of the mesenteric metastases, implying that the arterial branches come to be located closer together than normal, simulating hypervascularity (Fig. 7.14). The arterial branches or subbranches may also be encased or occluded depending on the severity of the fibrotic shrinkage and the vascular elas-

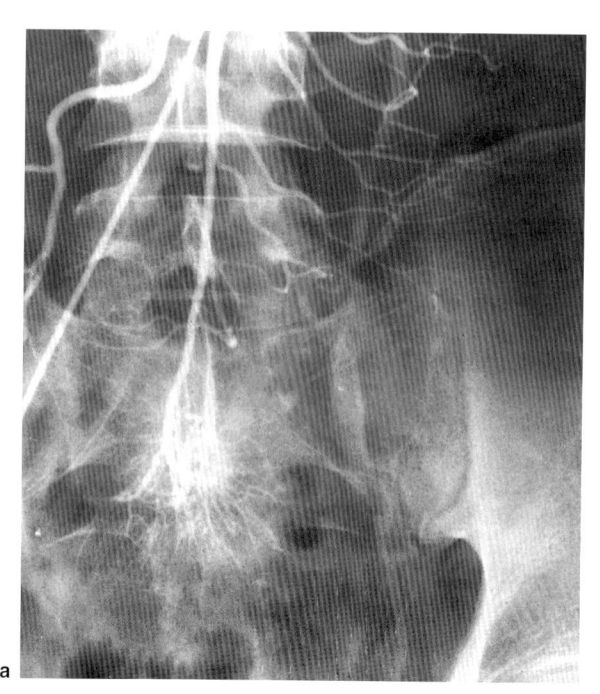

Fig. 7.14 Carcinoid syndrome in a 38-year-old patient. Angiography of the superior mesenteric artery shows shrinkage of the mesentery (a) with the ileal branches very close to each other and (b) the mesenteric metastasis staining intensively in the parenchymal phase; no early venous filling is seen

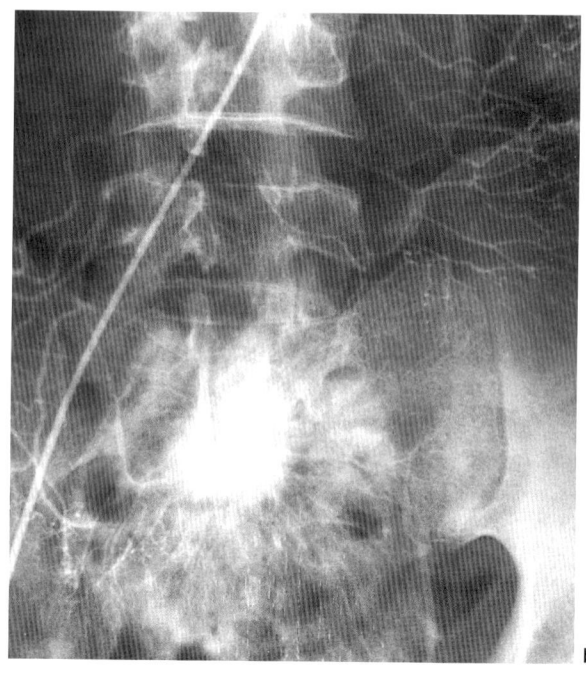

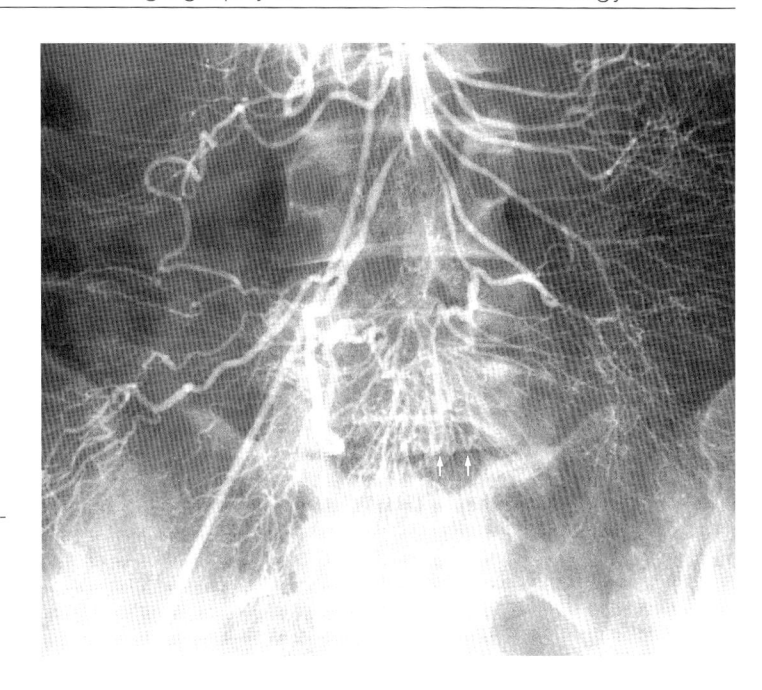

Fig. 7.**15** Carcinoid syndrome including insufficiency of both the tricuspid and the mitral ostea. Primary tumor not localized with small-bowel barium examination. Angiography shows encasement and occlusions of iliac arterial branches and collateral circulation via a proximal mesenteric arcade and an unimpaired terminal acrade (arrows)

tosis (Fig. 7.**15**). The vasa recta will sometimes radiate like spokes in a wheel toward the center of the retraction (Fig. 7.**16 b**), which may or may not show hyperdensity in the parenchymal phase at angiography (Figs. 7.**14 b** and 7.**16 b**). No newly formed arteries or neovessels seem to occur, but the fibrosis and the vascular elastosis may give the arteries an appearence simulating fibromuscular dysplasia (6) (Fig. 7.**16 a**), which is also a fibrous disease of the vascular wall. If all arterial arcades including that at the mesenteric junction are occluded, the blood supply to the vasa recta will be impaired and a bowel ischemia may supervene (Fig. 7.**17**). Intestinal gangrene may result from this impairment, either as pale or blue gangrene, depending on whether occlusion of arteries or veins predominates (26). Vascular elastosis is frequently found in advanced lesions associated with gangrene (10). Due to stenoses and occlusions of arteries, the an-

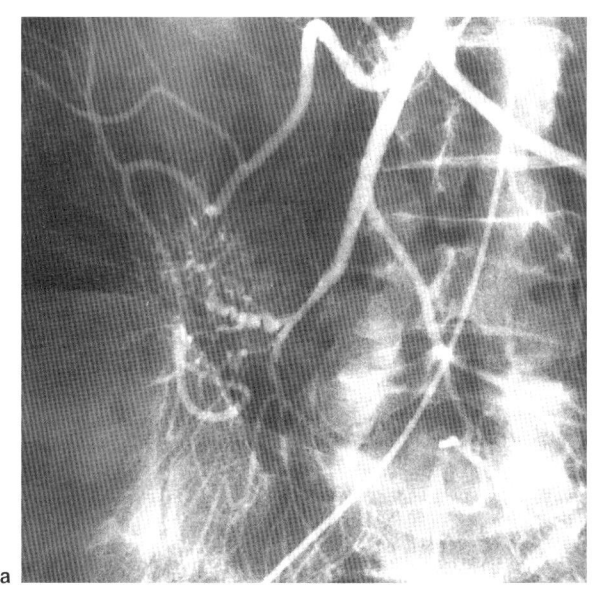

Fig. 7.**16** Anemia and blood in the stools in a 53-year-old patient. Barium studies of the colon and the small bowel negative. Angiography shows (**a**) encasement of arterial branches multiple membraneous stenoses simulating fibromuscular dysplasia and (**b**) the vasa recta arranged like spokes in a wheel because of shrinkage of the mesentery

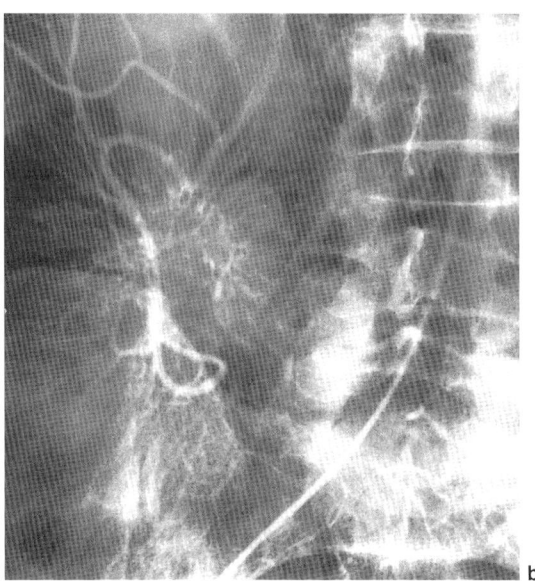

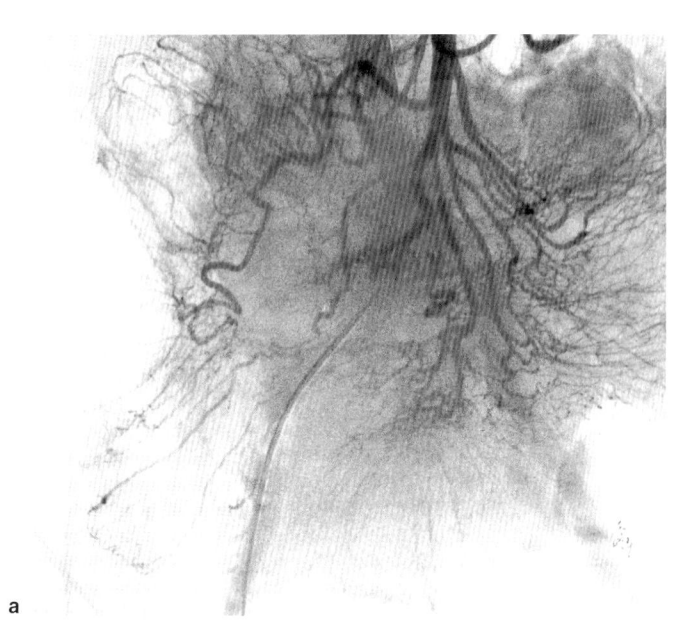

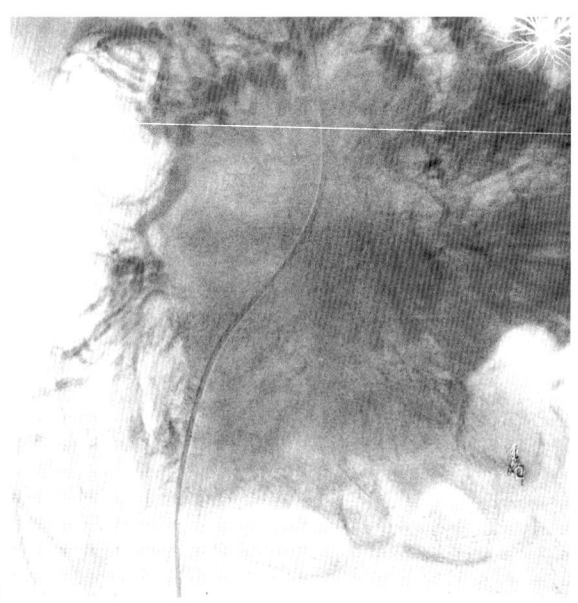

Fig. 7.**17** Midgut carcinoid tumor in a 82-year-old patient operated on 1 year earlier with an ileotransversostomi because of ileus due to an inoperable tumor in the ileocoecal region. Angiography because of relapsing attacks of abdominal pain shows (**a**) occlusion of arterial branches to the distal ileum where even the terminal arcades are occluded in a short segment of the ileum (**b**) occlusion of venous branches and collateral venous circulation. The severely impaired circulation both on the arterial and venous side indicates possible bowel ischemia

giography may often show corkscrew-like collateral arteries that should not be mistaken for neovessels (Fig. 7.**18**). Early filling of veins does not seem to occur even in cases in which the mesenteric metastases are hypervascular. On late films, widened venae recta and deficient filling of the draining venous branches may be found (Figs. 7.**17 b** and 7.**19 b**) that may be related to malabsorbtion (12, 13). Hypothetically, these dilated veins may be the source of intestinal bleeding.

The most frequent indication for mesenteric angiography is evaluation prior to elective surgery, aimed at resecting a primary tumor, removing obstructed or ischenic bowel and restoring the enteric passage (Fig. 7.**20**). Rarely, patients without known carcinoid disease may be referred for angiography because of slow gastrointestinal bleeding (Fig. 7.**16**).

Primary midgut carcinoid tumors are most frequently located in the terminal parts of the ileum. There seems to be no means of dealing with interventional radiology in primary tumors or mesenteric metastases.

Differential Diagnosis

These include other space-occupying lesions in the mesentery like lymphoma, tuberculosis of the gut, direct invasion of the mesentery from pancreatic cancer, and chronic sclerosing fibrous peritonitis.

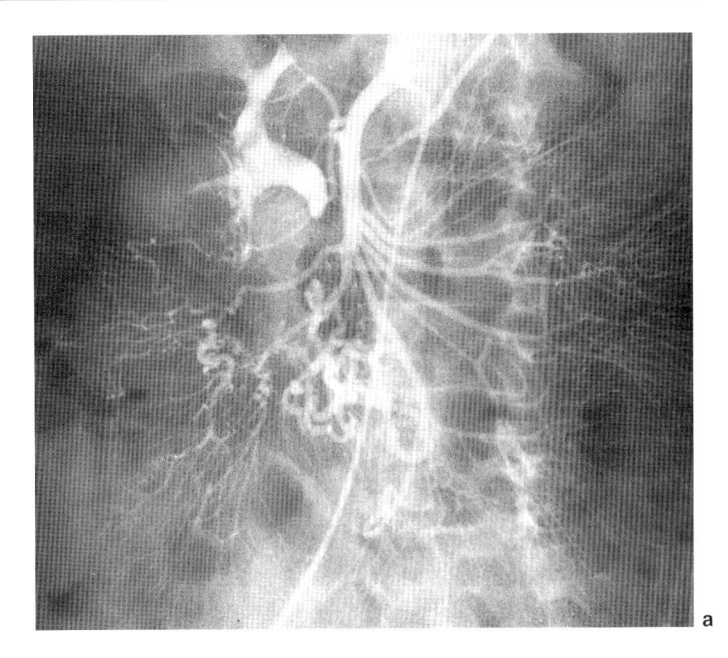

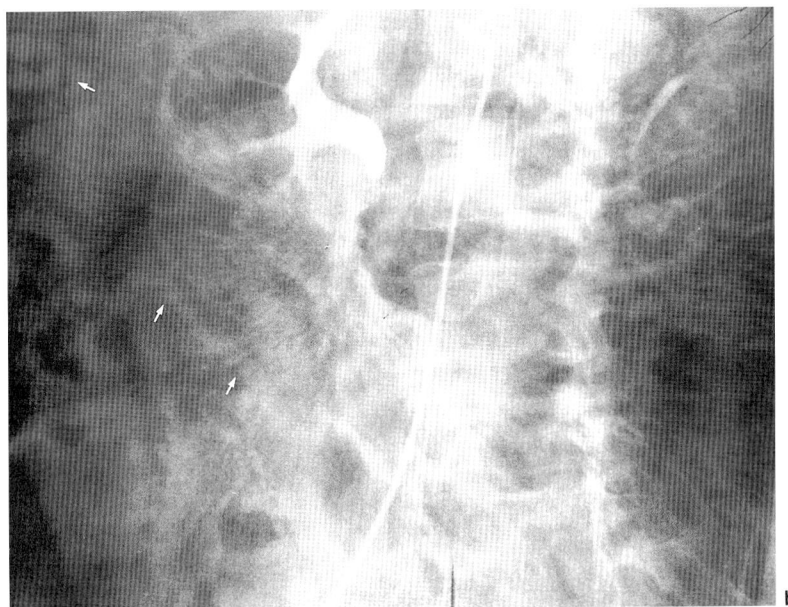

Fig. 7.**18** Superior mesenteric angiography in a 56-year-old patient with abdominal pain and blood in the stools. Barium investigation of the small bowel had indicated possible Crohn disease. Angiography because of GI bleeding shows (**a**) arterial occlusions with multiple corkscrew-like collateral arteries and (**b**) occlusion of the superior mesenteric vein causing a collateral venous drainage (arrows)

Liver Metastases

Liver metastases in patients with midgut carcinoid tumors frequently result in development of a carcinoid syndrome. These patients generally exhibit elevated levels of 5-hydroxyindole-acetic-acid (5-HIAA) in a 24 hour urine sample. The presence of liver metastases may be verified by ultrasound or CT or both. Before debulking surgery (17) or arterial embolization, angiography is indicated. It should include visualization of the celiac trunk and the superior mesenteric artery in order to detect variations in the normal anatomy, such as an origin of the right hepatic artery from the main mesenteric artery (16, 22). Carcinoid liver metastases are predominantly hypervascular, but hypovascular metastases are not unusual. They may be single or multiple, large or small (Figs. 7.**21**, 7.**22** and 7.**23**), neovessels can be seen and the metastases usually stain brightly against the liver parenchyma at angiography (Fig. 7.**22**, 7.**23**). The appearance of carcinoid liver metastases is, however, not angiographically different from other types of hypervascular liver metastases. There is generally no visible fibrosis or shinkage around these metastases in contrast to that which is seen in the mesenteric metastases (Figs. 7.**21** and 7.**22**). Whether this difference is due to cloning of cells with a tendency to

226   7 Carcinoid

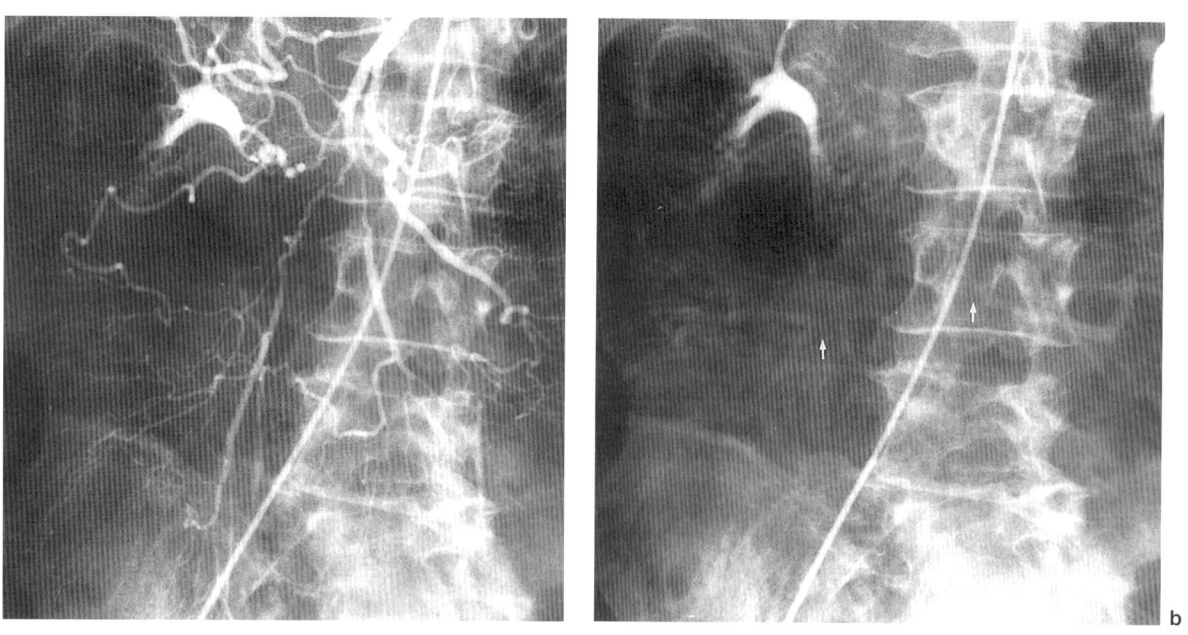

Fig. 7.**19** Mesenteric metastasis from a midgut carcinoid tumor in a 63-year-old patient who had the primary tumor resected from the distal ileum 5 years earlier. Angiography because of relapsing GI bleeding shows (**a**) mesenterial metastases with encasement of ileal and jejunal branches (**b**) no staining in the parenchymal phase, occlusion of ileal venous branches (arrows)

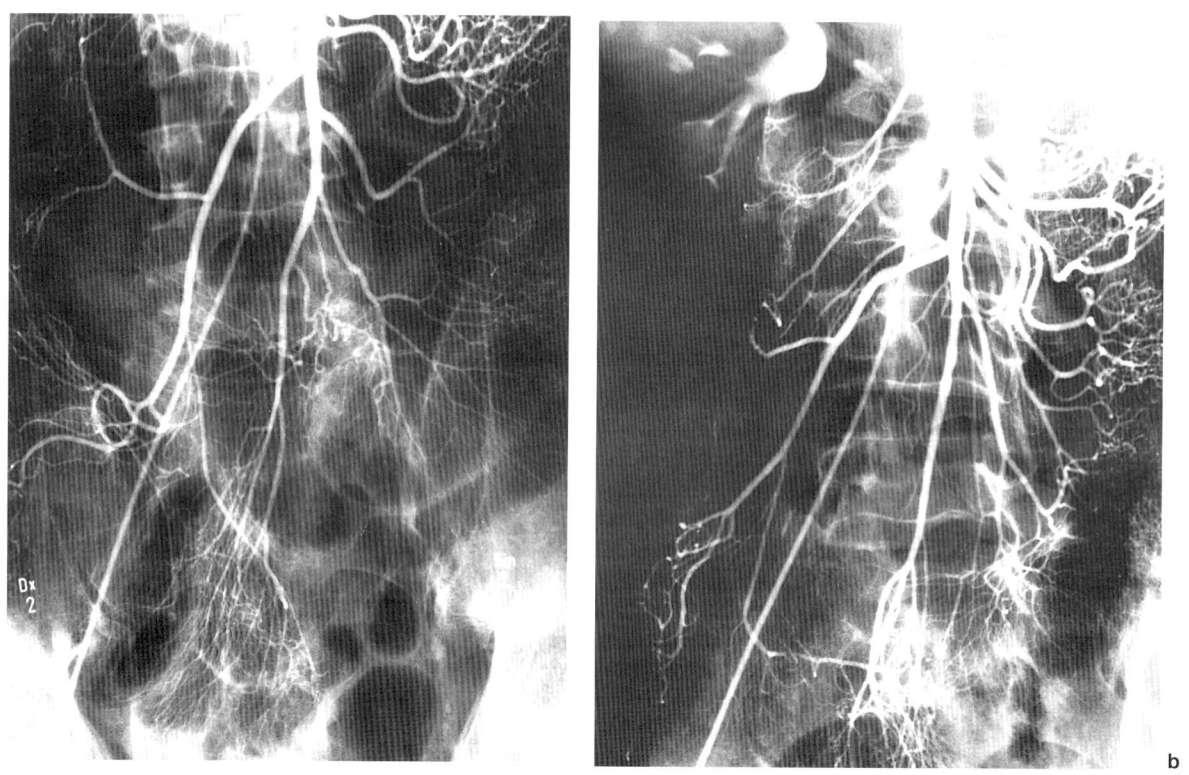

Fig. 7.**20**   Carcinoid syndrome in a 58-year-old patient with attacks of small bowel obstruction. Angiography shows (**a**) retraction of a segment of the proximal ileum and corkscrewlike arterial branches. (**b**) 3 months after operation with segmental resection and mobilization of the bowel

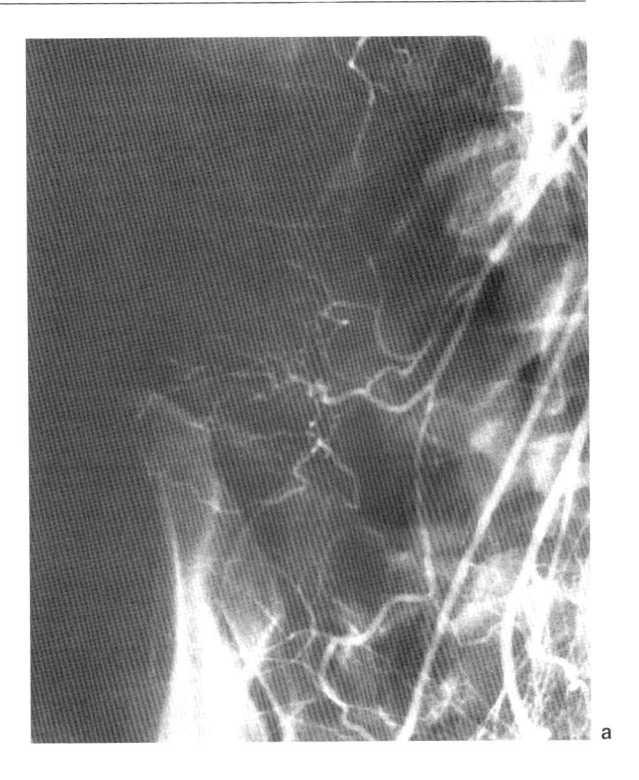

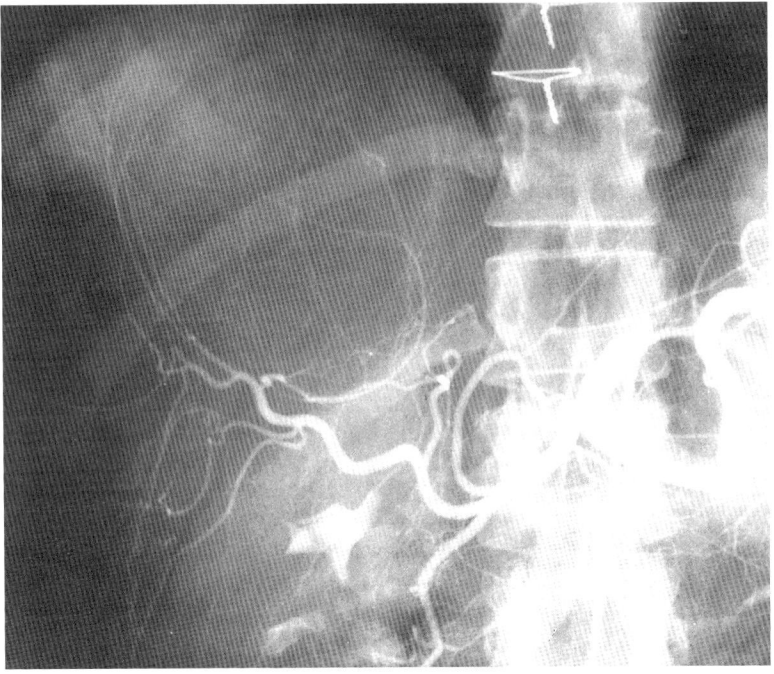

Fig. 7.21 Carcinoid syndrome in a 44-year-old patient. Angiography prior to resection of large solitary metastasis in the right liver lobe shows (**a**) rather discrete arterial abnormalities at the ileocaecal valve and (**b**) a large hypovascular solitary metastasis in the upper part of the right liver lobe

spread to the venous side, or if the liver reacts to carcinoid metastases differently from the mesenteric connective tissue has not been defined. Abdominal angiography in combination with the clinical symptoms and laboratory findings usually gives enough information for both diagnosis and treatment planning.

Interventional Radiology

The normal liver parenchyma has a dual blood supply with around 30% of the total blood flow from the hepatic artery and 70% from the portal vein. Liver tumors, on the other hand, receive their main nutritive

228 7 Carcinoid

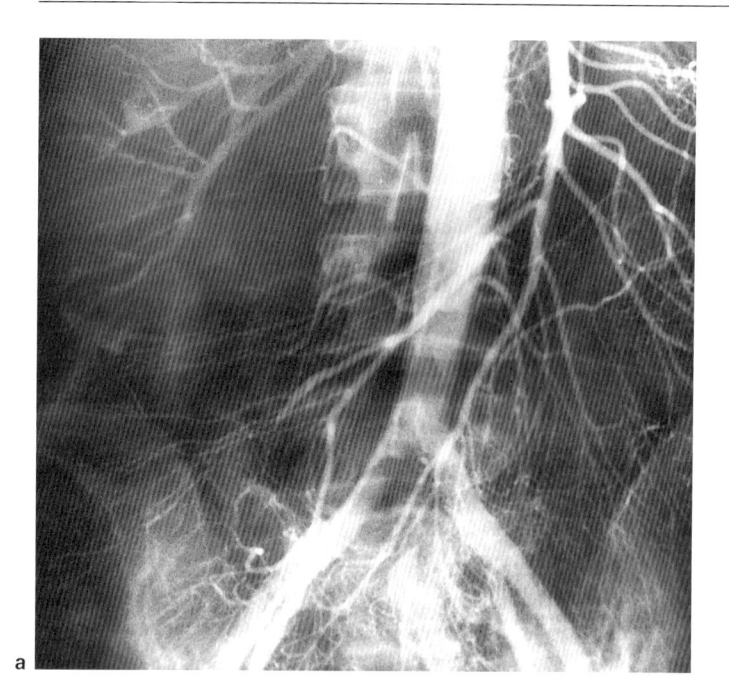

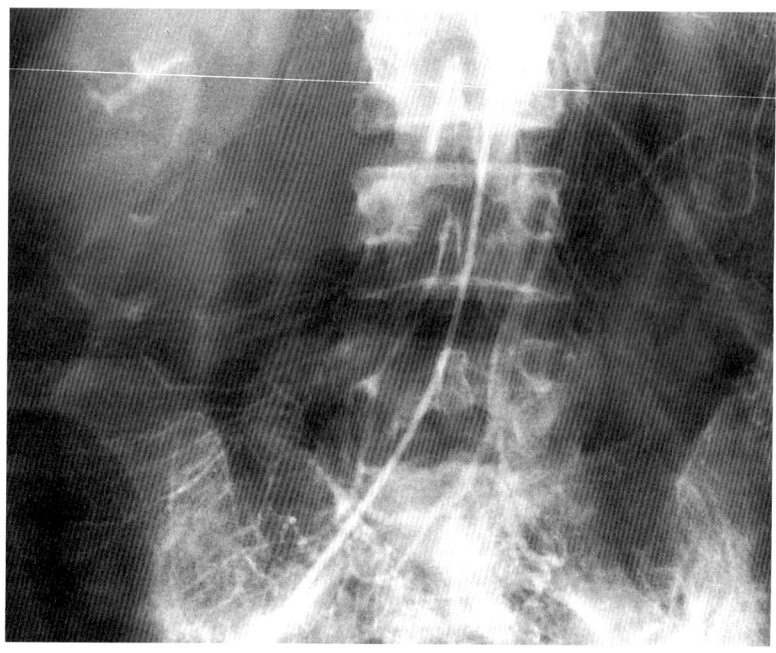

Fig. 7.**22** Carcinoid syndrome in a 44-year-old patient. Preoperative angiography before local resection of liver metastasis. Superior mesenteric angiography shows (**a**) encasement of an arterial arcade and (**b**) late arterial filling of the terminal arcade of a loop in the distal ileum. No neovascularity is seen. Hepatic angiography in the same patient shows (**c**) a large liver metastasis with neovascularity and (**d**) with intense parenchymal staining

blood flow from the hepatic artery (5). An arterial occlusion will therefore result in a severe ischemia in the hepatic tumor, whereas the normal liver parenchyma will be less ischemic because of the unaffected blood flow through the portal vein. This constitutes the basic concept for surgical ligation of the hepatic artery in patients with inoperable liver tumors (4). However, after proximal arterial occlusion, collateral circulation is soon established, and the clinical use of surgical ligation or proximal occlusion is limited. Possibly, intermittent arterial occlusion after hepatic sceletation may have a better effect (18).

Based on the same concept as surgical ligation of the hepatic artery, peripheral hepatic artery embolization (HAE) has been developed (1, 2, 7, 11, 18) and has become a widely accepted modality for radiological intervention in patients with liver metastases from carcinoid tumors. The advantage of HAE is that when collateral circulation develops, (23) it is less pronounced than after proximal occlusion. HAE should

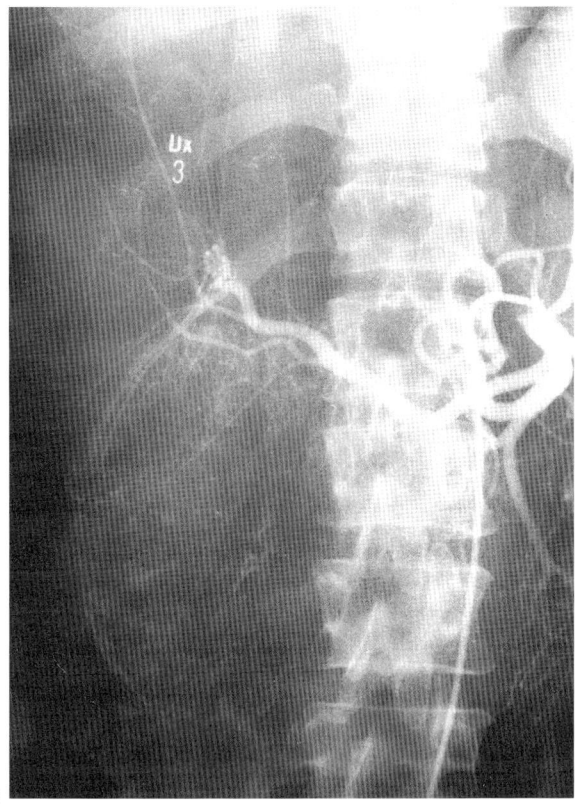

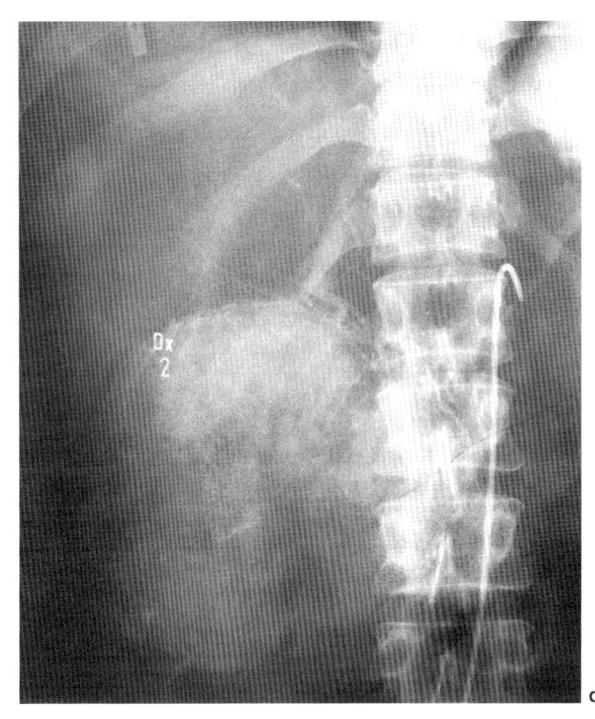

Fig. 7.**22c+d**

be considered a palliative treatment with a time-limited effect that will never cure the patient. It should be performed as a distal arterial embolization because proximal arterial occlusions are rapidly circumvented by collaterals (8).

Liquid embolization materials are not suitable for liver embolization because they may induce severe intrahepatic complications (9). Pieces of Gelfoam sponge, Gelfoam powder, or particles from polyvinyl alcohol (Ivalon) have all been used. Gelfoam powder is no longer commercially produced, and embolization with Gelfoam pieces is time consuming. At present, Ivalon with a particle size of 50–150 μm or 150–300 μm is the material of choice. The clinical response to embolization seems to be independent of the embolization material with a resulting significant decrease of hormone secretion from the tumor in around 80% and a significant reduction of tumor size in 50%. The duration of response varies from 6 months to several years, but the mean response lasts generally about 12 months. Earlier, both liver lobes were often embolized at the same time, but intense adverse reactions after total hepatic artery embolization may occur causing pain, fever, and sometimes life-threatening deterioration of the general condition (7, 15). HEA is mainly indicated in patients with liver metastases from a carcinoid tumor that is not suitable for surgical resection; the clinical symptoms should be progressive, disabling, and resistant to medical treatment with interferon and somatostatin analogs (14, 27).

Angiography including visulization of the portal vein is recommended as a study separate from the interventional procedure. The reason for this is that anatomy may often be complicated by anomalies and at least in these cases, the radiologist, the referring doctor, and the patient should have time to discuss possible risks and benefits of HAE.

Contraindications

Contraindications to embolization are portal vein occlusion, portal hypertension, and jaundice. In portal vein occlusion and portal hypertension, the normal liver parenchyma needs the arterial blood for oxygenation and in jaundice, dilated intrahepatic bile ducts may interfere with the portal circulation (21).

Preparation of the Patient

The patient should be well hydrated and given a continuous, slow i.v. infusion of saline. Another bottle should contain somatostatin analog, ready to give if severe carcinoid symptoms occur. The somatostatin

230 7 Carcinoid

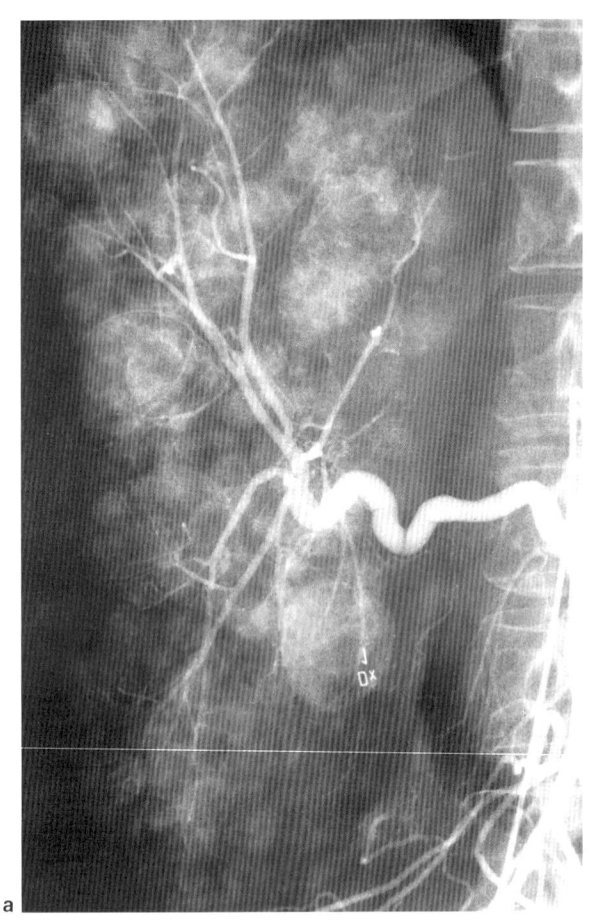

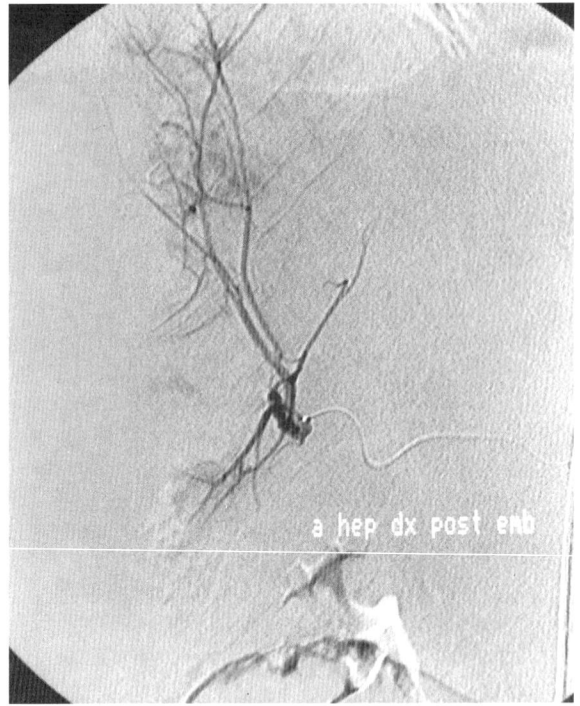

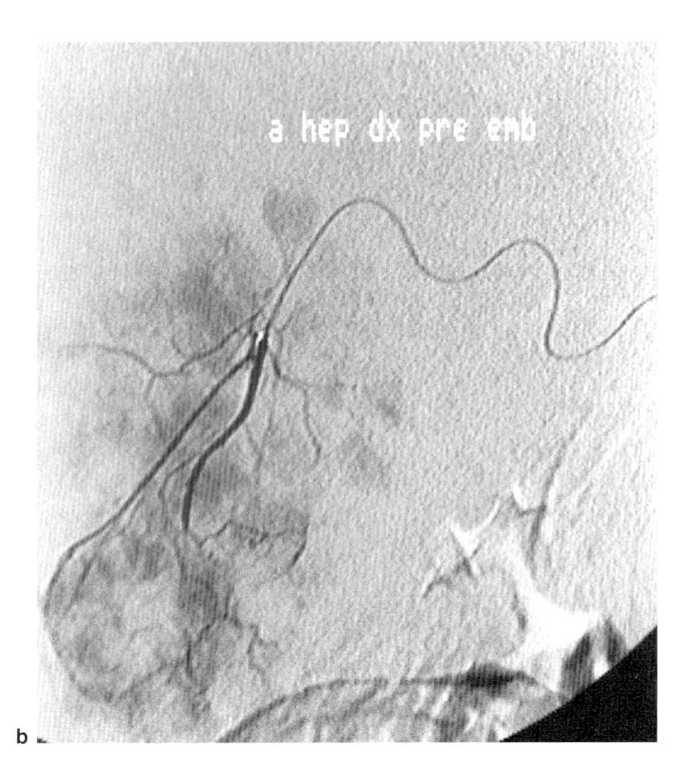

Fig. 7.23 Carcinoid syndrome including tricuspid insufficiency in a 62-year-old patient. (**a**) Superior mesenteric angiography shows a replaced right hepatic artery and multiple hypervascular liver metastases. (**b**) Superselective catheterization of segmental arteries to the posterolateral liver segment before and (**c**) 5 minutes after embolization with Ivalon

analog blocks the effect of hormones released during the embolization, but also reduces the hepatic arterial flow and should therefore, if possible, not be given until the embolization is finished. The majority of reports on HAE recommend that the patient be pretreated with antibiotics systemically. Some authors even recommend a mixture of antibiotics in the embolization material (2). Sterilization of the gut has also been used prior to embolization. It is always convenient for the patient to have a urethral catheter because forced diuresis will be medically induced during the first days after treatment (see below).

Embolization Technique

One of the reported complications of HAE is embolization of the cystic artery with concomitant gall bladder necrosis. With modern catheterization techniques, however, embolization peripheral to the origin of the cystic artery is possible. Thus, previously recommended preoperative cholecystectomy seems unnecessary.

The aim is always lobar embolization as opposed to total liver embolization. For most instances, conventional catheters and guidewires are sufficient. A good combination in our hands is a cobra-shaped, braided catheter with an outer diameter of 1.3 mm (Cordis) in combination with an angled, low-friction guidewire (Terumo). If the patient is catabolic and weak, fractionated embolization in one or two segmental arteries at a time with an interval of 4–6 weeks is prefered (Fig. 7.**23**). In such cases, a coaxial catheter system is very helpful (Tracker, Terumo, Ingenor). The embolic material is mixed with contrast medium and injected in small amounts during fluoroscopic control until blood flow has decreased to almost total arrest. When coaxial systems with a small inner lumen are used, particle size of 50–150 μm is recommended beause the bigger particles may obstruct the catheter lumen. Surprisingly small amounts of embolic material are needed to dearterialize a liver lobe and it is wise to use small syringes (2–5 mL). Peripheral HAE should never be combined with a proximal hepatic artery occlusion because of the risk of total liver infarction (24). The i. v. infusion of the somatostatin analog is started immediately after the embolization at a rate of 50–100 μg/h. After a control angiography to evaluate the effect of embolization, the catheter is withdrawn, and the patient is taken to an intensive care unit for 24 hours for pain treatment, hydration, and circulation control. To reduce the risk of renal tubular failure, the urine output should be kept at 2500–3000 mL/24 h during the first 2–3 days by appropriate administration of fluid and diuretics.

Even if the HAE is a palliative procedure, it is reported that patients previously embolized for carcinoid metastases respond better to various forms of medical treatment (11). The reason for this is unclear, but the finding puts HAE in a favorable light. The embolization may be repeated several times, but the efficiency seems to diminish with the number of embolizations directed against the same area of the liver, possibly due to the development of collateral circulation.

Adverse Reactions

Adverse reactions are related to the size of the embolized area of the liver. If both liver lobes are embolized adverse reactions are almost invariably most severe. Fever and abdominal pain occur regularly and last for 1–7 days after embolization. If the tumor necrosis is large, the split products from the necrosis may impair renal tubular function and result in renal failure (7, 15). This is best avoided by gentle embolization of one lobe or even of one or two segments of the liver at a time, with repeated embolizations at separate occasions within a 4–6-week interval.

With ultrasound, CT, and even with plain radiography, air may be seen in the embolized tumor during the first days after embolization. Usually, this phenomenon is harmless, and the finding should not be diagnosed as an abscess unless there is strong clinical evidence.

References

1. Allison DJ, Medlin IM, Jenkins WJ. Treatment of carcinoid liver metastases by hepatic artery embolization. Lancet. 1977;2:1323.
2. Allison DJ. Additional experience with hepatic embolization: Endocrine metastases. In: Clinical Radiology of the Liver. Ed. by Herlinger H, Lunderquist A, Wallace S, eds. Marcel Dekker, Inc. New York. 1985.
3. Antony PP, Drury RAB. Elastic vascular sclerosis of mesenteric blood vessels in argentaffin carcinoma. J Clin Pathol. 1970;23:110.
4. Bengmark S, Rosengreen L. Angiographic study of the collateral circulation of the liver after ligature of the hepatic arteries in man. Am J Surg. 1970;119:620.
5. Breedis C, Young G. The blood supply of neoplasms in the liver. Am J Pathol. 1954;30:969.
6. Boijsen E, Kaude J, Tylén U. Radiologic diagnosis of ileal carcinoid tumors. Acta Radiol. 1974;15:65.
7. Carrasco CH, Charsangajev C, Ajani J, Samaan NA, Richli W, Wallace S. The carcinoid syndrome: Palliation by hepatic artery embolization. AJR. 1986;147:149.
8. Chuang VP, Wallace S. Current status of thanscatheter management of neoplasms. Cardiovasc Intervent Radiol. 1980;3:256.
9. Doppman J. Bile duct cysts secondary to liver infarcts. Radiology. 1979;130:1.
10. Eckerhauser FE, Argenta LC, Strodel WE, Wheeler RH, Bull FE, Appelman HD, Thompson NW. Mesenteric angiopathy, intestinal gangrene, and midgut carcinoids. Surgery. 1981;90:719.
11. Hansen LE, Schrumpf E, Kolbensved AN, Tausjö J, Dolva LÖ. Recombinant a-2 interferon with and without hepatic artery embolization in the treatment of midgut carcinoid tumors. Acta Oncol. 1989;28:439.
12. Hudson HL, Margulis AR. The roentgen findings of carcinoid tumors of the gastrointestinal tract. AJR. 1964;91:833.
13. Kowlessar OD, Law DH, Sleisenger MH. Malabsorption syndrome associated with metastatic carcinoid tumor. Am J Med. 1959;27:673.
14. Kvols LK, Moertel CG, O'Connell MJ, Schutt AJ, Rubin J, Hahn RG. Treatment of the malignant carcinoid syndrome. Evaluation of a long-acting somatostatin analogue. N Engl J Med. 1986;315:663.

15 Löfberg AM, Lörelius LE, Eriksson B, Öberg K. Malignant neuroendocrine tumors of the gastrointestinal tract—Response to arterial embolization. Acta Oncol. [In press].
16 Lunderquist A. Arterial segmental supply of the liver. An angiographic study. Acta Radiologica Suppl. 1967:272.
17 Makridis C, Öberg K, Juhlin C, et al. Surgical treatment of midgut carcinoid tumors. World J Surg. 1990;14:377.
18 Nobin A, Månsson B, Lunderquist A. Evaluation of temporary liver dearterialization and embolization in patients with metastatic carcinoid tumor. Acta Oncol. 1989;28:419.
19 Qizilbash AH. Carcinoid tumours, vascular elastosis, and ischemic disease of the small intestine. Dis Colon Rect. 1977;20:554.
20 Reuter SR, Boijsen E. Angiographic findings in two ileal carcinoid tumours. Radiology. 1966;87:836.
21 Reuter SR, Chuang VP. The location of increased resistance to portal blood flow in obstructive jaundice. Invest Radiol. 1976;1:54.
22 Reuter SR, Redman HC, Cho KJ. Gastrointestinal angiography. Philadelphia: WB Saunders; 1986.
23 Stridbeck H, Lörelius LE, Reuter SR. Collateral circulation following repeat distal embolization of the hepatic artery in pigs. Invest Radiol. 1984;19:179.
24 Stridbeck H, Lörelius LE. Liver necrosis after hepatic dearterialization in pigs. Cardiovasc Intervent Radiol. 1985;8:50.
25 Williams ED, Sandler M. The classification of carcinoid tumours. Lancet. 1963;1:238.
26 Åkerström G, Makridis C, Johansson H. Abdominal Surgery in patients with midgut carcinoid tumors. Acta Oncol. 1991;30:547.
27 Öberg K, Norheim I, Lind E, et al. Treatment of malignant carcinoid tumors with human leukocyte interferon: Long term results. Cancer Treat Rep. 1986;70:1297.

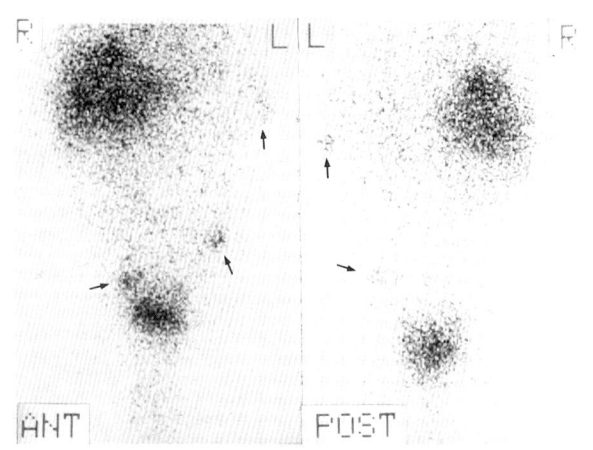

Fig. 7.**24** 76-year-old patient with multifocal carcinoid of the small bowels. I-131-mIBG scintigraphy 24 hours after injection shows residual activity in the bladder and liver. Note focally increased uptake in the abdomen due to multifocal tumor of the small bowels (arrows). Inhomogeneous liver uptake due to multiple intrahepatic metastases

Nuclear Medicine

U. Keske

Carcinoids are neuroendocrine tumors that arise from the enterochromaffin cells and are considered to be part of the APUD system (9). They occur principally in the submucosa of the intestine and main bronchi (7).

Imaging Technique

^{131}I or ^{131}I-MIBG, a guanethidine analog also used for adrenal medullary imaging, is used. Eighteen MBq of ^{131}I-MIBG or 370 MBq ^{123}I-MIBG are given intravenously (8). Patient preparation with Lugol's solution (strong iodine solution) (10 drops/day) or potassium perchlorate (300 mg/day) 1 day before and for 1 week after the administration of MIBG is necessary.

Radiation exposure for ^{131}I resp. ^{123}I-MIBG is 2 resp. 2.5 mGy for the liver, 5 resp. 3 mGy for the ovaries, 0.5 resp. 2 mGy for the whole body and 500 resp. 800 mGy for the adrenal medullary (8).

A large-field gamma camera should be used. Imaging of the thorax and abdomen in anterior and posterior views is performed 24, 48, and 72 hours after injection. Late scanning may improve visualization of hepatic metastases (5). Lateral views may be helpful. At least 50 000 to 100 000 counts per image are needed.

Scintigraphic Findings

Physiological tracer uptake is seen in the adrenal medulla and in organs with adrenergic innervation (salivary glands, spleen, myocardium), and also in excretory organs (liver, bowels, kidneys, and bladder). Kidney uptake is usually transient (3). Major locations of carcinoids are the stomach, duodenum, bronchus, jejunum and ileum, appendix (mostly asymptomatic), colon, and rectum (7). Tumor uptake is found in 59–73% of patients (4, Irvine). In a study by Hanson et al., (4) in 82 patients, pathologic uptake was seen more frequently in patients with elevated serum serotonin or, to a lesser extent, elevated urine 5-HIAA. Other authors found no correlation between urinary 5-HIAA levels and MIBG uptake (1, 5, 6). Mitgut carcinoids (ileum, cecum) seem to concentrate MIBG more readily than foregut carcinoids (pancreas, stomach, bronchus, see Feldman et al. [2]). MIBG uptake is not bound to the presence of the carcinoid syndrome (4).

Metastases are frequently found in the liver and may also show tracer uptake. Visualization of lymphomas is also possible (2).

Tracer uptake is also seen in pheochromocytomas, medullary carcinomas of the thyroid, neuroectodermal tumors (thymomas, oat cell carcinomas, ganglioneuroblastomas, and ganglioneuromas (3, 4, 9).

Treatment of malignant carcinoid tumors with a high MIBG uptake with large doses of ^{131}I-MIBG is possible (5).

References

1. Bomanji J, Levison DA, Zutarte J, Britton KE. Imaging of Carcinoid Tumors with Iodine-123 Metaiodobenzylguanidine. J Nucl Med. 1987;28:1907–1910.
2. Feldman JM, Blinder RA, Lucas KJ, Coleman E. Iodine-131 Metaiodobenzylguanidine Scintigraphy of Carcinoid Tumors. J Nucl Med. 1986;27:1691–1696.
3. Gross MD, Shapiro B, Thrall JH. Adrenal Scintigraphy. In: Gottschalk A, Hoffer PB, Potchen EH, eds. Volume 2. Diagnostic Nuclear Medicine. 2nd ed. Baltimore: Williams & Wilkins; 1988:815–882.
4. Hanson MW, Feldman JM, Blinder RA, Moore JO, Coleman RE. Carcinoid Tumors: Iodine-131 MIBG Scintigraphy. Radiology. 1989;17:699–703.
5. Hoefnagel CA, den Hartog Jager FCA, Taal BG, Abeling NGGM, Engelsman EE. The role of I-131-MIBG in the diagnosis and therapy of carcinoids. Eur J Nucl Med. 1987;13:187–191.
6. Jodrell M, Irvine AT, McCready VR, Woodcraft E, Smith IE. The use of ^{131}I-MIBG in the imaging of metastatic carcinoid tumors. Brit J Cancer. 1988;58:663–664.
7. Maton PN. The Carcinoid Tumor and the Carcinoid Syndrome. In: Becker KL, ed. Principles and Practice of Endocrinology and Metabolism. Philadelphia: Lippincott; 1990:1640–1643.
8. Montz R. Nebennieren und Nebenschilddrüse. In: Büll U, Hör G, eds. Klinische Nuklearmedizin. 1st ed. Weinheim: VCH Verlagsgesellschaft; 1987:125–132.
9. von Moll L, McEwan AJ, Shapiro B, et al. Iodine-131 MIBG Scintigraphy of Neuroendocrine Tumors Other than Pheochromocytoma and Neuroblastoma. J Nucl Med. 1987;28:979–988.

A Radiologist's View

A. Lunderquist

The early diagnosis of carcinoid tumors is hampered by the relative lack of symptoms in the early stage of the disease. The proportion of patients with symptomatic tumors is similar to that of patients with incidentally found tumors. Patients with symptoms have a significantly increased frequency of metastatic disease compared to patients with no symptoms (76% versus 7%) (1). Gastrointestinal hemorrhage is an uncommon symptom and not neccessarily related to the size of the tumor. Massive hemorrhage can be caused by very small primary tumors (2). Clinical presentation with abdominal pain, signs of intestinal obstruction or diarrhea occurs in about 40% of patients and may be an indication for small bowel enteroclysis. This examination can reveal a polypoid lesion or suggestion of an abdominal mass with signs of bowel strictures, adhesions, and edema. Carcinoid syndrome is an uncommon initial symptom (4%) and suggests hepatic metastases.

Because abdominal CT has become a rather common diagnostic procedure in patients with obscure symptoms, findings of small calcifications, mass lesions involving bowel loops and mesentery may also suggest a correct diagnosis without signs of liver metastases. The diagnosis can be strengthened with the aid of ^{131}I-MIGB scintigraphy, which has proven to be a sensitive procedure for the detection of intestinal carcinoid tumors. Liver metastases of carcinoid tumors may sometimes be difficult to reveal on CT because tumor attenuation may be almost identical to that of normal liver parenchyma, both on unenhanced and on enhanced scans (4). Negative CT results do not exclude liver metastases, which is why additional imaging methods such as ultrasound, MRI, angiography, or a combination thereof are useful. Enough experience has not yet been collected with MR in the diagnosis of carcinoid liver metastases. MR seems, however, to be slightly superior to CT in localizing the lesions. Not infrequently, angiography can demonstrate 2–3 mm liver metastases, which are not visible with other techniques.

Nonsurgical patients with carcinoid syndrome resistant to treatment with interferon or somatostatin analogs are usually referred to the interventional radiologists for HAE, a treatment that can markedly improve the patient's quality of life even if the tumor growth is only slightly retarded.

As pointed out by Lörelius, the embolic material should be small enough to be able to pass into 100–200 μm arterial branches, but not farther. For this purpose, Gelfoam or Ivalon powder has been used. The pliability of Gelfoam particles enables them to pass into vessels smaller than the actual size of the particle. Unfortunately, resorbable Gelfoam powder is no longer commercially available and nonresorbable Ivalon has to be used. If embolization performed with these materials is too heavy, arterial branches to the peribiliary plexa will become obliterated, and damage to the bile ducts similar to sclerosing cholangitis can be produced (5). Already a smaller amount of embolic materials, if mixed with cytotoxic drugs, can produce this damage (6). During the last few years, tumor treatment with arterial embolization with a mixture of Lipiodol and cytotoxic drugs has been used. When this mixture is injected into the hepatic artery, a large proportion of the oil passes immediately through the peribiliary plexa into the portal vein. Sinusoidal perfusion is then blocked by Lipiodol in the peripheral portal and the arterial branches. Arterial pressure is the only propulsive force to clean the vessels of oil, a procedure that takes several hours (7). If embolization with the Lipiodol mixture is followed by more proximal embolization with Ivalon, clearing of the sinusoids will be markedly retarded, and parenchymal necrosis will follow. A combination of intra-arterial Lipiodol embolization and chemotherapy has not yet been reported as a treatment of carcinoid liver metastases, but it is important to know possible side effects if such a treatment is tried.

References

1 MacGillivray DC, Snyder DA, Drucker W, ReMine SG. Carcinoid tumors: The relationship between clinical presentation and the extent of disease. Surgery. 1991;110:68.
2 Miller GA, Borten MM. Primary carcinoid tumor of the ileum associated with massive gastrointestinal haemorrhage. Aust N Z J Surg. 1991;61:645.
3 Adolph JMG, Kimmig BN, Georgi P, zum Winkel K. Carcinoid tumors: CT and I-131 metaiodo-benzylguanidin scintigraphy. Radiology. 1987;164:199.
4 Sako M, Lunderquist A, Owman T, Mårtensson H, Nobin A. Angiographic and computed tomographic appearance of secondary carcinoid of the liver. Cardiovasc Intervent Radiol. 1982;5:90.
5 Makuuchi M, Sukigara M, Mori T, et al. Bile duct necrosis: Complication of transcatheter hepatic arterial embolization. Radiology. 1985;156:331.
6 Ludvig J, Kim CH, Wiesner RH, Krom RA. Floxuridine-induced scerlosing cholangitis: An ischemic cholangiopathy? Hepatology. 1989;9:215.
7 Kan ZX, Ivancev K, Hägerstrand I, Chuang VP, Lunderquist A. In vivo microscopy of the liver after injection of Lipiodol into the hepatic artery and portal vein in the rat. Acta Radiol. 1989;30:419.

8 Multiple Endocrine Neoplasia

Endocrinology

K. Öberg

Multiple endocrine neoplasia is an inherited disorder of the neuroendocrine cell system. Two distinct entities can be recognized. MEN type I which ist the coexistence of hyperplasia and of neoplasia of the anterior pituitary gland, the parathyroids, and endocrine pancreas. MEN type II ist a genetically determined coexistence of pheocromocytomas and thyroid medullary carcinoma with or without hyperparathyroidism. A subgroup of MEN type II is called type II B or type III, which includes medullary thyroid carcinomas, marfanoid features, mucosal neurinomas, intestinal gangliomatosis, and medulated corneal nerve fibers.

Multiple Endocrine Neoplasia Type I (MEN I)

The first detected association of two MEN I lesions was reported by Erdheim in 1903 (1). However, it was not until 1954 that it was reported again when Wermer described a family in which the father and four of nine siblings were affected by tumors in two or more endocrine glands (Wermer's syndrome) (2). The MEN I syndrome ist an autosomally inherited disease with somewhat varying penetrance that affects half of the family members, equally in both sexes. Several hypotheses of the pathogenesis of the MEN I syndrome have been proposed, but the most attractive is currently the two mutation model of oncogenesis by Knudson (3). The first mutation occurs in germ cells, is present in all cells, and is followed by a second mutation, which occurs in somatic cells and represents an elimination of the normal allele ("wild type" allele). This hypothesis has been tested by using restriction fragment lengths polymorphis analysis (RFLP), and we have thus been able to locate a specific deletion to chromosome 11 locus q13 also called PYGM locus. This genetic defect might represent a loss of a tumor suppressor gene (4, 5).

Clinical Features

The actual prevalence of MEN I is difficult to assess because endocrine abnormalities can be asymptomatic. However, estimated prevalences are 0.02–0.2/1000 (6). Among unselected patients with HPT, about 18% are associated with the MEN I syndrome. 54% with Zollinger–Ellison syndrome, and 4% of insulinomas display a concomitant MEN I trait. In a series of 1500 pituitary tumors subjected to neurosurgery 2.7% occurred in the setting of MEN I (7). The clinical presentation of MEN I syndrome depends largely on the glands involved and whether or not the lesions hypersecrete symptom-causing hormones.

Parathyroid Lesion

The parathyroid lesion includes multicentric chief cell hyperplasia or adenomas and is the most common finding, present in 87–97% of necropsies (8, 9). The parathyroid glands are virtually always involved in patients with MEN type I and have been suggested to constitute the presenting lesions in the MEN I trait (10). Symptoms of HPT in MEN I are similar to those in sporadic cases, and although asymptomatic hypercalcemia is common, the diagnosis of HPT is confirmed by findings of hypercalcemia associated with an inappropriately elevated serum PTH level. Treatment of HPT involves surgical ablation of all glands with immediate autotransplantation of about 50–60 mg parathyroid tissue (11).

Pancreatic Lesion

The reported prevalence of pancreatic involvement in MEN I-affected individuals varies between 30% (screening materials) and 82% (necropsy materials) (6, 8, 9). However, recently in a ten year prospective screening study in four kindreds including 80 individuals, we demonstrated 75% penetrance of islet cell disease and 90% for primary HPT, which equals the prevalence of autopsy studies (12). Furthermore, age at presentation of MEN I trait averaged 18 years. Pancreatic endocrine involvement was recognized at a mean age of 25 years and constituted the presenting lesion in a majority of the patients. This represents a lowering of the "detection age" by about two decades (12).

Pancreatic lesions are multicentric and consist of different stages of endocrine cell proliferation; hyperplasia, adenomas, and carcinomas (Fig. 8.1). The clinical symptoms are dependent on the particular hormone production in the lesions. Even though the pancreatic endocrine tumors may secrete several peptides, one of them is usually predominant and associated with a specific syndrome. Most frequent of the classic endocrine syndromes seen in MEN I pancreatic tumor patients is the Zollinger–Ellison syndrome with gastritis and recurrent ulcer disease due to gastrin-producing tumors and hypoglycemic symptoms due to insulinoma (8, 13, 14). Other peptides involved in different combinations are vasoactive intestinal polypeptide (VIP), pancreatic polypeptide (PP), glucagon, somatostatin, and calcitonin (14). The diagnosis of pancreatic endocrine tumors is confirmed by findings of elevated basal peptide levels or specific stimulation or supression tests (Table 8.1) (12, 13, 14, 16).

Due to the multiplicity of the pancreatic endocrine lesion in MEN I, the only curative treatment available is total pancreatectomy. However, this procedure is rarely indicated, and instead partial resections and enucleations of lesions in the pancreas are applied. Symptomatic therapy by medication comprises histamine receptor blocking agents or inhibitors of the proton pump of parietal cells for Zollinger–Ellison syndrome, diazoxide in hypoglycemic patients, and long-acting somatostatin analogs (12, 14). For malignant and for recurrent pancreatic disease, chemotherapy with streptozocin, or treatment with interferon has been applied with promising results (14, 15).

It is important to realize that when Zollinger–Ellison syndrome is present in a patient with MEN type I, the increased gastrin secretion might be related to endocrine pancreatic lesions or to concomitant duodenal neuroendocrine tumors (carcinoids), or both (17).

Pituitary Lesion

Reported prevalences of lesions in the anterior pituitary are largely determined from reviewing MEN I necropsy cases in the literature, which range from 50–66% (8, 9). In a retrospective study from the Mayo Clinic, 27% of MEN I pituitary tumors subjected to surgery were micro-adenomas, and the remaining 73% were macroadenomas (7). Furthermore, it was concluded that the MEN I-associated pituitary adenomas are more often endocrinologically functional and display multiple hormone production. Tumors devoid of significant immunoreactivity for known pituitary hormones (Null cell adenomas) were observed in 7%. In comparison to pituitary adenomas occuring in the general population, the MEN I pituitary lesions were more frequently growth hormone and prolactin immunoreactive or both. Clinically, prolactinomas are most common with or without amenorrhea (10, 16). Diagnosis depends on endocrine assessment and detection of tumor mass. The management policies of MEN I pituitary lesions have largely been the same as those for sporadic pituitary adenomas, although no systematic evaluation of these issues has been reported.

Other Lesions

Adrenal cortical involvement is very common in patients with MEN I and ranges from 36–41% in large necropsy series (8, 9). Little clinical significance has been ascribed to the MEN I adrenal lesions because they are almost invariably nonfunctional except for a few cases of adrenocortical carcinomas. The lesions often consist of bilateral, difuse hyperplasia as well as microadenomas and macroadenomas (8, 18). The mesodermally derived adrenal cortex ist steroid hormone producing in contrast to the peptide hormone production of other involved organs in the MEN I complex. The adrenal cortical lesions, although rather frequent, do not display loss of gene locus 11q13 and thus, do not represent a "true" MEN I lesion (19). In agreement with the findings in sporadic cases of adrenocortical carcinoma, the genome showed loss of constitutional heterozygocity for the alleles of 17p, 13q, 11p, and 11q. The benign adrenal lesions retained heterozygocity for the MEN I locus chromosome 11q13. Pancreatic endocrine tumors were present in all the MEN I individuals with adrenal

Table 8.1   Biochemical screening program for MEN I

Hematology (hemoglobin, leukocyte and platelet count)
Sedimentation rate
Blood glucose
Albumin-correted total serum calcium
Serum creatinin
Serum sodium
Serum potassium
Serum aspartate aminotransferase
Serum alanine aminotransferase
Serum PTH
Serum prolactin
Serum GH (+ Serum IGF-1)
Serum insulin
Plasma proinsulin
Plasma C peptide
Serum pp
Serum gastrin
Serum calcitonin
Plasma glucagon
Plasma somatostatin
Plasma VIP
Serum HCG subunits α and β
Meal stimulation test

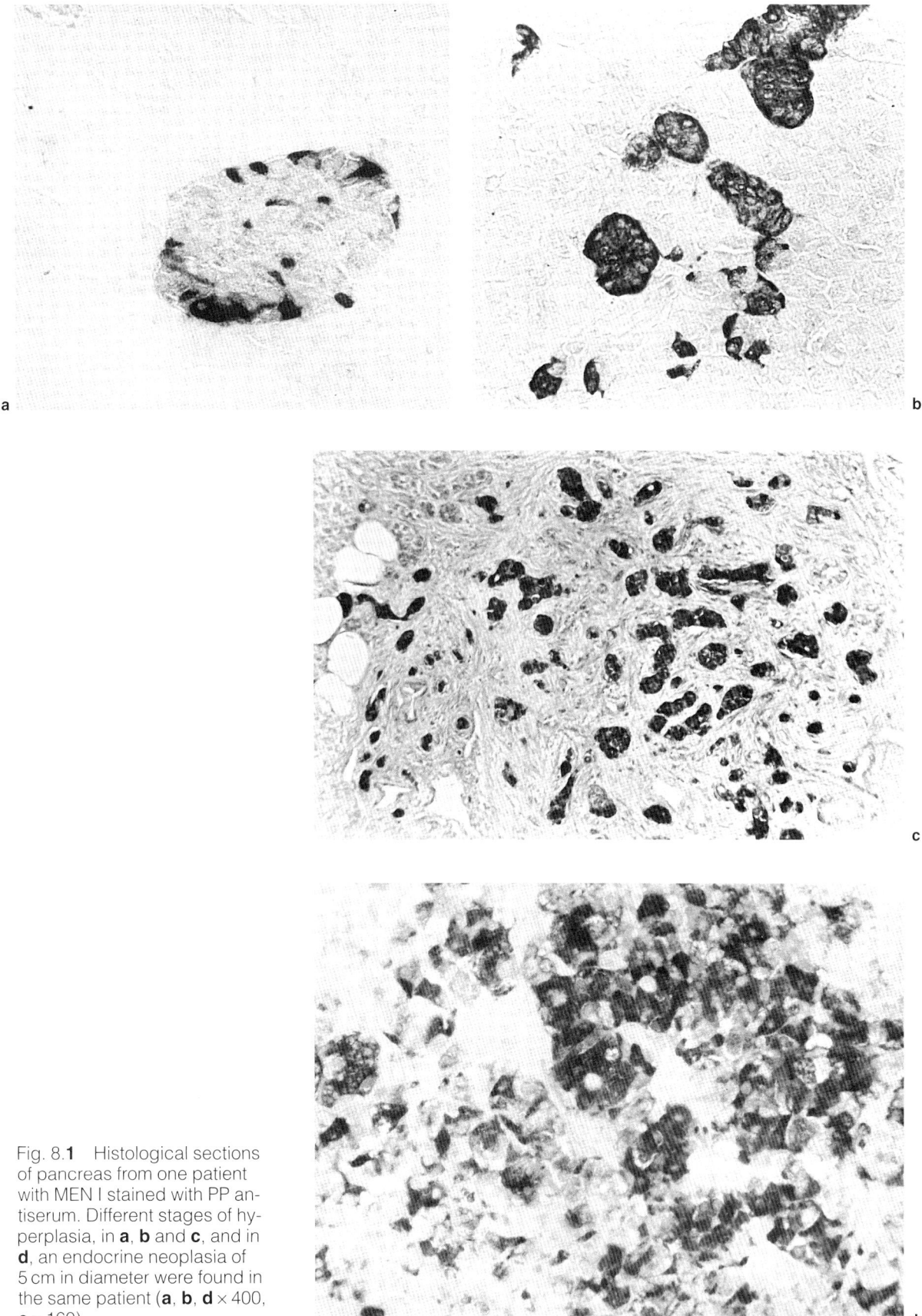

Fig. 8.1 Histological sections of pancreas from one patient with MEN I stained with PP antiserum. Different stages of hyperplasia, in **a**, **b** and **c**, and in **d**, an endocrine neoplasia of 5 cm in diameter were found in the same patient (**a**, **b**, **d** × 400, **c** × 160)

involvement, which might indicate some relation between these two MEN I lesions (19).

Thyroid disease, with an inconsistent pattern of involvement, has also been reported in MEN I patients (thyroid adenoma, coloid goiter, carcinoma, and thyrotoxicosis) (8, 9, 18). Furthermore, in the same papers, findings of lipomas, foregut carcinoids (bronchial, thymic, duodenal, or gastric), and pinealomas have also been reported.

Biochemical Diagnosis

A biochemical screening program for MEN I is listed in Table 8.1. The meal stimulation test has been particularly useful in the screening for involvement of the endocrine pancreas in families with MEN type I (20). By using this mixed meal stimulation test that measures secretion of PP and gastrin, we demonstrated an abnormal secretion pattern for a median of 4 years previous to radiological detection of any endocrine pancreatic lesion. For genetic determination, high molecular DNA was isolated from tumor tissue and corresponding leukocytes (peripheral blood). The DNA were then analyzed using the Southern blot method applying radiolabelled DNA probes. Using the suggested screening battery for various peptide hormones, the sensitivity of different tumor markers in nonprospectively and prospectively diagnosed pancreatic endocrine tumors is listed in Table 8.2.

Prognosis

The prognosis of MEN I depends on several factors but can generally be denoted as good in comparison with other potentially malignant diseases. Involvement of the endocrine pancreas is the most life-threatening lesion. An assessment of survival rates in patients with sporadic endocrine tumors compared to those that occur as part of the MEN I trait showed a significantly longer survival for the MEN I patients with an average of 15 years from diagnosis (14).

Table 8.2 Sensitivity of tumor markers among patients with prospectively and nonprospectively diagnosed pancreatic endocrine tumors

	Nonprospective (%)	Prospective (%)
Serum PP	67	67
Serum gastrin	67	22
Serum proinsulin	58	56
Serum insulin	46	56
Serum HCG α/β	26/33	11/0
Plasma glucagon	27	37
Plasma VIP	20	0
Meal test	100	75

Multiple Endocrine Neoplasia Type II (MEN II)

MEN II, or Sipple syndrome, is a genetically determined entity of disorders involving multiple endocrine glands (21). Most common are multiple bilateral adrenal pheocromocytoma, medullary carcinoma of the thyroid, and HPT or both either due to parathyroid hyperplasia or adenoma. A variant of MEN II, also called II B or MEN III, includes association of neurofibromatosis with pheocromocytoma, marfanoid features, mucosal neuromas, and intestinal ganglioneuromas (22). The condition of MEN II is autosomally dominantly inherited with varying degree of penetrance. Recently, a specific genetic deletion has been located on chromosome 10 (23).

Medullary Carcinoma of the Thyroid

Medullary thyroid carcinomas are the most frequent lesions found in MEN II. About 25% of cases of medullary thyroid carcinoma are familial (24). Approximately 5–10% of all thyroid carcinomas are of the medullary type. These tumors may either exist alone or with other tumors as part of the MEN II syndrome. The clinical manifestations of this tumor are remarkably disperse (24, 25). In early stages, and particulary during screening procedures in MEN II families, most of the affected members are completely asymptomatic. Only 50% of MEN II gene carriers will have presented symptoms by the age of 55 because clinical penetrance of the MEN II gene is incomplete (26). In later stages, the patient may manifest neck mass, watery diarrhea, flushing, peptic ulcer disease, hypertension, and hypercalcemia (25).

As a malignancy of thyroid C cells, the tumors always secrete calcitonin and calcitonin gene-related peptide (CGRP), or both. Other ectopically produced hormones may be ACTH, VIP, somatostatin and serotonin (25). Patients with medullary carcinoma of the thyroid show elevated basal levels of calcitonin in the plasma. In patients with early disease and small adenoma or hyperplasia of the C cells, administration of calcitonin secretagogs such as calcium or penta-gastrin are necessary to demonstrate the presence of excessive C cell function (26, 27). The penta-gastrin stimulation test has proved to be particularly useful in the screening of MEN II families (28). It is important to note that calcitonin may be ectopically produced by endocrine pancreatic tumors and lung tumors also and may thus be a part of the MEN I syndrome instead of MEN II (14).

In MEN II families, early screening for medullary thyroid carcinoma and early surgery will prevent death and distressing symptoms due to metastatic or local invasive diseases (29). Even after severe metastasizing, the medullary thyroid carcinoma of the MEN II syndrome seems to run a more indolent course than the sporadic tumors. Neither radiotherapy nor chemotherapy (doxorubicin) have demonstrated any significant antitumor effect. Somatostatin analog may sometimes ameliorate flushing and diarrhea.

Pheocromocytoma

The prevalence of pheocromocytoma in MEN II is difficult to determine because of the difficulty of diagnosing pheocromocytoma. The tumor often remains asymptomatic, and even provocative tests often fail (30). More than 50 percent of patients with MEN type IIa will eventually have adrenal medullary abnormalities (31). The affected MEN II members often present bilateral adrenal pheocromocytoma (31). The clinical presentation is not different from sporadic cases with pheocromocytoma and hypertension, which are the most common clinical features of this illness (30). In early stages, the hypertension may not be manifest with sporadic attacks may occuring at intervals of days, weeks, or months. Other features are headache, excessive sweating, pallor, or flushing. Sudden onset of tachycardia, palpitations, or arryhtmia is quite common and may be provoked by physical exercise (30). In addition to hypertension, increased concentration of free fatty acids and glucose related to catecholamine excess, can be noticed.

The diagnosis is based on typical clinical symptoms and biochemical testing. However, most patients do not present distinct clinical symptoms or abnormalities in catecholamine excretion until they have an adrenal tumor that can be radiologically verified (31). Past efforts using stimulatory agents, histamine, or glucagon to diagnose pheocromocytoma in MEN II have been unsuccessful and are potentially dangerous (32). Catecholamines in the urine and analysis of norepinephrine and adrenaline in plasma during attacks is widely applied (30). Under normal circumstances, the diagnosis of pheocromocytoma may be either confirmed or excluded on the basis of the analysis of a single 24 hour urine collection assayed for catecholamines, metanephrines, or vanilylmandelic acid (VMA). This holds true if the patient is significantly hypertensive during the period of collection (30). However, in early stages it is quite difficult to diagnose pheocromocytomas by analyzing basal urine catecholamine excretion. A bicycle exercise test measuring plasma epinephrine may distinguish patients with pheocromocytoma from healthy subjects. Recently, determination of a plasma glycoprotein, chromogranin, secreted along with catecholamines has proved to be quite efficient and may also detect catecolamine "negative" patients (34). Furthermore, determination of neuropeptide Y (NPY) can be helpful in the early diagnosis of pheocromocytoma (35).

Treatment is based on surgical resection of the pheocromocytoma. In sporadic cases of pheocromocytoma with unilateral lesions, adrenalectomy is quite common, but in MEN II patients with bilateral lesions, partial resections of the medullary part of the adrenals has been recommended to avoid adrenal insufficiency (B. Hamberger, personal communication, 30).

Parathyroid Disease

Parathyroid involvement occurs in 10–20% of family members proved to have MEN II (32, 36). Parathyroid involvement in MEN II is similar to that observed in MEN I and includes adenomas and hyperplasia of single or multiple parathyroid glands or both (32). HPT is not as common in MEN II as in MEN I, and the diagnosis is based on the presence of hypercalcemia and increased PTH levels.

MEN IIb (MEN III)

This condition is an uncommon variant of MEN II, in which medullary thyroid carcinoma and pheocromocytoma are associated with several other abnormalities including a characteristic facies, ganglioneuromatosis of the bowel, and a marfanoid body habitus. Medullary thyroid carcinoma commonly presents earlier and is more aggressive than in MEN IIa.

Biochemical Screening Program

Table 8.3 presents the suggested screening program for the various MEN II lesions.

Summary

Today, both the diagnosis of MEN types I and II can be diagnosed at an early stage by biochemical testing. Early involvement of various endocrine glands can be unveiled by analyzing various hormones, which can be further improved by stimulatory tests. Genetic screening using the RFLP method can now be per-

Table 8.3 Biochemical screening program for MEN II

Hematology (hemoglobin concentration, leukocyte, platelet count)
Blood glucose
Albumin-corrected total serum calcium
Serum creatinine
Serum PTH
Serum calcitonin (pentagastrin stimulated)
Plasma CGRP
Plasma chromogranin A + B
Plasma NPY
Plasma noradrenaline, adrenaline (during attack or after exercise)
Urine catecholamines (including, metanephrines, VMA, dopamine)

formed in MEN I but not yet in MEN II. When genetic counceling programs are ready for clinical use, the number of family members for biochemical testing can be significantly reduced.

References

1. Erdheim J. Zur normalen und pathologischen histologie der glandula thyroidea, parathyroidea und hypophysis. Beitr Pathol Anat. 1903;33:158–236.
2. Wermer P. Genetic aspects of adenomatosis of endocrine glands. Am J Med. 1954;16:363–371.
3. Knudson AG. Mutation and cancer: Statistical study of retinoblastoma. Proc Natl Acad Sci USA. 1971;68:820–823.
4. Larsson C, Skogseid B, Öberg K, Nakamura Y, Nordenskjöld M. Multiple endocrine neoplasia type I gene maps to chromosome 11 and is lost in insulinomas. Nature. 1988;332:85–87.
5. Nakamura Y, Larsson C, Julier C. et al. Localization of the genetic defect in multiple endocrine neoplasia type 1 within a small region of chromosome 11. Am J Hum Genet. 1989;44:751–755.
6. Brandi ML, Marx SJ, Aurbach GD, Fitzpatrick LA. Familial multiple endocrine neoplasia type I: A new look at pathophysiology. Endocr Rev. 1987;8:391–405.
7. Scheithauer BW, Laws ER, Kovacs K, Horvath E, Randall RV, Carney JA. Pituitary adenomas of the multiple endocrine neoplasia type I syndrome. Semin Diagn Pathol. 1987;4:205–211.
8. Ballard HS, Frame B, Harsock RJ. Familial multiple endocrine adenomapeptic ulcer complex. Medicine (Baltimore). 1964;43:481–516.
9. Eberle F, Grün R. Multiple endocrine neoplasia type 1 (MEN I). Ergeb Inn Med Kinderheilkd. 1981;46:75–149.
10. Benson L, Ljunghall S, Åkerström G, Öberg K. Hyperparathyroidism presenting as the first lesion in multiple endocrine neoplasia type 1. Am J Med. 1987a;82:731–737.
11. Malmaeus J, Benson L, Johansson H, et al. Parathyroid surgery in the multiple endocrine neoplasia type 1 syndrome: Choice of surgical procedure. World J Surg. 1986;10:668–672.
12. Skogseid B, Eriksson B, Lundqvist G, et al.: Multiple endocrine neoplasia type 1 – A ten year prospective screening study in four kindreds. J Clin Endocrinol Metab. 1991;73:281–287.
13. Öberg, K, Wålinder O, Boström H, Lundqvist G, Wide L. Peptide hormone markers in screening for endocrine tumors in multiple endocrine adenomatosis type 1. Am J Med. 1982;73:619–630.
14. Eriksson B. Recent advances in the diagnosis and management of endocrine pancreatic tumors. Comprehensive summaries of Uppsala Disertations from the Faculty of Medicine. Acta Universitatis Upsaliensis. 1988;160:7–90.
15. Eriksson B, Öberg K, Alm G, et al. Treatment of malignant endocrine pancreatic tumors with human leukocyte interferon. Lancet. 1986;II:1307–1309.
16. Marx SJ, Winik AI, Santen RJ, Floyd JC, Mills JL, Green J. Multiple endocrine neoplasia type 1: Assessment of laboratory tests to screen for the gene in a large kindred. Medicine. 1986;65:226–241.
17. Pipeleers-Marichal M, Somers G, Willams G, et al. Gastrinomas in the duodenums of patients with multiple endocrine neoplasia type 1 and the Zollinger-Ellison syndrome. N Engl J Med. 1990;322:723–727.
18. Croisier JC, Azerad E, Lubetzki J. L'adénomatose polyendocrinienne. A propos d'une observation personelle et revenue de la litterature. Sem Hop Paris. 1971;47:494–525.
19. Skogseid B, Larsson C, Lindgren P-G, et al. Clinical and genetic features of adrenal lesions in multiple endocrine neoplasia type 1. J Clin Endocrinol Metab [In press].
20. Skogseid B, Öberg K, Benson L, et al. A standardized meal stimulation test of the endocrine pancreas for early detection of pancreatic endocrine tumors in multiple endocrine neoplasia type 1 syndrome: Five years experience. J Clin Endocrinol Metab. 1987;64:1233–1240.
21. Sipple JH. The association of pheocromocytoma with carcinoma of the thyroid gland. Am J Med. 1961;31:163–166.
22. Rashid M, Khairi M.RA, Dexter RN, Burzynski NJ, Johnson CC jr. Mucosal neuroma, pheocromocytoma and medullary thyroid carcinoma: multiple endocrine neoplasia type 3. Medicine. 1975;54:89–112.
23. Mathew CGP, Chin KS, Easton DF et al. A linked genetic marker for multiple endocrine neoplasia type 2A on chromosome 10. Nature 1987;328:527–528.
24. Saad RK, Ordonez NG, Rashid RK et al. Medullary carcinoma of the thyroid. A study of the clinical features and prognostic factors in 161 patients. Medicine. 1984;63:319–342.
25. Stewart AM, Levine RJ. Neuroendocrine tumor that secrete biologically active peptides and amines. Clin Endocrinol Metab 1977;6:719–743.
26. Ponder B. A. J, Coffey R, Gagel RF, Semple P, Ponder MA, Pembrey ME. Telenius-Berg M, Easton DF, Risk estimation and screening in families of patients with medullary thyroid carcinoma. Lancet. 1988;1:397–410.
27. Wells SA Jr., Baylin SB, Linehan WM, Farrell RE, Cox EB, Cooper CW. Provocative agents and the diagnosis of medullary carcinoma of the thyroid gland. Ann Surg. 1978;188:139–141.
28. Telenius-Berg M, Almqvist S, Berg B, et al. Screening for medullary carcinoma of the thyroid in families with Sipple's syndrome; evaluation of a new stimulation test. Eur J Clin Invest. 1977;7:7–16.
29. Telenius-Berg M, Berg B, Hamberger B et al. Impact of screening on prognosis in the multiple endocrine neoplasia type 2 syndromes; natural history and treatment result in 105 patients. Henry Ford Hosp Med J. 1984;32:225–232.
30. Engelman K. Pheocromocytoma: Clin Endocrinol Metab 1977;6:769–797.
31. Gagel RF, Tashjian AH Jr, Cummings T, et al. The clinical outcome of prospective screening for multiple endocrine neoplasia type 2a. N Engl J Med. 1988;318:478–484.
32. Melvin KEW, Tashjian AM Jr, Miller HH. Studies in familial (medullary) thyroid carcinoma. Rec Prog Horm Res. 1972;28:399–470.
33. Telenius-Berg M, Adolfsson L, Berg B, et al. Catecholamine release after physical exercise; a new provocative test for early diagnosis of pheocromocytoma in multiple endocrine neoplasia type 2. Acta Med Scand. 1987;222:351–359.
34. O'Connor DT, Deftos LJ. Secretion of chromogranin A by peptide producing endocrine neoplasms. N Engl J Med. 1986;314:1145–1151.
35. Lundberg JM, Hökfelt T, Hansen A, et al. Neuropeptide-Y-like immunoreactivity in adrenaline cells of adrenal medulla and in tumors and plasma of pheocromocytoma patients. Reg Pept. 1986;13:169–182.
36. Heath H III, Sizemore GW, Carney JA. Preoperative diagnosis of occult parathyroid hyperplasia by calcium infusion in patients with multiple endocrine neoplasia type 2a. J Clin Endocrinol Metab. 1976;43:428–435.

Imaging

L.-E. Lörelius

The role or radiology in MEN is to localize the tumor that, from the endocrinological point of view, evidently exists. Radiological efforts to find an endocrine tumor in a patient without obvious endocrine dysfunction are usually fruitless.

The radiological diagnosis in patients with MEN II syndrome is not different from that of patients with sporadic pheocromocytoma or medullary thyroid cancer.

For patients with MEN I syndrome, the tumor of the hypophysis and the parathyroid glands are diagnosed the same way as sporadic tumors, but when endocrine pancreatic tumors are indicated, special care must be taken. Most of the patients with MEN I in the first generation already had metastases when diagnosed (8). The goal today is to find the tumors in the siblings of these patients before the tumors spread. Therefore, many of the patients with possible endocrine pancreatic tumors are found when screening MEN I families for endocrine abnormalities. Long before clinical disease is manifested, provocation tests are able to detect endocrine abnormalities. At this stage, tumors should be small or maybe even more similar to cell hyperplasia, but larger tumors with low production of active hormones also occur. In addition to the problem of tumor size, is the high frequency of multiple tumors (Fig. 8.**2**). Small, possibly multiple, tumors in an abdominal organ surrounded by bowel gas are a real challange for the radiologist.

CT with i.v. contrast enhancement, ultrasound, and pancreatic angiography are basic investigations. The results of all these investigations are, however, often negative, especially in screening detected patients, and the sensitivity is not improved even if CT with intra-arterial contrast administration is used (1). Percutaneous transhepatic portography (PTP) has a better sensitivity (5) but is, on the other hand, more complicated both for the patient and for the radiologist. The value of MR has been limited in early stages of MEN I pancreatic lesions. The mere expectation of finding a small tumor might even be a reason why a large tumor can be overlooked (Fig. 8.**3**). In recent years intraoperative ultrasound has been reported to be the method of choice in patients with endocrine tumors of the pancreas (2, 3, 4, 7). The spatial resolution is very high, and tumors with only 2 mm diameter can be detected. The major disadvantage of intraoperative ultrasound is the invasiveness and therefore, some type of preoperative evaluation is needed.

For clinically manifest disease, we use ultrasound, CT with intravenous contrast enhancement and conventional angiography. If these investigations are negative, transhepatic portography with blood sampling from the pancreatic veins is performed. With a positive PTP, the patient can be operated on, preferably with intraoperative ultrasound available.

For screening-detected patients with positive endocrinology but without clinical disease, the situation is much more complicated. One side of the problem is possible malignant transformation of the tumor before detection. The other side is that if multiple tumors are found at operation spread out through the pancreas, the symptom-free patient runs the risk of losing most of his or her pancreas and possibly developing pancreatic insufficiency including diabetes. Because the mean age of the screening-detected patients is about 20 years lower than that of patients with clinical manifest disease (8), this postoperative pancreatic insufficiency might add 20 years of disease to the patient. It is therefore of utmost importance that these patients are evaluated thoroughly in a close collaboration between endocrinologists, surgeons, and radiologists. The schedule for radiological investiga-

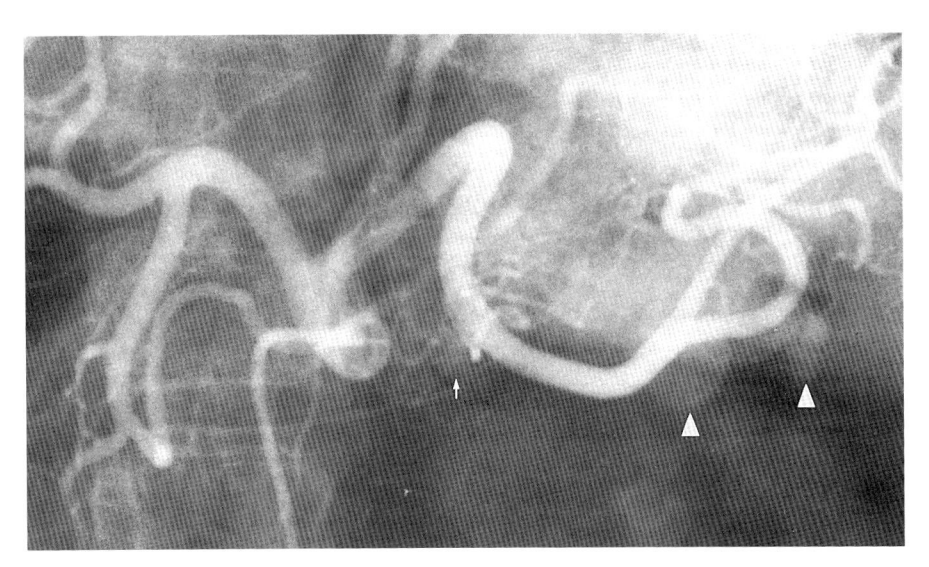

Fig. 8.**2** 56-year-old woman operated on for enucleation of an insulin-producing tumor in the tail of pancreas 14 years earlier, now with Zollinger–Ellison syndrome. Coeliac angiography shows two hypervascular tumors in the tail of pancreas (arrow heads). The patient was operated on (without intraoperative ultrasound) with resection of the pancreatic tail. Continuous symptoms induced reevaluation of the angiograms when a third, earlier overlooked, tumor was diagnosed (arrow). At reoperation, the tumor was found close to the border of resection

242   8 Multiple Endocrine Neoplasia

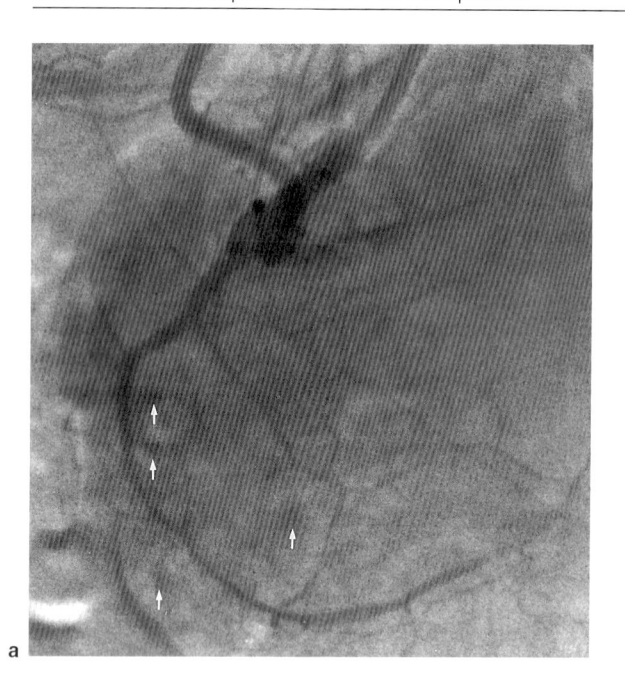

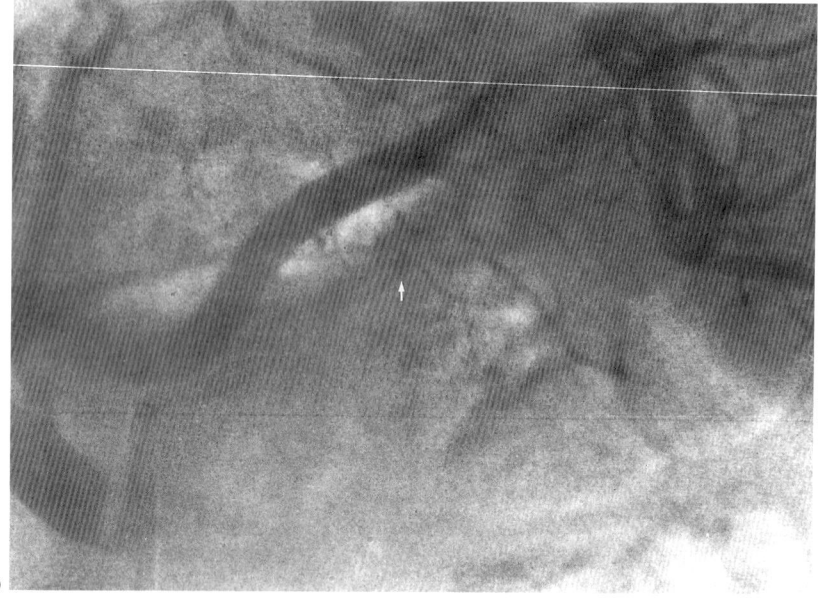

Fig. 8.3   36-year-old son of patient in Fig. 8.2 earlier operated on for prolactinoma of the hypophysis and hyperparathyroidism, now without clinical symptoms. Family screening indicated possible insulin producing tumor (**a**) Selective angiography of the gastroduodenal artery shows minor contrast densities in the head of pancreas (arrows) (**b**) similar minor contrast density in the tail of pancreas (arrow) (**c**) PTP indicated that the contrast densities were venous ectases and that the hormone release was from the tail. (**d**) Selective splenic angiography 2 years later shows a large possible tumor close to the spenic hilum. (**e**) CT directly after angiography and (**f**) during intra-arterial contrast injection shows a tumor with central necrosis to be located inside the tail. (**g**) In retrospect, the tumor had been obvious at CT 4 years earlier when it was interpreted as a cross-sectioned bowel. After resection of the tail of the pancreas, twelve minor tumors were found in the specimen together with the diagnosed tumor

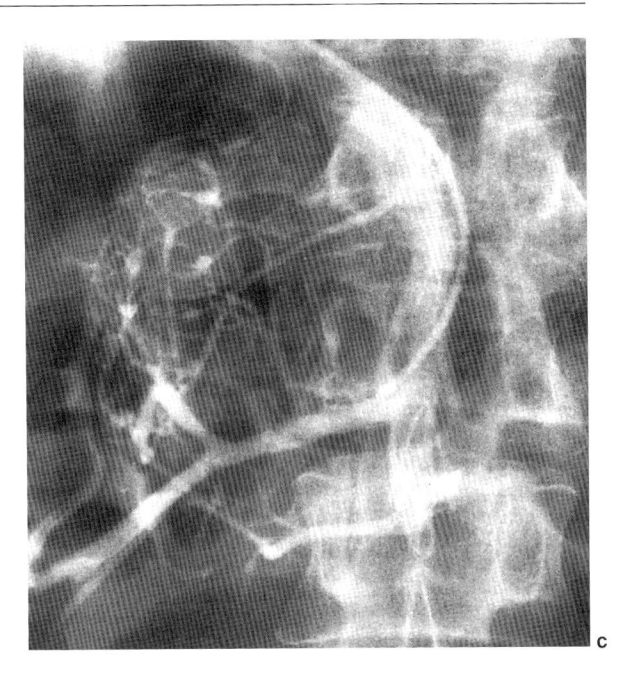

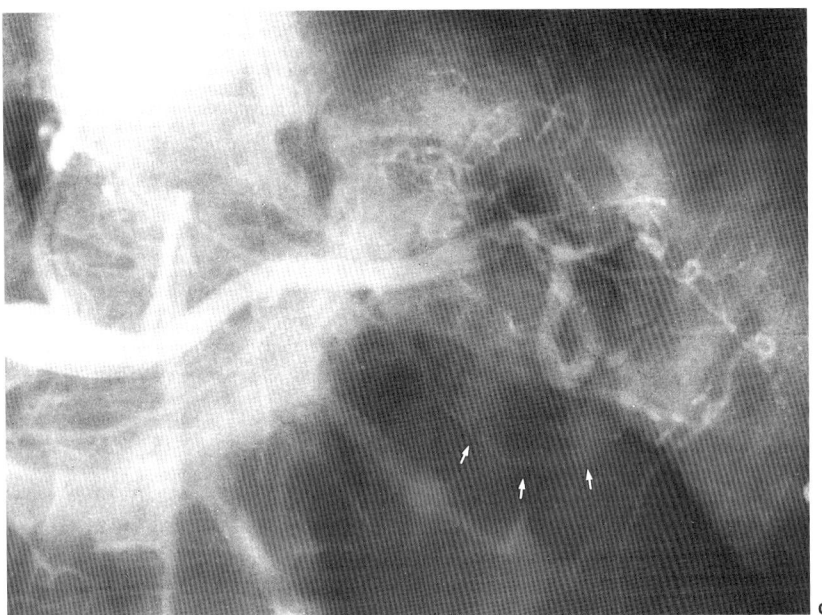

Fig. 8.**3c+d**

tions in our hospital is ultrasound, CT, and angiography every other year until a tumor is detected, or clinical symptoms are manifested. PTP is then performed, and the patient is thereafter operated on, and the tumor(s) are localized by intraoperative ultrasound. Changes in this schedule are often discussed, mainly because of the high penetrance of malignant degeneration in a patients family.

Until recently, no reliable scintigraphic technique was available for the detection of small pancreatic tumors. Promising results are however reported with a radiolabeled somatostatin analog "octreotide" that binds to the somatostatin receptors of most APUDomas. This technique gives not only the possibility to detect the tumor, but also gives information about the occurence of tumor cell receptors, which is a prerequisite for response to somatostatin therapy. This technique also offers the possibility of intracellular radiotherapy (6).

244　8　Multiple Endocrine Neoplasia

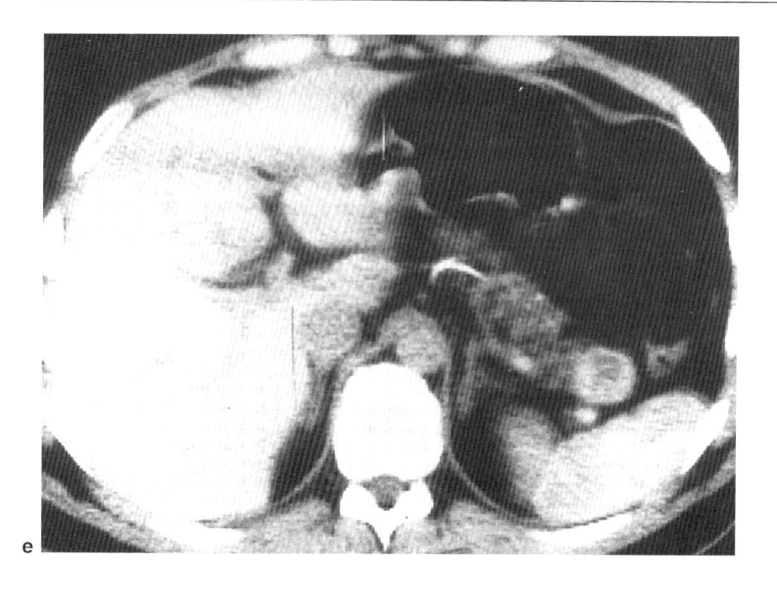

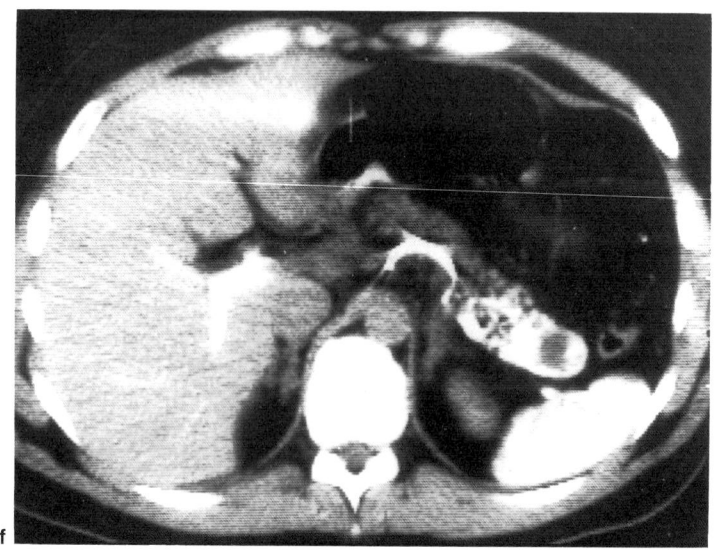

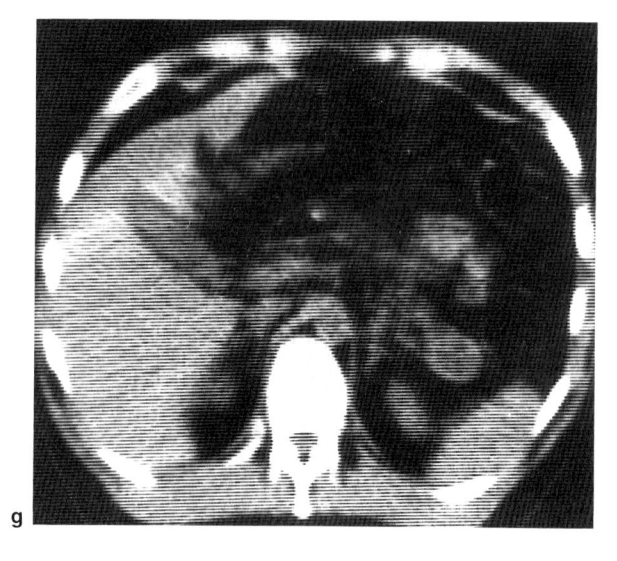

Fig. 8.**3e–g**

References

1 Ahlström H, Magnusson A, Grama D, Eriksson B, Öberg K, Lörelius LE. Preoperative localization of endocrine pancreatic tumors by intra-arterial dynamic computed tomography. Acta Radiol. 1990;31:171–175.
2 Galiber AK, Reading CC, Charboneau JW, et al. Localization of pancreatic insulinomas. Comparison of pre and intraoperative US with CT and angiography. Radiology. 1988;166:405–408.
3 Gigot JF, Gianello P, Dardenne AN, Pringot J, Detry R, Otte JB, Kestens PJ. Intraoperative ultrasonography in endocrine pancreatic surgery: preliminary results in 6 cases of insulinoma. JBR. 1986;69:57–62.
4 Grant CS, van Heerden JA, Charboneau JW, James EM, Reading CC. Insulinoma. The value of intraoperative ultrasonography. Arch Surg. 1988;123:843–848.
5 Ingemansson S, Lunderquist A, Lundqvist I, Lövdahl R, Tibblin S. Portal and pancreatic vein catheterization with radioimmunologic determination of insulin. Surg Gynecol Obstet. 1975; 141:705–711.
6 Lamberts SWJ, Hofland LJ, van Koetsveld PM, et al. Paralell in Vivo and in Vitro detection of functional somatostatin receptors in human endocrine pancreatic tumors: Consequences with regard to diagnosis, localization, and therapy. J Clin Endocrin. 1990; 71:566–574.
7 Norton JA, Cromack DT, Shawker TH, et al. Intraoperative ultrasonographic localization of islet cell tumors. A prospective comparison to palpation. Ann Surg. 1988;207:160–168.
8 Skogseid B, Eriksson B, Lundquist G, et al. Multiple endocrine neoplasia Type 1- A ten year prospective study in four kindreds. J Clin Endocrin. 1991;73:281–287.

9 Testis

Anatomy

J. Staudt

The testicles are paired organs that lie within the scrotal sac, which they reach at the end of the fetal period after their descent from the abdomen via the inguinal canal. The testicles have the size and shape of a small flattened chicken egg. The average size of the testicle in the adult is 4–5 cm in length, 2.4–3.5 cm in width, and 1.7–2.5 cm in depth. The left testicle descends further into the scrotal sac and is slightly larger than the right one. The testicles weigh between 25 g and 75 g each. Each testicle is covered by a thorough, firm tunica (albuginea) with a mirror-like outer surface, which, at the posterior face and at the upper pole, supports the fixation of the epididymis and of the neurovascular bundle (mediastinum testis), which offers a direct communication to the excretory ducts. Connective tissue septa run radially from the capsule to the mediastinum, giving the testicles their characteristic shape and architecture. The scrotal cave is located between the serosal layer of the tunica albuginea, also called 'lamina visceralis' or epiorchium, and the inner surface of 'lamina parietalis' or periorchium as the scrotal serosa. A small amount of serosal fluid lies within this space. The testicles are neighbored by the head and body of the epididymidis (Fig. 9.1).

The microscopic architecture of the testicles is determined by the testicular septulae, which extend from the capsule into the mediastinum and devide the organ into 250 lobuli. Each lobule contains two or three testicular canaliculi (tubuli seminiferi). Spermatogenesis takes place within the walls of those canaliculi. The mature spermatocytes lie close to the lumen of those canaliculi. The total length of all testicular canaliculi is approximately 300 m. The interstitial space between the tubuli is filled with reticular connective tissue, capillaries, and Leydig's cells, which are responsible for hormone production. The testicular canaliculi run out into the testicular net, from where they arbitrate into 12 descending canaliculi, which pass into the epididymidis (Fig. 9.2).

Due to the embryologic descent of the testis, the testicular artery originates from the abdominal aorta (rarely from the left renal artery) and runs into the

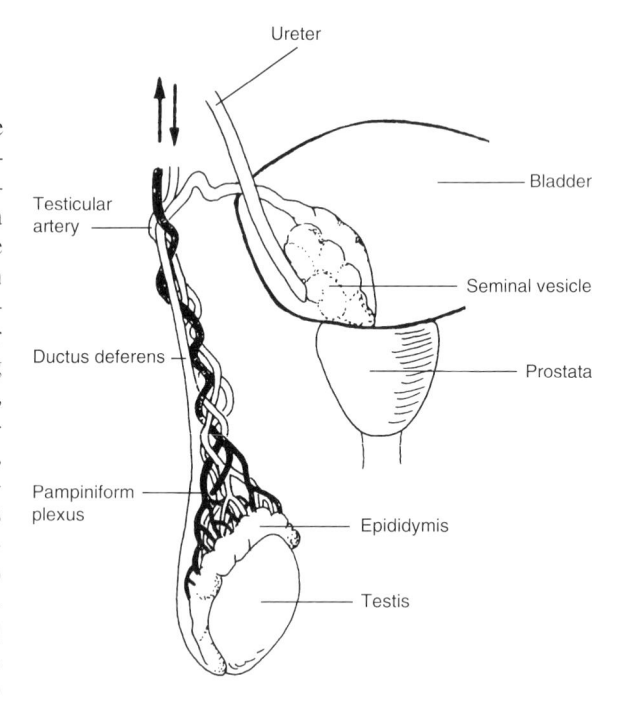

Fig. 9.1 Relation of the internal male genitalia

scrotum via the inguinal canal (rarely from the left renal artery). The lower part of the testicular artery is usually heavily coiled. After entering the mediastinum testis, the artery divides into two branches underneath the tunica albuginea with the blood flowing towards the mediastinum. After this mediastinal division, recurrent branches supply the testicular parenchyma.

The venous blood is drained by way of the septula toward the mediastinum, and also by way of collecting veins that follow a twisted course within the tunica albuginea from the surface to the mediastinum. Both venous plexuses join within the mediastinum and form the paminiform plexus. This plexus follows the spermatic cord through the inguinal canal, where the testicular vein originates at the level of the deep inguinal ring. The right testicular vein flows into the vena cava, whereas the left testicular vein flows into the left renal vein. Lymphatic vessels run along the pampiniform plexus. After passage through the deep

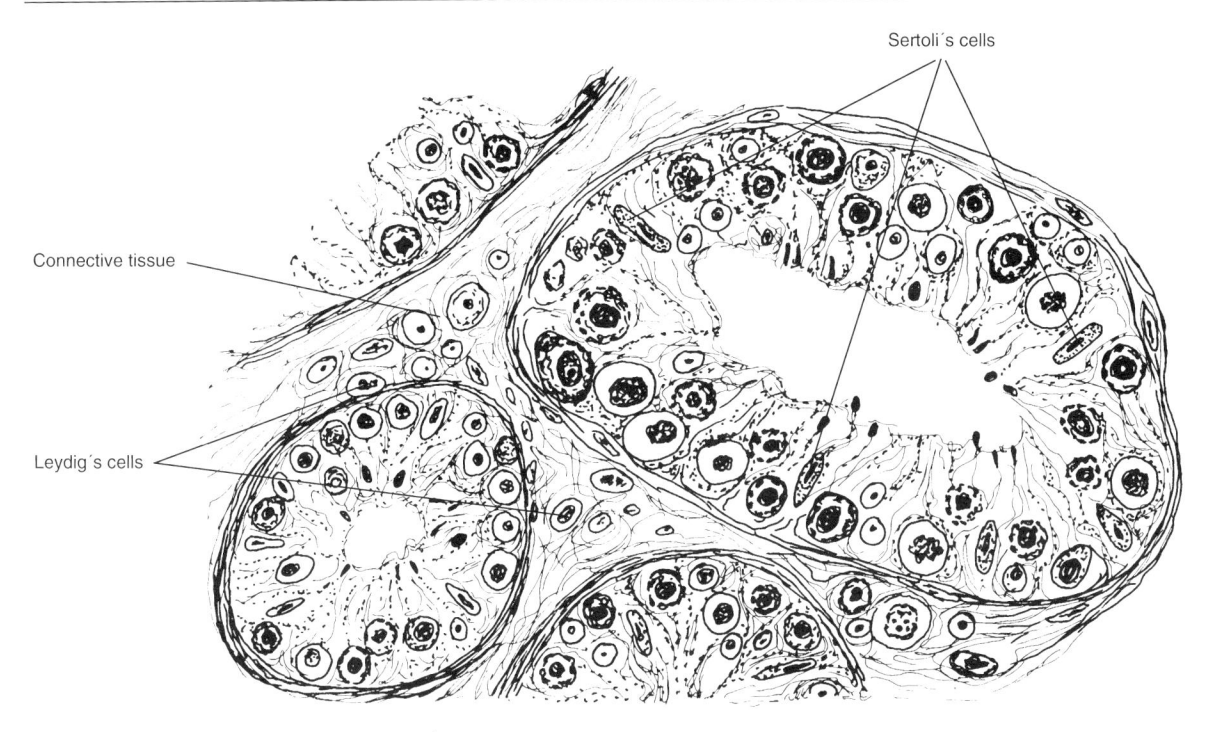

Fig. 9.2 Tubules with spermatogenesis

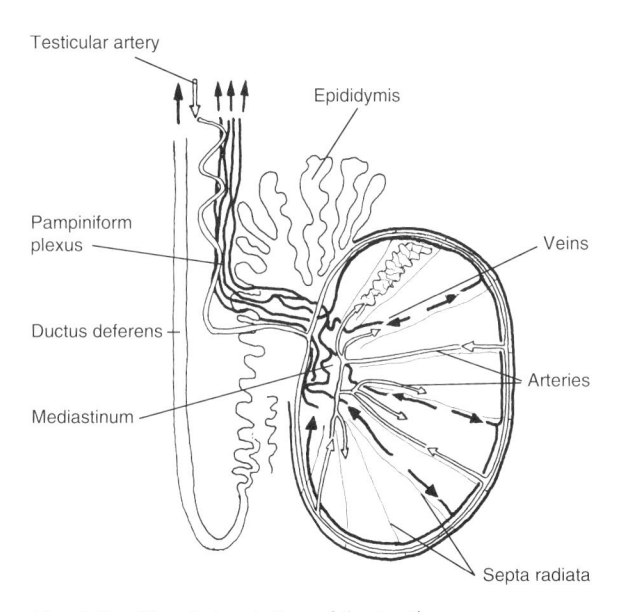

Fig. 9.3 Blood circulation of the testis

inguinal ring, they drain into pelvic lymph nodes or, as a side path, by way of scrotal veins into the inguinal lymph nodes (Fig. 9.3).

Endocrinology

F. Neumann and K.-J. Gräf

Physiology

Like the ovary, the testis is a bifunctional organ with an exocrine and an endocrine component. The testicular parenchyma consists of the seminiferous tubulus, in which spermatogenesis takes place; the androgen-producing Leydig's cells are located in the interstitial space.

The Leydig's cells of the testis are the main source of androgens. Only about 5% of circulating testosterone is of adrenal origin. Androgens are responsible for the anlage to the primary, and the development of the secondary sex characteristics. The main effects of androgens are summarized in Table 9.1. The figures for the physiological concentrations in serum and the daily production rates are shown in Table 9.2. Excretion occurs through the kidneys after glucuronidation and sulphatization. The main metabolites are androsterone and etiocholanolone. The early steps of androgen biosynthesis take place by way of squalene cholesterol and pregnenolone. Important intermediate steps are dehydroepiandrosterone and, in particular, progesterone and androstanedione. In many organs (e. g., the prostate) the actual biologically active androgen is not testosterone, but its reduced from 5 α-dihydrotestosterone (DHT). A small fraction of testosterone is converted into estradiol by the aromatase

Table 9.1 Sex-specific, metabolic, and other effects of androgens

Organ/function	Effect of androgens
Accessory sex glands (prostate, seminal vesicles)	Stimulation
Spermatogenesis	Maintenance (together with FSH)
Libido, potentia coeundi	Maintenance
Secondary male sex characteristics	Growth of facial hair, breaking of voice
Sexual differentation	Essential for development of male sexual organs
Bone maturation	Ossification (stop of longitudinal growth)
Skin and its appendages	Increase of thickness, stimulation of sebaceous glands
Lipids	Increase of high density lipoproteins
Protein metabolism	Anabolic effect
Erythropoiesis	Stimulation

Table 9.2 Testosterone synthesis, production rates, physiological concentrations, transport in blood

Sites of testosterone synthesis:	Testes (95%) Adrenal cortex (5%)
Daily production rate:	6–7 mg
Physiological concentrations in blood:	3–10 ng/mL
Circadian rhythm:	Highest values in the early morning
Annual rhythm:	Highest values in spring
Transport:	98% bound to SHBG (sex hormone binding globulin) and albumin Nonprotein bound 2%

enzyme complex, i. e., more than 90% of estrogens in men originate from the peripheral aromatization of androgens, e. g., in fatty tissue and muscle (Fig. 9.4, biosynthesis of sex hormones). The synthesis of androgens in the interstitial cells is stimulated by the pituitary.

Pituitary gonadotropin secretion is under the control of the hypothalamic releasing hormone GnRH (or LH-RH). LH stimulates the testicular production of testosterone. The adrenal secretion of androgens (mainly androstenedione and dehydroepiandrosterone or dehydroepiandrosterone sulphate) is regulated by ACTH. In turn, testosterone regulates the synthesis and release of the hypothalamic-releasing hormone via a negative feedback system (Fig. 9.5). More LH-RH is released at low testosterone concentrations thereby stimulating the pituitary secretion of LH and, subsequently, the synthesis of testosterone. When the latter reaches a certain level, the process is reversed.

Fig. 9.5 also shows the molecular mechanism of the action of testosterone. After incorporation in the cell, testosterone is reduced by the enzyme 5α-reductase to dihydrotestosterone (DHT) which, after binding to a specific receptor in the cell nucleus, sets in motion, by means of gene expression, transcription and translation processes.

Clinics

Puberty and Pubertal Disorders

The pubertal growth spurt is caused by the onset of sex hormone production (androgens in boys, estrogens in girls). The growth spurt lasts about 2 years. It starts at the age of 13 in girls and about 2 years later in boys. The process after ossification of the epiphysial cartilages in the long bones. The most suitable parameter for assessing the extent of pubertal maturity is the degree of skeletal maturity, which is determined radiologically. This parameter allows precise prediction of the anticipated final height. According to Tanner, five stages of puberty can be distinguished. Parameters are the development of pubic hair, in girls mammary development, and in boys penile and testis growth. A number of endocrine syndromes are associated with low final height (e. g., Ullrich–Turner syndrome).

Pubertas Tarda

Late puberty is present when the first secondary sex characteristics do not occur until after the age of 14 (girls) and 16 (boys). The differential diagnosis must rule out hypogonadism (boys) and primary amenorrhea (girls). The bone age determined radiologically in pubertas tarda does not correspond to the chronological age. Because, however, the start of puberty correlates more to bone age than to chronological age, determination of this parameter enables a precise prediction of when the onset of puberty can be expected.

Pubertas Precox

Secondary sex characteristics develop prematurely in all forms of precocious puberty. Precocious puberty is present when the onset of puberty occurs before the age of 6 in girls and 8 in boys. True pubertas precox can be caused by gonadotropin-producing pituitary tumors (very rare) or sex hormone-secreting tumors of the gonads (e. g., Leydig's cell tumors in boys, granulosa cell tumors in girls), or of the adrenal cortex.

Idiopathic pubertas precox occurs most frequently; girls are affected five times more often than boys. In this condition, bone age does not correlate to chronological age, i. e., skeletal maturation is accelerated. Ossification of the epiphysial cartilages and,

Endocrinology 249

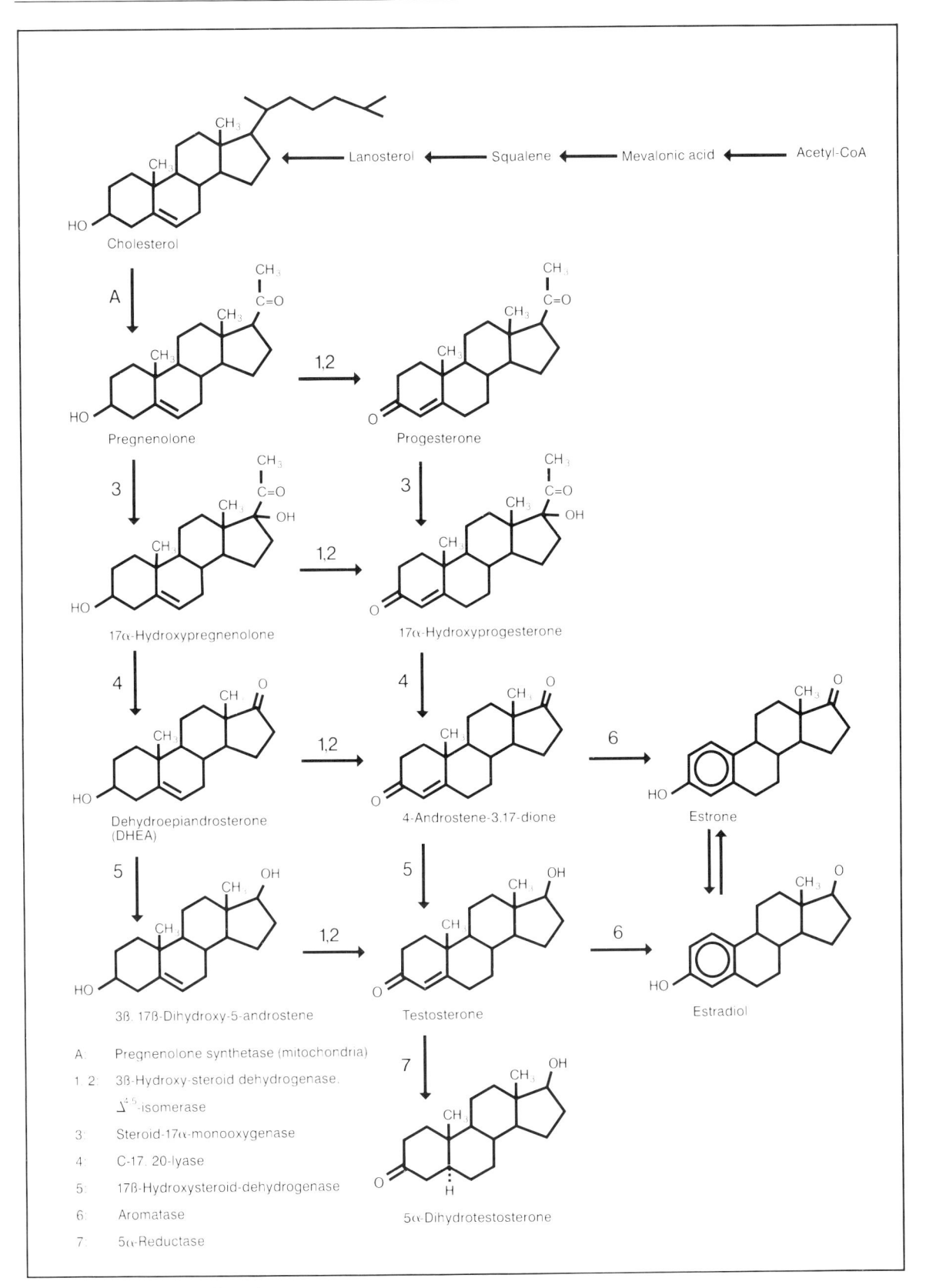

Fig. 9.4 Biosynthesis of sex hormones

Regulation of androgen biosynthesis and mechanism of androgen action

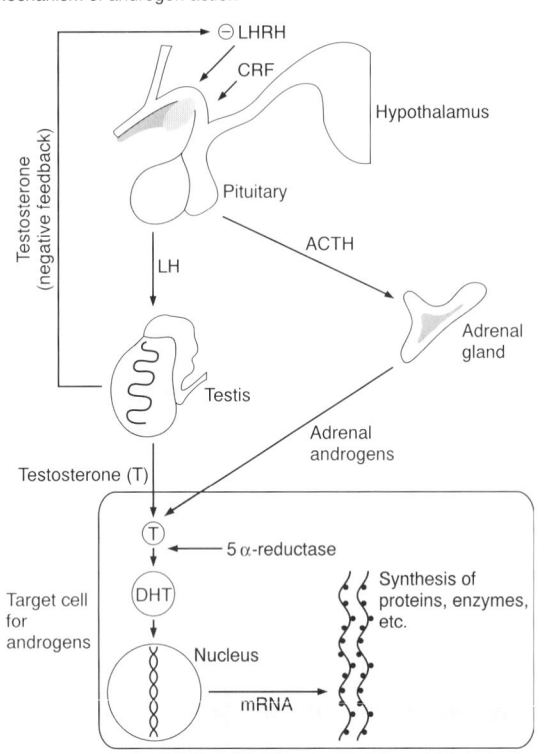

Fig. 9.5 Regulation of androgen biosynthesis and mechanism of androgen actions

Table 9.3 Normal values of semen parameter

Volume	>2.0 mL
pH	7.2–7.8
Concentration	$\geq 20 \times 10^6$ spermatozoon/ ejaculate
Motility	$\geq 50\%$ with progressive or $\geq 25\%$ with linear progressive movement 60 minutes after ejaculation
Morphology	$\geq 50\%$ normal
number of morphological normal sperms with progressive motility	$\geq 5 \times 10^6$/ejaculate
Vitality	$\geq 50\%$ alive (heads not stained red in the eosin test)
Leucocytes	$< 1 \times 10^0$/mL
Zinc (total)	$\geq 2,4$ µmol/ejaculate
Citric acid (total)	≥ 52 µmol/ejaculate
Fructose (total)	≥ 13 µmol/ejaculate
MAR-test*	10% of spermatozoos adherent to erythrocytes

* mixed antiglobulin reductions test

Table 9.4 Definition of disturbed spermatogenesis

Normozoospermia	Normal ejaculate as described in Table 9.3
Oligozoospermia	$< 20 \times 10^6$ spermatozoon/mL
Asthenozoospermia	$< 50\%$ with progressive or $< 25\%$ with linear progressive movement 60 minutes after ejaculation
Teratozoospermia	$< 50\%$ normally formed
Oligo–Astheno–Terato Spermia	Combination of the above mentioned disturbances
Azoospermia	No spermatomas in the ejaculate
Aspermia	No ejaculate

hence, cessation of longitudinal growth occur prematurely. If left untreated, final height is therefore drastically reduced. Radiological determination of the bone age also allows monitoring of the therapy.

Fertility Disorders

The many and various causes of fertility disorders can be dealt with only briefly here. Table 9.3 presents an overview of the normal values of the seminal parameters, and definitions of disturbed seminal parameters are given in Table 9.4. Fertility disorders can be caused by a deficiency of hormones (see the various reasons for hypogonadism), genetic defects, inflammations (e.g., mumps orchitis), liquefaction disorders, (i.e., functional disorders of the accessory sex glands (prostate, seminal vesicles), and others. Infertility is always present in bilateral cryptorchidism, and varioceles are often also associated with fertility disorders. Leydig's cell aplasia is associated with intersexuality because testosterone of the fetal testes is also essential to male differentiation. Patients with the "Sertoli cell only" syndrome do not display any gametes in the testes.

Other causes of male infertility are hyperthyroidism and hypothyroidism, congenital adrenal hyperplasia (see chapter 5), acquired or congenital obliterations in the region of the seminal ducts or epididymis, and iatrogenic disturbances of spermatogenesis due to a range of drugs such as barbiturates, spironolactone, reserpine, methyldopa, ketoconazole, tricyclic antidepressants, heroin, morphine, cocaine, amphetamines, and others. Disturbances of fertility—and sometimes also of potency—occur in diabetes mellitus, hyperprolactinemia, adrenocortical insufficiency, feminizing tumors (e.g., estrogen-producing Leydig's cell tumors of the testes), and in various nonendocrine severe illnesses. Phimoses of the penis and hypospadias can affect potentia coeundi and must be corrected surgically.

Hypogonadism is based on a deficient supply or effect of testosterone, for which there are many causes. Three basic causes can, however, be distinguished:

1. Disturbances in the hypothalamus–pituitary system, leading to a deficit of LH and, consequently, to insufficient synthesis of testosterone (secondary hypogonadism). Only in this form of hypogonadism can fertility be restored by treatment with gonadotropins (e.g., Kallmann syndrome).
2. The cause of the deficient production of testosterone lies in the testis itself (primary hypogonadism). It is often due to a chromosomal anomaly, e.g., in Klinefelter syndrome.
3. Another cause is an androgen receptor defect, which means that androgens are unable to have (sufficient) an effect on the target organ, e.g., in partial or complete "testicular feminization."

The main symptoms of primary and secondary hypogonadism are summarized in Table 9.5.

Congenital Anorchism, Monorchism

The presumed cause is infection or early torsion leading to complete degeneration of the testis. The HCG test must be performed in the differential diagnosis to rule out the presence of cryptorchidism.

Cryptorchidism

Undescended testis are found in 2–3% of newborns. In most of these children, the testes descend in the first 3 months of life. A distinction is made between abdominal cryptorchidism (testes are not visible or palpable) and inguinale testes (the testes are located in the inguinal canal). Descent is probably governed by tetosterone and the anti-Müller hormone. This is why cryptorchidism frequently occurs in testosterone deficiency in the fetal period, e.g., due to pituitary insufficiency (pituitary aplasia, Kallmann syndrome), enzyme defects of androgen biosynthesis, or receptor defects such as testicular feminization. Abnormalities in the upper urinary tract (e.g., hydronephrosis, renal hypoplasia) are found in about 10% of cryptorchid patients. There is a 30–40 times higher risk of testicular cancer if cryptorchidism remains uncorrected; this means, cryptorchidism has to be corrected as early as possible, primarily with hormones (HCG or GnRH), or by surgery.

Varicocele

Varicose dilatation of the spermatic veins (plexus pampiniformis) occurs in about 5% of all men, and is usually left sided. Insufficiency of the venous valves and congenital vessel wall damage have been discussed, among others, as causes. The varicocele is often associated with disturbances of spermatogenesis secondary to reduced perfusion and increased temperature in the testis. The diagnosis is made by palpation of the scrotum, Doppler sonography (venous reflux), and thermography (temperature increase). The disturbance of venous reflux can be eliminated by high ligature or radiological embolization of the spermatic vein.

The Most Common Endocrine Syndromes Associated inter alia with Infertility

Klinefelter Syndrome

Klinefelter syndrome is based on a chromosomal aberration. In the classic form, the karyotypic formula displays 47 XXY.

With an incidence of 1:500, Klinefelter syndrome is the most common form of hypogonadism. The guiding symptoms are: small, firm testes, infertility, and gynecomastia with elevated gonadotropin values (FSH > LH). This syndrome is often not diagnosed until after puberty, since the degree of virilization is usually normal, and libido and potency do not diminish in the early adolescence. Osteoporosis is a frequent complication in elderly, untreated patients as a result of reduced testosterone synthesis. Probably because of the almost obligatory gynecomastia, there is a 20 times higher risk of breast cancer. The gynecomastia is attributable to increased peripheral conversion of androgens to estrogens. Patients with Klinefelter syndrome who have low levels of testosterone have to treated by substitution with androgens throughout their lifetimes.

Kallmann Syndrome

Kallmann syndrome affects patients with hypogonadotropic hypogonadism associated with

Table 9.5 Symptoms of hypogonadism

Organ/function	Symptom
Testes	Small
Libido, Potentia coeundi	None or reduced
Spermatogenesis	Not initiated or cessation
Penis	Smal
Bones	Eunuchoid gigantism, osteoporosis
Muscles	Underdeveloped (atrophy)
Skin	Dry, thin skin, reduced sebum production
Hair	No facial hair growth, sexual hair female
Blood production (erythropoiesis)	Anemia

anosmism or hyposmism. The cause is a deficit of GnRH and, hence, of gonadotropins and testosterone. It is the second most frequent form of hypogonadism. The diagnosis is not generally made until puberty. Kallmann syndrome is readily distinguishable from pubertas tarda by the presence of anosmism.

Male Ullrich–Turner (Noonan) Syndrome

The male Ullrich–Turner, or Noonan, syndrome is rarely seen. Over 90% of the patients display the karyotype 46 XY. The guiding symptoms include a short neck, scutiform chest, anomalies of the ears, positional anomalies of the testes, and, usually, infertility. The syndrome is often associated with cardiovascular malformations such as atrial septum defects and stenosis of the aortic isthmus and pulmonary artery. About 50% of patients are mentally retarded. Androgen substitution is essential for the patient's lifetime.

Testicular Feminization ("Hairless Woman"), Complete Androgen Insensitivity

This syndrome is based on an androgen receptor defect, as a result of which all androgen-dependent steps of sexual differentiation fail to occur. Guiding symptoms are amenorrhea (absence of internal efferent genital tract), a blind-ending vagina, undescended testes (no scrotal anlage), and sparse sexual hair hence the name "hairless woman"). These patients live as women. Because of the high risk of developing tumors of the testes, orchiectomy should be performed at an age of approximately 18; thereafter, hormone replacement therapy with estrogens and progestogens should be offered.

Reifenstein syndrome (Incomplete Androgen Insensitivity)

These individuals show a spectrum of disorders due to an X-linked recessive trait. The clinical picture ranges from complete failure of virilization to almost complete masculinization. This variability lies in the degree of function of the androgen receptor. All individuals with this syndrome are infertile (azoospermia or oligozoospermia). Sex assignment is usually female. In this case orchiectomy should be performed because of the higher risk of tumors of the testes. If the gender identity is male, than feminization and gynecomastia occur after puberty (dominance of estrogens).

Rare Symptoms Associated with Hypogonadism

Imperato-McGinley Syndrome (5-α-reductase Deficiency)

In this form of incomplete male pseudohermaphroditism DHT-dependent structures are not developed normally. This syndrome is characterized by hypospadias, small prostate, and less facial and body hair. Usually, the gender is male. Androgen substitution is not necessary. It differs from the incomplete form of testicular feminization in that masculinization occurs at puberty because there is no reduced response to androgens.

Laurence–Moon–Biedl Syndrome

The main symptoms are oligophrenia, polydactylia, obesity, and retinitis pigmentosa. The probably hypothalamus-related hypogonadism is often associated with diabetes mellitus, diabetes insipidus, anal atresia, and heart defects. Neonates with this syndrome often display a micropenis and hypospadia. The cause is genetic (autosomal recessive trait).

Prader–Labhart–Willi Syndrome

The guiding symptoms include short stature, oligophrenia, scoliosis, hypoplasia of the dental enamel, cryptorchidism and, frequently, obesity as well. The hypogonadism is often associated with diabetes mellitus, and is believed to be caused by disturbed GnRH secretion. The genetic defect is usually located on chromosome 15. Life expectancy is reduced, and the syndrome cannot be diagnosed prenatally.

Testicular Tumors

Testicular tumors, with an incidence of 2–3 per 100 000, account for 1–2% of all malignant neoplasms in men; about 10% of testicular tumors are found in men with cryptorchidism. Germinal cell tumors account for 95% and Leydig's cell tumors for only 5% of testicular neoplasms. Germinal cell tumors are broken down further into seminomas (about 50%), embryonal cell neoplasms (about 30%), teratomas (about 10%), and chorionepitheliomas (about 2%).

Tumor indicators are β-HCG and α-fetoprotein. β-HCG is demonstrable in about 50% of patients with teratocarcinomas or embryonal cell tumors; α-fetoprotein is elevated in 70% of patients with nonseminomatous germinal cell tumors. The behavior of these markers can also be exploited to monitor the therapy. The therapeutic strategies depend on the tumor stage and the histological grading.

Prostatic Carcinoma

In the Western industrial countries, prostatic carcinoma is the second most frequent type of cancer in men. The etiology is unknown. That androgens must play a role is, however, proven by the fact that tumors of the prostate—either carinomas or hyperplasia—have never been observed in eunuchs or early castrates.

Prostatic acid phosphatase (PAP) and, even more specific, the prostate-specific antigen (PSA), are used as tumor markers. Increase of tumor markers under therapy is a sign of tumor progression. These markers are also measured to monitor therapy.

All diagnostic imaging procedures (X-ray, sonography, bone scintigraphy, and CT) are employed for tumor staging, which is important for therapeutic measures.

The final diagnosis is based on histology and biopsy material. The therapeutic strategy is androgen deprivation as first line treatment (orchiectomy, LHRH-analogs, antiandrogens, or combinations). About 80% of the patients will respond for about 2–3 years.

Benign Prostatic Hyperplasia (BPH)

BPH is the most common benign tumor in men. It affects more than half of all men older than 50 years. The hyperplasia can involve the stroma, epithelium, or both tissue components to varying degrees. The guiding symptoms are voiding complaints.

This hyperplasia originates from the periurethral glands of the inner zone. Although the etiology is unclear, it appears to be primarily a disease of the stroma. Because the stroma is also a target tissue for estrogens it is assumed, inter alia, that the androgen–estrogen imbalance, in favor of the estrogens, associated with increasing age causes stimulation of the fibromuscular stroma. The size of the prostate is determined by rectal palpation or sonography.

Tumors of the Seminal Vesicles, Epididymides, Vas Deferens, and Testicular Capsule

All these tumors are extremely rare, and the symptoms are uncharacteristic. In general, a diagnosis can be made only by exploratory surgery and histological examination of the biopsy material.

Tumors of the Penis

Squamous cell carcinomas of the penis are relatively rare and easy to diagnose. Inadequate sexual hygiene is believed to play a role in the etiology. Metastatic spread is mainly to the lung and liver.

References

1. Goodman Gilman A, Rall TW, Nies AS, Taylor R. The Pharmacological Basis of Therapeutics. 8th ed. Pergamon Press; 1990.
2. Greenspan FS, Forsham PH. Basic and Clinical Endocrinology. 2nd ed. Los Altos: Lange Medical Publications; 1986.
3. Speroff L, Glass RH, Kase, NG. Clinical Gynecologic Endocrinology and Infertility. 4th ed. Baltimore: Williams & Wilkins; 1989.
4. Nieschlag E, Behre HM, eds. Textbook of Endocrinology. 6th ed. Philadelphia: WB Saunders; 1981.
5. Grossman A, ed. Clinical Endocrinology, 1st ed. Oxford: Blackwell Scientific Publications; 1992
6. Wilson JD, Foster DW, eds. Williams Textbook of Endocrinology, 8th ed. Philadelphia. Saunders; 1992.
7. Niesellag E, Behre HM, eds. Testosterone Action Deficiency Substitution. Berlin. Springer; 1990

Ultrasound

P. Vassallo and J. Spiteri-Grech

Indications and Diagnostic Value of Testicular Ultrasonography

Due to their superficial location, the testicles are particularly suited for sonographic evaluation. The advent of high-resolution (5–10 MHz) ultrasound probes with optimized beam focusing, has opened a realm of new diagnostic possibilities for the evaluation of superficial organs.

The main indications for scrotal ultrasound include the following:

1. Scrotal pain
2. Acute or chronic scrotal swelling or a palpable scrotal mass
3. Difficulty palpating the testes (e.g., undescended testes, or in the presence of a varicocele)
4. History of late orchidopexy (after 10 years of age)
5. Follow-up of patients previously operated for a testicular neoplasm (particularly if serum tumor marker levels are elevated), or patients with recent episodes of orchitis to exclude the presence of an abscess, which would require surgery
6. Enlargement of inguinal or retroperitoneal lymph nodes of unknown etiology
7. Primary or secondary infertility and gynecomastia

The diagnostic value of high-resolution sonography alone and combined with clinical examination for the detection and characterization of scrotal disease has been assessed in several clinical trials. In one study with 284 cases followed over a 3-year period, Rifkin et al. reported a sensitivity of 98.5% for the detection of scrotal disease with high-resolution sonography

(1). In addition, the same group was able to correctly differentiate testicular from paratesticular disease in 99% of cases. London et al. described a sensitivity of 100% and a specificity of 99% for the detection and characterization of testicular tumors in 109 men with scrotal symptoms (2); Ultrasound provided clinically useful information in 53% of cases, and surgery could have been avoided in 8% of patients if ultrasound reports had been heeded. In their analysis of 230 patients over an 18-month period, Fowler et al. reported that 28% of testicular tumors detected by high-resolution ultrasonography had been missed on clinical examination (3), while Kronmann-Anderson et al. obtained positive predictive values of 33% with clinical examination alone, and of 53% with combined clinical and sonographic assessment for selecting between patients (n = 166) requiring surgical or conservative therapy (4).

Hamm et al. have shown that differentiation between testicular and epidydimal lesions was possible on the basis of clinical examination in 79%, and ultrasonography alone, in 98% of cases, while a correct characterization of the lesion was obtained in 72% on clinical examination and in 84% at sonography (5). The authors attribute the higher specificity of sonography to its capability to differentiate testicular from paratesticular lesions (sensitivity: 79% for clinical examination and 98% for ultrasound) with the former more likely to be malignant and the latter inflammatory.

Ultrasonography has not been shown to have any damaging effects on the testis. In order to generate a detectable increase in tissue temperature, sonographic wave energies at least a hundred times higher than those used for diagnostic purposes (approx. 10 mW/cm^2) are required (6). Other effects, such as microsomation and gas–body activation, have not been observed with normal exposure durations and wave energies (7).

Hardware and Examination Technique

To adequately evaluate the testes, high-resolution equipment with high-frequency sonographic probes (7.5–10 MHz) and optimal beam focusing are required. Although linear-array probes have been said to provide better resolution of near-field structures, we have obtained satisfactory images with sector probes, which can be more comfortably and intimately applied to the scrotum.

Due to severe reverberation and encoding artifacts occuring in regions immediately adjacent to the piezoelectric crystal arrays in the sonographic probe, the use of a short water path (0.5–1.0 cm) system between the skin and probe is highly recommended (8). In addition, the water path system also ensures minimal compression when examining painful testes. Earlier techniques employed water bath immersion of the testes, which allowed assessment without tissue compression or deformation, but precluded any simultaneous palpation during the examination (11).

Obtaining a relevant medical history and bimanual palpation of the testes and paratesticular structures prior to ultrasonography is an important part of the scrotal assessment, because correct interpretation of sonographic findings is frequently impossible without accurate clinical data. Recent or repeated urinary tract infections followed by acute scrotal pain and fever may prompt the diagnosis of secondary epididymo-orchitis, whereas a history of progressive painless swelling of the testis, possibly with weight loss and lethargy, should raise the possibility of neoplastic disease. Previous trauma or surgery to the scrotal region (e. g., orchidopexy), hormonal therapy, or systemic disease may also shed light on the nature of a scrotal lesion. Other factors such as impotence and infertility associated with small testes may suggest an endocrine disorder.

Clinical examination should be initiated with the patient in the recumbant position and in a warm environment to ensure adequate relaxation of the cremasteric and scrotal muscles. During inspection, differences in scrotal size as well as hair distribution, skin color and rugosity should be assessed. Bimanual palpation should determine testicular and epididymal position, volume, symmetry, consistency, and mobility within the scrotal sack, as well as scrotal temperature. Focal areas of tender or painless induration of the tunica albuginea are particularly important. Palpation of the epididymis is frequently unpleasant to the patient even in the absence of disease. The thickness and consistency of the vas deferens should also be assessed, particularly in patients with a history of epididymo-orchitis and infertility or both. Other conditions of the spermatic cord structures, such as testicular or spermatic varicoceles and inguinal hernias, are best assessed with the patient in the upright position performing Valsalva maneuver.

Ultrasonography should be initiated with the patient in the recumbant position and the penis held against the lower abdominal wall. Sonographic gel should be applied generously to the scrotum, because intervening air bubbles trapped by scrotal hair may severely impede adequate sonographic assessment. Particular care must be exercised in small children and neonates, because minimal manipulation, such as the application of sonographic gel or the probe may elicit a strong cremasteric reflex, which may retract the testis into the inguinal canal leading to false diagnoses of incomplete testicular descent. Gain and focus settings on the ultrasound machine are preferably performed on a longitudinal view of the uninvolved testis, which should be moderately echogenic at all distances from the sonographic probe.

Longitudinal scans showing the full extent of the testes and epididymis in each scrotal compartment, as well as transverse scans for comparison of both compartments, should be obtained. The length, width, and depth of the testes may be measured in order to calculate testicular volume (V = L × W × D × 0.65) (9). Small areas of induration detected on initial palpation should be evaluated by direct application of the sonographic probe. Testicular sonography in the upright position with Valsalva maneuver is also required, particularly when excluding a variocele or an inguinal hernia. The value of Doppler sonography for detecting retrograde flow in the spermatic cord veins in patients with varicoceles will be discussed later.

Simultaneous palpation of the testes during sonography also provides valuable information on lesions, which have been missed on initial clinical examination. Comparison to the opposite side during both clinical and sonographic examination may help confirm the presence or absence of scrotal abnormality.

Normal Ultrasonographic Appearance of the Scrotal Contents

The normal adult testis is avoid with longitudinal and transverse diameters of 3–5 cm and 2–3 cm, respectively and shows a homogeneously echogenic internal structure (Fig. 9.6): the rete and mediastinum testes cannot be delineated at sonography, whereas the tunica albuginea can only be appreciated when thickened by disease (10). The echogenicity of the testes provides a good background for the detection of testicular tumors and inflammatory lesions, which are generally hypoechoic (11).

The epididymis has smooth margins and a homogeneous echogenic internal structure similar to that of the testis. The head of the epididymis (globus major) is easily identified attached to the upper pole of the testis, whereas the epididymal body and tail (globus minor) are more difficult to locate on the dorsolateral aspect of the testis.

The testis and epididymis are surrounded by the tunica vaginalis, which consists of parietal and visceral layers normally separated by a few milliliters of serosal fluid (10). The two layers of the tunica vaginalis can only be differentiated in the presence of a hydrocele.

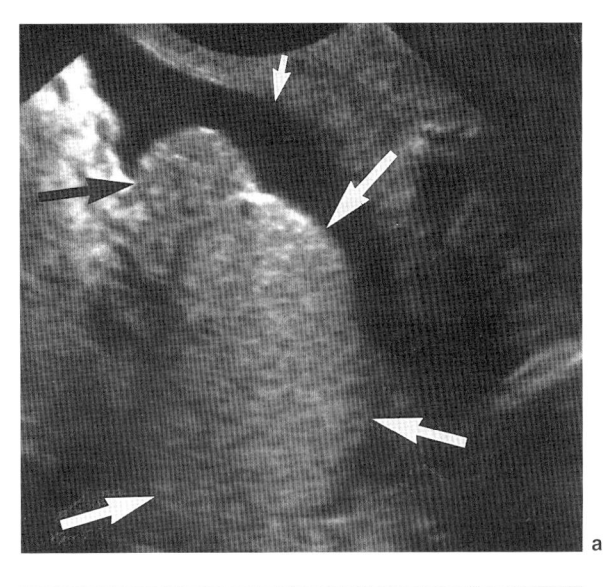

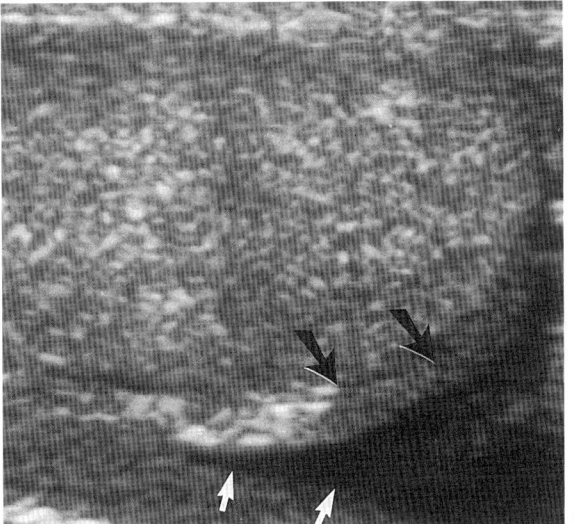

Fig. 9.6 Normal testis (longitudinal views): (**a**) The normal testis (large white arrows) and epididymal head (black arrow) are moderately echogenic. (**b**) The body and tail of the epididymis (black arrows) are located on the posterolateral aspect of the testis. Both cases have small hydroceles (small white arrows)

Congenital Anomalies of the Scrotum

Abnormal Migration

Abnormal migration of the testes from their embryological site of origin in the upper retroperitoneal region (urogenital tubercle) down to the scrotum results in two disorders of testicular location: arrested descent or ectopic location.

Arrested descent of the testes is by far the more common abnormality occuring in 2–3.4% of newborns (12). By 1 year of age, approximately 1.8% of infants require surgery for persisting abnormal testicular location associated with congenital inguinal hernia in 80% of cases (13). Undescended testes may be intraabdominal (8%), inguinal (63%), or prescrotal (24%). Possible ectopic locations of the testes include the extrafascial inguinal, perineal, femoral, or crural areas (14). Testicular retraction occuring during clinical or ultrasonographic examination, particularly in prepubertal males, may be difficult to differentiate from incomplete descent. Repeating the examination at a later date may help resolve this problem.

Complications of abnormal testicular location are azospermia (when bilateral), torsion, and malignant testicular tumors (especially germ cell tumors), which may occur even following surgical correction, particularly if performed after the age of 10 years (15). Malignant testicular tumors have been reported to occur 9–17 times more frequently in undescended testes (16, 17), and approximately 10% of all malignant testicular tumors occur in abnormally located testes. Torsion of an undescended testis in an adult is frequently associated with a testicular tumor, and the increased testicular size has been suggested to result in an increased tendency to torsion (5).

High-resolution ultrasound has been helpful in locating abnormally descended testes distal to the inner inguinal ring and for the detection of testicular tumors in these cases. The size and echo texture of a maldescended testis usually resembles the contralateral normal testis in the prepubertal years but shows a reduced volume and decreased echogenicity in later years, unless hormonal therapy has been administered, or early orchidopexy has been performed. When located in the inguinal canal (Fig. 9.7), the testis may appear somewhat flattened. Occasionally differentiating a pars infravaginalis gubernaculi from an atrophic undescended testis may pose problems. Visualization of a central echogenic band representing the mediastinum testis has been claimed to help in some cases (18).

Testis located proximal to the inner inguinal ring may be difficult to locate with sonography due to intervening gas-filled bowel loops. CT and MRI have been reported superior to ultrasound for the detection of intra-abdominal testes (19, 20). The absence of retroperitoneal fat in infants and small children makes locating retroperitoneal testes a difficult task with CT or MRI. Selective retrograde testicular phlebography has been also employed for testicular localization with success rates of 50–90% (21, 22, 23).

Table 9.6 Maldescended testes

Clinical findings:	Empty scrotum Abnormal testicular location (frequently inguinal)

Ultrasound findings:	Flattened oval testis
	  early: normal size/echogenicity
	  late: decrease in volume/echogenicity
	Inhomogeneity: suspect tumor
	Intra-abdominal location: CT or MRI

Complications:	Azospermia Torsion Tumor

Aplasia, Anorchia and Polyorchia

Abnormalities in number and size of testes have also been observed. **Aplasia** has been reported to occur in 4% of patients with maldescent and can only be reliably diagnosed at surgery, in which case a blind ending rudimentary vas deferens is identified. This abnormality has been attributed to intrauterine testicular torsion. Bilateral absence of the testes, or **anorchia**, has been reported in 0.6% of patients with maldescent (24). In addition to an empty scrotal sack, these patients also exhibit a micropenis, pubertas tarda, and an absent response of testosterone production to HCG stimulation. The absence of a testicle distal to the internal inguinal ring may be confirmed by ultrasonography in these cases. However other imaging methods or laparatomy may be required to exclude intra-abdominal testicular retention.

Polyorchia is a rare disorder reported in a total of 70 patients in the literature; this has been attributed to peritoneal folding resulting in segmentation of the primitive gonads in the upper retroperitoneal region (25, 26). Accessory testes and associated epidymes are generally hypoplastic and hypoechoic or iso-echoic; their resemblance to testicular tumors often makes resection unavoidable.

Macro- and Micro-orchia

Macro-orchia, or asymptomatic testicular enlargement, has been reported in mentally retarded individuals, particularly those with "fragile X"-linked syndrome (27, 28, 29, 30); these enlarged homogeneous echogenic gonads show an increased tendency to develop neoplasms. Macro-orchia also occurs in patients with acromegaly (Fig. 9.8) and prepubertal boys with hypothyroidism. Bilateral **micro-orchia** may be observed with disturbances of the hypothalamic–hypophysial–gonadal axis such as hy-

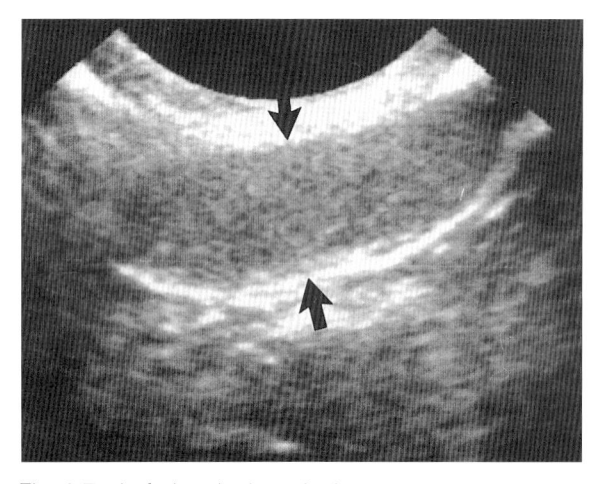

Fig. 9.7 Left inguinal testis in a prepubertal male (longitudinal view): The testis (black arrows) exhibits an echogenic internal structure and appears flattened within the narrow inguinal canal

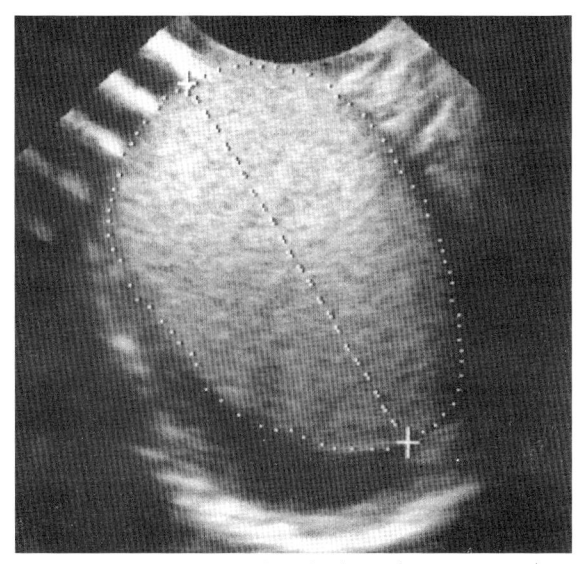

Fig. 9.8 Macro-orchia: Testicular volume was calculated to be 32 cm^3 in this patient with acromegaly (longitudinal view)

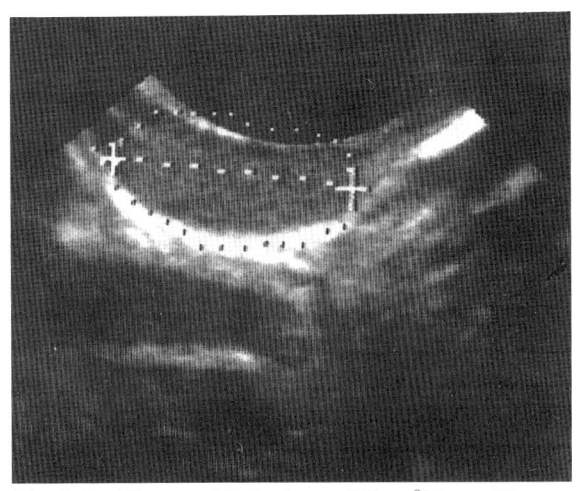

Fig. 9.9 Micro-orchia (volume 3.5 cm^3) in a 16-year-old patient with delayed puberty (longitudinal view)

pogonadotrophic hypogonadism and delayed puberty (Fig. 9.9).

Disorders of the Epididymis and Vas Deferens

Aplasia of the epididymis, epididymo-testicular dissociation and absence or atresia of the vas deferens are congenital anomalies that, if bilateral, are associated with infertility and normal secondary sexual development. These anomalies are more commonly seen associated with a maldescended testis. **Appendices of the epididymis or testis** are remnants of the mesonephric (Wolffian) and paramesonephric (Müllerian) ducts located at the upper poles of the epididymis and testis and are usually too small to be visualized on sonography unless a hydrocele is present; they may, however, undergo torsion and present as painful nodules at the upper pole of the testis or epididymis, which is hypoechoic and may show varying degrees of pedunculation on sonography. **Spermatoceles** are fluid-filled abberrant efferent ducts, which present as painless elastic nodules at the upper pole of the epididymis on palpation and appear as smooth, anechoic, occasionally multiloculated cysts on ultrasonography (Fig. 9.10); they may become acutely inflamed and present as painful nodules in the head of the epididymis. Although appendicular torsion and inflamed spermatoceles may be clinically indistinguishable from acute orchitis or testicular torsion, they can be readily identified by sonography (31).

Acute Scrotal Disease

The term "acute scrotum" is often used to refer to sudden or rapid onset of pain or swelling developing in

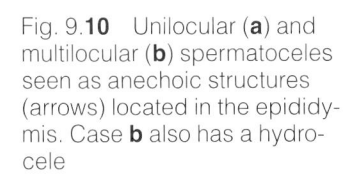

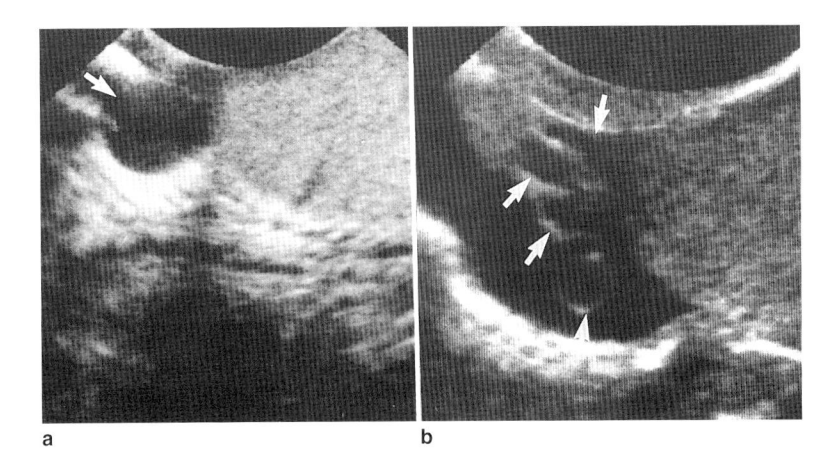

Fig. 9.10 Unilocular (**a**) and multilocular (**b**) spermatoceles seen as anechoic structures (arrows) located in the epididymis. Case **b** also has a hydrocele

one or both scrotal compartments. Acute conditions involving the testes include infections (Table 9.7), ischemia, trauma, and occasionally hydroceles.

Primary Orchitis

Primary orchitis, most often associated with mumps and thought to reach the testis by hematogenous spread, is frequently a subclinical condition and is more common in adults. In 18% of patients with clinical manifestations of **mumps,** orchitis with scrotal pain, swelling, and tenderness develops approximately 7 days after the onset of parotitis, and therefore poses no diagnostic problem. However, in 8% of cases, mumps orchitis occurs in the absence of parotitis. Primary orchitis has also been reported in association with **Henoch–Schönlein purpura** (32). Sonography may show diffuse testicular swelling and multifocal or diffuse areas of low echogenicity within the testicle with sparing of the epididymis (33, 34, 35), which usually resolve completely but may persist as smaller hypoechoic areas of fibrosis. These zones

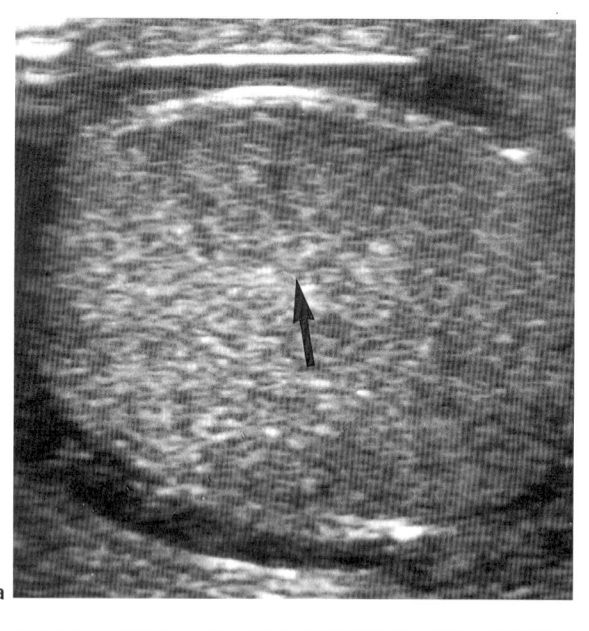

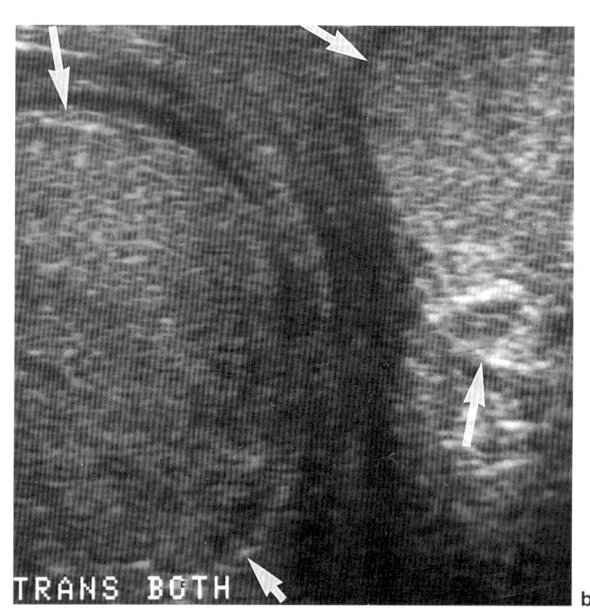

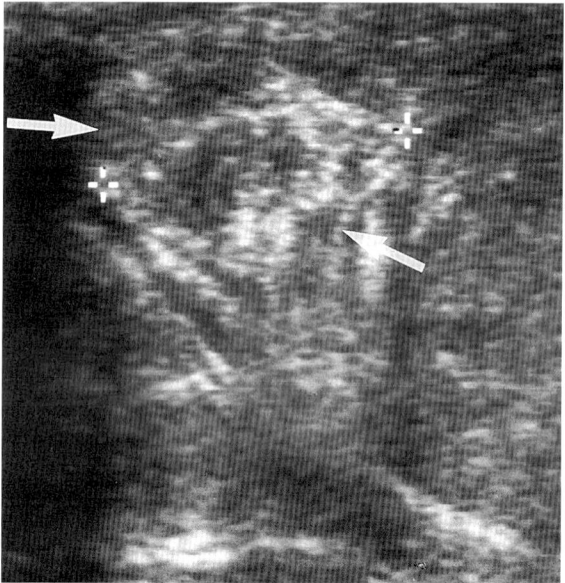

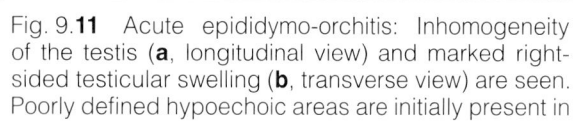

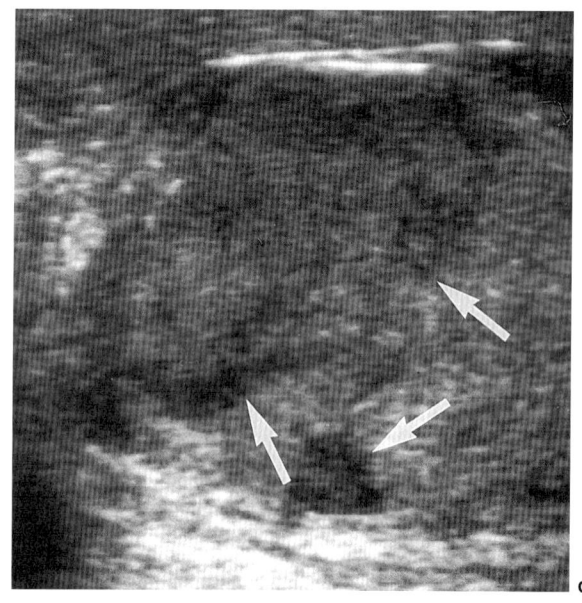

Fig. 9.**11** Acute epididymo-orchitis: Inhomogeneity of the testis (**a**, longitudinal view) and marked right-sided testicular swelling (**b**, transverse view) are seen. Poorly defined hypoechoic areas are initially present in the epididymis (**c**, longitudinal view), which are more extensive 10 days later (**d**, longitudinal view) in spite of antibiotic therapy

of fibrosis cause no symptoms, however, especially if single, would be difficult to differentiate from testicular neoplasms. Severe orchitis may result in atrophy with decrease in volume and echogenicity of the testis, and has been attributed to compartment syndrome.

Secondary Orchitis

In contrast, secondary orchitis is generally associated with **epididymitis (epididymo-orchitis)** and is usually the result of retrograde spread of a lower urinary tract infection with enterococci, *E. coli*, proteus, or pseudomonas by way of the vas deferens. Sexually-transmitted mycoplasma, chlamydial, and gonococcal infections also cause secondary orchitis. Granulomatous epididymo-orchitis, a much rarer condition, may occur with tuberculosis, syphilis, and sarcoidosis. Orchitis secondary to lymphatic or hematogenous spread from a perineal abscess may also occur. Isolated secondary orchitis (without epididymitis) is otherwise rare. The onset of secondary orchitis is heralded by scrotal pain, fever, erythema, swelling and tenderness, and is characterized by hypoechoic phlegmonous foci involving *both* the testis and epididymis, frequently in continuity at ultrasonography (Fig. 9.11). These findings are almost invariably associated with a hydrocele. Areas of decreased echogenicity and thickening in the scrotal wall may be present and may reflect scrotal involvement, which typically occurs by direct extension of disease from the testis (38). Although most epididymal and testicular lesions resolve completely following therapy, some may persist as a low grade infection with fibrosis and calcification **(chronic epididymo-orchitis)** (Fig. 9.12) or proceed to abscess formation (39) (Fig. 9.13). Chronic granulomatous diseases such as tuberculosis, syphilis, and sarcoidosis may take a chronic course with painless nodular thickening of the epididymis and vas deferens due to the presence of granulomas and testicular enlargement, swelling, and induration. At ultrasound, these granulomas appear as hypoechoic nodules located in the epididymis and along the course of the vas deferens (40). Abscess formation leading to fistula formation may occur with granulomatous orchitis (41).

Again, persisting hypoechoic granulomas or areas of fibrosis detected by ultrasound, particularly when limited to the testicle, may raise the suggestion of a testicular neoplasm.

Testicular Infarction

Idiopathic or primary testicular infarction is rare and has been reported in newborns. It has been suggested that the testicular artery thrombosis in these cases is the result of blood hyperviscosity due to neonatal polycythemia. Vasculitis and emboli have also been postulated as causes of primary testicular infarction. **Testicular infarction** is most commonly *secondary* to testicular torsion or an incarcerated inguinal hernia (42), although occasionally acute epididymo-orchitis may result in vascular thrombosis and testicular infarction due to compartment syndrome (36, 37, 43, 44). Patients with testicular infarction present with acute pain, swelling, and tenderness of the scrotum and occasionally fever, and may therefore be misdiagnosed as having acute orchitis. Ultrasonography shows diffuse testicular enlargement and focal or diffuse decrease in echogenicity, occasionally with anechoic areas due to hemorrhage (45, 36); these find-

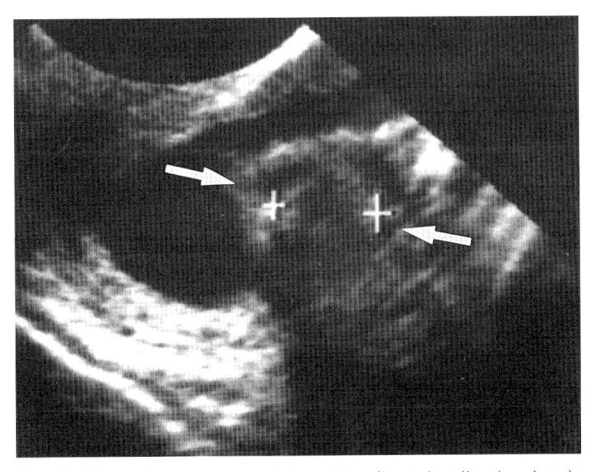

Fig. 9.**12** Chronic epididymitis (longitudinal view): Swelling and inhomogeneity of the epididymis in a middle-aged man, who was being evaluated for infertility and was otherwise asymptomatic. A small hydrocele is also present

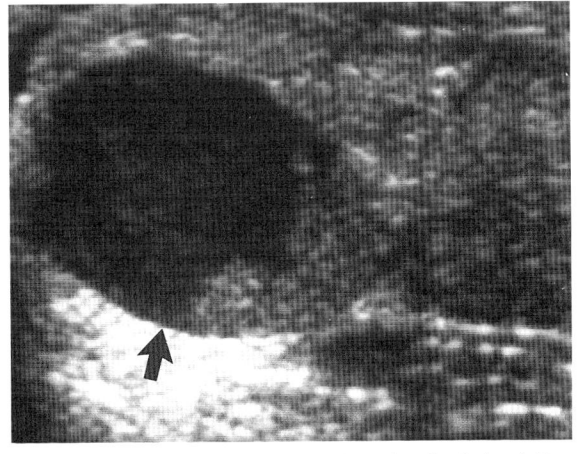

Fig. 9.**13** Epididymal abscess (longitudinal view): Enlarged epididymis containing an anechoic area (arrow) with some debris, which has sedimented

Table 9.7 Orchitis

Pathogenesis:
- Mostly secondary to retrograde spread of lower GU infection associated with epididymitis
- Primary: associated with mumps (rarely Henoch–Schönlein purpura): no epididymitis

Clinical findings:
- Acute: fever, severe local pain, swelling, erythema and tenderness. Testis and epididymis difficult to distinguish, hydrocele, fluctuation, pyuria/bacteruria
- Chronic: persistent testicular enlargement and possibly slight tenderness. Atrophy with decrease in size

Ultrasound findings:
- Acute: testicular enlargement, diffuse or multifocal hypoechogenic areas, anechoic areas due to abscess formation, hydrocele, occas. scrotal thickening
- Chronic: persistent testicular enlargement with hypoechoic areas of fibrosis, hypoechoic granulomas in epididymis. Later decrease in size due to atrophy

Table 9.8 Testicular tumors: histologic classification

Malignant			
Primary	Germ cell tumors	Seminoma
		Teratoma
		Embryonal carcinoma
		Yolk sac tumors
		Chorionic carcinoma
	Stromal tumors	Leydig cell tumors
		Sertoli cell tumors
	Lymphatic/Hemopoietic	Ac. lymphocytic leukemia
		Lymphoma
		Plasmacytoma
Metastatic	Prostatic cancer	
	Bronchial cancer	
	Renal adenocarcinoma	
	Malignant melanoma	
Benign	Epidermoids/ Dermoids	
	Teratomas	
	Malakoplakia	

ings are again not unlike those of acute orchitis (31) as is the testicular atrophy, which may ensue.

Testicular and Paratesticular Tumors

Benign tumors and **tumor-like lesions** such as epidermoids, dermoids, benign teratomas, and malakoplakia are rare (46, 47), as are syphilitic gummas.

Irrespective of age, most **malignant testicular tumors** (Table 9.8) are primary lesions originating within the testis. In the *adult,* germ cell tumors (particularly seminomas) (Fig. 9.14) are by far the more common ones, accounting for 95% of all primary testicular tumors (48). Stromal (Fig. 9.15) and lymphatic/hemopoietic (leukemia, lymphoma, or plasmocytoma) tumors are rare (49, 50, 51, 52, 53) as are testicular metastases (54).

In contrast, germ cell tumors account for only 60–75% of testicular tumors in *childhood,* with yolk sac tumors being the most common (50%) (55) followed by teratomas and leukemic infiltration (Fig. 9.16) (56, 57). Testicular neuroblastomas are only seen in the pediatric age group (58). Seminomas are rare in childhood.

Maldescent and contralateral testicular tumors have been reported to predispose to primary malignant testicular tumors (59, 60). "Primary" retroperitoneal or mediastinal germ cell tumors may be secondary to an occult or "burnt-out" germ cell tumor in the testes (61). In fact, a small fibrosed seminoma seen as a hypoechoic (62) or hyperechoic (63) scar at ultrasound may initially present with retroperitoneal lymph node metastases (64, 65), this being the most common form of spread.

Hormone-producing Leydig cell tumors frequently present with a clinical picture (Table 9.9) of virilizing syndrome of pubertas precox and gynecomastia; elevated estrogen, progesterone, androgen, or corticosteroid serum levels may be present in these patients (66, 67, 68). Serum α-fetoprotein levels may be raised with yolk sac tumors and β-HCG levels with chorionic carcinoma and in 33% of teratocarcinomas and yolk sac tumors.

Irrespective of histologic variety, most testicular tumors appear as areas of decreased echogenicity on ultrasound (65, 69, 70), which may be inhomogeneous and show irregular margins (71). Multifocal or bilateral lesions may occur, particularly with mixed-cell tumors and seminomas, and reflect the tendency of these lesions to arise within a more diffuse epithelial abnormality, possibly with dysplasia and multifocal carcinoma-in-situ (64). Anechoic zones of necrosis, hemorrhage, or cystic degeneration may be observed in larger tumors (72). Hyperechoic areas of fibrosis, calcification, ossification, and chondroid metaplasia may also occur within the tumor (72). Epidermoid (47) or dermoid cysts generally appear hypoechoic to anechoic centrally with a peripheral hyperechoic capsule and cannot be reliably differen-

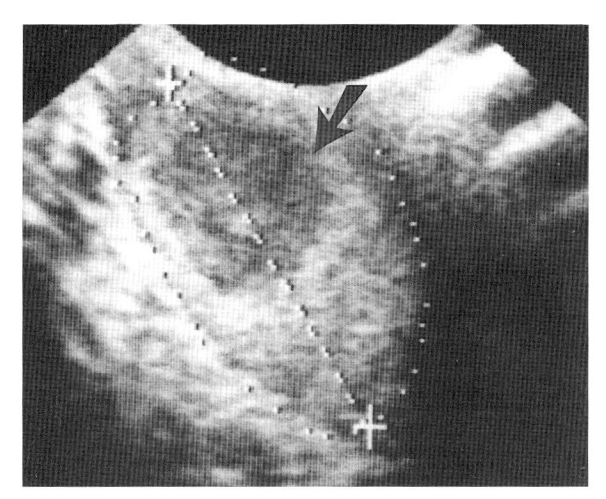

Fig. 9.**14** Seminoma (longitudinal view): Circumscribed inhomogenous hypoechoic area (arrow) in a normal-sized testis confirmed histologically to be a seminoma

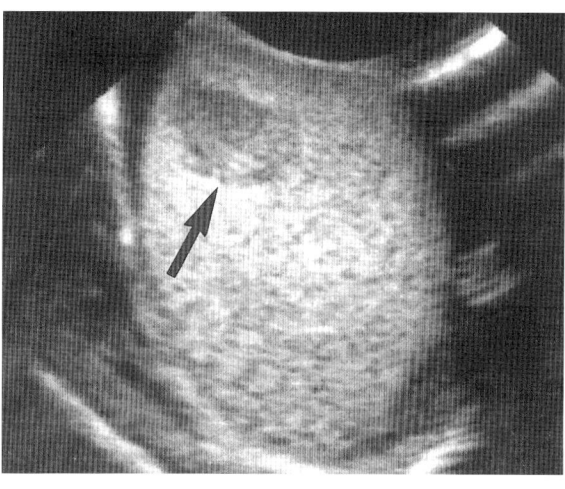

Fig. 9.**15** Leydig cell tumor (longitudinal view): Circumscribed hypoechoic area (arrow) in the upper pole of the testis confirmed histologically to be a Leydig's cell tumor, which was detected during evaluation for infertility. A small hydrocele is present

tiated from teratomas, which may be malignant particularly in the older age group (46, 73).

Decreased echogenicity of the epididymis and tunica albuginea reflect involvement by the tumor and are of no therapeutic consequence. On the other hand, involvement of the scrotal wall and seeding along the spermatic cord, also seen as areas of low echogenicity, should be carefully assessed. Hydroceles are frequent and do not necessarily signify extracapsular extension of disease.

Ultrasonic detection of a testicular lesion suggestive of neoplastic disease warrants evaluation for retroperitoneal lymph node metastases with CT or lymphography.

Primary tumors of the epididymis or spermatic cord are rare (74), and are more often benign than malignant. Benign tumors of the epididymis include adenomatoid tumors (75, 76, 77), which are seen in middle-aged men and are thought to arise from the mesothelium of the tunica vaginalis, and papillary cystadenoma, which is found associated with von Hippel–Lindau syndrome (78). Benign spermatic cord tumors include lipomas, fibromas, neurofibromas, myomas, hemangiomas, teratomas, and dermoids (79, 80, 81). Rhabdomyosarcoma of the epididymis or spermatic cord is a more common malignant tumor, which can occur at all ages; other malignant tumors of the epididymis or spermatic cord such as liposarcomas, primary carcinomas, leiomyosarcomas, lymphomas, and mesotheliomas are exceedingly rare (79, 82, 83, 84). Irrespective of histological type, epididymal and spermatic cord tumors usually present as slow-growing painless nodules, which are generally inhomogeneous and hypoechoic at sonography and may therefore

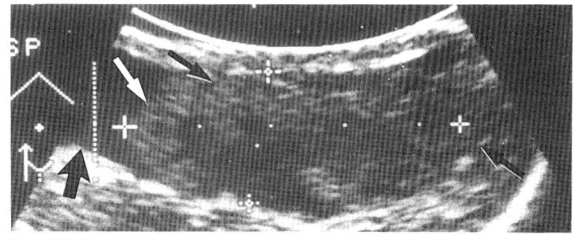

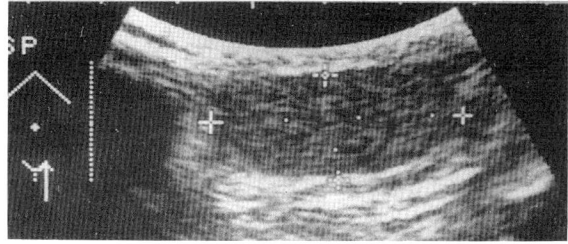

Fig. 9.**16** Leukemic infiltration of the testis (longitudinal views): A 6-year-old boy with newly diagnosed acute lymphoblastic leukemia developed right-sided testicular swelling and pain. (**a**) Ultrasonography showed a swollen inhomogenous testis (small black arrows) with poorly defined areas of low echogenicity, a small hydrocele (large black arrow) and a normal epididymis (white arrow). (**b**) After four weeks of treatment, the testis returned to normal size and became homogeneous. The hydrocele has resolved

closely resemble fibrotic nodules or granulomas of chronic epididymitis. Anechoic cystic areas may be present with teratomas and dermoids, whereas lipomas are generally hyperechoic and change their shape when compressed (85). Examination in the upright position and Valsalva maneuver may help

Table 9.9 Testicular tumors: diagnosis

Clinical findings:
- None
- Painless focal or diffuse induration or swelling
- Retroperitoneal lymph node enlargement (20–40% of cases at first diagnosis)
- Hematogenous metastases: late

Ultrasound findings:
- No lesion or hyperechoic scar
- Usually hypoechoic, inhomogenous, and poorly defined
- Anechoic zones of necrosis/hemorrhage/cystic degeneration
- Enlargement of epididymis, defect in tunica albuginea

Specific features:
- Most likely diagnosis: germ cell tumor
  Adult: seminoma; child: yolk sac tumor, or teratoma
- H/o neoplasm (bronchus, prostate, melanoma) or myeloproliferative disorder: metastases
- Enlarged mediastinal/retroperitoneal lymph nodes and no testicular lesion: occult or "burnt-out" seminoma
- Gynecomastia, pub. precox, virilizing syndrome: Leydig cell tumor
- Increased α-FP: yolk sac tumor
- Increased β-HCG: chorionic carcinoma

differentiate a spermatic cord lipoma from a hernial sac containing omentum.

Other Structural Abnormalities of the Testes

Hydroceles

The term hydrocele refers to a fluid collection separating the parietal and visceral layers of the tunica vaginalis. Hydroceles occur most commonly in the scrotum surrounding the testis and epididymis (testicular hydrocele), but may be located anywhere along the spermatic cord (spermatic hydrocele). **Congenital** hydroceles, due to a persistant processus vaginalis, usually resolve spontaneously within the first year of life with closure of the processus (86, 87, 88). Most **acquired** hydroceles occur secondary to acute orchitis, testicular trauma, or torsion and therefore present with acute pain in the scrotal compartment involved. Painless acquired hydroceles are known to occur with filarial infection due to lymphatic obstruction (89). Pyoceles are the result of direct extension of testicular infection, whereas hematoceles are seen following trauma and occasionally as a complication of Henoch–Schönlein purpura.

The main concern when evaluating patients with painless hydroceles is the possibility of an occult testicular neoplasm. In fact, 10% of hydroceles are due to testicular or spermatic cord neoplasms (45).

Hydroceles cause scrotal swelling, are elastic and fluctuant on palpation, and show positive transillumination. Ultrasonography shows anechoic fluid separating the testis and epididymis from the scrotal sac (Fig. 9.**17a**). The fluid is easily displaced by the examining probe and is best visualized at the periphery of the field. A congenital hydrocele can be followed through the inguinal canal and is best appreciated with the patient in the upright position. Chronic hydroceles may show septation (Fig. 9.**17b**) and debris or calcifications, which float around when the probe is moved.

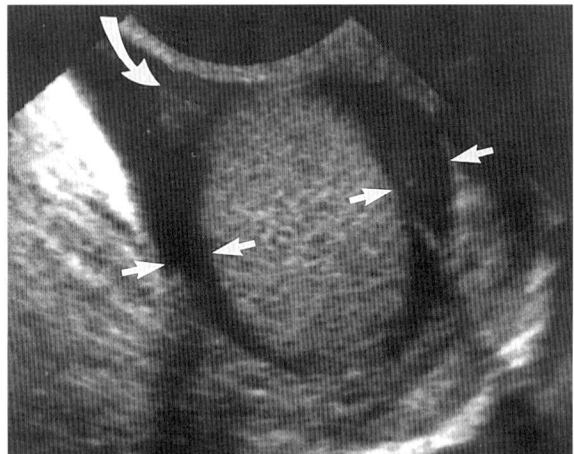

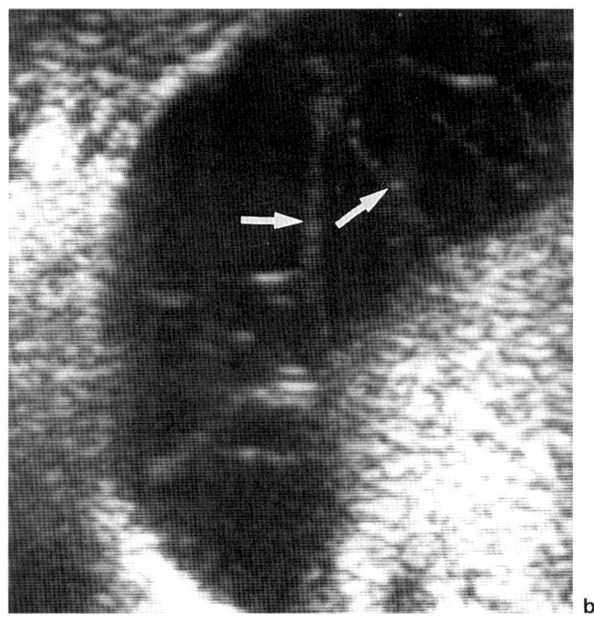

Fig. 9.**17** (**a**) Hydrocele (longitudinal view): Anechoic fluid (small white arrows) separating the scrotal wall from the testis and epididymis (curved arrow). (**b**) Chronic hydrocele (transverse view): Multiple separations (arrows) are present within the hydrocele

Spermatic cord hydroceles may present as hard, rubbery nodules, and in the presence of testicular atrophy, may be confused with an undescended testis. Ultrasonography, however, readily differentiates an anechoic hydrocele from a flattened hypoechoic inguinal testis with an epididymis.

Varicoceles

A varicocele consists of a dilated ("varicosed") portion of the pampiniform plexus of veins located in the scrotal wall, and may be unilateral (more commonly on the left side) or bilateral (90). **"Primary" varicoceles** are usually the result of incompetent venous valves within those veins, which drain the pampiniform plexus into the inferior vena cava on the right and into the left renal vein on the left. In these cases, the characteristic feature is their tendency to partially or completely empty with the patient in the recumbant position, and to become more prominent when the patient stands or performs the Valsalva maneuver. In contrast, **"secondary"** varicoceles are due to obstructed venous drainage either through external compression (e.g., enlarged retroperitoneal lymph nodes) or through venous occlusion (e.g., thrombus or intraluminal tumor extension frequently seen with renal adenocarcinoma). In this situation, the varicocele usually develops rapidly and may not drain when the patient lies down.

Varicoceles are found in 10–40% of men who are evaluated for infertility. In fact, increased scrotal temperature resulting from inefficient testicular cooling due to slow venous drainage has been postulated to adversely affect spermatogenesis (91).

Although many varicoceles may be visible and palpable as a mass of dilated ("wormlike") veins in the scrotal wall, correlative studies have shown ultrasonography to be much more sensitive, and that only about a third of varicoceles are detected clinically (92). Ultrasonography demonstrates a varying number of serpigenous tubular anechoic structures measuring 2 mm or more in diameter (Fig. 9.**18**), which increase in diameter when the patient stands or performs the Valsalva maneuver. The detection of clinically occult varicoceles in infertile patients has significant impact on their further treatment. With the introduction of duplex and color Doppler sonography, retrograde venous flow through the testicular veins can be evaluated. Positive venous reflux within the testicular veins in the extrainguinal portion of the spermatic cord, with the patient in the upright position or performing the Valsalva maneuver, has been shown to correlate well with the results of retrograde testicular venography (93) and has been found to be associated with impaired spermatogenesis and testicular atrophy (92, 94).

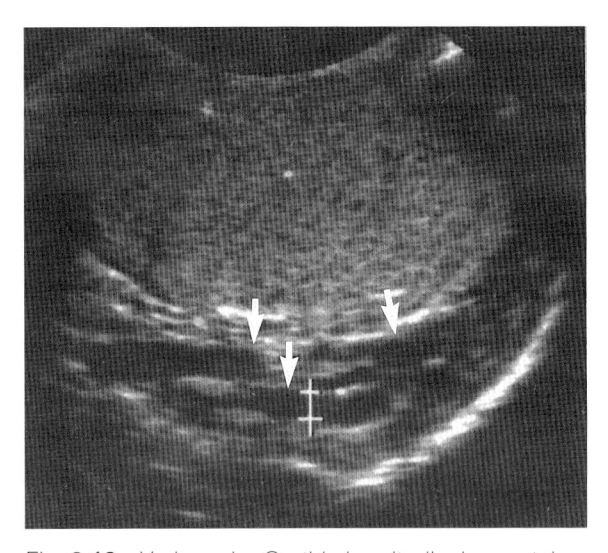

Fig. 9.**18** Varicocele: On this longitudinal scan taken with the patient lying down, the dilated veins of the pampiniform plexus are visualized as anechoic serpigenous structures (arrows) measuring 2.5 mm in diameter

Testicular Atrophy

Unilateral testicular atrophy is frequently observed following orchidopexy for incomplete descent or associated with a long-standing varicocele. Alternatively, it may develop as a complication of ischemia due to torsion or to compartment syndrome secondary to acute orchitis or following trauma.

Clinical findings include a small testicle, which usually has a soft consistency in contrast to the firm testes palpated in patients with Klinefelter syndrome. Ultrasonography demonstrates a small homogeneous hypoechoic testicle; the mediastinum testis is occasionally discernable in these cases (35, 45). Areas of capsular induration on palpation or hypoechoic foci on ultrasound should suggest malignant change, although fibrosis and infection may produce similar findings. Testicular volume can be assessed reliably by ultrasonography, as described above (95), and has been shown to directly correlate with testicular function (96).

Testicular Cysts

With the advent of testicular sonography, testicular cysts are more frequently detected (97, 98). They may be solitary or multiple. There are two forms of **solitary** cysts: **cysts of the tunica albuginea** (Fig. 9.**19a**), which are palpable and represent persistent portions of the ductus efferens (99, 100, 101), and nonpalpable, dysgenetic **central testicular cysts** (Fig. 9.**19b**), which are generally located close to the mediastinum testis (72). In contrast, **congenital cystic dys-**

264   9 Testis

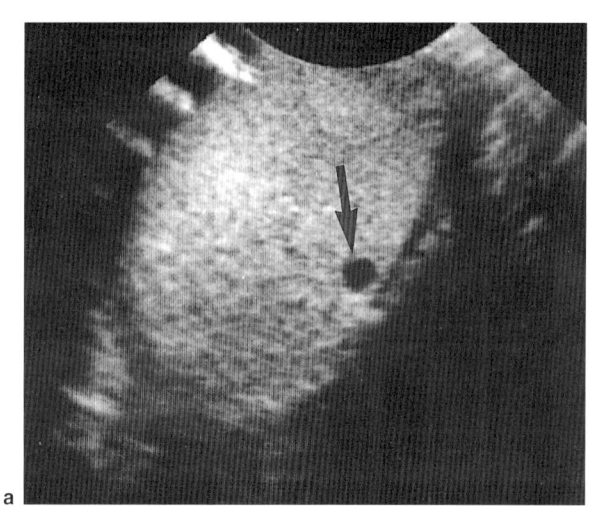

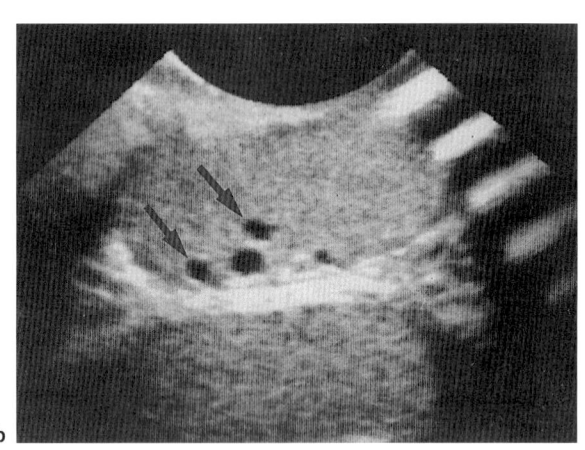

Fig. 9.**19** Testicular cysts: (**a**) A solitary cyst of the tunica albuginea (arrow) (longitudinal view). (**b**) Dysgenetic testicular cysts (arrows) are located further away from the capsule, usually within the area of the mediastinum testis (longitudinal view)

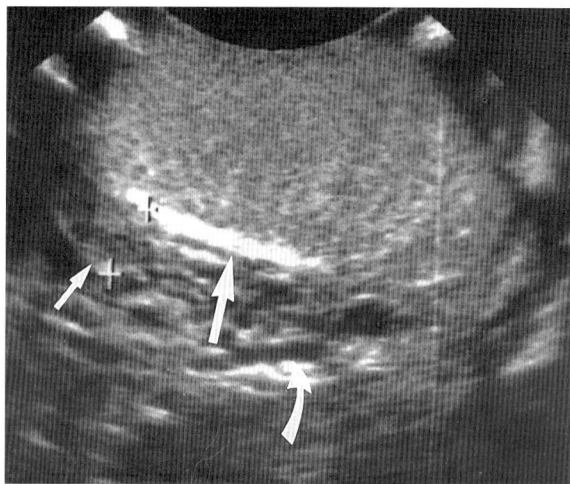

Fig. 9.**20** Thickening of the tunica albuginea: Longitudinal scan in a patient who was under evaluation for infertility, showing focal thickening of the tunica albuginea (large arrow), some thickening body of the epididymis (small arrow) and a varicocele (curved arrow)

plasia of the testis (102, 103) is seen with ipsilateral renal agenesis or dysplasia and is characterized by **multiple** cysts dispersed throughout the testes. At ultrasonography, cysts appear as discrete anechoic structures with some dorsal enhancement and no discernable capsule. Differentiating testicular cysts from cystic tumors (e. g., teratoma) may occasionally pose problems. A discrepancy between palpable size and sonographic measurements of a peripheral lesion or detection of an adjacent solid component to the lesion on ultrasonography suggest a testicular tumor.

Fibrosis and Calcification of the Tunica Albuginea

Although fibrous thickening of the tunica albuginea is said to occur following infection or trauma, frequently, no specific history is present. A painless area of testicular induration is noted on palpation. Ultrasound shows focal increased echogenicity and thickening of the tunica albuginea (Fig. 9.**20**) occasionally with dorsal shadowing due to calcification. Ultrasonographic examination of the testis should be performed from the side opposite the calcification to allow evaluation of subjacent testicular tissue free of shadowing.

Testicular Calcifications

Single or multiple calcifications of the testis may occur following infection or trauma (104, 105) and are seen as well-defined hyperechoic foci on ultrasound with dorsal shadowing occuring with larger lesions (Fig. 9.**21a**). With an appropriate history, and in the absence of a palpable mass or retroperitoneal lymph node enlargement, these lesions require no further evaluation. However, calcification may occasionally occur in a 'burnt-out' germ cell tumor and would require further evaluation, particularly in patients with a history of orchiopexy. **Testicular microlithiasis** is a rare, frequently idiopathic condition characterized by diffuse finely speckled, hyperechoic appearance of the testis (Fig. 9.**21b**); these fine, nonpalpable calcifications are located within the seminiferous tubules (106, 107). Similar diffuse fine testicular calcifications have also been reported following systemic chemotherapy.

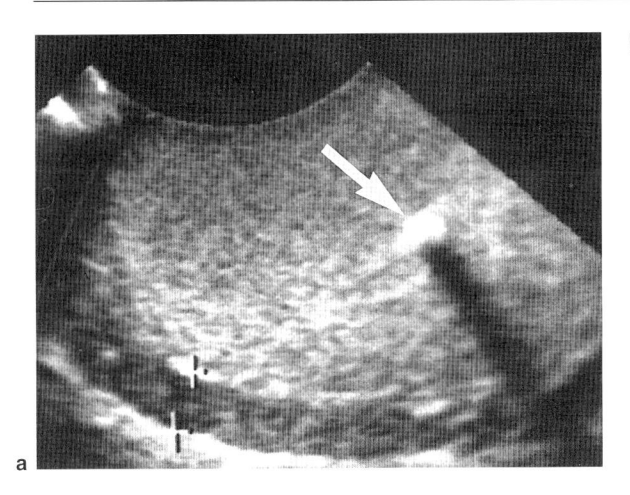

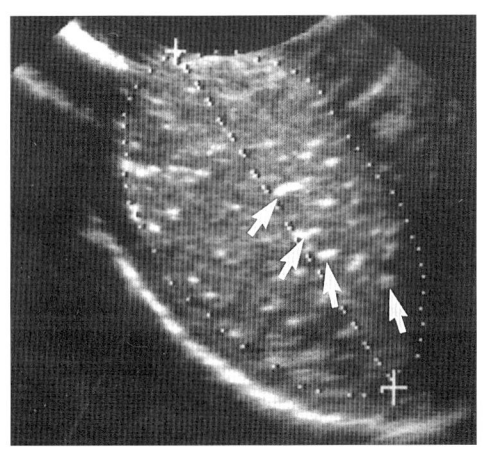

Fig. 9.21 Testicular calcifications: (**a**) Longitudinal scan showing a single parenchymal calcification (arrow) with dorsal shadowing. (**b**) Testicular microlithiasis in a patient who had received chemotherapy in the past: the longitudinal scan displays the speckled appearance of the testis (arrows) and no dorsal shadowing

Conclusion

Ultrasonography is capable of detecting scrotal abnormalities with a greater degree of accuracy than physical examination and plays a crucial role in evaluation of patients with suspected testicular disorders. However, due to the similarities in echostructure of different disease entities, characterization of a testicular lesion is often not possible based on sonographic findings alone. Fundamental problems, such as differentiating orchitis from a testicular neoplasm, can only be resolved through correlation with clinical findings. Thus, a coordinated, interdisciplinary approach is required to optimize the therapeutic impact offered by high-resolution ultrasonography in patients with testicular disease.

References

1. Rifkin MD, Kurtz AB, Pasto ME, Goldberg BB. Diagnostic capabilities of high-resolution scrotal ultrasonography: prospective evaluation. J Ultrasound Med. 1985;4(1):13–9.
2. London NJ, Smart JG, Kinder RB, Watkin EM, Rees Y, Haley P. Prospective study of routine scrotal ultrasonography in urological practice. Br J Urol. 1989;63(4):416–9.
3. Fowler RC, Chennells PM, Ewing R: Scrotal ultrasonography: a clinical evaluation. Br J Radiol. 1987;60(715):649–54.
4. Kromann Andersen B, Hansen LB, Larsen PN, et al. Clinical versus ultrasonographic evaluation of scrotal disorders. Br J Urol. 1988;61(4):350–3.
5. Hamm B. Sonographische Diagnostik des Skrotalinhalts: Lehrbuch und Atlas. Berlin: Springer; 1991:117–119.
6. American Institute of Ultrasound in Medicine (AIUM) (1984): Safety considerations for diagnostic ultrasound. Bioeffects committee.
7. Miller DL. A review of the ultrasonic bioeffects of microsonation, gas-body activation, and related cavitation-like phenomena. Ultrasound Med Biol. 1987;13(8):443–70.
8. Friedrich M. A simple attachment for superficial sonography (Einfache Vorlaufstrecke für die Nahbereichs-Sonographie). ROFO. 1987;146(2):223–31.
9. Doernberger V, Doernberger G, Eggstein M. Volumetrie des Hodens mittels Real-time-Sonographie. Ultraschall Med. 1986;7:300–303.
10. Leopold GR, Woo VL, Scheible FW, Nachtsheim D, Gosink B. High resolution ultrasonography of scrotal pathology. Radiology. 1979;131:719–723.
11. Friedrich M, Calaussen CD, Felix R. Immersion ultrasonography of scrotal and testicular pathology. Europ J Radiol. 1981;1:60–64.
12. Scorer CG, Farrington GH. Congenital anomalies of the testis. In: Harrison JH, Gittes RF, Perlmutter AD, Stamey TA, Walsh PC, eds. Campbell's Urology. 4th ed. Philadelphia: WB Saunders, 1979:1549–1565.
13. Kleinteich B. Klinische Problematik. In: Kleinteich B, Hadziselimovic F, Hesse V, Schreiber G, (eds). Kongenitale Hodendystopien. Leipzig: Thieme; 1979:15–76.
14. Dieckmann KP, Due W, Fiedler U. Perineale Hodenektopie. Urologe A. 1988;27:358–362.
15. Martin DC. Germinal cell tumors of the testis after orchiopexy. J Urol. 1979;121(4):422–424.
16. Wobbes T, Schrffordt Koops H, Oldhoff J. The relation between testicular tumors, undescended testes and inguinal hernias. J Surg Oncol. 1980;14(1)45–52.
17. Morrison AS. Cryptorchidism, hernia and cancer of the testes. J Natl Cancer Inst. 1976;56(4):731–733.
18. Rosenfield AT, Blair DN, McCarthy S, Glickman MG, Rosenfield NS, Weiss R. The pars infravaginalis gubernaculi: importance in the identification of the undescended testis. Am J Roentgenol 1989;153:775–778.
19. Wolverson MK, Houttuin E, Heiberg E, Sundaram M, Shields JB. Comparison of computed tomography with high-resolution real-time ultrasound in the localization of the impalpable undescended testes. Radiology. 1983;146:133–136.
20. Fritzsche PJ, Hricak H, Kogan BA, Winkler ML, Tanagho EA. Undescended testis: value of MR imaging. Radiology. 1987;164:169–173.
21. Wheeler MA. Selective testicular venography in abdominal cryptorchidism. J Urol. 1976;115:760–761.
22. Diamond AB, Meng CH, Kodroff M, Goldman SM: Testicular venography in the nonpalpable testis. Am J Roentgenol. 1977;129:129–135.
23. Greenberg SH, Ring EJ, Oleaga J, Wein AJ. Gonadal venography for preoperative localization of non-palpable testes in adults. Urology. 1979;13:453–455.
24. Levitt SB, Kogan SJ, Engel RM, Weiss RM, Martin DC, Ehrlich RM. The impalpable testis: a rational approach to management. J Urol. 1978;120:515–520.
25. Nacey JN, Urquhart Hay D: Polyorchidism. Br J Urol. 1987;59:280.
26. Rifkin MD, Kurtz, AB, Pasto ME, Goldberg BB. Polyorchidism diagnosed preoperatively by ultrasonography. J Ultrasound Med. 1983;2:93–94.

27. Hutton L, Rankin RM, Pozsinyi J. High-resolution ultrasound of macro-orchidism in mental retardation. J Clin Ultrasound 1985;13:19–22.
28. Nielsen KB, Tommerup N. Macroorchidism, mental retardation and the fragile X. N Engl J Med. 1981;305:1348.
29. Ruvalcaba RHA, Myhre SA, Roosen-Runga EC, Beckwith JB. X-linked mental deficiency megalotestes syndrome. JAMA 1977;238:1646–1650.
30. Turner G, Daniel A, Frost M. X-linked mental retardation, macro-orchidism and the Xq (27) fragile site. J. Pediatr. 1980;96:837–841.
31. Hoeg OM. Acute scrotum: how to distinguish between torsion of the testis, acute epididymitis and torsion of the appendix testis. Tidsskr Nor Laegeforen. 1988;108(17–18):1390–1392, 1423.
32. O'Regan S, Robitaille P. Orchitis mimicking testicular torsion in Henoch-Schonlein purpura. J Urol.1981;126:834.
33. Lentini JF, Benson CB, Richie JP. Sonographic features of focal orchitis. J Ultrasound Med. 1989;8:361–365.
34. See WA, Mack LA, Krieger JN. Scrotal ultrasonography: a predictor of complicated epididymitis requiring orchiectomy. J Urol. 1988;139:55–56.
35. Krone KD, Carroll BA. Scrotal ultrasound. Radiol Clin North Am. 1985;23:121–139.
36. Rencken RK, Du-Plessis DJ, De-Haas LS. Venous infarction of the testis as a cause of non-response to conservative therapy in epididymo-orchitis: a case report. S Afr Med J. 1990;78(6):337–338.
37. See WA, Mack LA, Krieger JN. Scrotal ultrasonography: a predictor of complicated epididymitis requiring orchiectomy. J Urol. 1988;139(1):55–56.
38. Rifkin MD, Kurtz AB, Pasto ME, et al. The sonographic diagnosis of focal and diffuse infiltrating intrascrotal lesions. Urol Radiol. 1984;6:20–26.
39. Mevorach RA, Lerner RM, Dvoretsky PM, Rabinowitz R. Testicular abscess: diagnosis by ultrasonography. J Urol. 1986;136:1213–1216.
40. Selikowitz SM, Schned AR: A late postvasectomy syndrome. J Urol. 1985;134:494–497.
41. Heaton ND, Hogan B, Michell M, Thompson P, Yates-Bell AJ. Tuberculous epididymo-orchitis: clinical and ultrasound observations. Br J Urol. 1989;64:305–309.
42. Grosfeld JL. Current concepts in inguinal hernia in infants and children. World J Surg. 1989;13(5):506–515.
43. Bird K, Rosenfield AT. Testicular infarction secondary to acute inflammatory disease: demonstration by B-scan ultrasound. Radiology. 1984;152:785–788.
44. Vordermark JS, Favila MQ: Testicular necrosis: a preventable complication of epididymitis. J Urol. 1982;128:1322–1324.
45. Hricak H, Filly RA. Sonography of the scrotum. Invest Radiol. 1983;18:112–121.
46. Schlecker BA, Siegel A, Weiss J, Wein AJ: Epidermoid cyst of the testis: a surgical approach for testicular preservation. J Urol. 1985;133:610–611.
47. Goldstein AMB, Mendez R, Vartgas A, Terry R. Epidermoid cysts of the testis. Urology. 1980;15:186–189.
48. Robbins SL, Cotran RS. Testis and epididymis. In: Robbins SL, Cotran RS. Pathologic Basis of Disease, 2nd ed. Philadelphia: WB Saunders; 1979:1216–1230.
49. Phillips G, Kumari-Subaiya S, Sawitsky A. Ultrasonic evaluation of the scrotum in lymphoproliferative disease. J Ultrasound Med. 1987;6:169–175.
50. Portalez D, Song MY, Marty MH, Joffre F. Ultrasonographic patterns of testicular non-Hodgkin's lymphoma. Eur J Radiol. 1982;2:222–225.
51. Rayor RA, Scheible W, Brock WA, Leopold GR. High resolution ultrasonography in the diagnosis of testicular relapse in patients with acute lymphoblastic leukemia. J Urol. 1982;128:602–603.
52. Levin HS, Mostofi FK. Symptomatic plasmocytoma of the testis. Cancer. 1970;25:1193–1203.
53. Campani R, Carella E, Moschini GL, Rugazzi E, Bossalini G, Quaretti P. US study of testicular plasmocytoma: a case report. Eng abstract. Radiol Med. 1990;79:247–248.
54. Dieckmann KP, Due W, Loy V. Intrascrotal metastasis of renal cell carcinoma. Case reports and review of the literature. Eur Urol. 1988;15:297–301.
55. Weißbach L, Altwein JE, Stiens R. Germinal testicular tumors in childhood. Eur Urol. 1984;10:73–85.
56. Klein EA, Kay R, Norris DG: Noninvasive testicular screening in childhood leukemia. J Urol. 1986;136:864–866.
57. Lupetin AR, King W, Rich P, Lederman RB: Ultrasound diagnosis of testicular leukemia. Radiology. 1983;146:171–172.
58. Casola G, Scheible W, Leopold GR. Neuroblastoma metastatic to the testis: ultrasonographic screening as an aid to clinical staging. Radiology. 1984;151:475–476.
59. Dieckmann KP, Boeckmann W, Brosig W, Jonas D, Bauer HW. Bilateral testicular germ-cell tumors. Report of nine cases and a review of the literature. Cancer. 1986;57:1254–1257.
60. Von der Maase H, Rorth M, Walblom-Jorgensen S, et al. Carcinoma-in-situ of contralateral testis in patients with testicular germ-cell cancer: study of 27 cases in 500 patients. Br Med J. 1986;293:1398–1401.
61. Shawker TH, Javadpour N, O'Leary T, Shapiro E, Krudy AG. Ultrasonographic detection of "burned-out" primary testicular germ cell tumors in clinically normal testes. J Ultrasound Med. 1983;2:477–479.
62. Gross GW, Rohner TJ, Lombard JS, Abrams CS. Metastatic seminoma with regression of testicular primary: ultrasonographic detection. J Urol. 1986;136:1086–1088.
63. Greist A, Einhorn LH, Williams SD, Donohue JP, Rowland RG. Pathologic findings at orchiectomy following chemotherapy for disseminated testicular cancer. J Clin Oncol. 1984;9:1025–1029.
64. Daugaard G, Von der Maase H, Olsen J, Rorth M, Skakkebaeck NE. Carcinoma-in-situ testis in patients with assumed extragonadal germ-cell tumours. Lancet II 1987;528–530.
65. Glazer HS, Lee JK, Melson GL, McClennan BL. Sonographic detection of occult testicular neoplasms. Am J Roentgenol. 1982;138:673–675.
66. Due W, Dieckmann KP, Loy V, Stein H. Immunohistological determination of oestrogen receptor, progesterone receptor, and intermediate filaments in Leydig cell tumors, Leydig cell hyperplasia, and normal Leydig cells of the human testis. J Pathol. 1989;157:225–234.
67. Einhorn LH. Treatment strategies of testicular cancer in the United States. Int J Androl. 1987;10:399–406.
68. Gabrilove JL, Nicolis GL, Mitty HA, Sohval AR. Feminizing interstitial cell tumor of the testis: personal observations and a review of the literature. Cancer. 1975;35:1184–1202.
69. Hendry WS, Garvie WH, Ah-See AK, Bayliss AP. Ultrasonic detection of occult testicular neoplasms in patients with gynecomastia. Br J Radiol. 1984;57:571–572.
70. Stoll S, Goldfinger M, Rothberg R, et al. Incidental detection of impalpable testicular neoplasm by sonography. Am J Roentgenol. 1986;146:349–350.
71. Schwerk WB, Schwerk WN, Rodeck G. Testicular tumors: prospective analysis of real-time US patterns and abdominal staging. Radiology. 1987;164:369–374.
72. Hamm B, Fobbe F, Loy V. Testicular cysts: differentiation with US and clinical findings. Radiology. 1988;168:19–23.
73. Berger Y, Srinivas V, Hajdu SI, Herr HW. Epidermoid cysts of the testis: role of conservative surgery. J Urol. 1985;134:962–963.
74. Schröder R, Hediger C. Paratestikuläre Tumoren. Schweiz Med Wochenschr. 1970;100:1281–1287.
75. Elsässer E. Epidymal tumors. Recent Results Cancer Res. 1977;60:163–175.
76. Fiedler U, Rost A, Gross UM. Tumoren des Nebenhodens. Urologe. 1977;A16:103–106.
77. Arcadi JA. Adenomatoid tumors in the tunica albuginea of the testis. J Surg Oncol. 1988;37(1):38–39.
78. Restrepo C. Surgical pathology of the male adnexa and diseases of the soft tissue. In: Javadpour N, Basky S, eds. Surgical pathology of urologic disease. Baltimore: Williams and Wilkens; 1987:247–260.
79. Hays DM. Rhabdomyosarcoma and other soft tissue sarcomas. In: Hays DM, ed. Pediatric surgical oncology. New York: Grune and Stratton; 1986:87–122.
80. Livolsi VA, Schiff M. Myxoid neurofibroma of the testis. J Urol. 1977;118(2):341–342.
81. Shental J, Fischelovitz J, Sudarsky M, Rizescu J. Hemangioma of the tunica albuginea testis. Eur Urol. 1982;8(6):370–371.

82. Fitzmaurice H, Hotiana MZ, Cricioli V. Malignant mesothelioma of the tunica vaginalis testis. Br J Urol. 1987;60(2):184.
83. McFaccen DW. Myxoid liposarcoma of the spermatic cord. J Surg Oncol. 1989;40(2):132–134.
84. Zwanger Mendelsohn S, Shreck EH, Doshi V. Burkitt lymphoma involving the epididymis and spermatic cord, sonographic and CT findings. Am J Roentgenol. 1989; 153(1):85–86.
85. Gooding GAW. Sonography of the spermatic cord. Am J Roentgenol. 1988;151:721–724.
86. Bousvaros A, Shamberger RC, Winter HS. Abdominal wall defects. In: Rudolph AM, ed. Rudolph's pediatrics. East Norwalk: Appelton and Lange; 1991:1040–1042.
87. Sasidharan P, Crankson S, Ahmed S. Fetal abdominoscrotal hydrocele. Am J Obstet Gynecol. 1991;165(5/1):1353–1355.
88. Achiron R, Amsel S, Zakut H. Prenatal ultrasonic diagnosis of congenital hydrocele and undescended testis: report of two cases. J Foetal Med. 1987;7(1–2):25–26.
89. Liu J, Wong S, Chen Z, Tu Z. Clinical manifestations of filariasis in fujian China. Trop Doct. 1992;22(3):104–106.
90. Demas BE, Hricak H, McClure RD. Varicoceles: radiologic diagnosis and treatment. Radiol Clin North Am. 1991;29(3):619–628.
91. Ali JI, Weaver DJ, Weinstein SH, Grimes EM. Scrotal temperature and semen quality in men with and without varicocele. Arch Androl. 1990;24(2):215–220.
92. Kupeli S, Arikan N, Aydos K, Aytac S. Multiparametric evaluation of testicular atrophy due to varicocele. Urol Int. 1991;46(2):189–192.
93. Petros JA, Andriole GL, Middelton WD, Picus DA. Correlation of testicular color Doppler ultrasonography, physical examination and venography in the detection of left vericocele in men with infertility. J Urol. 1991;145(4):785–788.
94. Nashan D, Behre HM, Grunert JH, Nieshlag E. Diagnostic value of scrotal sonography in infertile men: Report on 658 cases. Andrologia. 1990;22(3):387–395.
95. Behre HM, Nashan D, Nieschlag E. Objective measurement of testicular volume by ultrasonography: evaluation of the technique and comparison with orchidometer estimates. Int J Andro. 1989;12:395–403.
96. Takihara H, Cosentimo JM, Sakatoku J, Cockett ATK: Significance of testicular size measurement in andrology: II. Correlation of testicular size with testicular function. J Urol. 1987;137(3):416–419.
97. Gooding GAW, Leonhardt W, Stein R. Testicular cysts: US-findings. Radiology 1987;163:537–538.
98. Leung ML, Gooding GAW, Williams RD. High-resolution sonography of scrotal contents in asymptomatic subjects. Am J Roentgenol. 1984;143:161–164.
99. Kromann Andersen B, Hansen U, Iversen E, Jakobsen H. Benign cystic lesions of the tunica albuginea. Ann Chir-Gynaecol. 1987;76(2):133–135.
100. Mancilla JR, Matsuda GT. Cysts of the tunica albuginea, report of 4 cases and review of the literature. J Urol. 1975; 114:730–733.
101. Mennemeyer RP, Mason JT. Non-neoplastic cystic lesions of the tunica albuginea: an electron microscopic and clinical study of 2 cases. J Urol. 1979;121:373–375.
102. Cho CS, Kosek J. Cystic dysplasia of the testis: sonographic and pathologic findings. Radiology. 1985;156:777–778.
103. Nistal M, Regadera J, Paniagua R. Cystic dysplasia of the testis. Light and electron microscopic study of three cases. Arch Pathol Lab Med. 1984;108:579–583.
104. Martin B, Tubiana JM. Significance of scrotal calcification detected by sonography. J Clin Ultrasound. 1988;16:545–552.
105. Mitcheson HD, Conley G, Sant GR, Heaney JA, Sarno R, Doherty FJ. Tunica albuginea inclusion cysts and calcifications demonstration by ultrasound. 79th Annual Meeting of the American Urological Association, Inc. New Orleans, LA., USA, May 6–10th, 1984. J Urol. 1984;131(4 part 2):181a.
106. Mullins TL, Sant GR, Ucci AA, Doherty FJ. Testicular microlithiasis occurring in postorchiopexy testis. Urology. 1986;27:144–146.
107. Jaramillo D, Perez-Atayde A, Teele RL. Sonography of testicular microlithiasis. Urol Radiol. 1989;11:55–57.

MR Imaging

Y. S. Kang, M. J. Popovich, and H. Hricak

Various imaging modalities, including ultrasonography (1, 2), CT (3, 4), 99mTc scintigraphy (5), and testicular angiography (6), have been used to supplement the physical examination in the evaluation of scrotal contents. Although high-resolution ultrasound remains the imaging modality of choice in most clinical settings, MRI, the most recent major noninvasive imaging method, may be valuable in selected cases of testicular and extratesticular pathology (7–11). MRI provides superb soft-tissue contrast in multiple planes without the use of ionizing radiation.

Major Clinical Indications

Because of its relatively low cost, easy accessibility in an office setting, and efficient soft-tissue discrimination, ultrasound is the initial imaging study in the investigation of the testes and other scrotal contents in most clinical situations. MRI is used selectively as a problem-solving modality, when results of ultrasound or other preliminary studies are equivocal or suboptimal. Among the potential advantages of MRI compared to ultrasound are superior tissue characterization based on signal intensity analysis, large field of view imaging and less operator or patient habitus dependence. Specific indications for MRI include searching for undescended testes, and evaluating intratesticular disease when ultrasound is inconclusive or there is discrepancy between ultrasound and physical examination findings. MRI can also be used to distinguish between intratesticular and extratesticular disease, or to demonstrate the full extent of diffuse disease involvement.

Safety

The safety of MRI as it relates specifically to scrotal imaging has been studied (12). Although elevation in scrotal temperature by 0.2°C to 3°C was demonstrated during imaging, this is well below the level considered significant enough to cause permanent infertility (12).

Technique

The MR examination is usually performed with the patient supine; either the body coil or a surface coil can be used comfortably in this position. For high-resolution images, use of a surface coil, such as a circular 5-inch (12.5 cm) coil, is mandatory. Correct positioning of the surface coil is critical when imaging the scrotum. A towel is placed beneath the scrotum and over the thighs to prevent scrotal contents from falling between the legs, away from the coil. Then the coil is placed flat over a thin sheet of cloth covering the scrotum. The entire setup is well secured to the patient with tape. Because the whole assembly can be affected by breathing motion, use of a respiratory compensation technique is recommended.

A T1-weighted sagittal sequence is initially done as a localizer. Thin sections—4 mm, with 1- mm interslice gap, for example—are used. This is followed by a T2-weighted sequence, either conventional or fast spin echo, in any or all of three orthogonal planes. Two out of three planes are usually sufficient, and the choice of planes should be tailored to each particular case. A set of T1- and T2-weighted spin-echo sequences should give sufficient diagnostic information for most disease. However, if further tissue characterization is desired, special sequences can be employed, as in the rest of the body. A fat suppression technique can be used for high-signal tissues on T1-weighted images and indeterminate signal on T2-weighted images to distinguish between hemorrhage and fat. Gradient-echo images can be obtained for better evaluation of vascular structures. Contrast medium administration may help to further characterize in selected cases.

In a search for undescended testes, the body coil (or the head coil for infants) should be used for imaging of the pelvis, and if necessary for the lower abdomen. The bladder is emptied to prevent it from displacing inguinal structures. After a sagittal T1-weighted localizer, T1- and T2-weighted axial sequences are obtained from the bottom of the scrotum to above the seminal vesicles. A coronal T2-weighted sequence is optional if the testes are seen in the pelvis.

Anatomy

Details of the testicular and scrotal anatomy are discussed in a previous section in this chapter. A brief discussion of the anatomy necessary to understand the MRI appearance of normal scrotal contents follows.

The normal testis has a homogeneous texture, exhibiting medium signal intensity on T1-weighted images, and high signal intensity on T2-weighted images (Fig. 9.22). The tunica albuginea, a dense fibrous connective tissue capsule covering the testis, has low signal intensity on both T1- and T2-weighted images. Mediastinum testis, the invagination of the tunica albuginea into the testicular parenchyma, has similarly low signal intensity on all sequences. Often, low intensity thin linear structures extending from the mediastinum are seen representing fine septulae and dividing the testis into lobules, which in turn are composed of two to four convoluted seminiferous tubules. The rete testis, the straightened portion of seminiferous tubules near the mediastinum, can occasionally be seen and confused with a pathology lesion. The tunica vaginalis is an outpouching of the peritoneum enveloping each testis. A small amount of normal serous

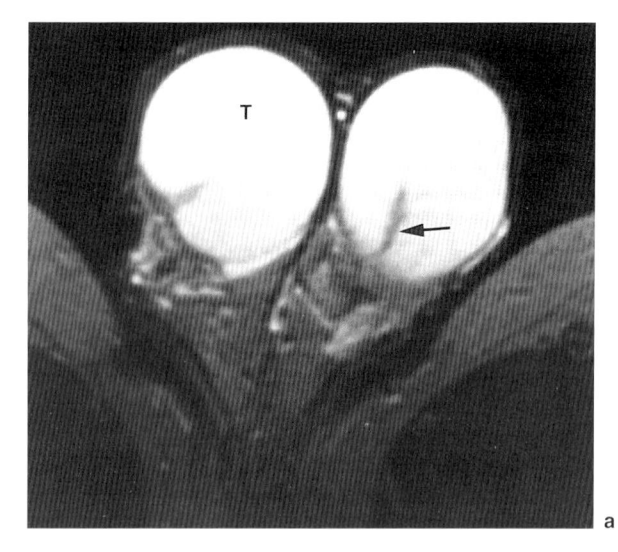

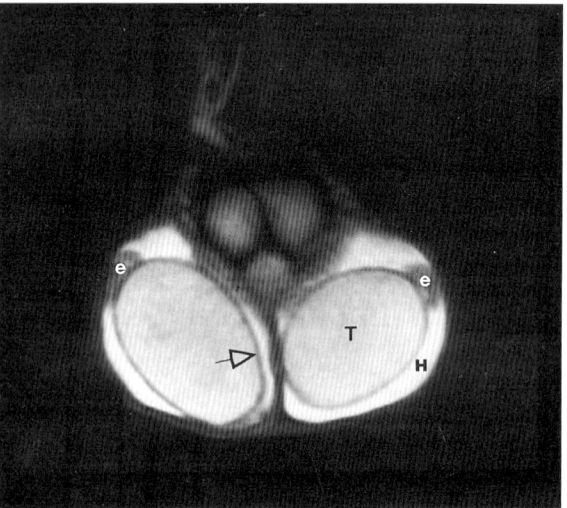

Fig. 9.22 Normal testis. (**a**) axial T2-weighted image, and (**b**) coronal T2-weighted image. The testis (T) has homogeneous high signal intensity on T2-weighted images. The intermediate signal intensity epididymis (e) is readily identified on T2-weighted images. The mediastinum testis (black arrow) is of low signal intensity, similar to the tunica albuginea (open arrow). A small amount of normal fluid (H) is seen between the two layers of tunica vaginalis

fluid can be seen between the two layers of the tunica vaginalis, which demonstrates low intensity on T1-weighted images and high intensity on T2-weighted images.

The epididymis, lying on the posterior aspect of the testis, is isointense or slightly hypointense on T1-weighted images and hypointense on T2-weighted images, relative to the testis. The epididymis can therefore be relatively easily distinguished from adjacent testicular tissue or fluid on T2-weighted images. The scrotal skin has medium to high signal intensity on T1-weighted images, and can be differentiated from the low-intensity dartos muscle just under the skin. This signal difference decreases on T2-weighted images. The envelope of the spermatic cord, formed by fascias and cremasteric muscles, is readily seen as a low-intensity ring within subcutaneous fat. Separate components within the spermatic cord (the testicular veins and pampiniform plexus, the testicular arteries and nerves, and the ductus deferens) are difficult to resolve below the level of the internal inguinal ring. However, the anatomic landmarks of the spermatic cord (the external ring, the inguinal canal, and the internal ring) are usually well demonstrated.

Pathology

Congenital Anomalies

Imaging can be helpful in the evaluation of rare congenital conditions affecting the testis, such as unilateral (monorchidism) or bilateral (anorchidism) absence, or duplication (polyorchia) (13). However, by far the most frequent indication for an imaging study in this group is the search for a nonpalpable undescended testis (14). An undescended testis is one of the most common genitourinary anomalies (15, 16) with a prevalence of 3.5% at birth for otherwise normal infants (higher for premature neonates). Because of a high rate of spontaneous descent, the prevalence decreases to 0.8% by 1 year of age. Bilateral involvement is seen in 10% of the cases. The clinical significance of this disorder is twofold. An undescended testis is associated with a variety of abnormalities (17), including an increased incidence of malignant neoplasms. Also, if left untreated, undescended testes have infertility rates of 100% for bilateral, and 60% for unilateral involvement (18). With successful surgery, the incidence of infertility decreases significantly.

In the past, preoperative localization has been performed with gonadal venography, CT, and ultrasound (19). MRI has more recently (20–23) shown the unique advantage of combining noninvasiveness, unparalleled soft-tissue contrast, absence of ionizing radiation, a large field of view, multiplanar capabilities, and relative operator independence. The diagnosis is based on demonstration of an elliptical mass seen along the expected path of testicular descent. The undescended testis may be in a high scrotal position (along the course of the spermatic cord, usually close to the external inguinal ring; Fig. 9.**23**), in the canalicular position (within the inguinal canal), or in the abdominal position (above the internal inguinal ring; Fig. 9.**24**). MRI has high sensitivity for detecting the testis in most of these locations except for the rare cases of high abdominal or truly ectopic positions.

Specific advantages of MRI as a problem-solving modality have emerged. First, the testis within the

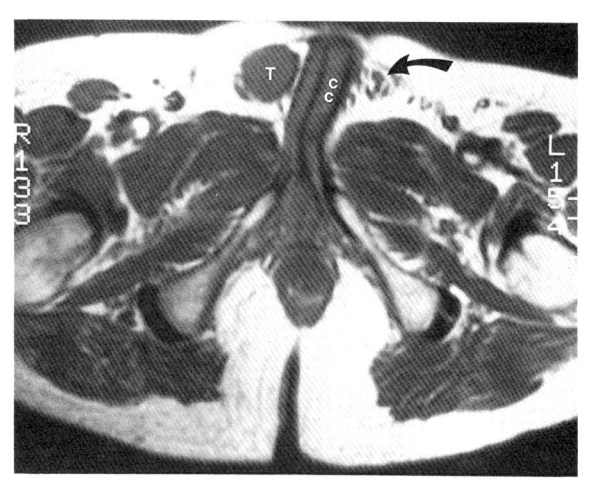

Fig. 9.**23** Undescended testis in a high scrotal position. Axial T1-weighted image showing a right undescended testis (T) along the course of the spermatic cord below the external inguinal ring. (cc) corpus cavernosum. (arrow) normal left spermatic cord

spermatic cord can be readily distinguished from inguinal lymph nodes (unlike in an ultrasound examination) (Fig. 9.**25**). Second, MRI can be used to differentiate between a true undescended testis and a retractile testis, which lies in the scrotum only intermittently and may occupy a high scrotal position secondary to contraction of the cremasteric muscle. While a retractile testis has normal volume and signal intensity, the undescended testis is usually small and may exhibit intensity lower than normal on T2-weighted images. Third, MR can be helpful in avoiding a recently reported imaging pitfall: the misdiagnosis of the remaining bulbous gubernaculum as an undescended testis (24). The gubernaculum shows low intensity on both T1- and T2-weighted images, whereas the testis exhibits higher intensity unless severe testicular atrophy and fibrosis have occurred.

MRI can also be valuable in the workup of patients with ambiguous genitalia (25, 26). Male pseudohermaphrodites (genetic males with decreased androgen production or end-organ sensitivity) often have undescended testes, which can be seen on MRI. In patients with mixed gonadal dysgenesis, usually a streak gonad or absent gonad on one side, and a testis on the other side are found. In true hermaphrodites, the most commonly found testicular–ovarian tissue combination is an ovotestis on one side and an ovary or testis on the other.

Inflammatory Processes

Acute epididymitis is the most common inflammatory lesion of the scrotum. Orchitis is usually associated with epididymitis. Rarely, isolated orchitis can be seen in a viral infection, typically mumps.

270   9 Testis

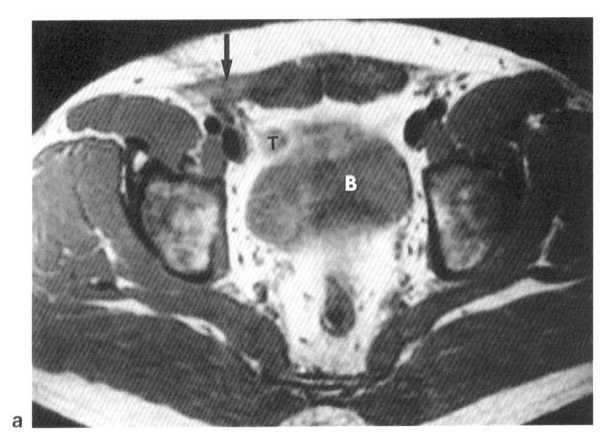

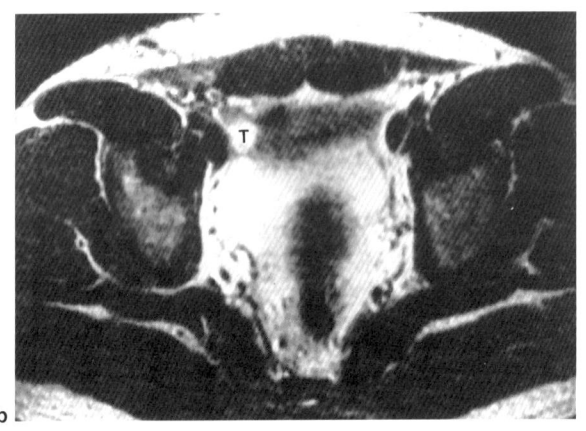

Fig. 9.24 Abdominal undescended testis. Axial (**a**) proton density, and (**b**) T2-weighted images. The testis (T) is seen above the level of the internal inguinal ring. Scar tissue (arrow) from previous unsuccessful surgery for localization is present. B = bladder

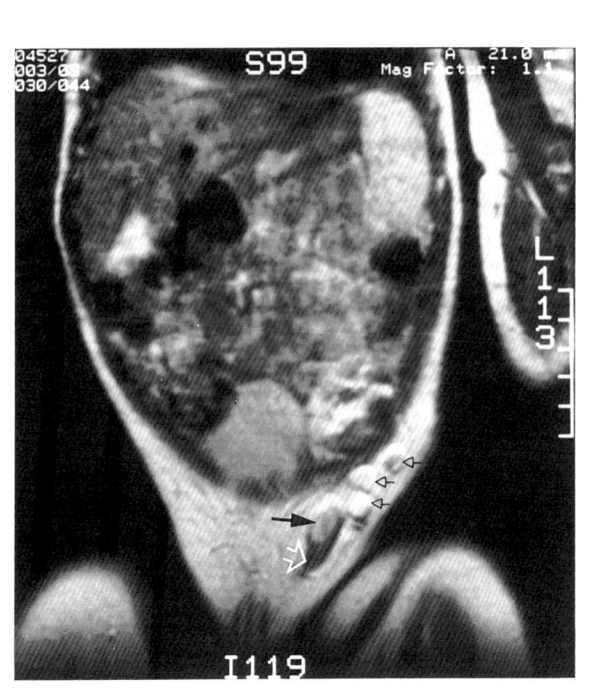

Prompt treatment of epididymo-orchitis is important because severe edema of scrotal contents can compromise blood flow to the testis leading to infarction. Potential complications also include a scrotal abscess and gangrene. Clinically, it is also important to differentiate acute epididymitis from acute torsion (27) or a testicular neoplasm. When the clinical diagnosis of epididymitis needs reinforcement by imaging, ultrasound is considered the primary approach, usually providing high diagnostic accuracy. MRI is a problem-solving modality used only when ultrasound is limited. An MRI diagnosis of epididymitis is based on finding an enlarged epididymis, which usually has low intensity on T2-weighted images except in some acute cases (Fig. 9.26). The inflammatory process often ascends along the spermatic cord and the ductus deferens. When epididymitis is accompanied by orchitis, the testis has areas of decreased intensity on T2-weighted images (Fig. 9.27). However, imaging findings alone are not thought to be sufficient to distinguish benign from malignant disease of the testis, although a recent study reports some promise in specificity of MRI findings in orchitis: areas of ill-defined heterogeneous but predominantly low signal intensity within the testis (27). Other associated MRI findings include scrotal skin thickening, a reactive hydrocele, and in the case of abscess formation, presence of air.

Torsion

Torsion of the spermatic cord usually has developmentally predisposing factors such as absent or defective fixation by the gubernaculum, a long mesorchium, or an entwined cremasteric muscle (28). Failure to detect

Fig. 9.25 Undescended testis with adjacent lymphadenopathy. Coronal T2-weighted image demonstrating the left undescended testis (black arrow) in a high scrotal position. The mediastinum testis is seen as a linear structure of low signal intensity within the testis, while the gubernaculum (open white arrow) is located inferior to the testis. High intensity inguinal lymphnodes (small open black arrows) are readily distinguished from the testis

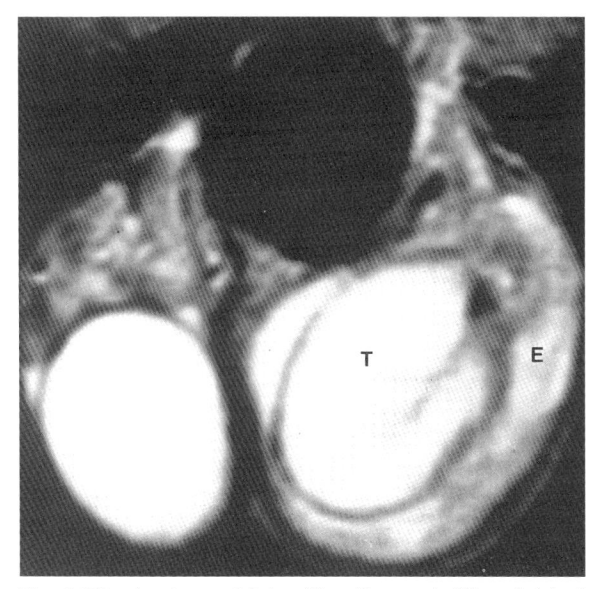

Fig. 9.**26** Acute epididymitis. Coronal T2-weighted image showing a diffusely enlarged epididymis (E) of heterogeneous high signal intensity, an atypical appearance that can be seen in the acute phase. The left testis (T) remains of normal high signal intensity with no evidence of involvement by an inflammatory process

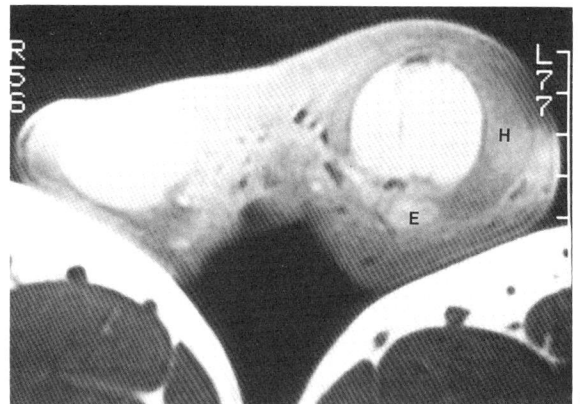

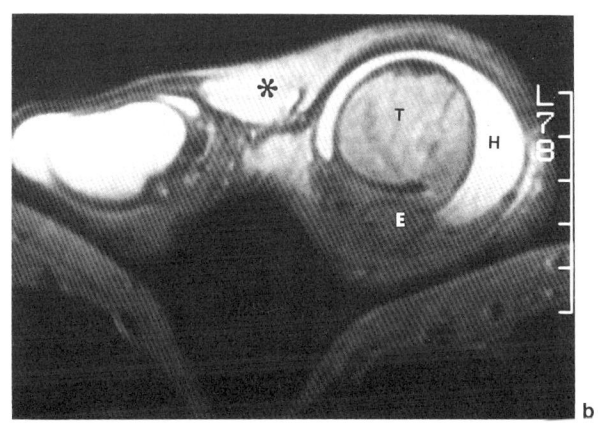

Fig. 9.**27** Epididymitis with associated orchitis. Axial (**a**) proton density, and (**b**) T2-weighted images. The left epididymis (E) is enlarged and of low signal intensity on the T2-weighted image. The ipsilateral testis (T) has relatively lower signal intensity on the T2-weighted image. Also noted is thickening and higher signal intensity of the scrotal skin on the left (*). H = reactive hydrocele

torsion early (within the first 24 hours) in most cases leads to irreversible loss of testicular viability. Clinical distinction from epididymitis can be difficult. Dynamic and static Tc-DTPA scintigraphy, and more recently color Doppler sonography, are the mainstays of radiological diagnosis. The exact clinical role of MRI is currently not defined. In an animal model, the acutely torsed testis may demonstrate enlargement and diffusely heterogeneous signal intensity on T2-weighted images (29). In intermittent torsion, high signal intensity on both T1- and T2-weighted images has been demonstrated, corresponding to the histologically found diffuse subacute hemorrhage (Fig. 9.**28**). In chronic torsion, decreased intensity on T2-weighted images appears to be a consistent feature (27, 29). Additional findings distinguishing torsion from epididymitis include a torsion knot and whirlpool pattern of the spermatic cord, and in chronic cases, decreased cord vascularity and small testicular size. ^{31}P MR spectroscopy has detected marked decrease in ATP and PM (phosphomonoester) levels with a concomitant increase in inorganic phosphates, which may be characteristic of torsion (Fig. 9.**29**) (30).

Neoplasm

The majority (over 95%) of primary testicular tumors are malignant (31, 32). Although testicular cancer accounts for only 1% of all cancers in men, it is the most common cancer in men aged 15–34 years (33). In the vast majority of the cases (over 90%) testicular cancers are of germ cell origin. The four principal histological patterns are: seminoma, embryonal carcinoma, teratoma, and choriocarcinoma (34). Serum markers associated with certain germ cell tumors have aided in their evaluation (32). Of disseminated nonseminomatous germ cell tumors, approximately 40% have elevated alpha-feto protein (AFP), and 75% demonstrate elevated HCG; 85% have one or both markers elevated. HCG is elevated in 10% of seminomas, and AFP is never elevated in a pure seminoma. Non–germ cell malignant tumors are most commonly lymphoma (5% of all testicular neoplasms, and the most common tumor in patients older than 50 years). The testes may also be involved in acute lymphocytic leukemia. Metastases to testes from melanoma, carcinoma of the prostate, lung,

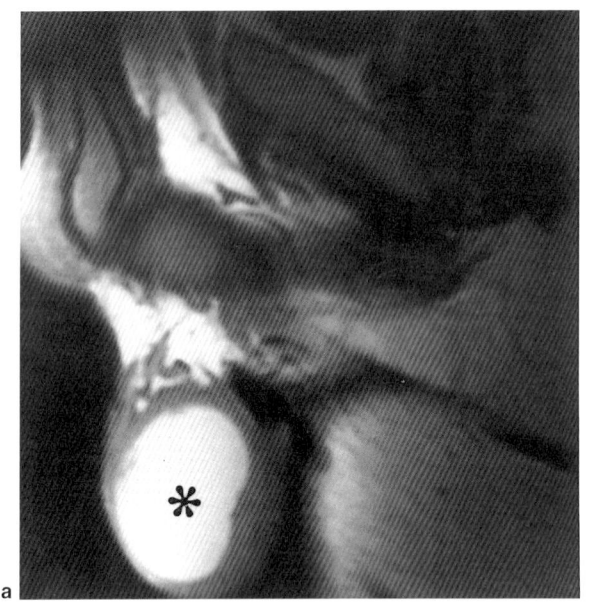

272   9 Testis

Fig. 9.28 Intermittent testicular torsion. (**a**) sagittal T1-, and (**b**) coronal T2-weighted images. The left testis (*) is mildly enlarged, and shows high signal intensity on both images consistent with testicular hemorrhage. (T) normal right testis. H = hydrocele. Arrow = spermatic cord

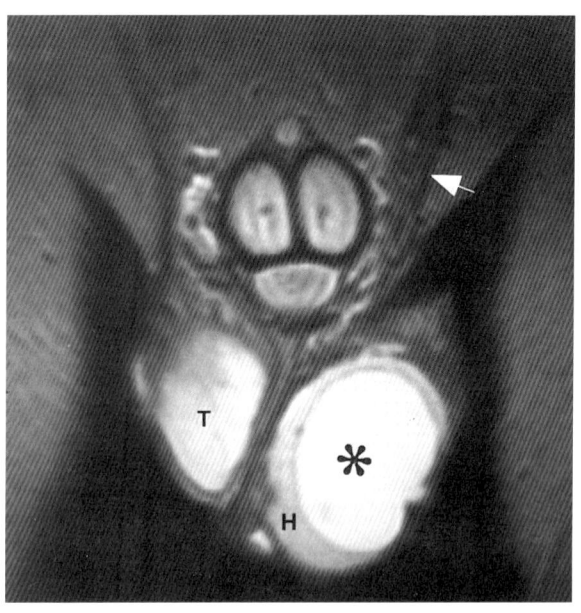

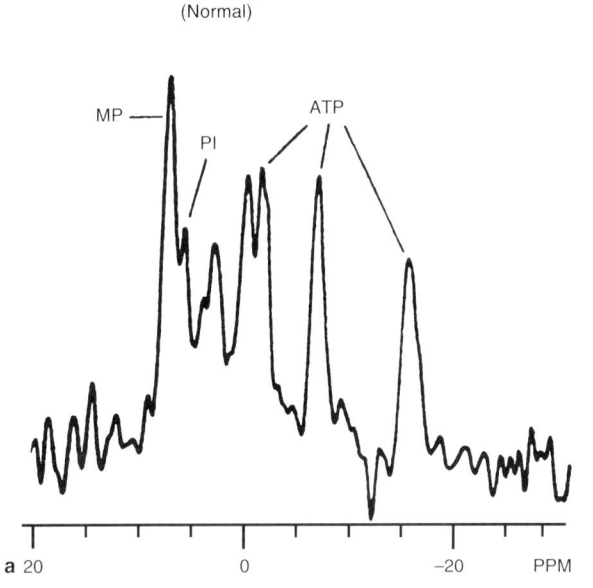

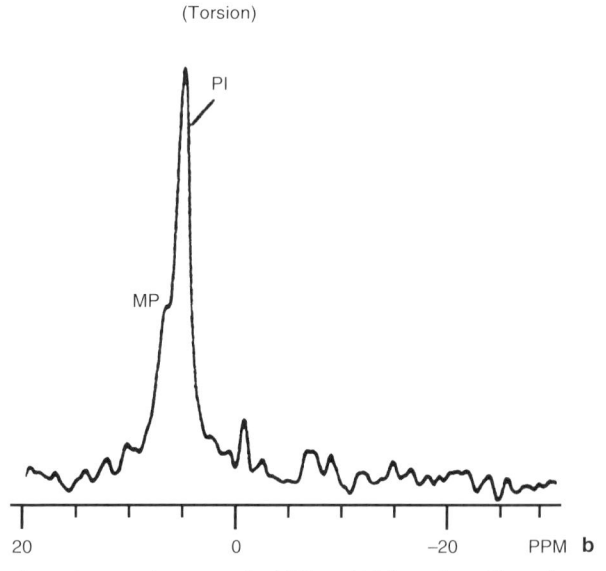

Fig. 9.29 Spectroscopy in acute torsion. ^{31}P MR spectra in (**a**) normal testis, and (**b**) testis with acute torsion, show a decrease in ATP and PM peaks with an increase in Pi. (Reprinted with permission from ref. 45)

gastrointestinal tract, and kidney have been documented (34). Other related, rare malignancies such as adenocarcinoma of the rete testis (35), and juxtatesticular tumors such as mesothelioma have been reported. Benign tumors are mostly (90%) of non-germ cell origin, arising from Leydig's or Sertoli cells, or connective tissue stroma (31, 32). Benign epidermoid cysts can also occur (31, 32).

Ultrasound is the primary diagnostic imaging modality for a suggested testicular tumor (1, 2, 36). Ultrasound and MRI have similar accuracy for evaluation of a localized testicular lesion. However, when ultrasound is technically suboptimal, MRI should be the next study of choice. MRI may be particularly helpful in localizing diffuse infiltrative disease or a process involving both testes.

Certain patterns of MR appearance of malignant testicular tumors have been found (7, 9, 10, 11, 37), and it has even been suggested that the signal intensity and degree of heterogeneity may correlate to a specific histological type of tumor (38). Seminomatous tumors are reported to be isointense on T1-weighted and homogeneously hypointense on T2-weighted images relative to adjacent normal testicular tissue (Fig. 9.30). However, exceptions frequently exist. A seminoma demonstrating medium signal intensity on T1-weighted images and heterogeneous high signal intensity on T2-weighted images is shown in Fig. 9.31. Acute bleeding into a seminoma can cause heterogeneous high signal intensity on both T1- and T2-weighted images (Fig. 9.32).

A nonseminomatous tumor usually exhibits heterogeneous signal intensity (Fig. 9.33) and can show a low signal margin toward normal testicular tissue, which corresponds to a fibrous capsule seen on histological examination. A secondary malignancy of the testis similarly causes decrease in signal intensity on T2-weighted images. When a benign epidermoid cyst is suggested by ultrasound, the cystic nature can be confirmed by MRI. Testicular cysts are sharply out-

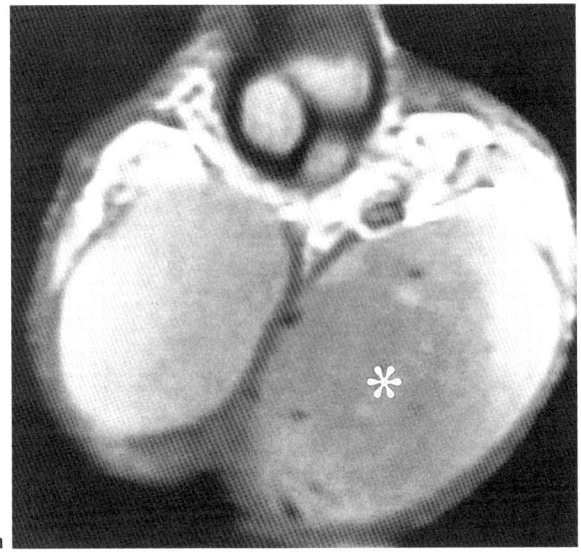

Fig. 9.30 Seminoma of the left testis. Coronal (a) T1- and, (b) T2-weighted images. The large left testicular tumor (*) has low signal intensity on the T2-weighted image, contrasting with the high signal intensity of uninvolved testicular parenchyma (T)

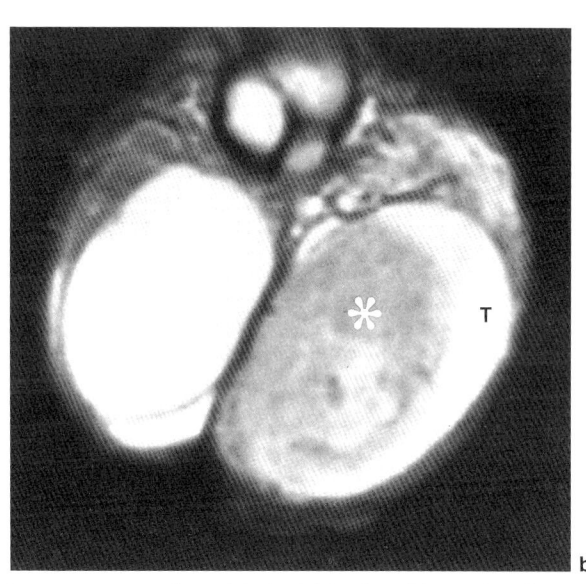

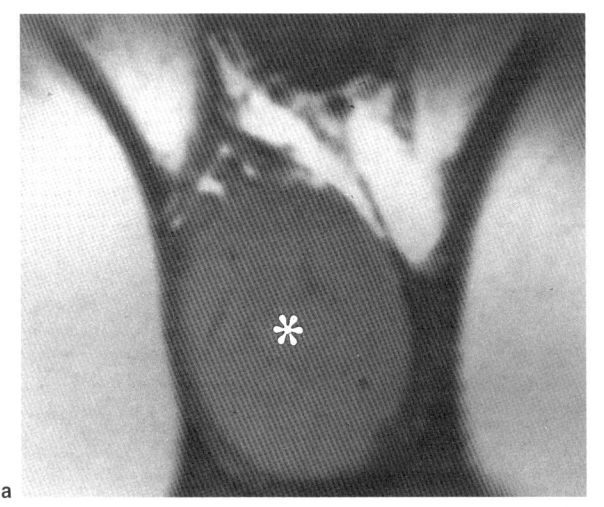

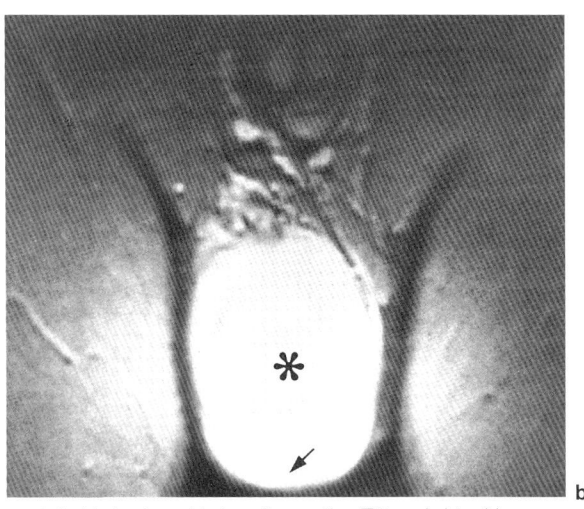

Fig. 9.31 Seminoma infiltrating the entire right testis. Coronal (a) T1-weighted, and (b) T2-weighted images. The tumor (*) has low signal intensity on T1-, and moderately high signal intensity on the T2-weighted image. Arrow = tunica albuginea

274   9 Testis

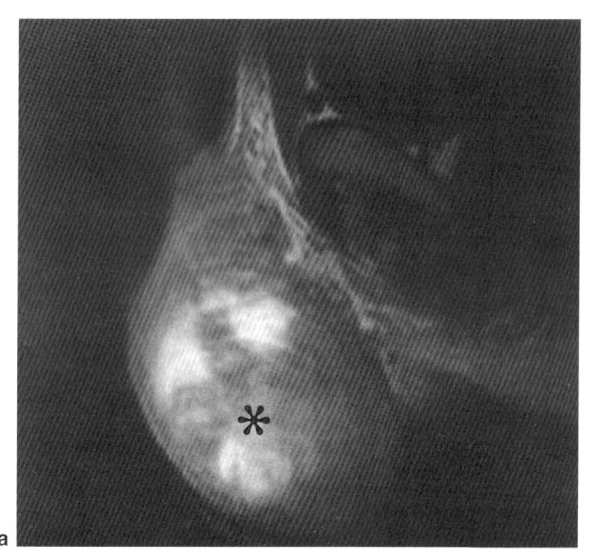

Fig. 9.32 Acute hemorrhage into a seminoma of the left testis. (**a**) sagittal T1-, and (**b**) coronal T2-weighted images. The tumor (*) exhibits heterogeneous signal intensity on both sequences, with areas of high signal intensity representing hemorrhage. T = normal right testis. (Reprinted with permission from 45)

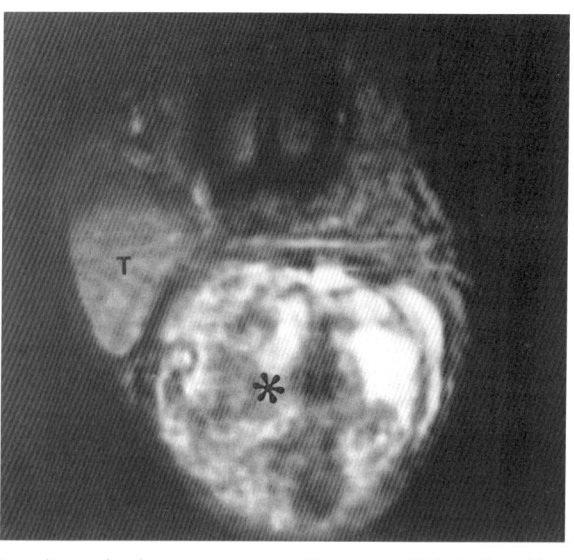

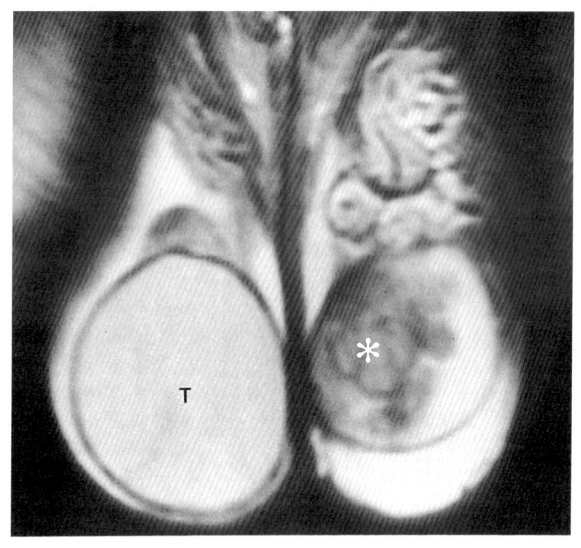

Fig. 9.33 Embryonal cell carcinoma. Coronal T2-weighted image demonstrating heterogenous signal intensity of the testicular tumor (*). T = normal right testis

lined and show homogeneous low and high intensity on T1- and T2-weighted images, respectively (Fig. 9.34). However, high protein content within the cyst may render the diagnosis somewhat difficult. The overall current MR specificity for the histological composition of a focal lesion should be considered relatively low.

Despite its generally superb soft-tissue discrimination, MR appears to be no more accurate than ultrasound for local tumor staging (7). When a low-intensity tumor is in proximity to the tunica albuginea, which consistently exhibits low signal intensity, the extent of involvement can be difficult to assess (7). Also, concomitant inflammatory changes in the spermatic cord can result in a false-positive interpretation of tumor extension. Detection of lymph node metastasis is essential for overall testicular cancer imaging. This can be done initially with CT or MRI with equivalent efficacy. In patients with previous lymph node dissection, MR is preferred as a follow-up study, because unlike CT, surgical clip artifacts do not significantly degrade image quality.

Miscellaneous

Testicular Prosthesis

Prostheses are commonly placed in patients with congenitally absent or surgically removed testes for cosmetic or psychological reasons. Older prostheses contain viscous fluid and are hard on palpation. On MR they demonstrate low signal intensity on both T1- and T2-weighted images (Fig. 9.35) and should not be mistaken for a homogeneous pathologic process replacing normal tissue. Newer prostheses are made of solid elastomer, and are similar to normal testicular tissue in consistency as well as MR signal intensity: medium on T1-weighted images and high on T2-weighted images. These can often be distinguished from normal tissue by a prominent chemical shift artifact at the tissue–prosthesis interface and also by absence of other scrotal or spermatic cord structures (39).

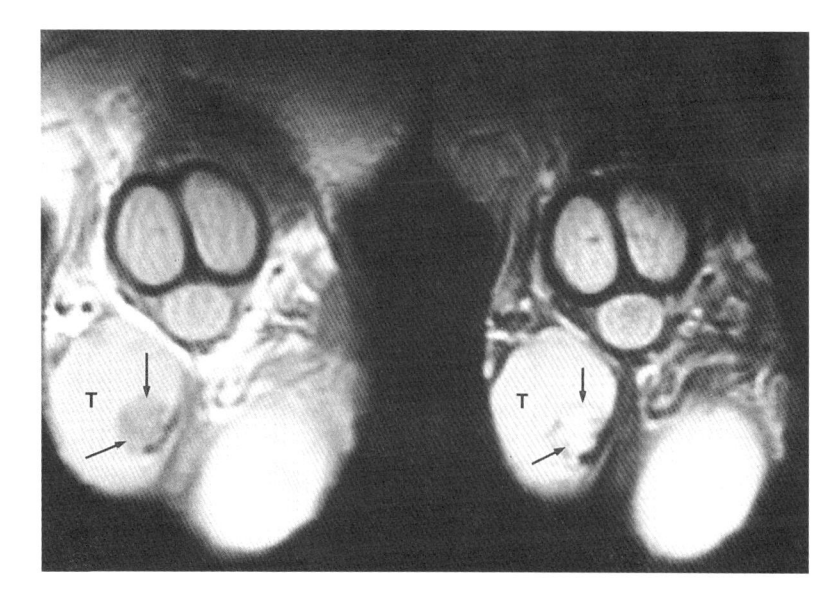

MR Imaging 275

Fig. 9.34 Epidermoid cyst of the right testis. Coronal proton density, and (**b**) T2-weighted images. A well-defined cyst (arrows) within the testis (T) exhibits signal intensity typical of a cystic lesion

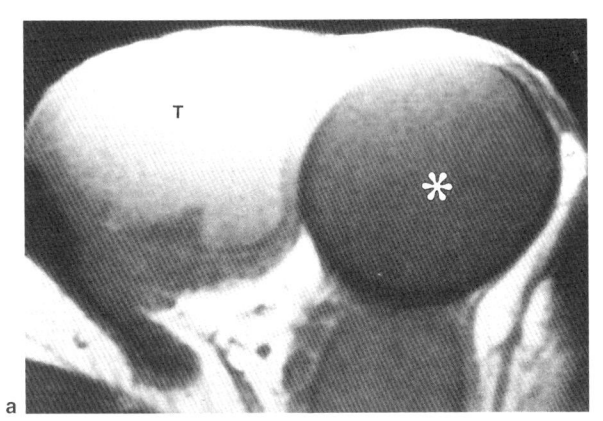

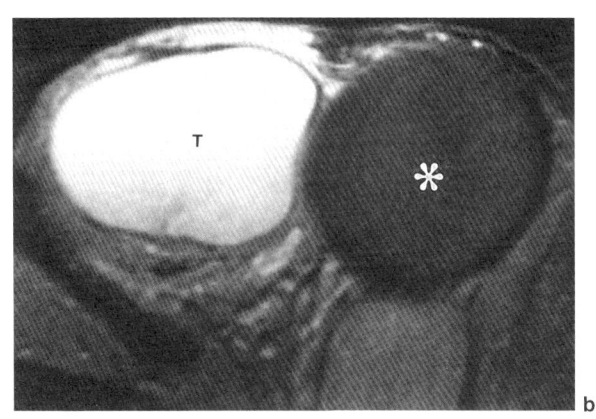

Fig. 9.35 Left testicular prosthesis. Axial (**a**) T1-, and (**b**) T2-weighted images. This older prosthesis (*) exhibits low signal intensity on both sequences. T = normal right testis

Vasculitis

Vasculitis of the testis is rare and usually occurs in patients with systemic disorders such as polyarteritis nodosa, rheumatoid arthritis, and Henoch–Schönlein purpura (40). Infarction, hemorrhage, and eventual atrophy of the testis may occur. In a recently described case, MR findings consisted of multiple, ill-defined peripherally located foci of low signal intensity within the testis, consistent with infarcts (Fig. 9.36) (41). Secondary findings include a hypervascular spermatic cord, hydrocele, and decreased testis size.

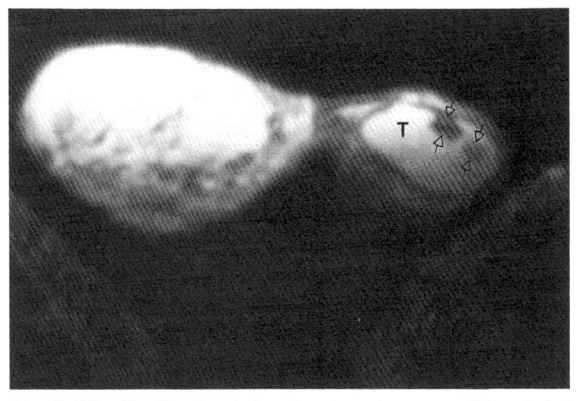

Arteriovenous Malformation (AVM)

AVM occurs in a variety of organ systems, and cases involving the scrotum have been reported. Patients

Fig. 9.36 Testicular infarcts due to vasculitis. Axial T2-weighted image showing several focal areas of low signal intensity (arrows) in the periphery of the left testis. Note also the testis (T) is small

typically present with a swollen scrotum containing engorged vascular channels that may bleed. As in other organs, MRI lends itself readily to studying the extent of the vascular malformation and changes in surrounding soft tissues. Contiguous images in multiple planes also allow careful evaluation of possible involvement of the testes, corpora cavernosa, or corpus spongiosum (Fig. 9.37). MRI offers excellent assessment before treatment (surgery or embolization) as well as convenient post-therapy evaluation.

Fluid Collections and Benign Scrotal Masses

Extratesticular fluid collections, such as a hydrocele, hematocele, and pyocele, can present as scrotal masses. A hydrocele is excessive fluid accumulated between the visceral and parietal layers of the tunica vaginalis (28). It can form from a congenital defect or develop secondary to a variety of causes including epididymo-orchitis, torsion, trauma, or a neoplasm. On MR, a hydrocele has low signal intensity on T1-weighted images and high signal intensity on

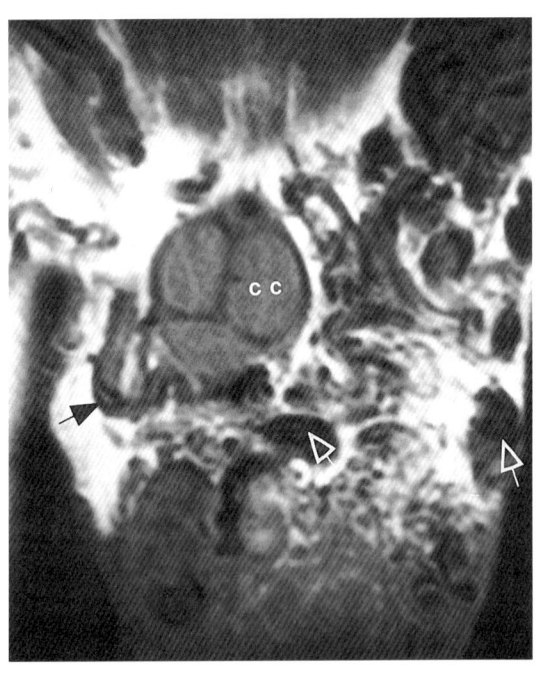

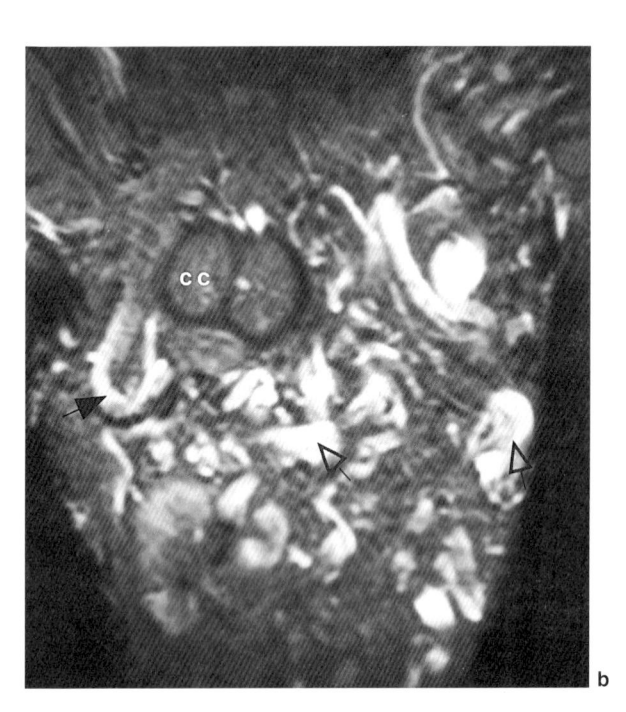

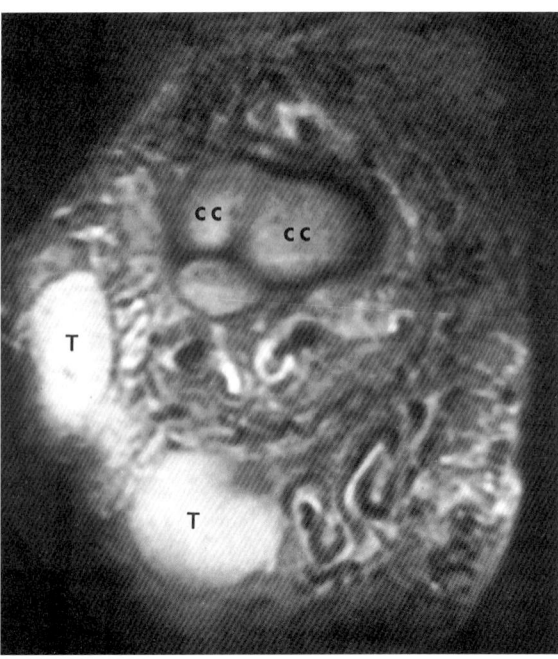

Fig. 9.**37** AVM of the scrotum. Coronal (**a**) T1-weighted, and (**b, c**) gradient-echo images. Numerous enlarged vascular channels (arrows) with flow void are seen on T1-weighted images. High signal intensity within these vessels on gradient-echo images confirm the presence of blood flow. The testes (T) or the corpora cavernosa (cc) are not involved

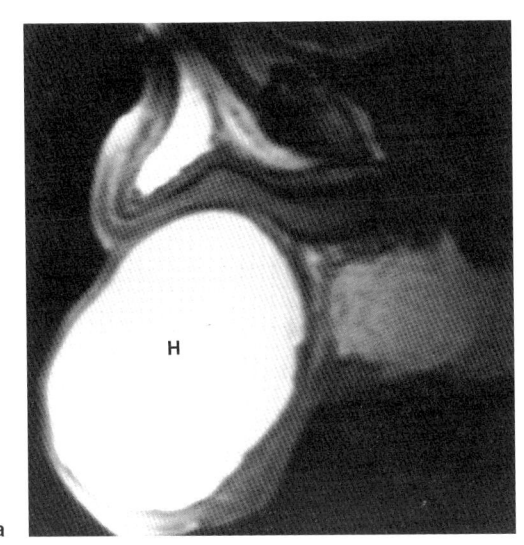

Fig. 9.**38** Chronic hematocele. (**a**) Sagittal T1-, and (**b**) axial T2-weighted images. The hematocele (H) shows high signal intensity on both images, consistent with subacute hemorrhage. The compressed right testis (T) is seen on the axial image. * = normal left testis

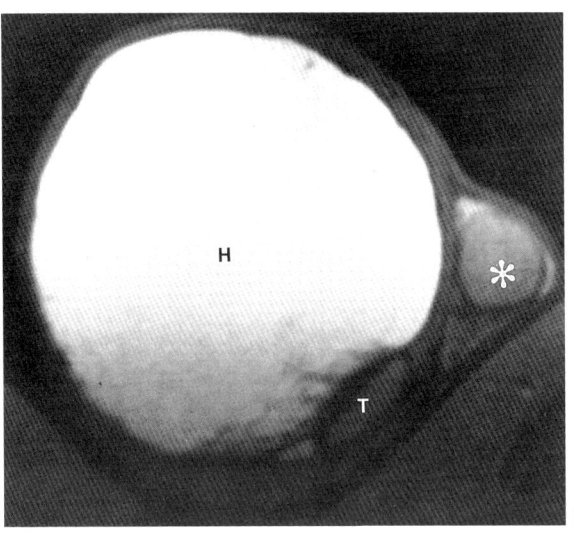

T2-weighted images (7). A hydrocele is easily distinguished from the testis on either T1- or T2-weighted images. A hematocele contains blood products and usually develops as a result of trauma. The presence of a hematocele is easily diagnosed by MRI. A hematocele misdiagnosed on ultrasound as probable hernia is shown in Fig. 9.**38**. Low-level echoes were nonspecific on ultrasound, and floating debris were misinterpreted as bowel contents. The MR signal is characteristic of subacute hemorrhagic fluid.

A pyocele is a hydrocele containing infected debris as a complication of epididymo-orchitis. In a pyocele, multiloculations and septations are often seen within the fluid collection. The septa and debris are usually better seen on T2-weighted images.

A spermatocele is a retention cyst of small tubules containing sperm (42); an epididymal cyst typically occurs in the head of the epididymis. These two entities have an identical appearance on MR imaging and show variable signal intensity depending on the protein or cellular content (9).

A varicocele, a dilatation of testicular veins, can be primary or idiopathic, or can result from proximal venous obstruction (for example in the presence of an abdominal mass) (42, 43). Ultrasound and venography have proven useful in diagnosing and delineating varicoceles. In selected cases, embolization of a varicocele has resulted in successful treatment of infertility. On MRI, a group of serpentine vessels superior to the testis in the region of the epididymal head and the spermatic cord are seen. Because of relatively slow flow, intraluminal signal can be detected on spin-echo images; in fact, increased signal intensity is often seen on T2-weighted images, especially if a flow compensation technique, such as gradient moment nulling is used. A flow-sensitive gradient-echo sequence may help confirm the presence of engorged veins.

A scrotal hernia can also present as an enlarged scrotum. Tissue characteristics of hernia contents—air and fluid within bowel loops, and mesenteric fat—are readily displayed on MR images (Fig. 9.**39**). In addition, the course of the herniation along the inguinal canal is easily depicted, especially on axial or coronal imaging planes. A case of meconium hernia misdiag-

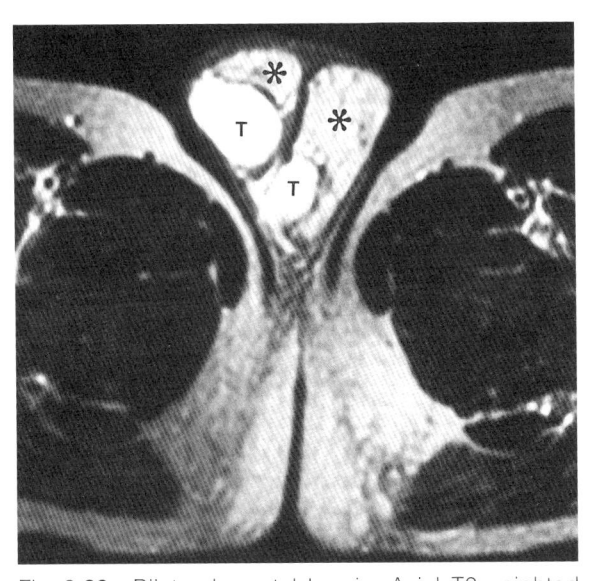

Fig. 9.**39** Bilateral scrotal hernia. Axial T2-weighted image showing fat (*) extending into the scrotal sac. Normal testes (T) are identified adjacent to the herniated fat

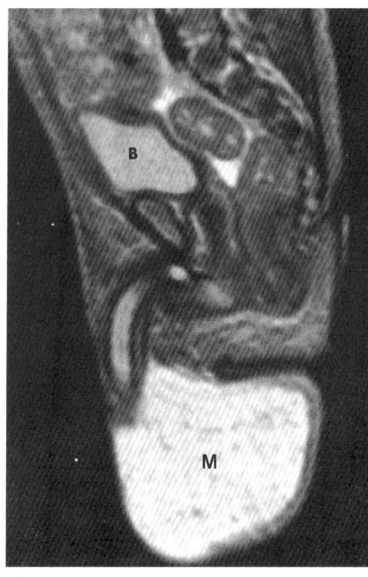

Fig. 9.**40** Large meconium hernia in a newborn. Sagittal T2-weighted image demonstrating marked enlargement of the scrotal sac by high signal intensity meconium (M). B = bladder

nosed clinically and on ultrasound as a testicular mass is shown in Fig. 9.**40**.

Summary

In summary, the ultrasound examination is sufficient in most patients with either intratesticular or extratesticular disease. MRI should be used only in selected cases in which ultrasound is limited, when there is a discrepancy between the physical examination and ultrasound findings, or when further characterization of the fluid content or disease extent will impact patient treatment.

References

1 Hricak H, Filly RA. Sonography of the scrotum. Invest Radiol. 1983;18:112–121.
2 Benson CB, Doubilet PM, Richie JP. Sonography of the male genital tract. Review Article, AJR. 1989;153:705–713.
3 Husband JE, Hawkes DJ, Peckham MJ. CT estimations of mean attenuation values and volume in testicular tumors: A comparison with surgical and histologic findings. Radiology. 1982;144:553–558.
4 Marincek B, Brutschin P, Triller J, Fuchs WA. Lymphography and computed tomography in staging nonseminomatous testicular cancer: Limited detection of early stage metastatic disease. Urol Radiol. 1983;5:243–246.
5 Holder LE, Melloul M, Chen DCP. Current status of radionuclide scrotal imaging. Semin Nucl Med. 1981;11:232–249.
6 Coalsaet BLRA. Varicocele syndrome, Venography determining the optimal level for surgical management. Radiology. 1981;140:266.
7 Thurnher S, Hricak H, Pobiel R, Carroll P, Filly RA. Imaging the testis: Comparison between MR imaging and US. Radiology 1988;167:631–636.
8 Cramer MC, Schlegel EA, Thueroff JW. MR imaging in the differential diagnosis of scrotal and testicular disease. Radiographics. 1991;11:9–21.
9 Baker LL, Hajek PC, Burkhard TK, et al, MR imaging of the scrotum: Normal anatomy. Radiology. 1987;163:89–92.
10 Rholl KS, Lee JKT, Ling D, et al. MR imaging of the scrotum with a high-resolution surface coil. Radiology. 1987; 163:99–103.
11 Seidenwurm D, Smathers RL, Lo RK, et al. Testes and scrotum: MR imaging at 1.5 T. Radiology 1987;164:393–398.
12 Shellock FG, Rothman B, Sarti D. Heating of the scrotum by high-field strength MR imaging. AJR. 1990;154:1229–1232.
13 Baker LL, Hajek PC, Burkhard TK, et al. Polyorchidism: Evaluation by MR. Case Report. AJR. 1987;148:305–306.
14 Friedland GW, Chang P. The role of imaging in the management of the impalpable undescended testis. AJR. 1988; 151:1107–1111.
15 Rajfer G, Walsh PC. Testicular descent: Normal and abnormal. Urologic Clin North Am. 1978;5:223–235.
16 Kogan SJ. Cryptorchidism. In: Kelalis King B, ed. Clinical Pediatric Urology, 2nd ed. Philadelphia: WB Saunders; 1985:864–887.
17 Fallon B, Welton M, Hawtrey C. Congenital anomalies associated with cryptorchidism. J Urol. 1982;127:91–93.
18 Kogan SJ. Cryptorchidism and infertility: An overview. Dial Pediatr Urol. 1981;4:2–3.
19 Weiss RM, Carter AR, Rosenfield AT. High resolution real-time ultrasonography in the location of the undescended testis. J Urol. 1986;135:936–938.
20 Fritzsche PJ, Hricak H, Kogan BA, et al. Undescended testis: Value of MR imaging. Radiology. 1987;164:169–173.
21 Miyano T, Kobayashi H, Shimomura H, et al. Magnetic resonance imaging for localizing the nonpalpable undescended testis. J Pediatr Surg. 1991;26(5):607–9.
22 Zobel BB, Vicentini C, Masciocchi C, et al. Magnetic resonance imaging in the localization of undescended testes. Europ Urol. 1990;17:145–148.
23 Kier R, McCarthy S, Rosenfield AT, et al. Nonpalpable testes in young boys: Evaluation with MR imaging. Radiology. 1988;169:429.
24 Rosenfeld AT, Blair DN, McCarthy S, et al. The pars infravaginalis gubernaculi and associated structures. An imaging pitfall in the identification of undescended testis. AJR. 1989;153:775.
25 Secaf E, Nuruddin R, Hricak H, et al. Evaluation of ambiguous genitalia with MRI (work in progress). Radiol Soc North Am. Suppl to Radiology. 1989;371.
26 Togashi K, Nishimura K, Itoh K, et al. Vaginal agenesis: Classification by MR imaging. Radiology. 1987;162:675–677.
27 Trambert MA, Mattrey RF, Levine D, et al. Subacute scrotal pain: Evaluation of torsion versus epididymitis with MR imaging. Radiology. 1990;175:53–56.
28 Lierse W. Testis. In: Applied Anatomy of the Pelvis. Berlin: Springer; 1984:188–198.
29 Tzika AA, Moseley ME, Hricak H, et al. Comparison of MR imaging and P-31 MR spectroscopy in a rat model of testicular torsion. Presented at the 75th Scientific Assembly and Annual Meeting of the Radiological Society of North America, Chicago: Radiological Society of North America; 1989.
30 Chew W, Hricak H, Carroll P, Clinical utility of P-31 MR spectroscopy in the evaluation of human testicular abnormalities. Presented at the 75th Scientific Assembly and Annual Meeting of the Radiological Society of North America. Chicago: Radiological Society of North America; 1989
31 Mostofi FK. Testicular tumors, Epidemioligic, etiologic and pathologic features. Cancer. 1973;32:1186.
32 Einhorn LH, Crawford ED, Shipley WU, et al. Cancer of the testes. In: DeVita VT, Jr, Hellman S, Rosenberg SA, eds. Volume 1: Cancer Principles and Practice of Oncology. 3rd ed. Philadelphia: J. B. Lippincott; 1989:1071–1098.
33 Silverberg E. Cancer in young adults (ages 15 to 34). Cancer 1982;32:32.
34 Mostofi FK, Price EP Jr. Tumors of the male genital system. In: Atlas of tumor pathology. Fascicle 8, Series 2. Washington, D. C.: Armed Forces Institute of Pathology; 1973.
35 Smith SJ, Vogelzang RL, Smith WM, Moran MJ. Papillary adenocarcinoma of the rete testis: sonographic findings. AJR. 1987;148:1147–1148.

36 Benson CB. The role of ultrasound in diagnosis and staging of testicular cancer. Semin Urol. 1988;6:189–202.
37 Thomsen C, Jensen KE, Giwercman A, et al. Magnetic resonance: In vivo tissue characterization of the testes in patients with carcinoma-in-situ of the testis and healthy subjects. Intern J Androl. 1987;10:191–198.
38 Johnson JO, Mattrey RF, Phillipson J. Differentiation of seminomatous from nonseminomatous testicular tumors with MR imaging. AJR 1990;154:539–543.
39 Semelka R, Anderson M, Hricak H. Prosthetic testicle: Appearance at MR imaging. Radiology. 1989;173(2):561–562.
40 Gondos B, Wong TW, Non-neoplastic diseases of the testis and epididymis. In: Murphy W, ed. Urologic Pathology. Philadelphia: WB Saunders; 1989:284.
41 Hayward I, Trambert MA, Mattrey RF, Saltzstein, Demby AM. Case report: MR imaging of vasculitis of the testis. JCAT. 1991;15(3):502–504.
42 Bunce PL. Scrotal abnormalities. In: Glenn JF, ed. Urologic Surgery. New York: Harper and Row; 1975:232.
43 Gonda RL, Karo JJ, Fonte RA, et al. Diagnosis of subclinical varicocele in infertility. AJR 1987;148:71–75.
44 Hricak H, Carrington BM. MRI of the Pelvis: A Text Atlas. London: Martin Dunitz; 1991:343–381.

A Surgeon's View

R. Friedrichs and R. Nagel

Before the introduction of sonography and MRI into clinical practice, the diagnosis of scrotal and testicular disease was based on history, clinical examination, and surgical exploration alone.

Testicular Tumors

The diagnosis of a testicular neoplasm is made in 97% of cases by the urologist's palpation alone. This means that an inguinal exploration with high ligation of the spermatic cord, which is usually combined with intraoperative frozen section diagnosis, is mandatory. Subsequent orchiectomy and excision of the spermatic cord is performed after histologic confirmation by frozen section diagnosis. It is generally accepted that orchiectomy performed promptly after the onset of testicular symptoms not only helps reduce mortality from testicular cancer but also has a major effect on its morbidity by reducing the need for systemic chemotherapy or major surgery (1).

Approximately 20% of testicular tumors are clinically misdiagnosed as simple hydroceles because of the formation of a secondary hydrocele. Therefore, it is important to carefully investigate the testis for an underlying neoplasm, especially in young men (2). The method of choice for evaluation of unclear testicular masses is scrotal sonography (3). The major benefit of scrotal sonography is the identification of intratesticular as opposed to extratesticular abnormalities (4, 5). The majority of intratesticular abnormalities will prove to be malignant (4). In the era of general availability of testicular sonography, the misdiagnosis factor should be reduced substantially. MR imaging may be an adjunct in suggestive cases.

In a series of 29 testicular neoplasms, the most common finding was a hypoechogenic mass (72%) with one or more hyperechogenic foci (66%). Thirty-one percent had diffuse echotextural change. The margins of the mass varied from sharp to indistinct (6). Sonography cannot accurately identify histological cell type (4) although seminomas are usually homogeneous, hypoechoic masses in contrast to nonseminomatous tumors, which contain cystic areas or dense, highly hyperechoic foci that may be caused by calcification, cartilage, bone, or fibrosis (7).

Milner and Blease (8) examined whether scrotal sonography reduces the need for orchiectomy in the clinically malignant testis by investigating 15 patients in which a firm, clinical diagnosis of testicular malignancy was made. In all cases, orchiectomy was performed. Scrotal sonography rejected the diagnosis of malignancy in seven cases with subsequent histological proof of benignity. The nature and extent of the benign disease was such that orchiectomy was considered to be the most appropriate method of treating the patient. The authors concluded that with a clinical diagnosis of malignancy, sonography should not alter management.

Before inguinal exploration, a synchronous, impalpable tumor in the contralateral testis should be excluded by testicular sonography and documented for follow up (10, 11, 13) because synchronous occurrence of bilateral testicular tumors is found in 0.5% (9).

Current diagnostic procedures and treatment regimens of malignant germ cell tumors of the testis, especially cisplatin-containing regimens, produce high complete response rates and cure in 95% of patients (10–12). Therefore, the frequency of second (subsequent) testicular tumors is increasing. Second testicular tumors occur in 2,8% of patients in the follow up (9). Subsequent tumors may occur after long-term intervals of 10 years or more (13), requiring long-term follow-up by self-palpation and testicular sonography of the remaining testis (14).

An increasing number of nonpalpable second testicular tumors found by routine use of sonography in the follow-up has been described (15). In one of six patients with bilateral testicular tumors seen at our institution, the second tumor was diagnosed by routine sonography during the follow up (10). The earlier the diagnosis is made, the better the prognosis for the patient (16). In carefully selected cases, organ-preserving tumor excision may be performed in patients with sonographically detected tumors (17).

More than 175 Leydig's cell tumors of the testis had been described until 1979. In the adult, feminization predominates, consisting of gynecomastia, decreased sexual libido, and contralateral testicular atrophy. Serum LH and serum FSH are decreased, and serum and urinary estrogens are increased in adults. Leydig's cell tumors in children are benign, whereas metastasis to the liver, bone, lungs, and lymph nodes is found in 10% of tumors in adults for up to 9 years after removal of the primary tumor (5). Recently, a case of synchronous, nonpalpable, bilateral Leydig's cell tumors that were detected only by sonography was described (18).

Definite evaluation and treatment protocols have not been established so far for sonographically detected, nonpalpable testicular masses in patients who have no history of testicular tumor. It has been recommended that such cases with negative serum tumor markers, normal chest radiographs, and normal abdominal sonography should be followed by serial imaging (19).

The case of a 23-year-old man with a metastatic germ cell tumor and normal findings on testicular physical examination, but with multiple circular echogenic foci on testicular sonography has been described. Orchiectomy revealed intratubular germ cell neoplasia with testicular microlithiasis that correlated with the sonographic finding of multiple circular echogenic foci (20). It was concluded that testicular sonography is mandatory in cases of unclear metastatic disease in young men and in cases when a retroperitoneal germ cell tumor is suggested (21). MRI may be helpful in suggestive cases.

Imaging, especially sonography, is useful in the evaluation of clinical findings that cannot be evaluated by palpation alone. Unnecessary exploration may be avoided by using sonography and MRI (22) in selected cases. Imaging can help in the differential diagnosis of malignant tumors of the testis, but can not replace surgical and histological exploration of the testis when a testicular tumor is suggested (4, 8).

Acute Scrotum

The problem in acute scrotum is the differential diagnosis of epididymitis and orchitis versus torsion. Testicular torsion means that the spermatic cord is twisted, disrupting arterial flow. The torsion must be corrected within 6 to 8 hours to prevent irreversible testicular damage. Testicular torsion usually occurs at the age of 10 to 14 years, but may also be observed in newborns and in young men up to the age of 30 years. The patient usually has acute onset of scrotal (and abdominal) pain and scrotal swelling. Clinically, a torsion may be misdiagnosed as incarcerated hernia, ureteral colic, or appendicitis (23).

For differential diagnosis, it is important that epididymitis, which rarely occurs before the age of 15 years, usually presents with fever after puberty; abdominal pain is usually not found (23). Good results of color Doppler sonography in the evaluation of the acute scrotum have been reported (24–26). If color Doppler sonography or MRI is performed in these patients to determine the value of this technique, it must not lead to a delay of the exploration. At present, irrespective of the results of imaging studies, if the urologist strongly suspects testicular torsion, scrotal exploration is mandatory in order to salvage the ischemic testis.

Testicular sonography may give important additional information for the evaluation of testicular trauma. The intact testis can often be treated conservatively, whereas a ruptured testicle requires surgical intervention (3).

Conclusion

From the urologist's point of view, testicular sonography is the most important diagnostic procedure for imaging of the testis. Because of the wide availability, low cost, and short examination time, sonography remains the imaging technique of first choice for testicular disease. MRI may be valuable in selected cases of testicular and extratesticular disease. If a tumor is suggested, an inguinal exploration has to be performed by the urologist. Furthermore, imaging is not reliable enough to replace operative exploration in patients with suggested torsion.

References

1 Wishnow KI, Johnson DE, Preston WL, Tenney DM, Brown BW: Prompt orchiectomy reduces morbidity and mortality from testicular carcinoma. Brit J Urol. 1990;65:629–633.
2 Vick CW, Bird KI, Rosenfield AT, Richter J, Taylor KJW. Sonography of the scrotal contents. Urol Radiol. 1982;4:147–153.
3 Rifkin MD. Scrotal sonography. Urol Radiol. 1987;9:119–126.
4 Marth D, Scheidegger J, Studer UE. Ultrasonography of testicular tumors Urol Int. 1990;45:237–240.
5 Friedrichs R, Rübben H, Lutzeyer W. Differential diagnosis of rare testicular tumors. Eur Urol. 1986;12:217–223.
6 Grantham JD, Charboneau JW, James EM et al. Testicular neoplasms: 29 tumors studied by high-resolution US. Radiology 1985;157:775–780.
7 Schwerk WB, Schwerk WN, Rodeck G. Testicular tumors: prospective analysis of real-time US patterns and abdominal staging. Radiology. 1987;164:369–373.
8 Milner SJ, Blease SCP. Does scrotal sonography reduce the need for orchiectomy in the clinically malignant testis? Brit J Radiol. 1990;63:263–265.
9 Reinberg Y, Manivel JC, Zhang G, Reddy PK. Synchronous bilateral testicular germ cell tumors of different histologic type. Pathogenetic and practical implications of bilaterality in testicular germ cell tumors. Cancer. 68:1991;1082–1085.
10 Friedrichs R, Haslberger K, Drossel HC, Nagel R. Diagnose und Therapie bilateraler Hodentumoren. Urologe A. 1990; A36.
11 Friedrichs R, Sudhoff F, Fischer R, Nagel R. Kontralaterale Zweittumoren des Hodens nach Chemotherapie des Ersttumors. Urologe A. 1992; A93.
12 Schwabe HR, Herrmann R, Mathew M., et al. Langfristige Toxizität der Polychemotherapie bei kurativ behandelten Hodenkarzinomen. Dtsch Med Wschr. 1992;117:121–126.
13 Dieckmann KP, Boeckmann W, Brosig W, Jonas D, Bauer HW. Bilaterale testikuläre Keimzelltumoren. Bericht über 9 Fälle und Literaturübersicht. Akt Urol. 1986;17:25–29.
14 Hoekstra HJ, Wobbes T, Sleyfer DT, Koops HS. Bilateral primary germ cell tumors of testis. Urology. 1982;19:152–154.
15 Csapo Z, Bornhof C, Giedl J. Impalpable testicular tumors diagnosed by scrotal ultrasonography. Urology. 1988;32:549–552.

16 Scheiber K, Ackermann D, Studer UE. Bilateral testicular germ cell tumors: a report of 20 cases. J Urol. 1987;138:73–76.
17 Weißbach L. Ist eine organerhaltende Operation des Hodentumors gerechtfertigt? Urologe A. 1993;32:49–52.
18 Corrie D, Norbeck JC, Thompson IM et al. Sonography detection of bilateral Leydig cell tumors in palpable normal testes. J Urol. 1987;137:747–748.
19 Corrie D, Mueller EJ, Thompson IM. Management of ultrasonically detected nonpalpable testis masses. Urology 1991; 38:429–431.
20 Kragel PJ, Delvecchio D, Orlando R, Garvin DF. Ultrasonographic findings of testicular microlithiasis associated with intratubular germ cell neoplasia. Urology. 1991;37:66–68.
21 Burt ME, Javadpour N. Germ-cell tumors in patients with apparently normal testes. Cancer. 1981;47:1911–1915.
22 Schultz-Lampel D, Bogaert G, Thüroff JW, Schlegel E, Cramer B. MRI for evaluation of scrotal pathology. Urol Res. 1991;19:289–292.
23 Nagel R, Borgmann V. Urologische Ursachen eines akuten Abdomens. In: Beger HG, Kern E, hrsg. Akutes Abdomen, Stuttgart: Thieme; 1987:183–201.
24 Krieger JN, Wang K, Mack L. Preliminary evaluation of color doppler imaging for investigation of intrascrotal pathology. J Urol. 1990;144:904–907.
25 Zoeller G, Ringert R-H. Color-coded duplex sonography for diagnosis of testicular torsion. J Urol. 1991;146:1288–1990.
26 Dewire DM, Begun FP, Lawson RK, Fitzgerald S, Foley WD. Color doppler ultrasonography in the evaluation of the acute scrotum. J Urol. 1992;147:89–91.

10 Ovary

Anatomy

J. Staudt

In the mature woman, the ovary has a flat oval shape and is about 4 cm long, 2 cm wide, and 1 cm deep. In the menopausal woman, the ovary becomes smaller. It is positioned at the lateral wall of the pelvis in the ovarian fossa between the external and internal iliac arteries. Its peritoneal covering (mesovarium) is fixed together by elastic fibers at the upper pole by the ligamentum suspensorium ovarii and at the lower pole by the ligamentum ovarii proprium (Fig. 10.1). Physiologically, it serves two purposes: formation and release of the oocytes and the production of hormones.

The microscopic architecture of the ovary consists of the external peritoneal covering as the germinal epithelium and the fibrous capsule (tunica albuginea) underneath. The fibrous capsule extends as a connective tissue network, i.e., ovarian stroma, into the inner part of the ovary. In general, the ovary consists of the cortical zone with follicles in different stages of maturity and lutein corpora, and of the medullary zone, which contains mainly blood and lymphatic vessels as well as nerves within its network.

The ovarian artery originates from the aorta, caudally to the renal artery. The artery follows the ligamentum ovarii suspensorium. In rare cases, the artery for the left ovary originates from the left renal artery. The artery enters the ovary at the hilum where it forms an anastomosis with the ovarian branch from the uterine artery (branch of the internal iliac artery). Venous drainage takes place via the pampiniform plexus located within the lig. suspensorium ovarii. Whereas the right ovarian vein drains directly into the inferior vena cava or indirectly into the pelvic veins including the uterine veins, blood from the left ovary

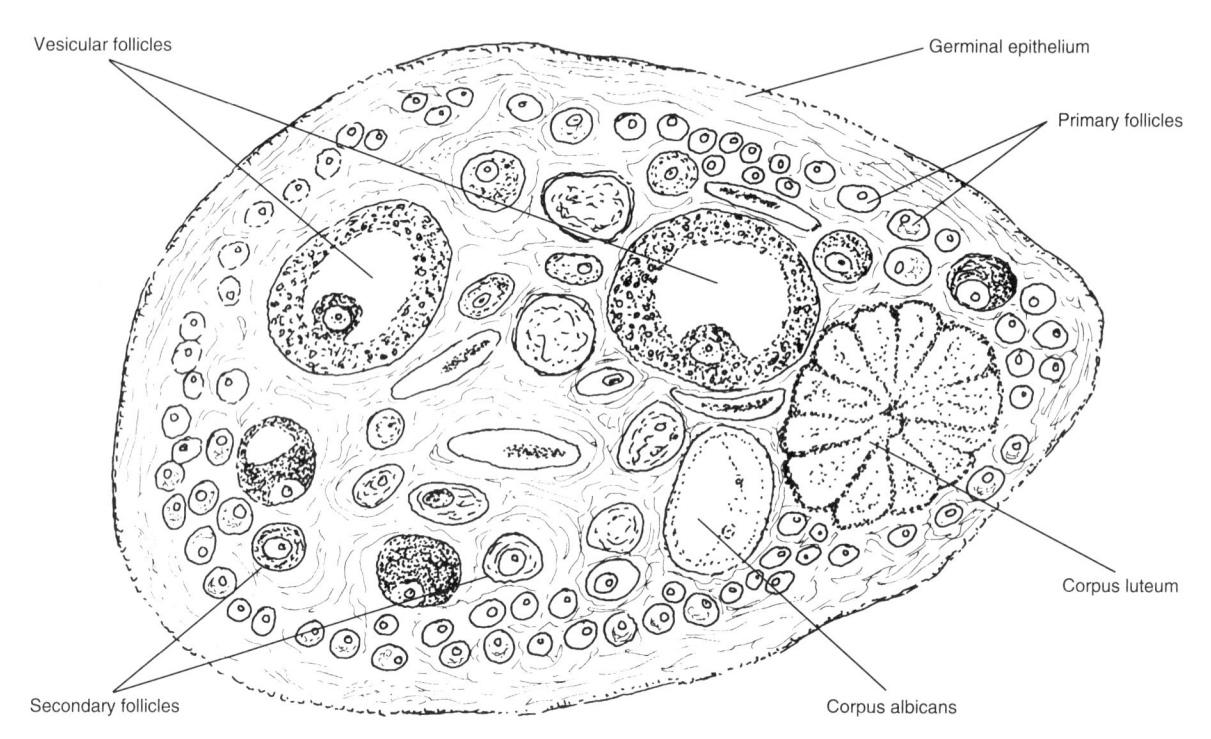

Fig. 10.1 A section through the ovary

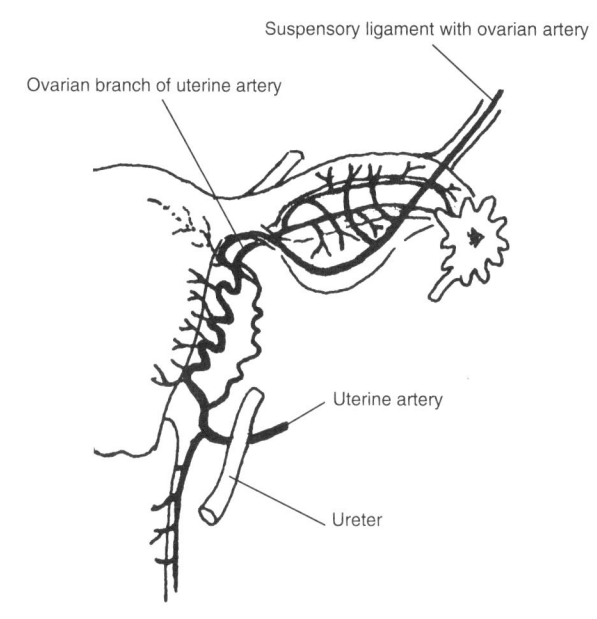

Fig. 10.2 The blood supply of the female reproductive organs (posterior view)

drains into the left renal vein (Fig. 10.2). The major lymphatic drainage of the ovary takes place along the mainstream from the ovary to the lumbar lymph nodes (Nn. lymphatici lumbales dextri et sinistri). The minor part of the lymphatic drainage passes along the parauterine lymph nodes to the internal iliac lymph nodes. The latter have connections to the superficial inguinal lymph nodes by way of the ligamentum teres uteri.

Endocrinology

F. Neumann and K.-J. Gräf

Physiology

Like the testis, the ovary is an incretory (hormone-producing) organ and is the main source of the female sex hormones, estrogens and progesterone. All processes of female reproduction are regulated by the synergistic interaction of estrogens and progesterone; in general, estrogens have more of a proliferative effect in the target organs, whereas progesterone has more of a differentiating effect.

The biosynthesis of estrogens and progesterone in the ovaries is regulated by the two pituitary gonadotropins LH and FSH. Gonadotropin secretion is stimulated by the hypothalamic releasing hormone GnRH, which is secreted in a pulsatile manner with a peak every 90–120 minutes. LH stimulates above all the synthesis of progesterone in the corpora lutea and of androgens primarily in the theca cells surrounding the follicles. Estrogens arise in the granulosa cells of the follicle from androgenic precursur molecules under the influence of the aromatase enzyme complex. The activity of the aromatase in the granulosa cells is FSH dependent (Fig. 10.3).

In the blood, estrogens are bound to transport proteins—primarily to SHBG and albumin.

Progesterone is present in free form to the extent of only 2–3%. It is bound mainly to albumin, CBG (corticosteroid-binding globulin) and SHBG.

The plasma concentrations and production rates of estrone, estradiol, and progesterone in the various phases of the cycle are shown in Table 10.1. The half-life of estrone is about 90 minutes. Excretion takes places through the kidneys after glucuronidation or sulphatization. The main metabolite is estriol. The half-life of progesterone is only 20 minutes. The main metabolite is pregnandiol.

Figs. 10.4 and 10.5 depict the hormonal situations in the cycle and during pregnancy.

The functional axis hypothalamus–pituitary–ovary works on the principle of the thermostat, i.e., the secretion of GnRH is usually dependent on the current concentration of estrogens and progesterone in the blood. The lower the concentration, the more GnRH and, consequently, the more gonadotropins are released. Conversely, an increased concentration of estrogens and progesterone leads to cessation, or reduction, of the secretion of GnRH and, hence, of gonadotropins as well (see also Chapter 2).

The extent to which an ovarian peptide hormone (inhibin) also specifically inhibits pituitary FSH secretion has not yet been fully clarified. When a particular hormonal constellation is present—i.e., when there is a deficit of progesterone—estrogens exert a positive feedback effect on the pituitary release of gonadotropins (particularly LH).

In the follicular phase of the cycle, a relatively spontaneous release of estrogens into the blood that lasts several hours occurs in the mature follicle. This estrogen peak induces a peak in LH secretion which, in turn, triggers ovulation (see also Fig. 10.4).

The main physiological and metabolic effects of the estrogens and progesterone are summarized in Tables 10.2 and 10.3.

Clinics

Puberty and Disorders of Puberty

Cf. Chapter 9 Endocrinology

Ovarian Agenesis and Dysgenesis

The ovaries are absent or contain only connective tissue cords instead of oogonia. A gene defect is usually present (e.g., Ullrich–Turner syndrome). Secondary sex characteristics are poorly developed, if at all; gonadotropins (particularly FSH) are increased as in menopause (no negative feedback).

284 10 Ovary

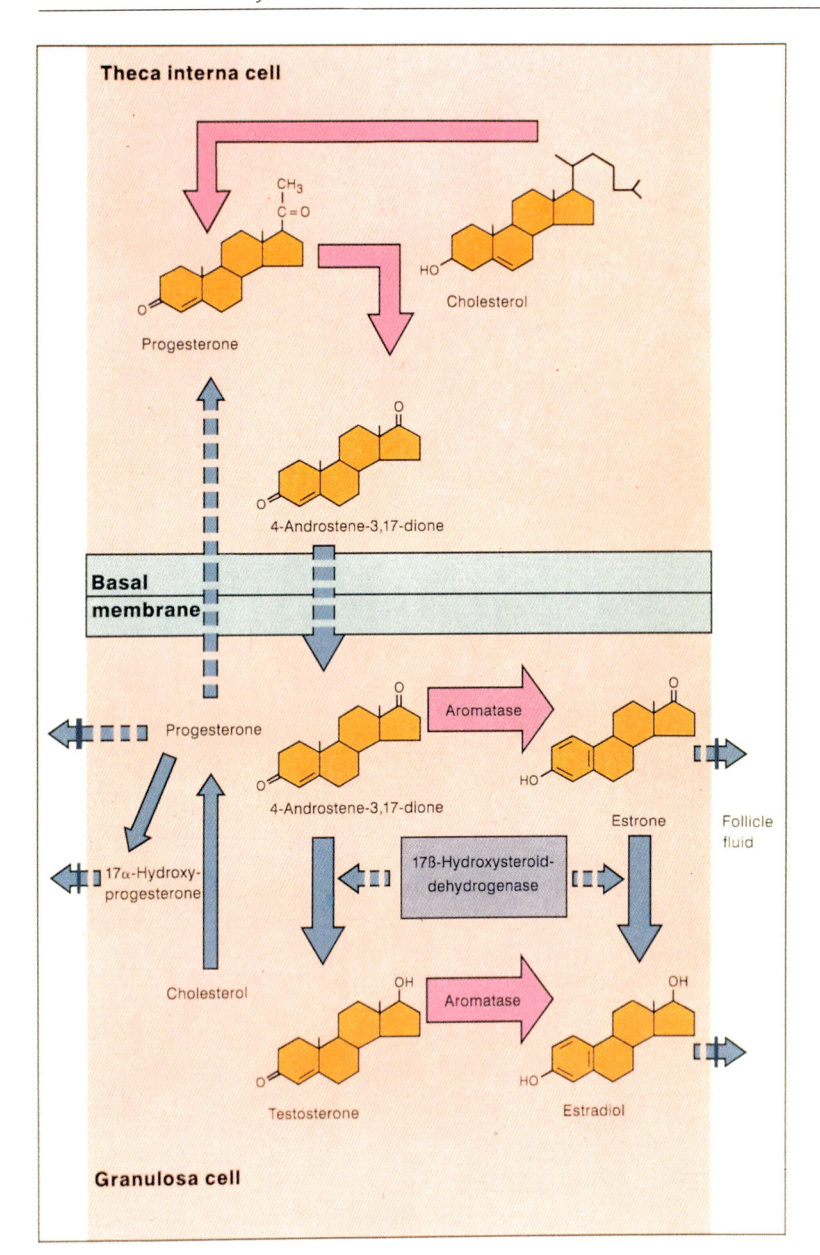

Fig. 10.3 Progesterone and estrogen biosynthesis in the ovary. LH stimulates the synthesis of androgens in the theca cells (androstenedione and testosterone). The synthesis of estrogens from androgenic precursor molecules (estrone arises from androstenedione, estradiol from testosterone) is catalyzed in the granulosa cells of the follicle by an aromatase enzyme complex. (Cf. also Fig. 9.4 in the chapter 9 for the biosynthesis of steroids)

Table 10.1 Plasma concentration and production rate of estradiol, estrone, and progesterone in the different phases of the cycle

		Plasma concentration (ng/dL)	Production rate (mg/day)
Estradiol	Early follicular phase	0.005	0.08
	Late follicular phase	0.03 – 0.08	0.5 – 1
	Middle luteal phase	0.02	0.3
Oestrone	Early follicular phase	0.005	0.1
	Late follicular phase	0.015 – 0.03	0.3 – 0.7
	Middle luteal phase	0.1	0.2 – 0.3
Progesterone	Follicular phase	0.1	2
	Luteal phase	1.1 – 1.3	25

Endocrinology 285

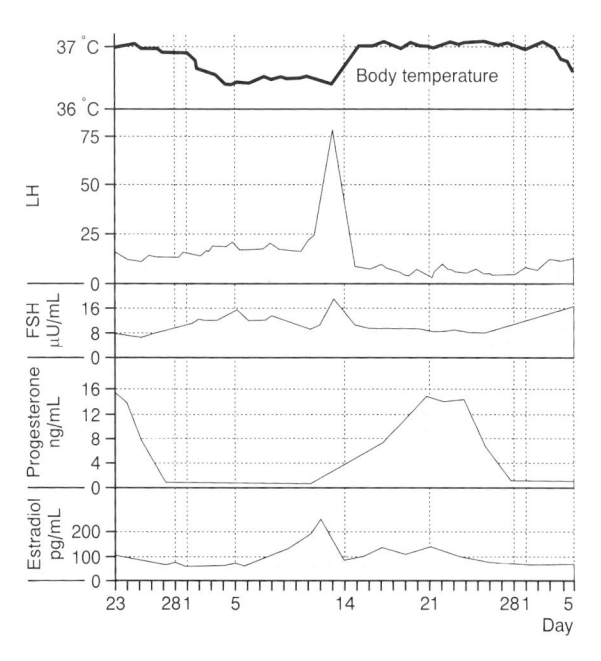

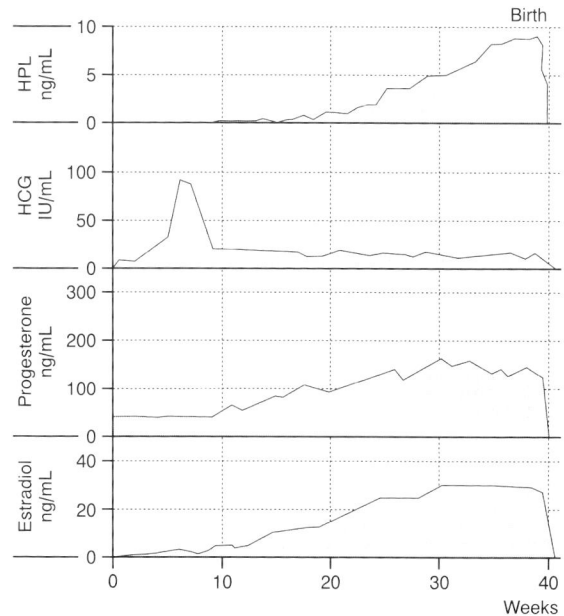

Fig. 10.**4** Hormonal situation in the menstrual cycle. In the first half of the cycle, the oocyte matures under the influence of FSH (primarily) and LH. The mid-cycle increase of estradiol triggers the ovulation-inducing LH peak (positive feedback). Progesterone begins to rise shortly before ovulation and achieves its highest concentrations in the second half of the cycle. If pregnancy does not occur, the corpus luteum perishes and the progesterone level falls

Fig. 10.**5** Serum hormone concentrations during pregnancy. HCG (human chorionic gonadotropin) is demonstrable just a few days after conception. HCG maintains the synthesis of progesterone in the corpus luteum. Maximum values are measured in the 5th–6th week of pregnancy. The HCG level falls when the synthesis of progesterone is taken over by the placenta (at about 3 months). Progesterone and estradiol increase continuously during pregnancy to fall again sharply at delivery. HPL (human placental lactogen) is a peptide hormone with growth hormon-like properties. Its level likewise increases dramatically particularly in the phase of greatest growth of the foetus. A decrease of progesterone, estradiol, or HPL signals an acute threat to the pregnancy and usually leads to a miscarriage

Table 10.**2** Some sex-specific effects of estrogens and progesterone

Organ	Estrogens	Progesterone
Vagina	Increased glycogen incorporation, increase of the karyopyknotic index (increased anuclear cells in vaginal smears)	Massive shedding of immature cells, decrease of the karyopyknotic index
Cervix	Dilation of the os uteri, mucus increased, spinnbar/fern-like crystallization. Promotion of spermatozoal ascension on estrogen dominance at the time of ovulation	Constriction of the os uteri and cervix, cervical secretion sparse, viscous, markedly cross-linked, not spinnbar
Uterus	Growth of all layers, in particular endometrial proliferation, increase of contractility and, hence, of responsiveness to, e.g., oxytocin	Mucosal transformation with glandular growth, formation of spiral arteries, quiesence, so-called progesterone block, reduced responsiveness to contraction-inducing stimuli (e.g., oxytocin)
Tubes	Increase of motility and secretion, delay of egg transport (not certain)	Reduced secretion and change of composition
Breast	Stimulation, particularly of duct growth and stroma (breast tension)	Gland growth, formation of gland vesicles (alveoli)

Table 10.3 Some metabolic and other effects of estrogens and progesterone

Effect on	Estrogens	Progesterone
Calcium metabolism	Promotion of absorption and of incorporation in bone	–
Lipids	Influence in favor of high density lipoproteins (HDL)	–
Transport proteins for sex, adrenocortical and thyroid hormones	Stimulation of the synthesis of SHBG and TBG	–
Capillaries	Dilation	–
Melatonin content of the skin	Increase (e.g., linea alba, areola)	–
Protein-anabolic effect	Yes	–
Distribution of body fat	Redistribution, increased deposition in the pelvic, thigh and breast region	–
Longitudinal growth	Arrest of longitudinal growth through ossification of the epiphyseal cartilages of the long bones	–
Basal body temperature	–	Increase from 36.5 °C to 37 °C
Insulin response	–	Decrease
Sodium reabsorption	–	Reduction
Ventilation (respiratory center)	–	Increase

Amenorrhea

Amenorrhea is present when menstruation fails to occur for more than 3 months. If menstruation has not occurred by the age of 15 years, the diagnosis is primary amenorrhea; otherwise, it is secondary. There can be different reasons for amenorrhea. The diagnosis follows a step-up scheme (WHO). The following are just some examples:

The progesterone test (induction of withdrawal bleeding) is negative in the presence of an estrogen deficit.
In hypothyroidism, the TRH test induces an exaggerated increase of FSH.
Increased testosterone or an increased LH–FSH ratio is indicative of the syndrome of polycystic ovaries (see below).
Increased gonadotropins (particularly FSH) signal ovarian insufficiency or the start of menopause.
Reduced gonadotropin values are an indication of disturbances in the hypothalamo–pituitary region (e.g., tumors, particularly prolactinomas).
Amenorrhea with increased prolactin values suggests a hypothalamic disturbance of GnRH pulsatility.
Amenorrhea in anorexia nervosa is also of hypothalamic origin (GnRH deficiency).

Anomalies (agenesis, obliteration) of the efferent genital tract, e.g., absence of the uterus, tubes, tubal obliteration, closed hymen, must also be considered in primary amenorrhoea. The Rokitanski–Küster–Hauser syndrome (see below) is also associated with primary amenorrhea.

In rare cases, secondary amenorrhea can be caused by antibodies to steroid producing cells (autoimmune disease). Exogenous factors (e.g., irradation and cytostatics) can likewise cause amenorrhea. Amenorrhea can be associated with severe illnesses also. The Sheehan syndrome, which sometimes occurs after complicated deliveries, must be mentioned. Head injuries leading to pituitary stalk lesions can also induce amenorrhea. The PCO syndrome, the adrenogenital syndrome, anorexia nervosa (underweight), prolactin-producing tumors and tumors of the hypothalamus, should also be mentioned. All the conditions are or can be accompanied by amenorrhea.

That amenorrhea is frequent in female athletes was mentioned as long ago as 100 B.C. by Soranus of Ephesus in his work "On the Disease of the Women." If intensive training begins before puberty, the onset of the menarche can be delayed by more than 3 years. Women with little overall body fat are most affected.

Polycistic Ovary Syndrome (PCO)

PCO syndrome is probably the most frequent endocrine disturbance in women. Diagnosis is made with increasing frequency not in the least as a result of the introduction of sonography. The guiding symptoms are signs of androgenization such as hirsutism (in about 70% of these patients), amenorrhea and anovulation (in about 50%) and overweight (in about

Endocrinology

PCOD: The "Vicious Circle"

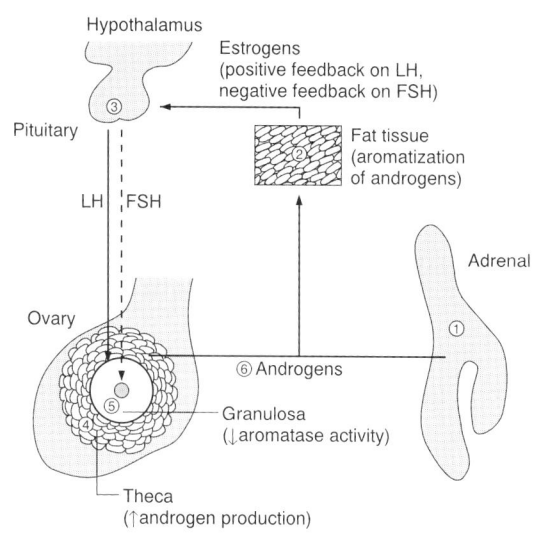

Fig. 10.6 The polycystic ovarian syndrome
The "vicious circle":
1. Start of the "vicious circle": Probably initiated by excessive androgen production by the adrenals and/or ovaries at puberty
2. Aromatization of androgens, e.g., in fatty tissue, results in increased estrogen levels
3. Estrogen exert a positive feedback on LH and a negative feedback on FSH synthesis and secretion. Results: High LH and low FSH concentrations, respectively
4. LH leads to excessive androgen production by theca cells
5. FSH is needed for aromatase activity in granulosa cells. Owing to the low levels of FSH, androgens cannot be converted into estrogens by granulosa cells
6. Excessive amounts of androgens are released into the circulation—the "vicious circle" is perpetuated

40%). The ovaries are enlarged and display follicular cysts. Fibrosis of the capsule and stroma is demonstrable. The etiology of this endocrine disorder is shown schematically in Fig. 10.6.

Idiopathic Hirsutism

5-α-reductase activity is frequently increased in what is known as idiopathic hirsutism. As a result, increased amounts of testosterone (including those in the skin and androgen-dependent cutaneous appendages) are converted to dihydrotestosterone (the most potent androgen). The consequences are similar to those in the PCO syndrome (see also Chapter 5).

Ovarian Hyperthecosis

Ovarian hyperthecosis, a hyperplasia of luteinized paraluteal cells, leads to ovarian insufficiency and hirsutism because of increased production of testosterone, progesterone, and 17-α-hydroxyprogesterone. Pronounced hyperinsulinism and simultaneous insulin resistance are characteristic of this disease. In contrast to PCO syndrome, gonadotropin levels are slightly raised, if at all. Ovariectomy is the therapy of choice.

Adrenogenital Syndrome (AGS)

This syndrome is based on various enzyme defects of glucocorticoid synthesis (primarily 21-hydroxylase). Since no or biologically only slightly active glucocorticoids are produced, the secretion of ACTH is increased by way of counterregulation, resulting in adrenal hyperplasia with increased adrenal secretion of androgens. Owing to the increased production of androgens, the hypothalamus–pituitary–ovarian axis is also blocked (inhibition of gonadotropin secretion), and women become amenorrhoic. The guiding symptom is hirsutism. This also applies to late-onset AGS, in which the enzyme defect does not display any clinical effects until after puberty (see Chapter 5).

Cushing Syndrome

This syndrome can have various causes, e.g., adrenal tumors, ACTH-producing tumors of the pituitary or of other regions (e.g. the mediastinum) (see Chapters 2 and 5).

Hyperprolactinemia (Galactorrhea-Amenorrhea Syndrome)

This syndrome can be of iatrogenic origin (several drugs stimulate prolactin secretion), but it is often due to a prolactin-producing tumor of the pituitary (see Chapter 2).

Ullrich–Turner Syndrome

With an incidence of about 1 : 3.000, this syndrome is one of the most common congenital endocrine symptoms associated with infertility. The syndrome is based on genetic defects (mainly Karyotype 45X0, but various other mosaics like 45X0/46XX). Guiding symptoms are short stature, gonadal dysgenesis, amenorrhea, scutiform chest, anomalies of the kidneys and efferent urinary tract, hanging angle of the mouth, often aortic isthmus stenosis, and disturbances of ocular motility. Gonadotropins are increased (no feedback from ovarian steroids).

Swyer Syndrome

Patient's with gonadal dysgenesis (Karyotype XX and XY) have a normal female internal and external genitalia with functionless rudimentary gonads. In contrast to Turner syndrome, gonadal dysgenesis is not associated with small stature.

Rokitanski–Küster–Hauser Syndrome

This syndrome has the anatomical cause of primary amenorrhea. The guiding symptoms are the absence of, or a hypoplastic vagina and no or only rudimentary communication between uterus and vagina. The diagnostic demonstration of the efferent urinary tract is important because malformations of the kidneys and ureters are frequently also present.

Kallmann Syndrome in Women

This is a very rare condition that is associated with anosmism or hyposmism (see Chapter 9). The male to female ratio is 5 : 1.

Endometriosis

Endometriosis is defined as the aberrant occurrence of endometrial tissue outside the uterus that is still subject to the cyclical processes of transformation and degeneration. These fragments of endometrial tissue can occur on the ovaries, tubes, sacrouterine ligaments, the serosa of the Douglas pouch, the roof of the bladder, and the vagina, as well as outside the minor pelvis on the intestines, and elsewhere. The etiology is largely unknown. It is estimated that endometriosis occurs in about 2% of all women of fertile age. The symptoms are not particularly specific and depend on the location of the endometriotic foci: pain in the sacral and inguinal region, on sexual intercourse, voiding complaints, hematuria, dysmenorrhea. The main diagnostic procedure is laparoscopic endoscopy, if possible complemented by histology.

Glandular Cystic Endometrial Hyperplasia

This is defined as excessive proliferation of the endometrium with gland formation and secondary prolonged follicular persistence in most cases (estrogen dominance). The most common symptom is irregular and prolonged bleeding (dysfunctional bleeding). It is believed that endometrial carcinoma may develop from glandular cystic hyperplasia if it remains untreated.

Ovarian Carcinoma

The incidence of ovarian carcinoma increases with increasing "ovulatory age" (10–15 new cases/100 000 women/year). This is defined as the phase in the life of a woman in which ovulatory cycles are not suppressed by pregnancy, lactation, or the use of oral contraceptives. Estrogen and progesterone receptors can be demonstrated in some malignant ovarian tumors; some granulosa and paraluteal cell tumors display gonadotropin receptors, i.e., they are stimulated by gonadotropins. For classification of ovarian tumors see Table 10.**4**. Hirsutism develops very quickly in the very rare cases of androgen-producing Sertoli-Leydig's cell tumors in women. Granulosa and paraluteal cell tumors secrete mainly estrogens. Chorionepitheliomas, which are very rare, produce HCG.

Ovarian carcinoma is usually diagnosed late and the symptoms are nonspecific (vaginal bleeding, lower abdominal pain). Endometriosis must be ruled out by differential diagnosis. The diagnostic procedure of choice is transvaginal sonography supplemented by histology and CT (for staging). The prognosis depends on the type of tumor, the grade of malignancy, and the stage of the disease. Most important is the risk evaluation postoperatively in accordance to the FIGO classification. The 5-year survival rate in the low-risk group is approximately 90%, in the high-risk group, about 50%.

Uterine Myomas (Uterus Myomatosus)

These are benign nodes with smooth muscles which first appear after the onset of sexual maturity. Their in-

Table 10.**4** Classification of ovarian tumors

I.	Epithelial tumors a Serous tumors b Mucinous tumors c Endometrioid tumors d Clear Cell (mesonephroid) tumors e Brenner tumors f Mixed epithelial tumors g Undifferentiated carcinomas h Unclassified epithelial tumors
II.	Stromal tumors a Granulosa stromal cell tumors b Androblastomas, Sertoli-Leydig cell tumors c Gynandroblastomas d Unclassified stromal tumors
III.	Lipid cell tumors
IV.	Germinal cell tumors a Dysgerminoma b Endodermal sinus tumor c Embryonal carcinoma d Polyembryoma e Chorionepithelioma f Teratoma g Mixed forms
V.	Mixed germinal cell tumors and stromal tumors a Pure gonadoblastomas b Mixed with dysgerminoma or other germinal cell tumors
VI.	Connective tissue, non-ovary-specific tumors
VII.	Unclassified tumors
VIII.	Secondary (metastatic) tumors
IX.	Tumor-like changes

cidence is reported to be 5% of all women, and their growth is stimulated by oestrogens. Myomas can easily be diagnosed by sonography.

Endometrial Carcinoma

Like mammary carcinoma, endometrial carcinoma belongs to the estrogen-dependent tumors. With an incidence of about 20/100 000 women/year, it accounts for 10% of all malignant tumors in women. Risk factors are obesity (increased production of estrogens from androgenic precursor molecules in fatty tissue), prolonged cycle disturbances with anovulation (no progesterone effect and, thus, absence of menstruation, e.g., in PCO syndrome), and replacement therapy with estrogens in menopause without the addition of a progestogen.

70% of the tumors are adenocarcinomas. Symptoms occur late and are not very characteristic: e.g., pain, ascites, uremia. Abnormal PAP smear and curettage usually provides information helpful to the diagnosis. Various diagnostic procedures are used for tumor staging: X-ray, ultrasound, and particularly CT of the pelvis and abdomen. In the initial phase, the differential diagnostic demarcation from glandular cystic endometrial hyperplasia is difficult.

Cervical Carcinoma

With an incidence of about 30/100 000 women/year, this is the most common form of genital cancer. Etiologically, deficient sexual hygiene of the partner and frequent change of partner are believed to be causative or promoting factors. Over 90% of lesions are squamous cell carcinomas. Due to screening programs, cervical carcinoma is usually diagnosed in the stage of precancerosis (PAP staining of smears). The symptoms are discharge, postcoital bleeding, and, in later stages, pain. The main prognostic criterions are the size of the tumor lesion and the lymphatic and hematogenic spread.

Vaginal Carcinoma, Vulvar Carcinoma

Vaginal carcinomas are rare (1% of all malignant genital tumors) and consist almost exclusively of squamous cell carcinomas. The main symptoms are bleeding and bloody discharge (almost exclusively postmenopausal).

Vulvar carcinomas are also rare, (3% of all genital cancers) and also occur almost exclusively postmenopausally. They are mostly squamous cell carcinomas.

References

1 Goodman Gilman A, Rall TW, Nies AS, Taylor R. The Pharmacological Basis of Therapeutics. 8th ed. New York: Pergamon Press; 1990.
2 Greenspan FS, Forsham PH. Basic & Clinical Endocrinology. 2nd ed. Los Altos: Lange Medical Publications; 1986.
3 Speroff L, Glass RH, Kase NG. Clinical Gynecologic Endocrinology and Infertility. 4th ed. Baltimore: Williams & Wilkins; 1989.
4 Williams RH, ed. Textbook of Endocrinology. 8th ed. Philadelphia: WB Saunders; 1992.
5 Rabin D, McKenna TJ, eds. Clinical Endocrinology and Metabolism – Principles and Practice. Dietschy JM, ed. Vol 9: Science and Practice of Clinical Medicine. New York: Grune & Stratton; 1982.
6 Grossmann A, ed. Clinical Endocrinology, 1st ed. Oxford: Blackwell Scientific Publications; 1992.

MR Imaging

S. K. Stevens

Major Clinical Indications

MRI is becoming an increasingly useful modality for the detection and evaluation of ovarian masses (1–10). Although ultrasound remains an excellent screening examination for the initial evaluation of ovarian lesions, it is operator dependent and may be inadequate for staging pelvic malignancies (11, 12). CT has improved spatial resolution when compared to ultrasound and is currently being used not only to detect and characterize pelvic lesions but also to stage ovarian carcinoma (10, 13, 14). Potential limitations of CT include restriction of imaging to the transaxial plane and suboptimal soft-tissue contrast. Recent experience with MRI has shown that its multiplanar imaging capacity, excellent soft-tissue contrast, and large field of view may offer specific advantages over either ultrasound or CT in evaluating ovarian lesions (15).

The ability of MRI to demonstrate uterine zonal anatomy on T2-weighted images for example, makes it particularly useful in differentiating adnexal masses from those arising in the uterus (2). Precise localization of pelvic lesions is particularly important in evaluating pregnant patients with masses, which on ultrasound are of uncertain origin (16, 17). MRI is also useful in facilitating lesion characterization. Specific MRI features that are diagnostic of such benign cystic lesions as endometriomas and teratomas, as well as benign solid lesions such as ovarian fibromas have recently been described (18–25). Preoperative differentiation of benign from malignant lesions is also possible in many instances using MRI, and is facilitated by the use of the intravenous contrast medium Gd-DTPA (7, 8). Early experience with MRI suggests that it may also be helpful in the preoperative staging of ovarian carcinoma (7).

Imaging Techniques

Imaging Sequences

When evaluating the ovaries, a combination of both T1- and T2-weighted spin-echo sequences is recommended for optimal tissue characterization and anatomic delineation. T1-weighted images provide the necessary contrast between neoplasms and adjacent pelvic fat, and are also necessary to characterize hemorrhagic and fat-containing lesions. Adenopathy is optimally displayed on T1-weighted images. T2-weighted images, on the other hand, are required for superior tissue characterization, which is not provided on T1-weighted images. The ovaries are more easily identified on T2-weighted images than on T1-weighted images due to the bright signal intensity of ovarian follicles on the former. Uterine zonal anatomy is also best depicted on T2-weighted images.

Gd-DTPA-enhanced T1-weighted images contribute to lesion characterization by facilitating differentiation of cystic from solid lesions and depicting intratumoral architecture (regions of tumor necrosis, nodularity, or vegetations). In patients with ovarian malignancies, Gd-DTPA is useful in identifying peritoneal implants, the presence of omental pathology, anhd extraperitoneal extent of disease (7, 8).

Fat-saturation MRI hass been shown recently to be useful in differentiating hemorrhagic from fat-containing pelvic lesions, and may be used as a problemsolving sequence in differentiating endometriomas and other cystic hemorrhagic masses from teratomas (23, 24). Gradient-recalled echo techniques are usually reserved for differentiating adenopathy from flowing blood in adjacent iliac vessels. The role of fast spin-echo and fast gradient-recalled echo imaging techniques in evaluating adnexal disease is currently under investigation. Whether these imaging sequences will eventually replace standard T2-weighted spin-echo images remains to be seen.

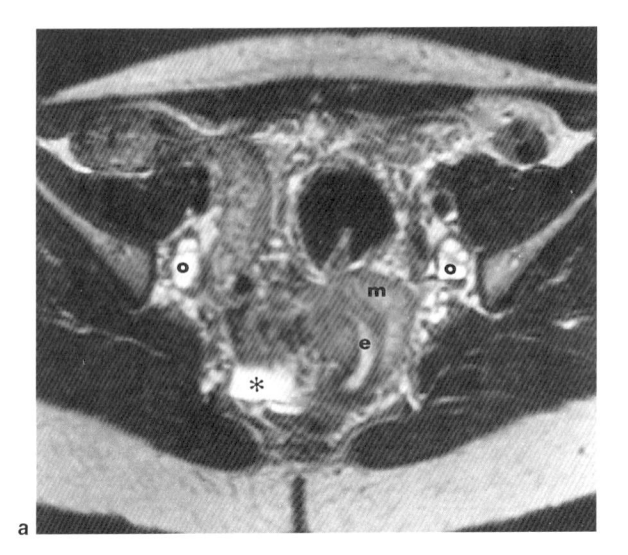

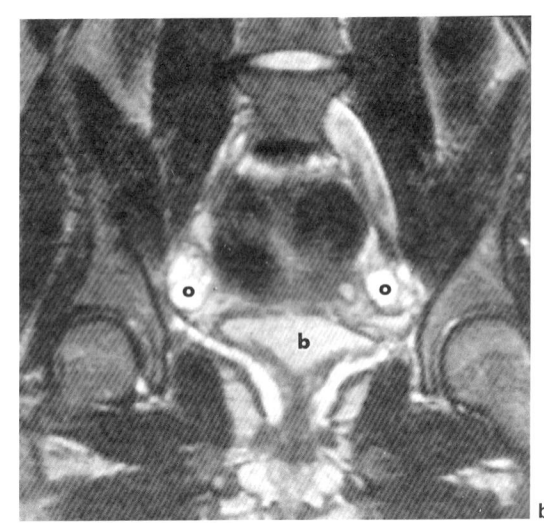

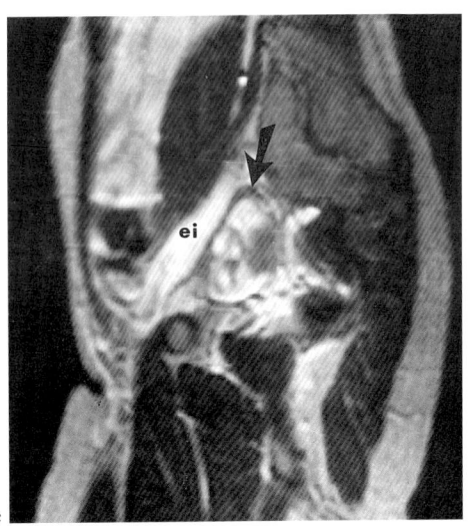

Fig. 10.**7** Normal ovaries. (**a**) transaxial T2-weighted fast spin-echo (4000/90 effective TE, 8 echo train length), (**b**) coronal T2-weighted (2000/70), and (**c**) sagittal T2-weighted (2000/80) images (1.5 T). The ovaries (o) have multiple bilateral high signal intensity follicular cysts that are well demonstrated in all three planes. A landmark for identifying the ovaries in the sagittal plane is their position inferior to the common iliac bifurcation (arrow). The myometrium (m) and endometrium (e) are also well seen. A small amount of fluid (*) is identified in the culde-sac. b = bladder, ei = external iliac vein

Imaging Planes

A combination of transaxial and coronal, or transaxial and sagittal planes is recommended for evaluating the adnexa (Fig. 10.7). The transaxial and coronal planes will most accurately display the normal ovaries in their expected position on either side of the uterus attached to the posterior aspect of the broad ligament. Most ovarian abnormalities are readily appreciated in the transaxial plane although the coronal plane is a useful adjunct in depicting ovarian pathology and evaluating congenital anomalies of the uterus, cervix, or vagina. Scanning from the level of the symphysis pubis to at least the level of the renal hila on T1-weighted transaxial images is necessary to evaluate the retroperitoneum for the presence of adenopathy and hydronephrosis or both.

In the sagittal plane, the ovaries are readily identified inferior to the landmark of the common iliac bifurcation. This plane is often the most useful in differentiating a collection of ovarian cysts from a hydrosalpinx. The sagittal plane also affords improved evaluation of the presacral space and determination of extraperitoneal extent of disease.

MRI Appearance of Normal Ovaries

Childhood and Premenarchal

At birth, the human ovary measures an average of 1.28 × 0.42 × 0.28 cm (length × width × height) and weighs approximately 0.12 g. The ovary enlarges throughout infancy and childhood so that by the time of puberty it has reached the size, weight, and shape of the adult ovary. The increase in size and weight is due to increases in the amount of stroma, the size of individual follicles, and the number of follicles (26, 27). Active follicular growth and atresia are seen throughout childhood in approximately 90% of ovaries, particularly after age 6 or 7 (28). Within the first year of life ovaries that have failed to descend normally may be found above the pelvic brim, and those that have descended too far may be found within the inguinal canal (29).

On MRI, normal childhood ovaries are of low to medium signal intensity isointense with muscle or uterus on short TR/TE (T1-weighted) sequences. On long TR/TE sequences (T2-weighted) the ovaries have signal intensity equal to or greater than fat (Fig. 10.8). Follicles are more easily identified on T2-weighted images.

Reproductive Age

The adult ovary is ovoid in shape and measures approximately 3–5 cm × 1.5–3 cm × 0.6–1.5 cm with an average weight of 5–8 g (30). Although histologically, the ovaries contain an outer cortex, an inner medulla, and a hilus, these zones are not appreciated on MRI. The signal intensity of adult ovaries on T1- and T2-weighted spin-echo images is similar to that of the premenarchal female. Follicular structures are best appreciated on either T2-weighted or gadolinium-enhanced T1-weighted images (Fig. 10.7). Normal ovaries have been identified on MRI in 87–96% of reproductive age women when thin slices are used and when the plane of imaging is either coronal, transverse, or a combination of transverse and sagittal (2, 31).

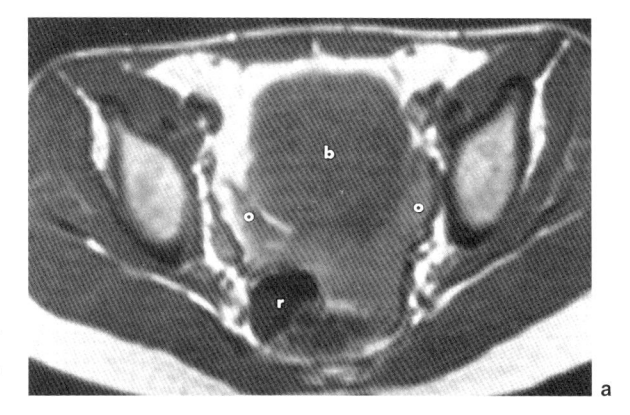

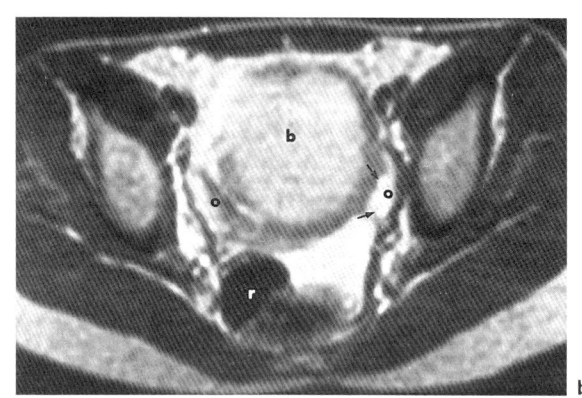

Fig. 10.8 Normal ovaries in a 7-year-old girl. (**a**) proton density (1000/30), and (**b**) T2-weighted (1000/70) images (1.5 T). The ovaries (o) have intermediate signal intensity on the proton density image and are isointense with fat on the T2-weighted image. A few small follicles (arrows) are identified in this patient. b = bladder, r = rectum

Postmenopausal

The postmenopausal ovary is approximately one-half the size of that of the reproductive age woman. Follicles are usually absent although on occasion they may persist for several years after cessation of menses (26). On MRI postmenopausal ovaries are usually low to medium signal intensity isointense with uterus on both T1- and T2-weighted images. They may have signal intensity similar to that of reproductive age women, however. Postmenopausal ovaries may be difficult to identify, not only because of their smaller size, but also because of the absence of high signal intensity follicles on T2-weighted images. Both ovaries have been detected on MRI in only 47% of postmenopausal women (2).

Ovarian Pathology

Disorders of Sexual Differentiation

The noninvasive multiplanar nature of MRI makes it an excellent modality for the evaluation of disorders of sexual differentiation. Used in conjunction with chromosomal, cytogenetic, hormonal, and biochemical analysis, MRI may help characterize abnormal and variable anatomy associated with patients with ambiguous genitalia.

True Hermaphroditism

True hermaphrodites have both testicular and ovarian tissue that may exist either separately or combined in an ovotestis (32). The most common carrier types in true hermaphroditism are 46XX (60%), 46XY (12%), and mosaic (28%). Location of the gonad is influenced by the type of gonadal tissue present. Specifically, gonads with a large amount of ovarian tissue are usually located in an ovarian position, whereas gonads that contain testicular tissue or a combination of ovarian and testicular tissue are more commonly located in the scrotum, inguinal region, or in the internal inguinal ring (32). Most patients have ambiguous genitalia usually in the form of a small phallus or enlarged clitoris.

In true hermaphroditism, a fallopian tube is adjacent to an ovary and an epididyms or vas deferens is adjacent to a testis. Gonads have an increased incidence of germ cell tumors, particularly gonadoblastoma (2.6%) (32). Uteri, if present, are often abnormal, as these patients have an increased incidence of unicornuate uterus (10%), absent cervix (14%), and uterine hypoplasia (46%) (32).

When radiologic evaluation of true hermaphroditism is requested, it usually is for morphologic display of the uterus and vagina, prostate gland and penis, or localization of the gonads (Fig. 10.9) (33). Sagittal films are needed for evaluation of the uterus, prostate, and penis; transverse sections are needed for localizing the gonads and demonstrating the vagina (34).

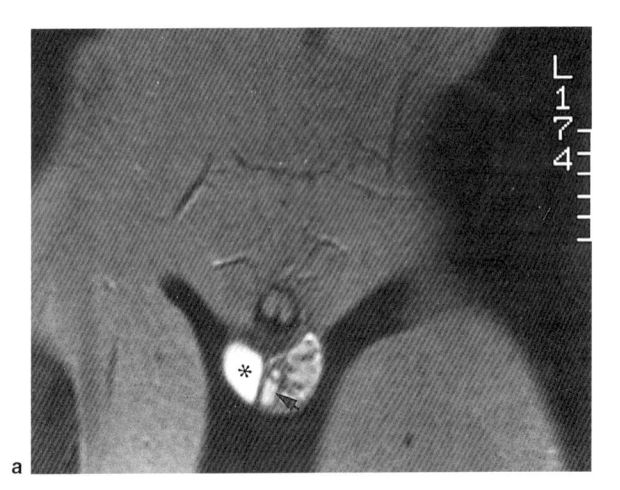

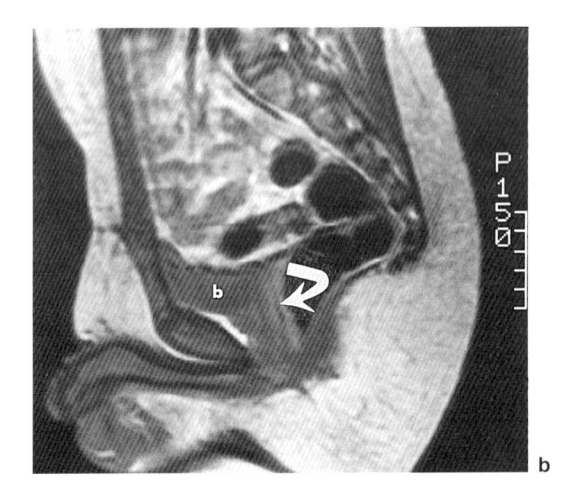

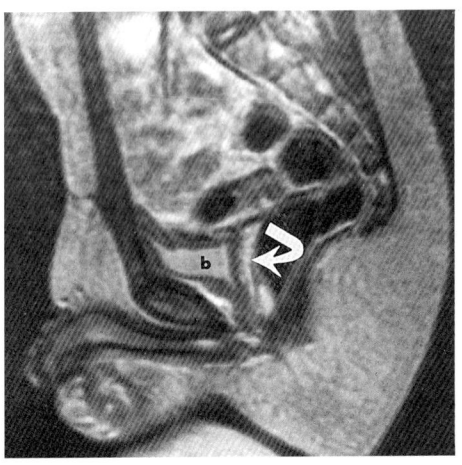

Fig. 10.9 True hermaphrodite. (a) T2-weighted coronal image shows a gonad within the left scrotal sac (arrow) which on biopsy contained both testicular and ovarian tissue with ovarian germ cells. A small hydrocele (*) is noted on the right. (b) proton density (2200/20), and (c) T2-weighted (2200/70) (1.5 T) images show a rudimentary Müllerian remnant (arrow) posterior to the bladder (b). (Reprinted with permission from reference 33)

Pseudohermaphroditism

Pseudohermaphrodites are individuals in whom the gonadal sex differs from the genital sex. Male pseudohermaphrodites are 46XY and usually have gonads that are testes but have female external genitalia, whereas female pseudohermaphrodites are 46XX, have ovarian gonads, and have masculinized external genitalia (32, 35).

Male pseudohermaphroditism. Causes of male pseudohermaphroditism include deficient androgen formation, defects in androgen action (end-organ androgen insensitivity), lack of müllerian duct regression, and Leydig's cell hypoplasia. The most common type is testicular feminization, an X-linked trait due to a qualitative or quantitative deficiency of androgen receptor protein. In the complete form, the external genitalia are female. The condition is rarely diagnosed before puberty unless an inguinal hernia is discovered. Primary amenorrhea is the most common complaint leading to the diagnosis. Testes are cryptorchid and located in the inguinal canal, pelvis, or rarely the labia. Usually the cervix and uterus are absent as are the epididymides, vasa deferentia, seminal vesicles, and prostate. Testes in patients with testicular feminization have an increased incidence of Sertoli cell adenomas and seminomas. The risk of testicular malignancy in patients with testicular feminization reaches 33% by age 50 (32).

MRI is useful in confirming the absence of a uterus as well as demonstrating the location of the testes. Immature testes are difficult to differentiate from immature ovaries on MRI as both may have medium signal, intensity on T1-weighted images and medium to high signal intensity to T2-weighted images. The anatomy of the vagina and presence or absence of a uterus and cervix are consistently displayed on MR images. Sagittal and transaxial imaging are essential (34, 36, 37). A finding that has been reported on T2-weighted images in patients with testicular feminization is the presence of an outer rim of medium signal intensity surrounding the gonads. This presentation often differentiates the gonads from lymph nodes (37).

Female pseudohermaphroditism. Female pseudohermaphroditism results from relative androgen excess in utero in an individual who is 46XX and has two ovaries (32). Pseudohermaphroditism may either be due to the adrenogenital syndrome, maternal ingestion of progestins or androgens, or maternal virilizing tumors such as pregnancy luteomas (32). The most common cause of female pseudohermaphroditism is AGS (congenital adrenal hyperplasia) due to 21-hydroclylase deficiency. The uterus, fallopian tubes, and ovaries are usually normal in these patients, although external genitalia are often masculinized (35). Early diagnosis is paramount because normal reproductive function is often possible after appropriate hormonal treatment has been instituted. On MRI, an immature

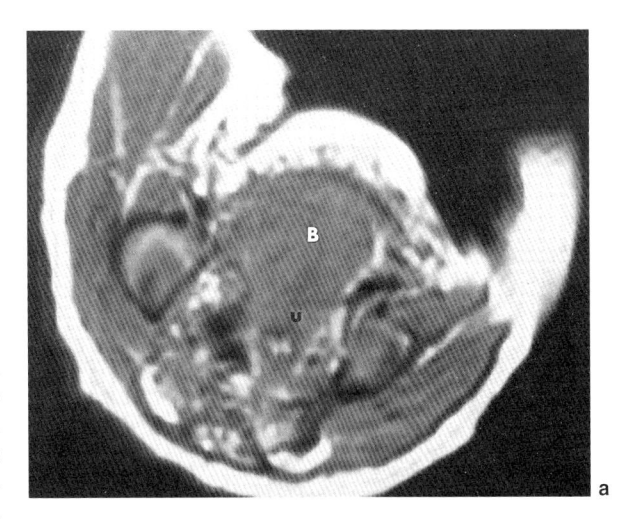

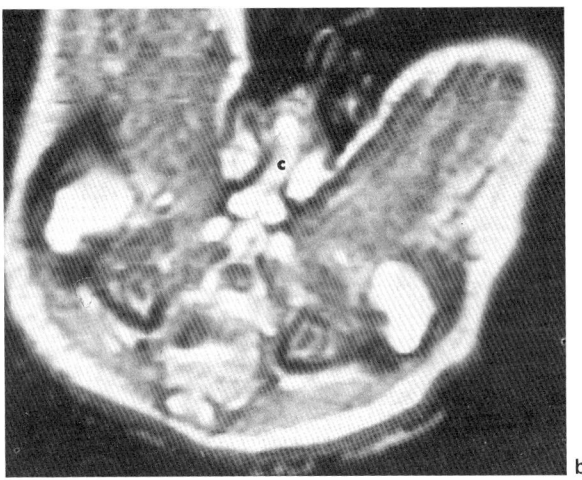

Fig. 10.**10** Three-week-old with ambiguous genitalia. Transaxial (**a**) proton density (2000/20) and (**b**) T2-weighted (2000/70) (1.5 T) images. A small uterus (u) with normal zonal anatomy as well as clitoromegaly (c) are seen. B = Bladder. (Reprinted with permission from reference 33)

uterus, clitoral hypertrophy, or the presence of a common urogenital sinus may be seen (Fig. 10.**10**).

Gonadal Dysgenesis

Gonadal dysgenesis is divided into three types: pure gonadal dysgenesis, mixed gonadal dysgenesis, and gonadal dysgenesis combined with growth retardation and somatic anomalies (Turner syndrome) (38). In pure gonadal dysgenesis the carrier type is either 46XX with female phenotype or 46XY with female phenotype and virilization. Both types have bilateral streak gonads.

In mixed gonadal dysgenesis, the carrier type is usually mosaic 45X/46XY. Patients have persistent müllerian duct structures (uterus and fallopian tubes), an abnormal testis, and a contralateral streak gonad

(32). Neonates usually have ambiguous genitalia. A palpable testis may bulge through an indirect inguinal hernia, descend completely into the labioscrotal fold, or remain intra-abdominal. Although the gonad that descends is usually a testis, the streak gonads are usually intra-abdominal. Approximately one-third of patients with mixed gonadal dysgenesis develop gonadoblastomas, and approximately 30% of gonadoblastomas are overgrown by a malignant germ cell tumor, usually dysgerminomas (32).

Turner syndrome is a disorder in which sexually immature phenotypic females have short stature, various congenital anomalies, and streak gonads. The carrier type is 45X0 (35). The external genitalia, vagina, and uterus in Turner syndrome patients are usually normal, although infantile. The gonads are fibrous streaks approximately 2–3 cm in length located in the position normally occupied by the ovary. Although germ cell tumors are rare in these patients due to the paucity of germ cells, epithelial neoplasms have been reported (39). There is also an increased incidence of endometrial carcinoma in patients who have had long-standing estrogen therapy to foster development of female secondary sexual characteristics (40).

On MRI, the sagittal and transverse planes are valuable in depicting the small uterus and streak gonads (Fig. 10.11). Gonads demonstrate low to intermediate signal intensity on T1-weighted images and may be isointense with, or slightly lower in signal intensity, than fat on T2-weighted images. Locating abnormal gonads in these patients is occasionally difficult due to the absence of high signal intensity follicles on T2-weighted images. When abnormal high signal in-

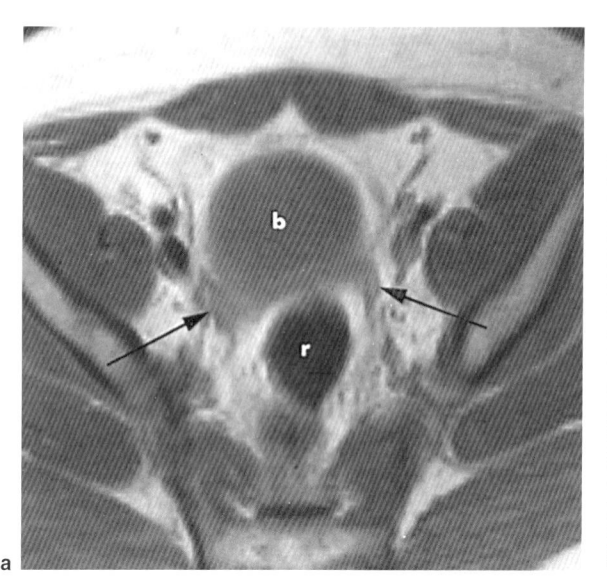

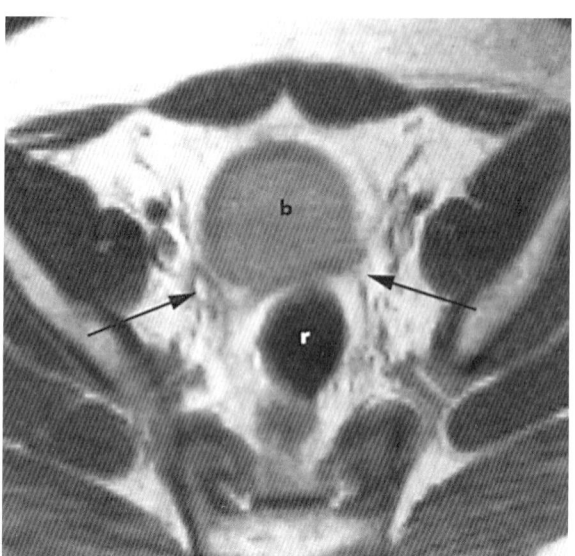

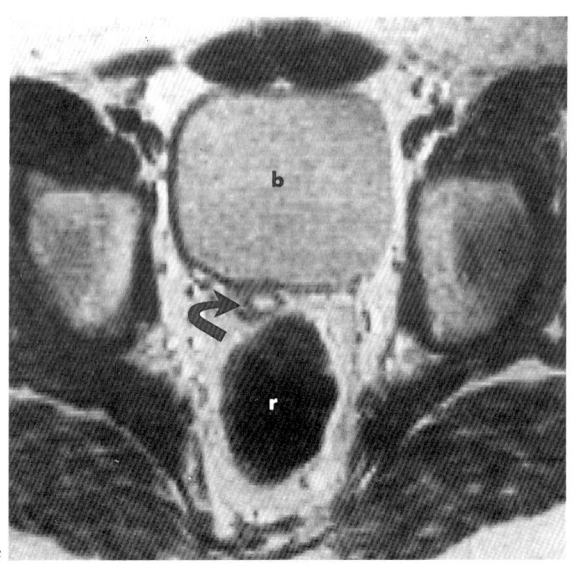

Fig. 10.11 Turner syndrome. Transaxial (a) proton density (2000/30), and (b), (c) T2-weighted (2000/60) (.35 T) images. Bilateral streak ovaries (straight arrows) are seen as well as a hypoplastic infantile uterus (curved arrow) in this 16-year-old woman. r = rectum, b = bladder

tensity is identified in an enlarged gonad, the possibility of an associated neoplasm such as gonadoblastoma should be considered (37).

Endometriosis

Endometriosis refers to the presence of endometrial tissue ectopically located outside the uterus. It is most common in women between the ages of 30 and 40 and has been reported to affect as many as 40% of infertile women (41, 42). An increased incidence of endometriosis is seen in patients who have müllerian duct anomalies with obstructed uterine drainage.

Endometriosis is usually limited to the pelvis although lesions in remote body sites have been reported (43, 44). The most common areas of involvement in decreasing order of frequency include the ovaries, uterine ligaments, cul-de-sac, pelvic peritoneum covering the uterus, fallopian tubes, rectosigmoid, and bladder (45). Endometriotic foci involving the pelvic peritoneal surfaces are multiple and frequently surrounded by dense fibrous adehsions. They may enlarge to produce nodules, cysts, or both. Endometriotic cysts (endometriomas) most commonly involve the ovaries. They are bilateral in one-third to one-half of patients, and although they may range from a few millimeters to several centimeters in size, they rarely exceed 15 cm. If larger, the presence of a neoplasm arising within the cyst should be excluded because this complication has been documented in 0.3–0.8% of patients with ovarian endometriosis. The most common malignancies arising from ovarian endometriomas are endometrioid carcinoma and clear cell carcinoma (45).

On pathologic examination, endometriomas typically have a fibrotic wall of variable thickness and are commonly covered by dense fibrous adhesions that may result in fixation to adjacent structures. Cyst contents consist of semifluid, chocolate-colored material. On occasion, endometriomas may appear as multiple polypoid masses that fill the pelvis and simulate a malignant tumor. In addition, abscess formation in an endometrioma that has undergone bacterial infection is a rare but notable complication (45).

On MRI, endometrial implants usually demonstrate signal intensity similar to that of normal endometrium on T1- and T2-weighted images (Fig. 10.12). Because endometrial implants can exhibit various degrees of hemorrhage due to hormonal stimulation, however, implants may demonstrate a spectrum of appearances dependent on the age of the hemorrhage. Specifically, low signal intensity on T1- and T2-weighted images due to deoxyhemoglobin or hemosiderin, high signal intensity on T1-weighted images and low signal intensity on T2-weighted images due to intracellular methemoglobin, or bright signal intensity on both T1- and T2-weighted images due to extracellular methemoglobin in subacute hemorrhage

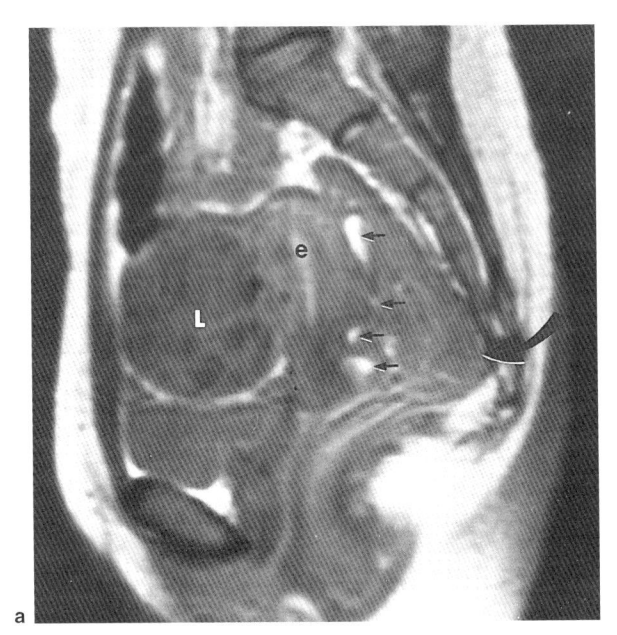

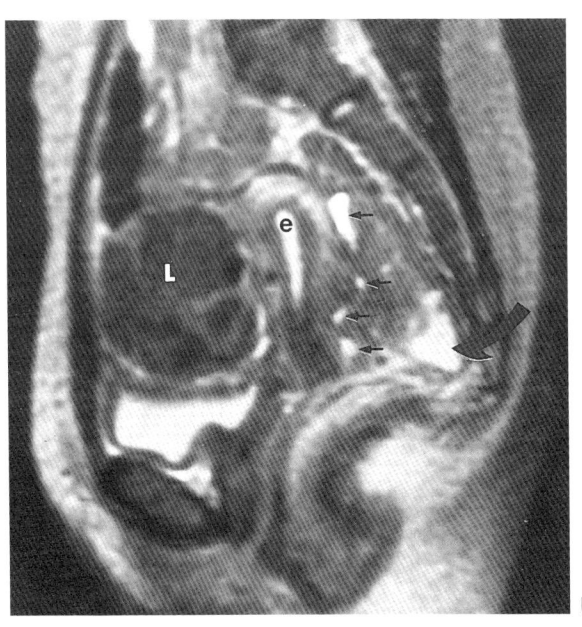

Fig. 10.12 Intraperitoneal and extraperitoneal endometrial implants. Sagittal (**a**) proton density (2000/20), and (**b**) T2-weighted (2000/20) images. High signal intensity intraperitoneal implants are identified along the uterine serosal surface and in the cul-de-sac (small arrows). Extraperitoneal endometrial implant with intermediate signal intensity on the proton density image and high signal intensity on the T2-weighted image within the presacral region (curved arrow) was found to be adherent to the rectum. e = endometrium, L = leiomyoma. (Reprinted with permission from reference 15)

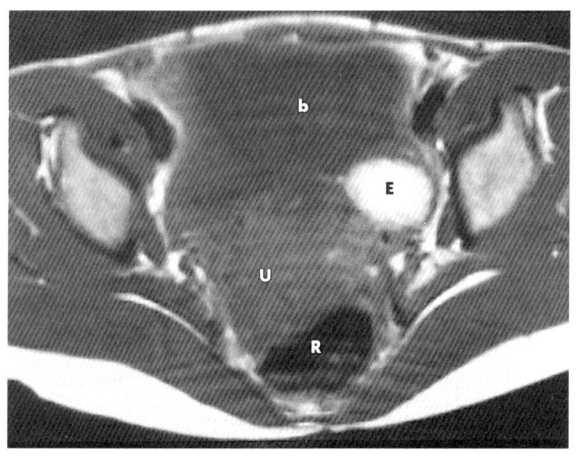

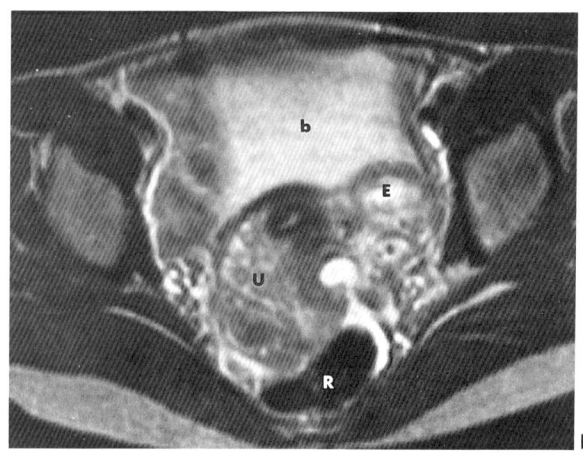

Fig. 10.**13** Left ovarian endometrioma with adhesions. Transaxial (**a**) T1-weighted (700/20), and (**b**) T2-weighted (2000/70) (1.5 T) images show that the endometrioma (E) has an indistinct margin with the uterus consistent with adhesions. Shading is noted within the endometrioma on the T2-weighted image. U = Uterus, R = rectum, b = bladder

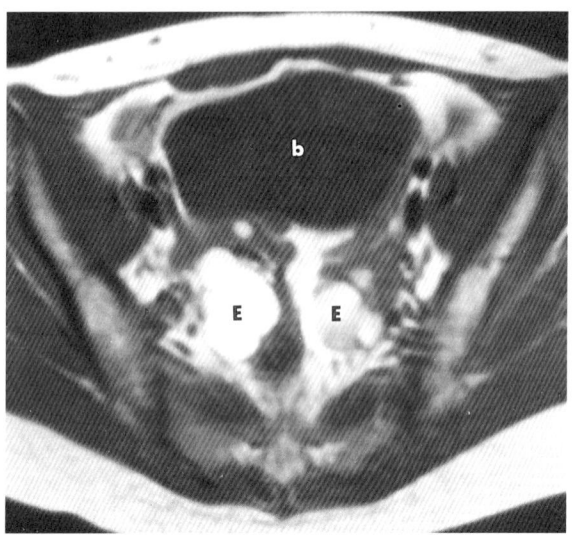

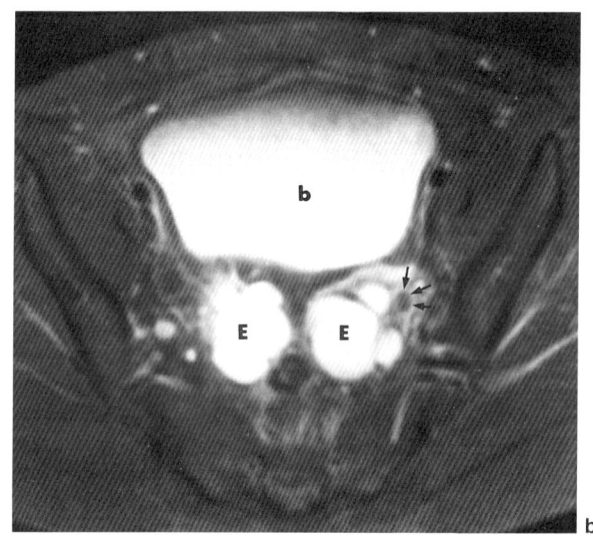

Fig. 10.**14** Bilateral endometriomas, transaxial plane. (**a**) T1-weighted (700/20), and (**b**) gadolinium-DTPA-enhanced T1-weighted (700/20) fat saturation images (1.5 T). On the fat saturation image, the multilocular endometriomas (E) remain of bright signal intensity. A small left follicular cyst is seen after gadolinium administration (small arrows). b = bladder

may be seen (18–21). MRI has been shown to be particularly useful in detecting extraperitoneal implants (vaginal fornix, rectovaginal ligament, urinary bladder, and presacral region); however, it cannot accurately depict intraperitoneal endometrial implants and ovarian endometrial adhesions in all patients (19). These limitations indicate that MR imaging cannot replace laparoscopy in the diagnosis and staging of endometriosis.

Although the MRI appearance of endometrial implants is variable, characteristic MRI findings suggestive of endometriomas have been reported. These include: a) a hyperintense cyst on T1-weighted images that demonstrates shading on T2-weighted images (Fig. 10.**13**, or b) a lesion consisting of multiple hyperintense cysts on T1-weighted images regardless of signal intensity on T2-weighted images (21). Additional findings contributing to the diagnosis of endometrioma include the presence of a thick fibrous capsule and adhesions to surrounding organs. Rarely, layering due to a hematocrit effect is seen in endometriomas (20). Following administration of Gd-DTPA, enhancement of the endometrial cyst wall and any areas of focal thickening or nodularity may be seen (Fig. 10.**14**). Presence of the latter suggests the possibility of underlying malignancy. Occasionally, the signal intensity of endometriomas on unenhanced MR images resembles that of teratomas. Fat-saturation imaging is useful in differentiating between these two entities (23, 24).

Nonneoplastic Cysts

Solitary Functional Cysts (Follicle Cyst and Corpus Luteum Cyst)

Follicle cyst. Follicle cysts range from 3 to 8 cm in diameter, are thin walled, and unilocular. They are usually asymptomatic; however, spontaneous rupture can occur. These cysts infrequently undergo torsion or infarction. Follicular cysts in childhood may be associated with isosexual precocity, and during the reproductive years, with menometrorrhagia and anovulation (46).

Corpus luteum cyst. Corpus luteum cysts are similar in size and appearance to follicle cysts. They occur during the reproductive years and are less common than follicle cysts.

Most follicle and corpus luteum cysts regress spontaneously within two months. Oral contraceptive pills may be prescribed to accelerate the involution of functional cysts. Failure to regress may require operative removal (46). On MRI, functional cysts are well circumscribed and homogeneous with a smooth, barely perceptible wall (Fig. 10.**15**). They have low signal intensity on T1-weighted images and high signal intensity on T2-weighted images. Occasionally functional cysts may be hemorrhagic and difficult to differentiate from endometriomas (19, 20). Following administration of Gd-DTPA, functional cysts demonstrate enhancement of a barely discernible or very thin peripheral wall isointense with surrounding ovarian tissue. The low signal intensity cyst contents remain of low signal, thereby resulting in increased conspicuity.

Theca-Lutein Cysts

Theca-lutein cysts result from high levels of HCG or an increased sensitivity of theca cells to HCG. In one-third to one-half to cases theca-lutein cysts are found in association with hydatidiform mole and choriocarcinoma. Maternal virilization, ascites, or hydrothorax may be present. Theca-lutein cysts are also seen in patients treated with ovulation inducing agents such as gonadotropins or clomiphene. Cysts can grow to more than 25 cm in size, are often bilateral, and may contain intracystic hemorrhage. They spontaneously regress as the HCG level falls and the ovaries return to normal size. Complications include torsion or rupture with hemorrhage (46). The MRI ap-

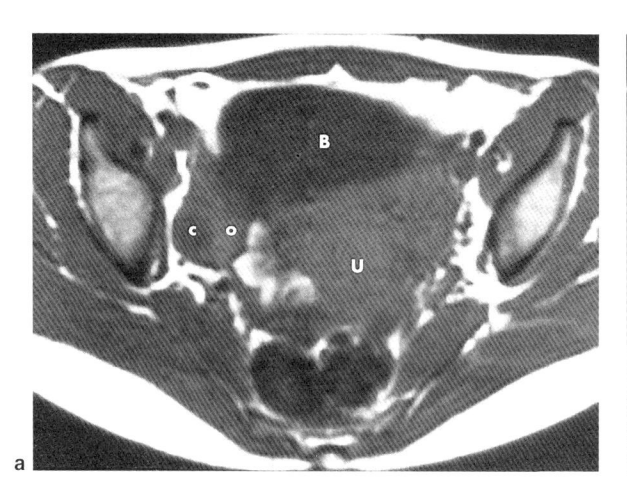

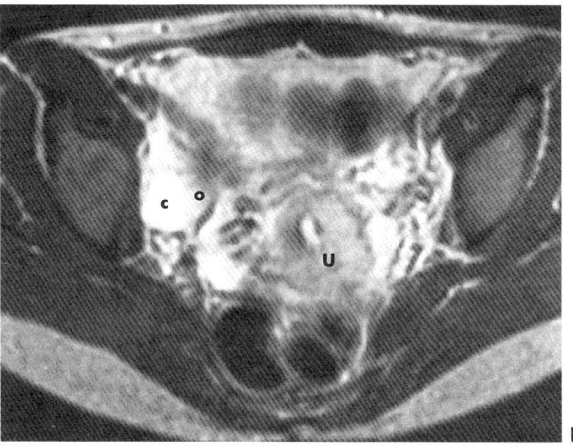

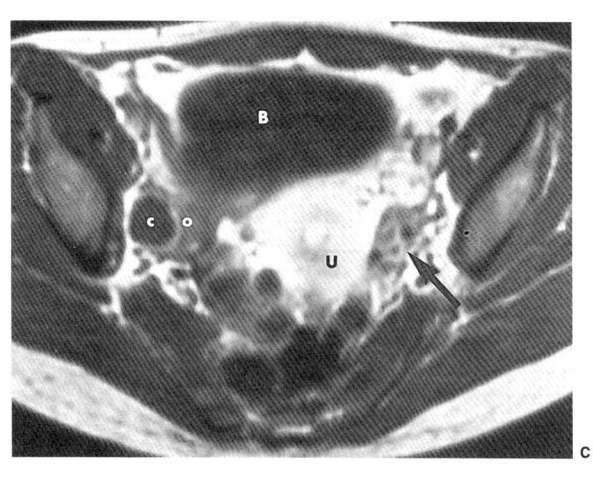

Fig. 10.**15** Bilateral follicular cysts, transaxial plane. (**a**) T1-weighted (550/20), (**b**) T2-weighted (2000/70), and (**c**) gadolinium-enhanced T1-weighted (550/20) images (1.5 T). Right follicular cyst (c) has low signal intensity on T1-weighted images, high signal intensity on T2-weighted images, and a thin peripheral wall that enhances after gadolinium administration. Enhancing adjacent ovarian tissue (o) should not be mistaken for a thick cyst wall. After i. v. administration of gadolinium-DTPA, increased conspicuity of small follicular cysts often results (arrow). U = uterus, B = bladder

pearance of theca-lutein cysts is similar to that of functional cysts.

Polycystic Ovarian Disease

Polycystic ovarian disease (PCOD), as originally described by Stein and Leventhal in 1935, consists of four clinical features: obesity, oligomenorrhea or amenorrhea, infertility, and hirsutism (47). The disease has been estimated to involve 3.5–7% of the female population and can be familial. The precise etiology remains unknown although PCOD is characterized by an alteration in the pattern of normal steroid feedback resulting in abnormal ovarian steroid secretion, inappropriate gonadotropin secretion, hyperandrogenemia, and increased peripheral conversion of androgens to estrogens (48, 49).

Patients with PCOD may exhibit manifestations of unopposed estrogen stimulation including endometrial hyperplasia and endometrial carcinoma. The endometrial carcinomas are usually well-differentiated adenocarcinomas, and many are reversible with progesterone therapy or by ovulation induction. Other associated abnormalities in patients with PCOD include hyperprolactinemia in 27% and galactorrhea in 13% (48).

Ovaries in patients with PCOD are two to five times normal size, although size may be normal. Numerous unruptured follicles are situated beneath a thickened white cortex. There is hypertrophy of the capsule and central ovarian stroma (50, 51).

On MRI, the characteristic appearance of polycystic ovaries consists of multiple small peripheral cysts demonstrating low signal intensity on T1-weighted images and high signal intensity on T2-weighted images adjacent to abundant low signal intensity central stroma (Fig. 10.16) (51, 52). T2-weighted images are useful in evaluating the uterus, which may be hypoplastic (although zonal anatomy is usually preserved), for potential endometrial carcinoma.

Stromal Hyperthecosis and Stromal Hyperplasia

Stromal hyperthecosis and hyperplasia refer to focal luteinization and proliferation of the ovarian stroma. When stromal proliferation is excessive it is said to be hyperplastic, and in some young women with stromal hyperplasia it is sufficiently pronounced causing enlargement or displacement of follicles and other structures. The abnormal stromal cells produce androgens resulting in masculinization that may be severe. The ovaries are usually enlarged and either solid or partly cystic. Clinical and pathological features often overlap with those of PCOD except that hyperthecosis produces masculinization. Patients with stromal hyperplasia and hyperthecosis also have an increased incidence of endometrial hyperplasia and endometrial carcinoma (48). Unlike patients with polycystic ovaries however, patients with hyperthecosis usually do not respond to treatment with clomiphene or ovarian wedge resection. The MRI appearance of the ovaries in patients with stromal hyperthecosis and hyperplasia may be either normal or similar to that of patients with polycystic ovarian disease (Fig. 10.17).

Ovarian Tumors

Tumors of the ovary may be either benign or malignant. Approximately 80% are benign and occur in young women between the ages of 20 and 45. Malignant tumors, on the other hand, are more commonly found in older women between 40 and 65 years of age (53). Among cancers of the female genital tract, the incidence of ovarian cancer ranks third behind only car-

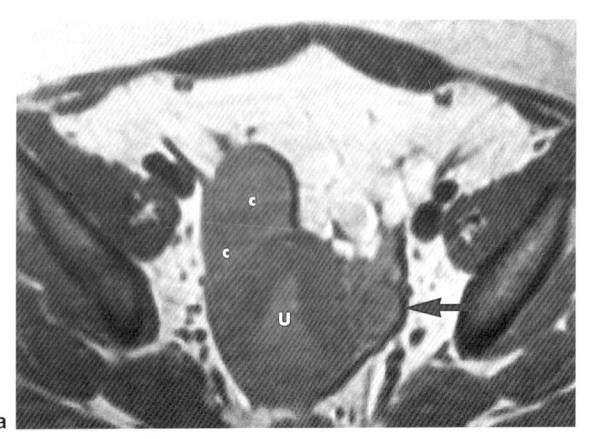

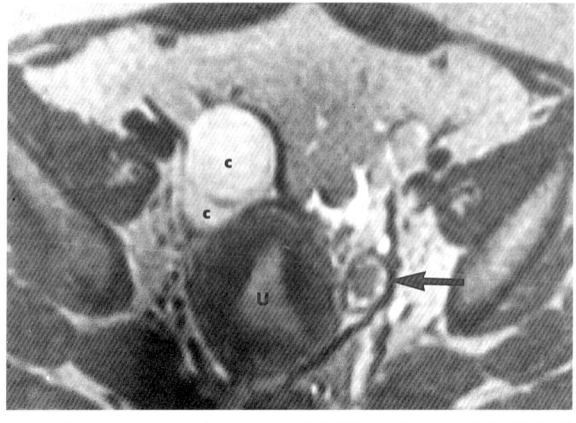

Fig. 10.**16** Polycystic ovarian disease. Transaxial (**a**) proton density (2100/20), and (**b**) T2-weighted (2100/70) images at 1.5 T. Left ovary (arrow) is of normal size and contains multiple peripheral high signal intensity cysts surrounding central low signal intensity stroma. The right ovary also contains multiple cysts (c), although these are larger than the cysts on the contralateral side. The uterus (U) in this patient is of normal size with preservation of the zonal anatomy

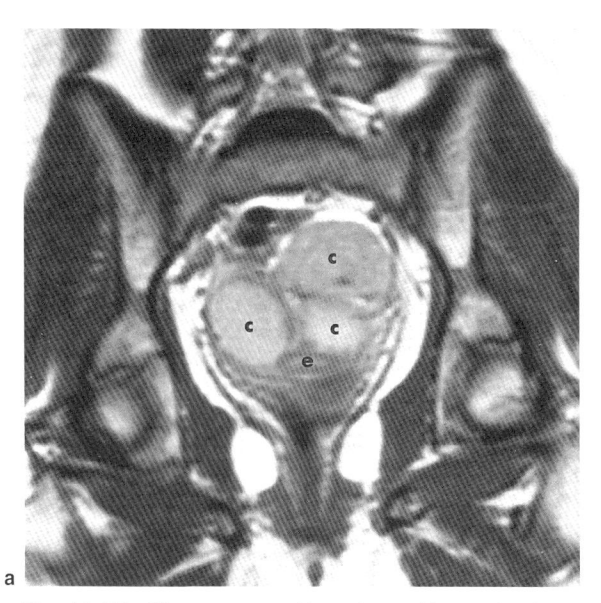

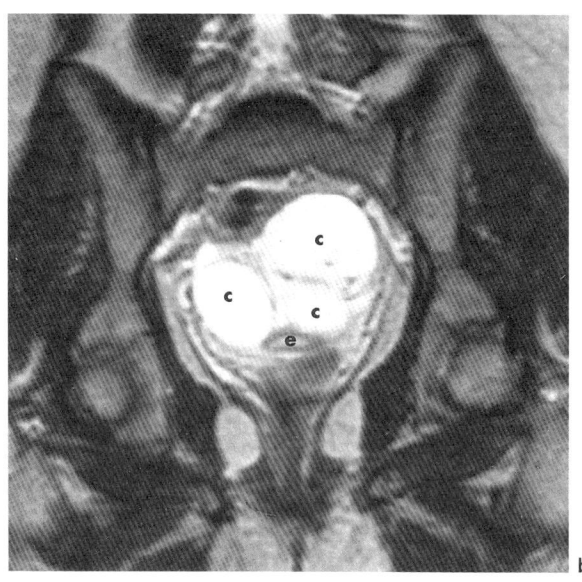

Fig. 10.17 Sixteen-year-old patient with ovarian hyperthecosis and stromal hyperplasia. Transaxial (**a**) proton density (2000/30), and (**b**) T2-weighted (2000/80) images (1.5 T). Multiple bilateral ovarian cysts (c) are seen causing ovarian enlargement. In addition, a small hypoplastic uterus with normal zonal anatomy is noted. e = endometrium

Table 10.5 FIGO Staging of Ovarian Carcinoma L55

STAGE I	Tumor limited to the ovaries	STAGE III	Tumor involving one or both ovaries with peritoneal implants outside the pelvis and/or positive retroperitoneal or inguinal nodes. Superficial liver metastasis equals Stage III. Tumor is limited to the true pelvis but with histologically proven malignant extension to small bowel or omentum
Stage Ia	Limited to one ovary; no ascites present; no tumor on external surface; capsule intact		
Stage Ib	Limited to both ovaries; no tumor on external surfaces; capsules intact		
Stage Ic	Stage Ia or Ib but with tumor on surface of one or both ovaries; or with capsule rupture; or with ascites present containing malignant cells or with positive peritoneal washings	Stage IIIa	Tumor grossly limited to the true pelvis with negative nodes but with microscopic seeding of abdominal peritoneal surfaces
		Stage IIIb	Tumor of one or both ovaries with histologically confirmed implants of abdominal peritoneal surfaces none exceeding 2 cm in diameter. Nodes are negative
STAGE II	Growth involving one or both ovaries with pelvic extension		
Stage IIa	Extension and/or metastases to the uterus/tubes		
Stage IIb	Extension to other pelvic tissues	Stage IIIc	Abdominal implants greater than 2 cm in diameter and/or positive retroperitoneal or inguinal nodes
Stage IIc	Tumor either Stage IIa or IIb, but with tumor on surface of one or both ovaries; or with capsules ruptured; or with ascites present containing malignant cells or with positive peritoneal washings	STAGE IV	Growth involving one or both ovaries with distant metastases. If pleural effusion is present, there must be positive cytology to allot a case to Stage IV. Parenchymal liver mets equals Stage IV

cinoma of the cervix and endometrium. Risk factors include nulliparity and family history. An increased incidence of ovarian cancer exists in industrialized countries and in patients with gonadal dysgenesis (53). The current classification of ovarian tumors is according to the WHO schema, which is based on the cell or tissue of origin. Most tumors arise from one of three ovarian components: a) the surface coelomic epithelium, b) the germ cells, and c) the stroma of the ovary, including the sex cord (54). The staging of ovarian carcinoma is according to the International Federation of Gynecology and Obstetrics (FIGO). Criteria presented in Table 10.55.

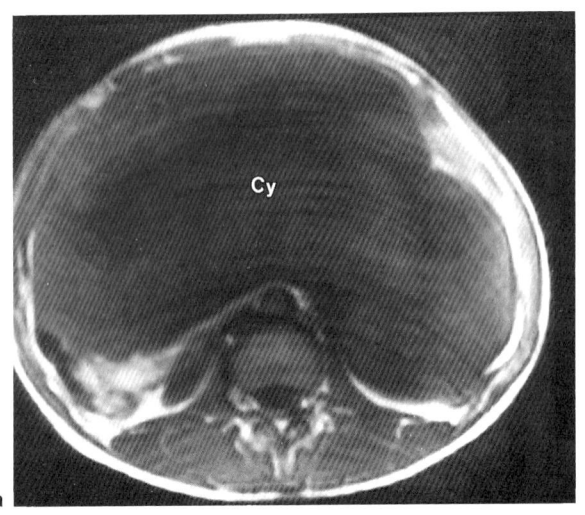

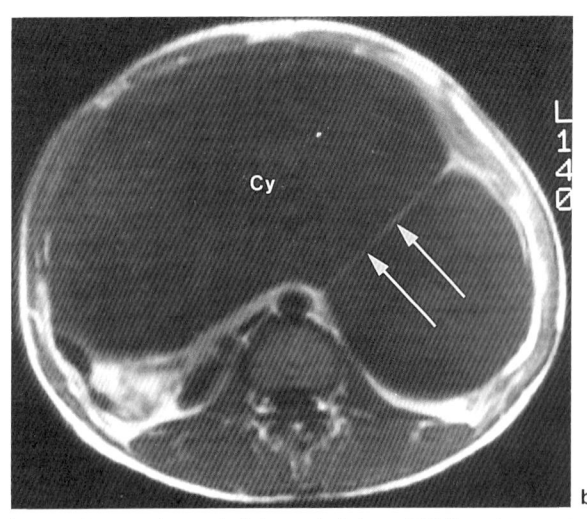

Fig. 10.**18** Serous cystadenoma, transaxial plane. (**a**) unenhanced, and (**b**) gadolinium-DTPA-enhanced T1-weighted (700/20) 1.5 T images show a large cystic mass (Cy) with a single enhancing septum (arrows) best appreciated on the gadolinium-enhanced image

Tumors of Surface Epithelium (Common Epithelial Tumors)

Tumors of the surface epithelium constitute approximately two-thirds of all primary ovarian neoplasms and nearly 90% of all malignant ovarian tumors (56). The major types include serous, mucinous, endometrioid, undifferentiated, and clear cell tumors. Each histologic type may be categorized into benign, malignant, and tumors of low malignant potential.

Serous tumors. Sixty percent of serous tumors are benign, 25% malignant, and 15% represent tumors of low malignant potential (53). Serous cystadenomas are usually cystic, unilocular, large, and are lined by a characteristic tall columnar epithelium (Fig. 10.**18**). They often contain projections, and 25% of papillary serous tumors have psammoma bodies (round microscopic calcifications due to degenerative changes). Cystadenocarcinomas tend to have larger and more numerous papillary projections, more complex multiloculation, and more complex solidification of spaces. Ca-125 antigen is commonly associated with nonmucinous borderline and malignant epithelial ovarian tumors, particularly those of the serous and endometrioid types. Bilateral ovarian involvement is seen in approximately two-thirds of borderline and malignant serous tumors (50).

Mucinous tumors. Mucinous tumors are slightly less common than the serous forms and account for approximately 25% of all ovarian neoplasms. 80% are benign, 10–15% are borderline, and 5–10% are malignant (53). Mucinous tumors may roughly resemble serous cystadenomas and cystadenovarcinomas; however, these tumors are more apt to be unilateral, larger, and the characteristic lining of these lesions consists of characteristic tall columnar epithelial cells with prominent mucin vacuoles. Five to 10% of mucinous tumors contain cystic teratomas or Brenner tumors and 2–5% are complicated by pseudomyxoma peritonei (Fig. 10. **19**) (53, 56). Mucinous tumors often produce carcinoembryonic antigen (CEA), and rarely may produce enough gastrin to cause Zollinger–Ellison syndrome (50).

Endometrioid tumors. These tumors account for 20% of ovarian neoplasms, and most are carcinomas. The name is derived from the histological pattern closely resembling that of uterine endometrial adenocarcinoma. Endometrioid carcinomas are often partly cystic with prominent solid areas. Fifteen to 30% of endometrioid carcinomas are accompanied by a carcinoma of the endometrium, although it is not thought that one represents metastatic spread from the other (53).

Clear cell tumors. The appearance of clear cell tumors is often a combination of solid and cystic components similar to endometrioid carcinoma. The cytoplasm of the large epithelial cells contains abundant glycogen. Ten percent are bilateral. Clear cell carcinomas of the ovary may occur in association with endometriosis or endometrioid carcinoma of the ovary (53).

MR imaging of epithelial tumors. On MRI the appearance of ovarian tumors is varied and depends not only on histologic type, but also on whether the lesion is benign or malignant. Benign tumors such as serous and mucinous cystadenomas are usually unilocular or multilocular thin-walled cystic lesions with a smooth outer surface and few septa or nodules. They usually have low signal intensity on T1-weighted images and high signal intensity on T2-weighted but may have high signal intensity on both T1- and T2-weighted images if they contain mucin or hemorrhage. Layering

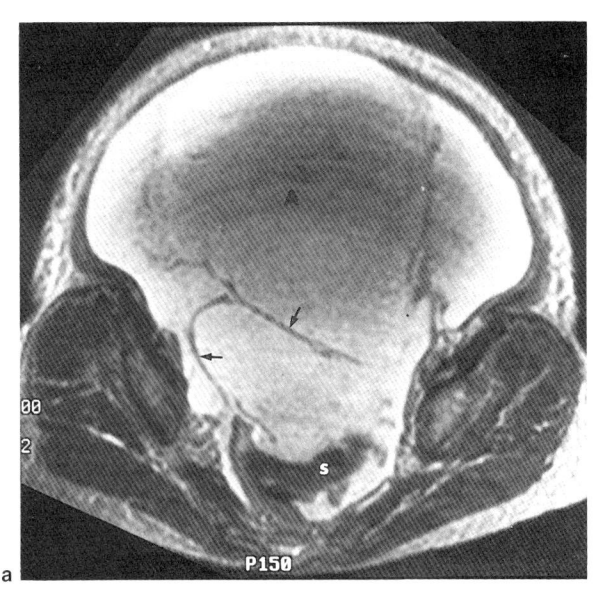

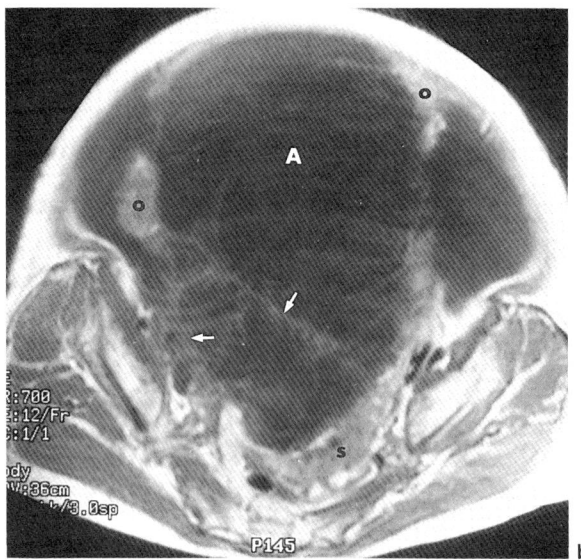

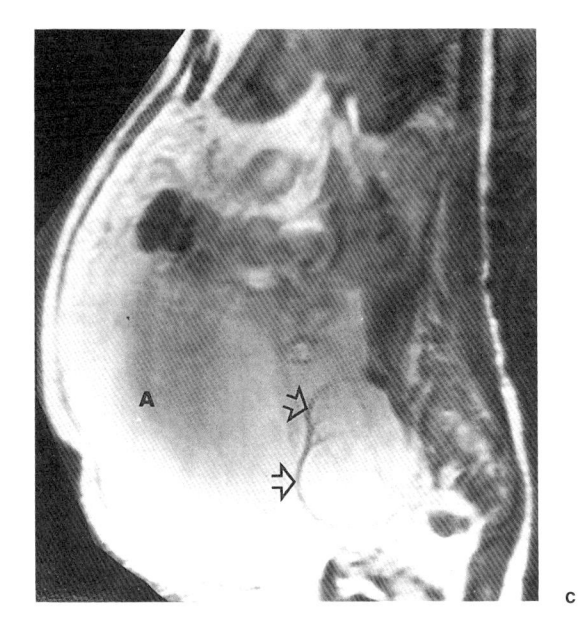

Fig. 10.**19** Pseudomyxoma peritonei associated with a nonmalignant mucinous ovarian neoplasm. Transaxial (**a**) T2-weighted (2000/80), (**b**) gadolinium-enhanced T1-weighted (700/12), and sagittal (**c**) T2-weighted fast spin-echo (3000/85 effective TE, 16 echo train length) images (1.5 T). A large amount of mucinous ascites (**a**) is seen in association with multiple linear strands (short arrows). The multilocular cystic masses involving the ovaries that represented pseudomyxoma ovarii are best appreciated on the fast spin-echo T2-weighted image (open arrows). The enhancing linear strands and omental involvement are best appreciated after gadolinium administration. s = sigmoid

or fluid–fluid levelsl may be seen (1–4, 7, 8, 10). Septations and regions of nodularity are best demonstrated on either T2-weighted or Gd-DTPA-enhanced T1-weighted images (Fig. 10.**18**) (7, 8).

In contrast to benign epithelial lesions, malignant epithelial tumors are usually large (greater than 4 cm) and may be either solid or cystic. Solid masses usually demonstrate low to intermediate signal intensity on T1-weighted images and high signal intensity on T2-weighted images unless complicated by areas of hemorrhage and necrosis or both. Like their benign counterparts, malignant neoplasms containing proteinaceous or hemorrhagic fluid may have bright signal intensity on both T1- and T2-weighted images. Cystic ovarian neoplasms usually have thick walls or septa (greater than 3 mm) and contain vegetations or regions of nodularity. As with benign lesions, these findings are best demonstrated on either T2-weighted or Gd-DTPA-enhanced T1-weighted images (Fig. 10.**20**). Gd-DTPA expedites lesion characterization by facilitating assessment of intratumoral architecture. Gadolinium is also useful in determining wall thickness, the presence and thickness of septations, identifying vegetations or regions of nodularity, and depicting tumor necrosis (7, 8).

In staging ovarian neoplasms, MRI is capable of determining extent and location of disease within the pelvis including involvement of adjacent organs (uterus, bladder, rectosigmoid) (Figs. 10.**21** and 10.**22**), retroperitoneal spread, and disease pelvic side-

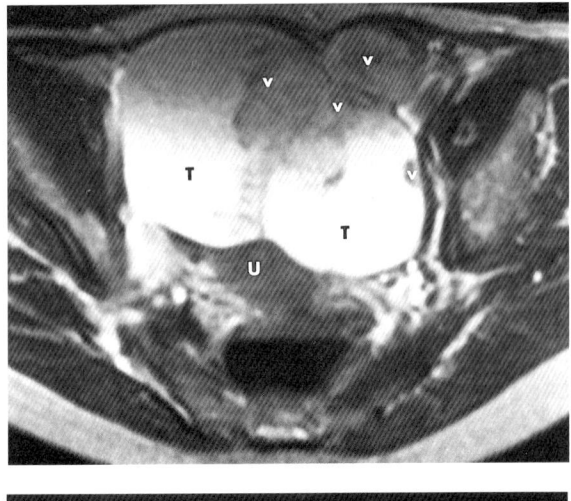

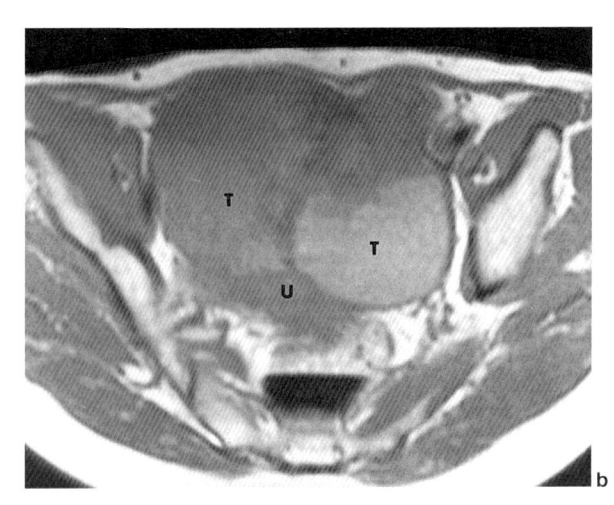

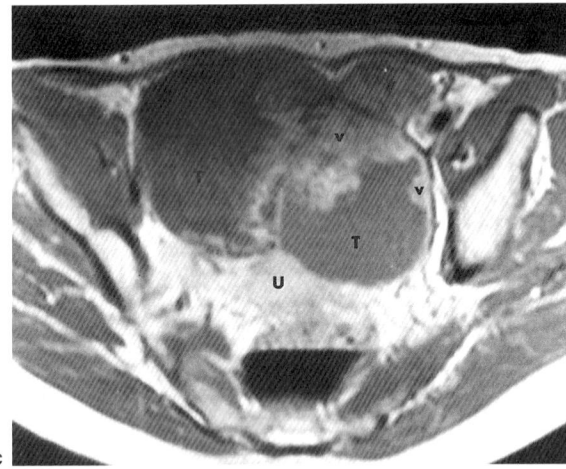

Fig. 10.**20** Ovarian endometrioid carcinoma, transaxial plane. (**a**) T2-weighted (2000/80), (**b**) T1-weighted (700/20), and (**c**) gadolinium-enhanced T1-weighted (700/20) 1.5 T images show bilateral cystic ovarian tumors (T) with large, solid, enhancing intracystic vegetations (v). U = uterus

wall invasion. Intra-abdominal disease including the presence of ascites, omental deposits, and peritoneal implants is also readily assessed on MRI. Ascites uncomplicated by hemorrhage usually demonstrates low signal intensity on T1-weighted images and high signal intensity on T2-weighted images. Diffuse omental disease and peritoneal implants larger than 1 cm in size are best seen after gadolinium administration (Figs. 10.**23** and 10.**24**), although small peritoneal implants less than 1 cm in size remain difficult to detect. Distant metastases to the liver, umbilicus, or bone may also be appreciated (Figs. 10.**22** and 10.**25**) (7). Preliminary work suggests that the MRI detection rate for pelvic and retroperitoneal lymphadenopathy equals that of CT (Fig. 10.**26**) (57).

Although the preoperative differentiation of benign from malignant lesions remains difficult, preliminary experience with MRI suggests that the following criteria are strongly suggestive of a malignant lesion: 1. size greater than 4 cm, 2. solid or predominantly solid lesion, 3. wall thickness greater than 3 mm, 4. septa greater then 3 mm, vegetations, or nodularity, and 5. necrosis. Ancillary criteria associated with malignant lesions include: 1. involvement of adjacent pelvic organs or extension to the pelvic sidewall, 2. peritoneal, mesenteric, or omental disease, 3. ascites, and 4. adenopathy. The current preoperative characterization sensitivity of adnexal lesions using unenhanced T1- and T2- weighted images and gadolinium-enhanced T1- weighted MR images is reported to be 95%. Staging accuracy is 75% (7).

Germ Cell Tumors

Germ cell tumors comprise 20% of all ovarian tumors and represent the second largest group of ovarian neoplasms after the epithelial tumors. They are encountered at all ages, but are most frequent from the first to sixth decades. In children and adolescents, over 60% of ovarian neoplasms are of germ cell origin, and one-third are malignant. In adults, the vast majority (95%) are benign cystic teratomas (58). The most common germ cell tumors include teratomas, dysgerminomas, endodermal sinus tumors, embryonal carcinoma, and choriocarcinoma. Mixed forms also occur in any possible combination. Gonadoblastoma is a tumor

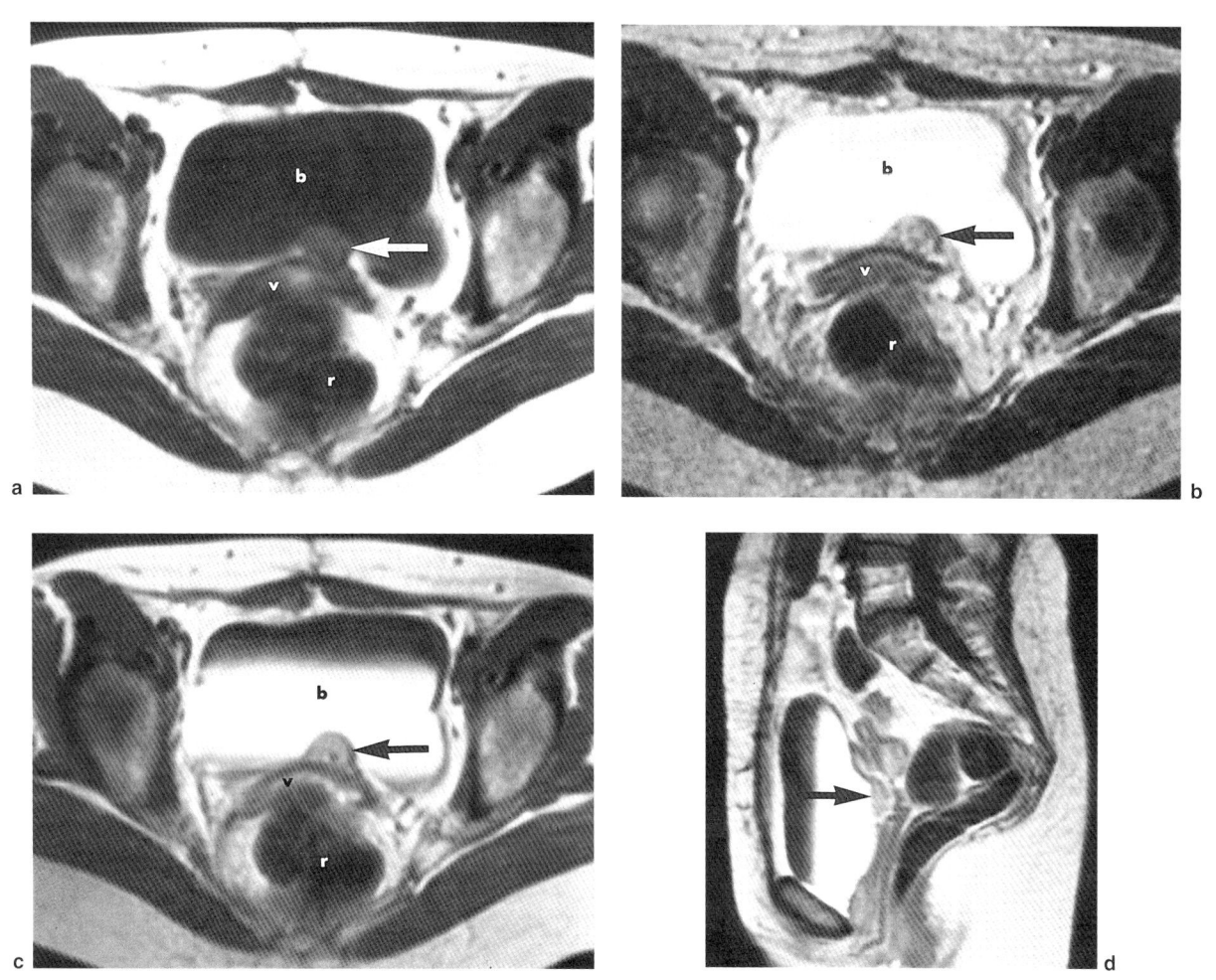

Fig. 10.**21** Bladder implant in patient with ovarian carcinoma. Transaxial (**a**) T1-weighted (700/20), (**b**) T2-weighted (2000/80), and (**c**) gadolinium-enhanced T1-weighted (700/20) images. (**d**) Sagittal gadolinium-enhanced T1-weighted (700/20) image (1.5 T). A metastatic implant (arrow) along the posterior bladder wall is identified on all pulse sequences but is most easily seen following gadolinium administration. b = bladder, v = vagina, r = rectum

composed of both germ cells and sex cord–stromal derivatives.

Teratomas. Teratomas are divided into three categories: 1. mature (benign), 2. immature (malignant), and 3. monodermal or highly specialized (struma ovarii and carcinoid) (53). Ninety-nine percent consist of cystic and mature forms (dermoid cysts). Mature cystic teratomas are almost always benign although 1–2% may undergo malignant change, usually to squamous cell carcinoma (59). Most cystic teratomas are 5–10 cm in size and 10–15% are bilateral. They are usually unilocular cysts that contain ectodermal, mesodermal, and endodermal structures, although ectoderm is the predominant element. Arising from the wall of these tumors is often a nodule composed of a mass of tissue known as a dermoid plug or Rokitansky protuberance. It is within this area that a variety of tissues including bone or teeth may be found. Complications of cystic teratomas include torsion (16%), rupture (1%), autoimmune hemolytic anemia, and rarely, infection or virilization (59).

In contrast to the much more common mature cystic teratoma, immature teratomas are composed of immature or embryonal tissues derived from the three germ cell layers. These tumors constitutre less than 1% of ovarian teratomas and occur most commonly in the first two decades of life. They are usually unilateral but may coexist with a benign cystic teratoma in the opposite ovary. These tumors are usually large, bulky, form adhesions to surrounding structures, grow rapidly, and have a poor, 5-year survival (50, 53, 58).

Monodermal or highly specialized teratomas include stroma ovarii and carcinoid. Stroma ovarii is a

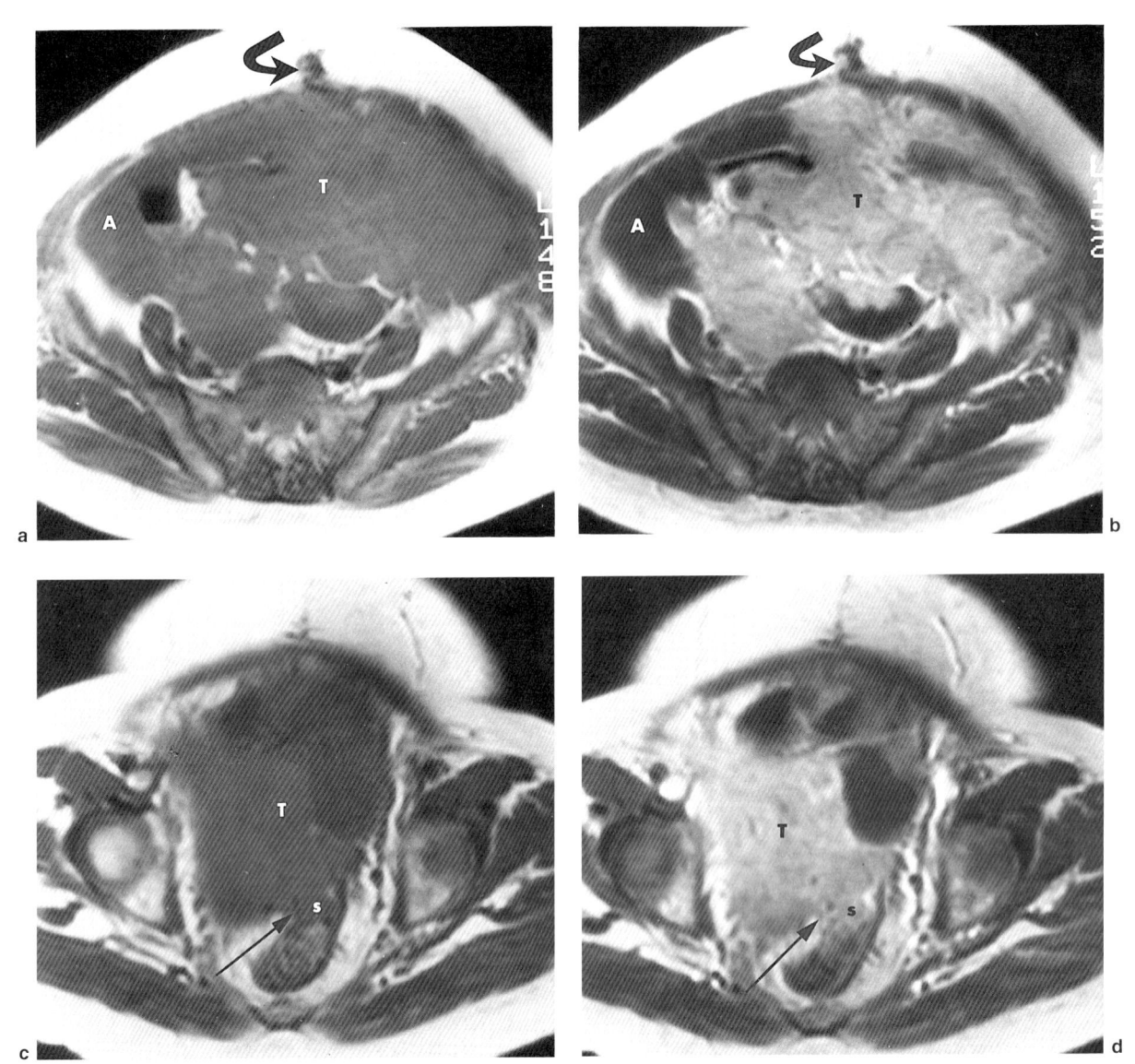

Fig. 10.22 Clear cell carcinoma with sigmoid invasion and metastasis to the umbilicus, transaxial plane. Unenhanced (**a**), (**c**), and gadolinium-DTPA-enhanced (**b**), (**d**), T1-weighted (600/20) images (1.5 T). The solid portion of the tumor (T) as well as its distinction from adjacent ascites (A) is best appreciated after gadolinium administration. The umbilical metastasis (curved arrow) is not well seen on the unenhanced T1-weighted image. Invasion of the sigmoid colon (s) is appreciated on both the unenhanced and enhanced sequences (straight arrow)

teratoma composed either entirely or predominantly of thyroid tissue and occurs in 2.7% of ovarian teratomas (58). The ovarian thyroid tissue may develop adenomas, chronic thryoiditis, and follicular or papillary carcinoma. Clinical hyperthyroidism or even thyrotoxicosis have been reported (58).

Primary carcinoid tumor of the ovary is rare (200 cases reported) (59). This tumor usually arises in gastrointestinal or respiratory epithelium within a mature cystic teratoma. Ovarian carcinoids are more frequently associated with the carcinoid syndrome (50%) than intestinal carcinoids because blood from the ovary flows directly into the systemic circulation and does not pass through the liver where serotonin is inactivated (58). Ovarian carcinoids grossly resemble mature cystic teratomas. The tumors grow slowly, and metastases are rare (59).

On MRI, teratomas usually demonstrate some component of signal intensity paralleling that of subcutaneous fat on T1- and T2-weighted images (2–4, 7–9, 60). Signal characteristics may vary however, depending on the amount of calcification, hair, and

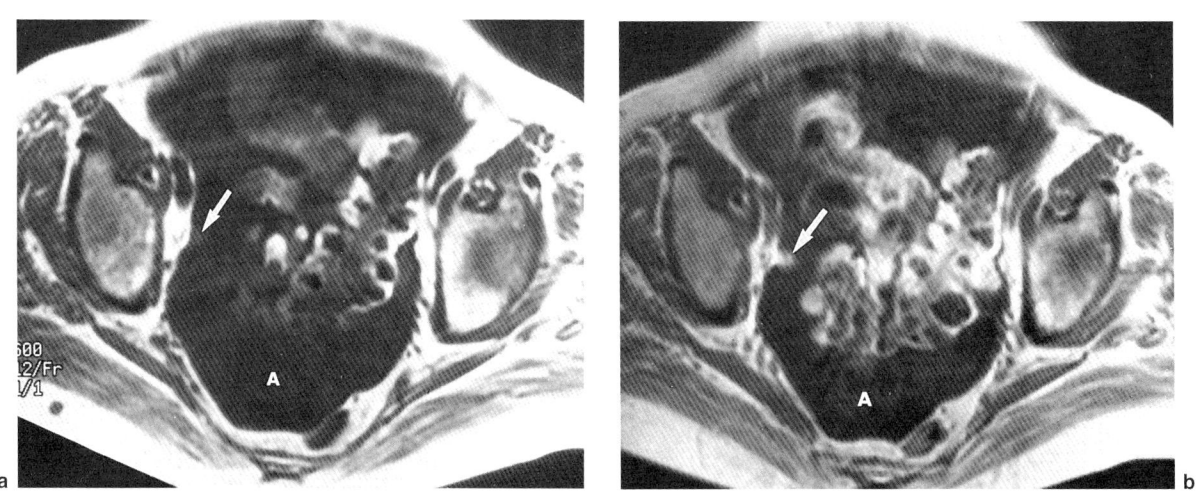

Fig. 10.23 Peritoneal implant and ascites in patient with ovarian carcinoma. Transaxial (**a**) unenhanced and (**b**) enhanced T1-weighted (600/12) images (1.5 T). The small 1-cm peritoneal implant (arrow) was only identified on the gadolinium-enhanced image. A = ascites

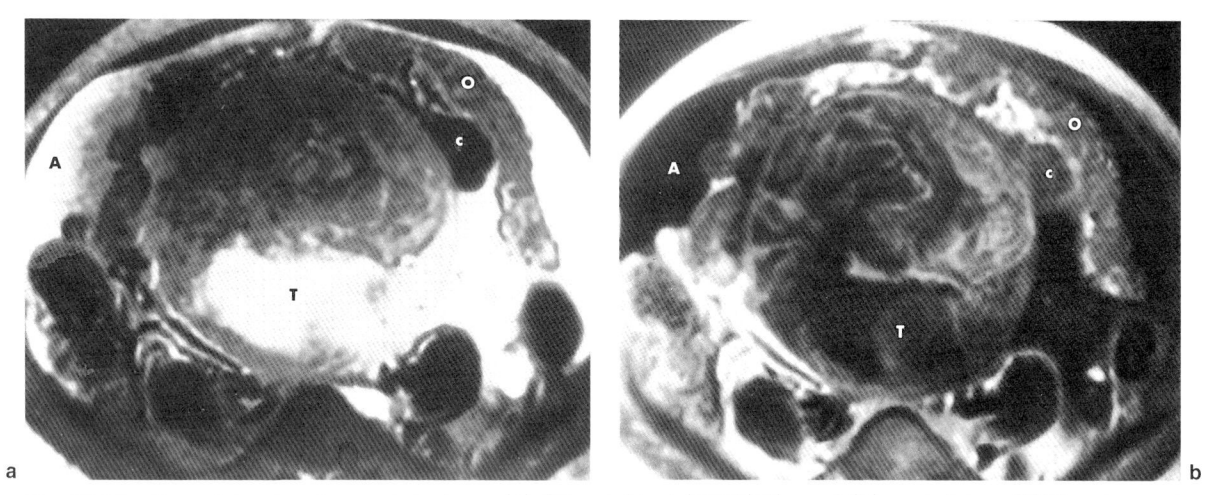

Fig. 10.24 Omental cake, transaxial plane. (**a**) T2-weighted (2000/70), and (**b**) gadolinium-DTPA-enhanced T1-weighted (700/20) images (1.5 T). The omental cake (O) lies anterior to the transverse colon (c) and is draped over the large cystic ovarian tumor (T). On the gadolinium-enhanced image, diffuse omental enhancement is seen. On pathologic examination, the omentum was completely involved by tumor. A = ascites

fibrous tissue present. Gravity-dependent layering or floating debris, Rokitansky nodules, fat–fluid levels, and globular calcification assist in the diagnosis of cystic teratoma (22). Hemorrhage has been reported within these lesions (3). On MRI the presence of a chemical shift artifact at fat–fluid interfaces within teratomas is characteristic, when seen (Fig. 10. **27**); however, as presence of chemical shift artifact depends on several factors, including the shape of the lipid–water interface, orientation along the section select gradient, and imaging parameters selected, it may not always be identified (Fig. 10.**28**) (23, 61). Fat-saturation imaging has been shown to be useful in characterizing teratomas when diagnosis is difficult using standard T1- and T2-weighted spin-echo images. Preliminary experience suggests that fat-saturation MRI is particularly efficacious in differentiating teratomas from cystic hemorrhagic adnexal lesions (Fig. 10.**29**) (23, 24). Gd-DTPA administration will enhance the wall and dermoid nodule in benign cystic teratomas. Solid components of immature teratomas may also demonstrate enhancement following in-

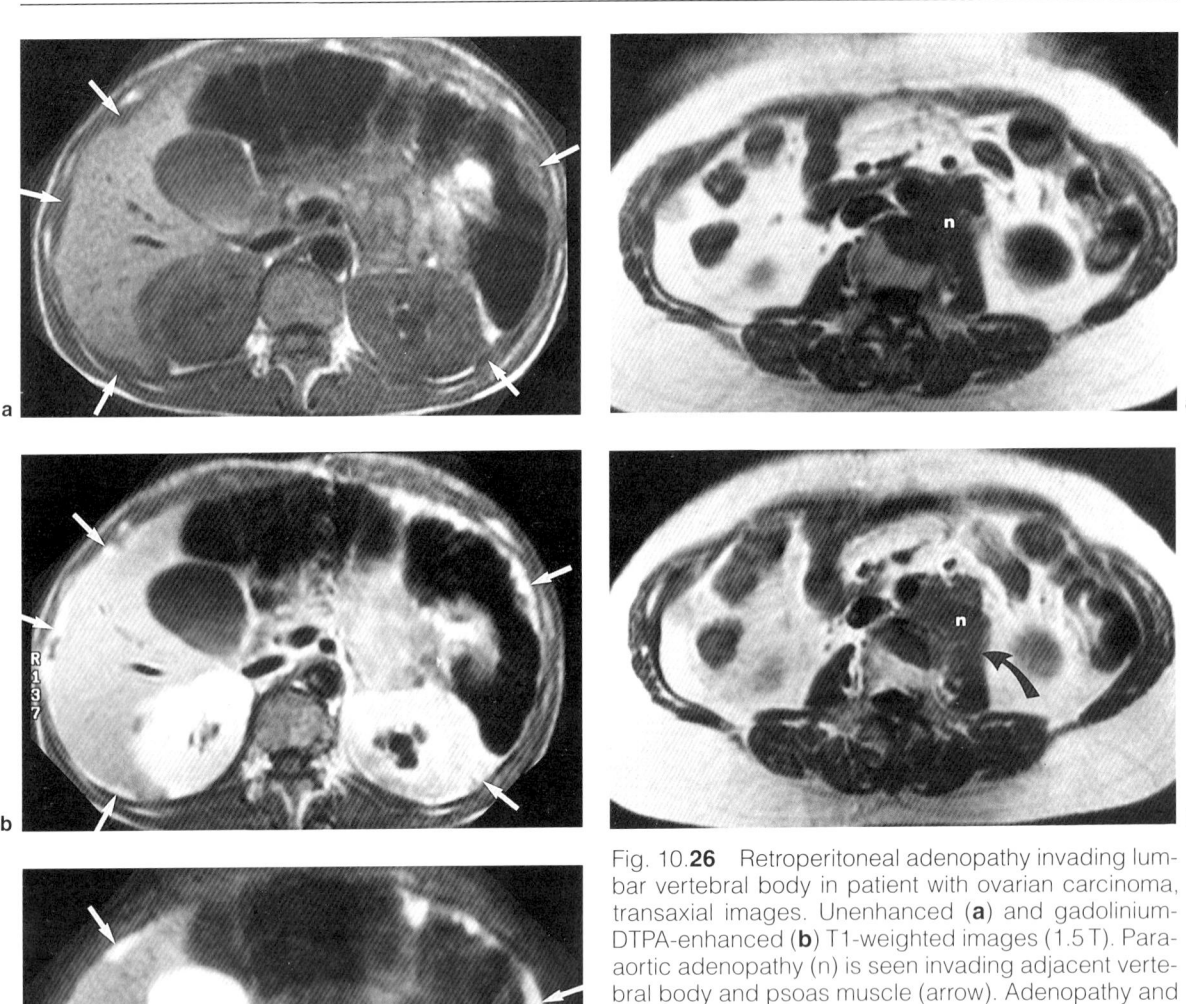

Fig. 10.25 Peritoneal and hepatic capsular metastases from mucinous ovarian adenocarcinoma, transaxial plane. (**a**) T1-weighted (300/12), (**b**) gadolinium-enhanced T1-weighted (600/12), and (**c**) fat-saturation T2-weighted (2400/70) images (1.5 T). Low-signal-intensity peritoneal and hepatic capsular metastases enhance with gadolinium (small arrows). They are most conspicuous on the T2-weighted fat-saturation image

Fig. 10.26 Retroperitoneal adenopathy invading lumbar vertebral body in patient with ovarian carcinoma, transaxial images. Unenhanced (**a**) and gadolinium-DTPA-enhanced (**b**) T1-weighted images (1.5 T). Para-aortic adenopathy (n) is seen invading adjacent vertebral body and psoas muscle (arrow). Adenopathy and invaded portions of psoas muscle enhance following gadolinium administration. (Reprinted with permission from reference 15)

travenous contrast medium administration (Fig. 10.30) (7, 8).

Dysgerminoma. Dysgerminoma is the most common malignant germ cell tumor, and 80% of patients are under 30 years of age at the time of diagnosis. There is an increased incidence of dysgerminomas in patients with pseudohermaphroditism, gonadal dysgenesis, and gonadoblastoma (53, 58, 59). These tumors are lobulated, solid, and are histologically identical to the classic seminoma of the testis. Fifteen percent are bilateral. In 6–8% of dysgerminomas there are collections of syncytiotrophoblastic giant cells that produce HCG (58). Dysgerminoma is extremely radiosensitive and curable with radiotherapy even in the presence of metastases (50).

MR Imaging 307

Fig. 10.**27** Cystic teratoma, transaxial plane. (**a**) proton density (2000/30), and (**b**) T2-weighted (2000/80) images (1.5 T). Dermoid nodule (n) within cystic teratoma (T) contained calcification. Atypical chemical shift artifact is noted along the periphery of the lesion (short arrows). b = bladder

Fig. 10.**28** Thirty-two-year-old woman with struma ovarii and polycystic ovarian disease. Sagittal (**a**) proton density (2000/30) and (**b**) T2-weighted (2000/80) images. Transaxial (**c**) T2-weighted (2500/80) image (1.5 T). The large cystic left ovarian mass with septations and focal area of nodularity was found to be a large ovarian teratoma containing thyroid elements, or struma ovarii (St). The central nodule (curved arrow) contained the greatest quantity of thyroid tissue. The right ovary (o) contained multiple small, high signal intensity, peripherally located cysts surrounding low-signal-intensity central stroma compatible with polycystic ovarian disease. (Reprinted with permission from reference 15)

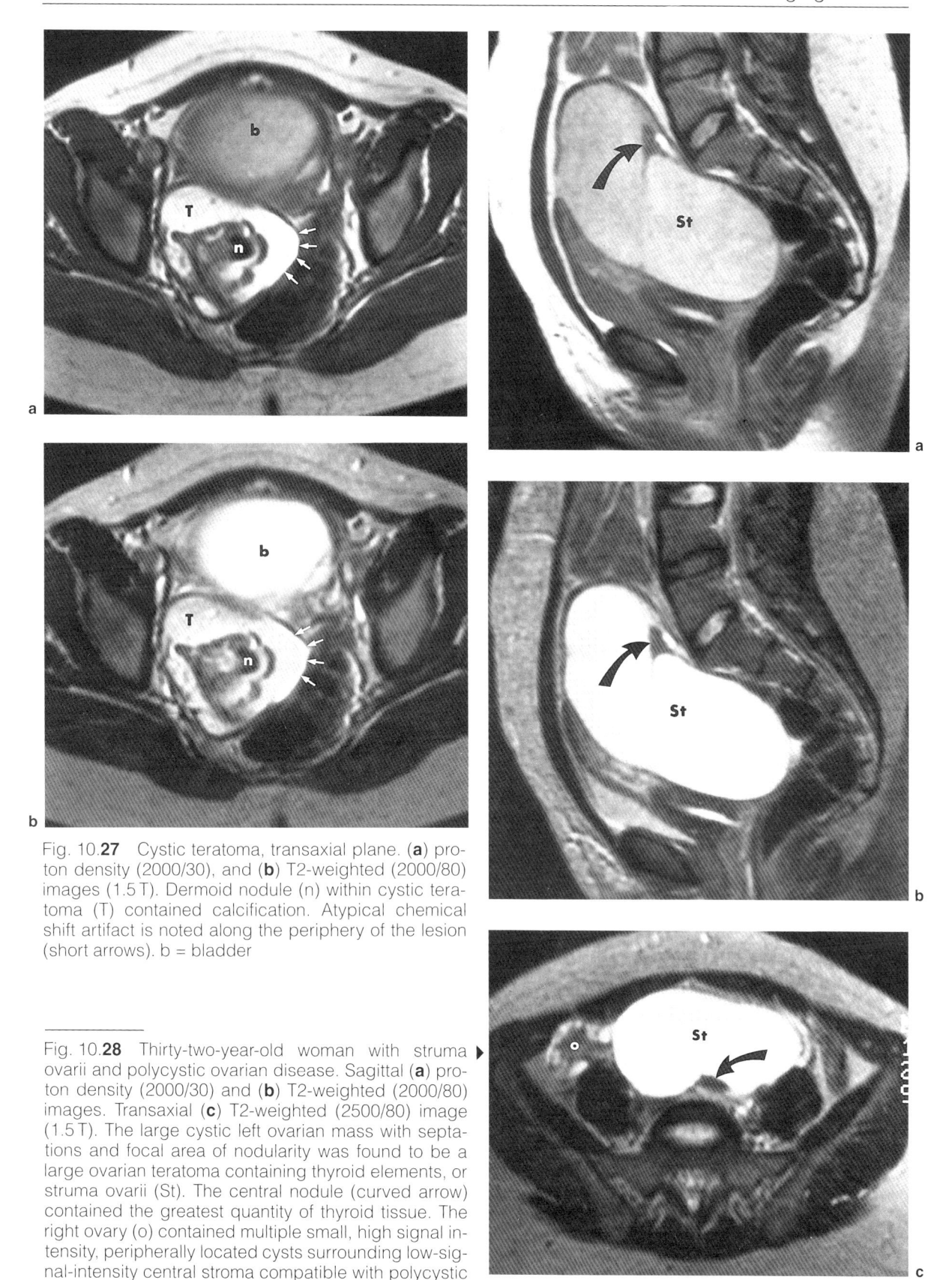

308 10 Ovary

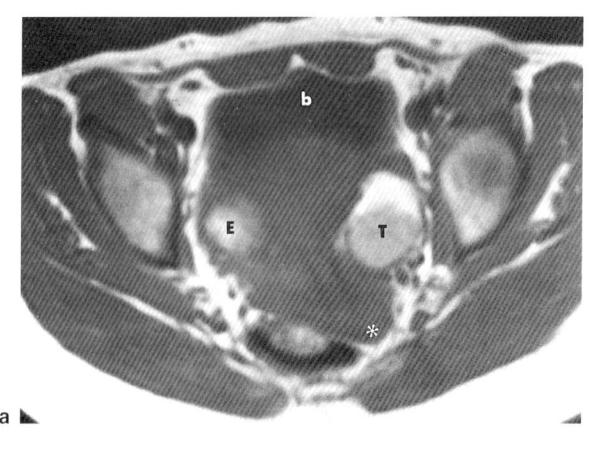

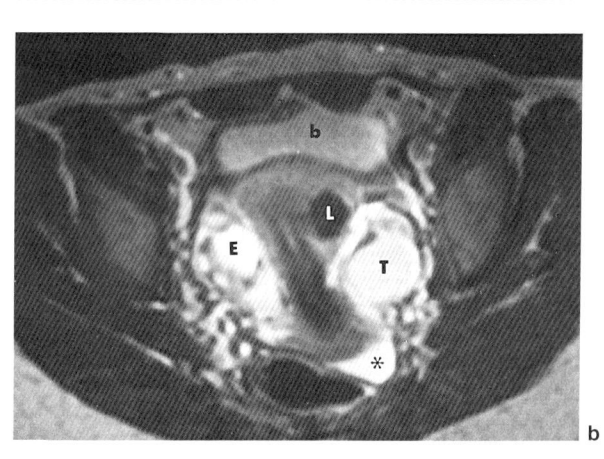

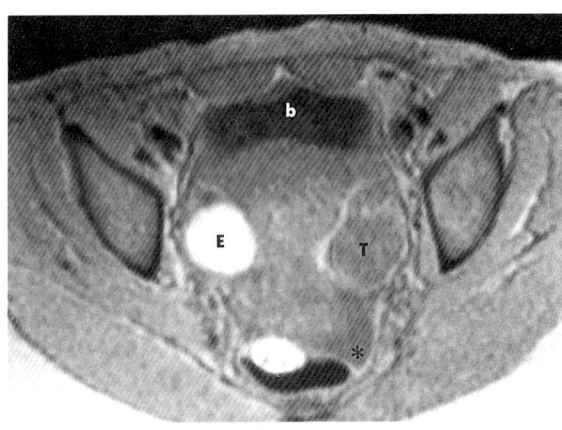

Fig. 10.**29** Thirty-year-old patient with right adnexal endometrioma and left adnexal cystic teratoma, transaxial plane. (**a**) T1-weighted (600/12), (**b**) T2-weighted (2000/80), and (**c**) T1-weighted fat saturation (700/10) images (1.5 T). The right adnexal endometrioma (E) has signal intensity equal to fat on the T1-weighted image and greater than fat on the T2-weighted and fat-saturation images. The left adnexal cystic teratoma (T), on the other hand, has some components isointense with fat on all pulse sequences including the fat-saturation sequence. (*) cul-de-sac fluid

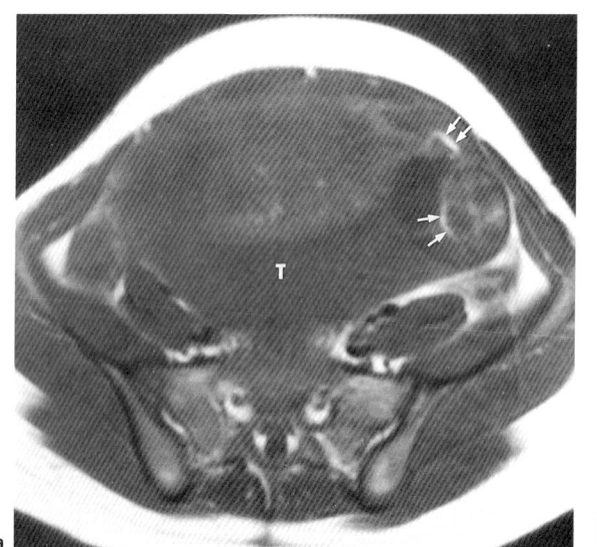

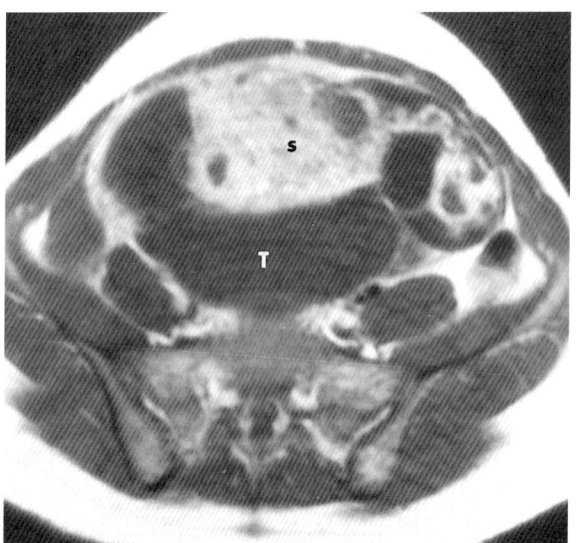

Fig. 10.**30** Immature teratoma containing glial elements, transaxial plane. (**a**) unenhanced, and (**b**) gadolinium-DTPA-enhanced T1-weighted (600/20) images (1.5 T). Tiny foci of high signal intensity similar to that of subcutaneous fat are seen on the unenhanced T1-weighted image (arrows). Following gadolinium-DTPA administration, the large solid portion (s) of the immature teratoma (T) enhances

Endodermal sinus tumor. Endodermal sinus tumor is one of the most malignant neoplasms arising in the ovary and occurs almost exclusively in children and young women with an average age of 20 years. Most tumors are large (3–30 cm in diameter), round or globular, firm, smooth, and lobulated. They contain areas of hemorrhage and cystic or gelatinous change. Endodermal sinus tumours are not usually associated with endocrine symptoms unless the tumor is combined with choriocaricnoma (mixed germ cell tumor). Endodermal sinus tumors are associated with elevated levels of serum AFP. AFP is synthesized in the yolk sac, liver, and upper gastrointestinal tract during fetal life and is elevated in patients with endodermal sinus tumors and mixed germ cell tumors containing endodermal sinus tumors (58). AFP is useful as a diagnostic test in patients with endodermal sinus tumor and is also of value in monitoring the results of therapy.

Embryonal carcinoma. Ovarian embryonal carcinoma is usually combined with other neoplastic germ cell elements to form part of a mixed germ cell tumor. Only 15 cases of embryonal carcinoma of the ovary have been reported (58, 59). The median age at diagnosis is 15 years. Tumors are usually solid with foci of necrosis and hemorrhage in the larger lesions. They may produce both AFP and HCG. Premenarchal girls may undergo precocious puberty, and adults may develop abnormal vaginal bleeding. Nearly all patients have a positive pregnancy test. Treatment is surgical resection and combined chemotherapy (54).

Choriocarcinoma. Nongestational ovarian choriocarcinoma is a very rare neoplasm and the majority of tumors are admixed with other neoplastic germ cell elements. They occur in children and young adults and secrete HCG. Children often show evidence of isosexual precocious puberty and uterine bleeding. These tumors are usually unilateral, solid, and hemorrhagic. Choriocarcinomas are highly malignant and unlike gestational choriocarcinoma, do not respond well to treatment with methotrexate. Surgery and combination chemotherapy are the treatments of choice (54, 58).

Gonadoblastoma. Gonadoblastoma occurs almost entirely in patients with pure gonadal dysgenesis, mixed gonadal dysgenesis, or male pseudohermaphroditism. Eighty percent of patients are phenotypic females, and the remainder are phenotypic males with cryptorchidism, hypospadias, and female internal secondary sex organs. Sixty percent of females show some evidence of masculinization.

Gonadoblastomas consist of germ cells intimately mixed with sex cord elements. Tumors are usually small, and are bilateral in one-third of cases. The gonad from which the tumor arises is usually a streak or a testis. Gonadoblastomas are solid and usually smooth or slightly lobulated. They may contain calcific granules or be almost completely calcified. Although gonadoblastomas themselves are benign, in 50% of cases gonadoblastoma is overgrown by a dysgerminoma. Treatment of choice is bilateral excision of the gonads except in the rare patient who has a normal ovary on the contralateral side (59).

MRI of germ cell tumors. The majority of germ cell tumors are benign cystic teratomas and have the MRI findings described above. The remaining germ cell tumors have a varied appearance, but are often solid lesions containing cystic areas or hemorrhage (Fig. 10.31). The clinical history, physical findings, age, and hormonal status including the presence or ab-

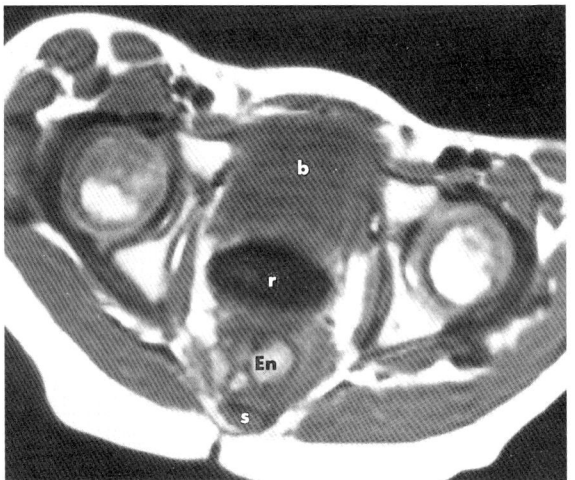

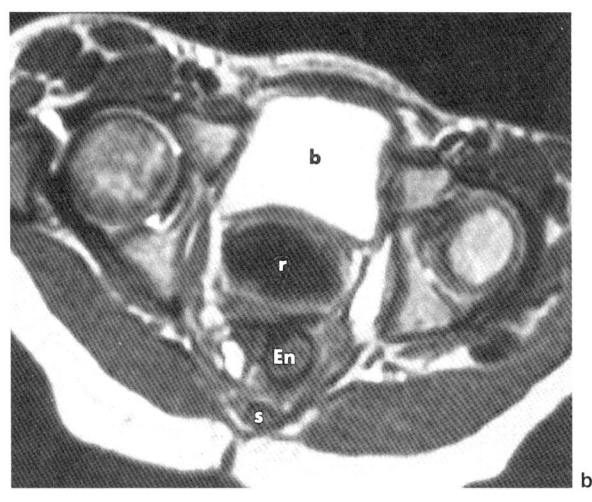

Fig. 10.**31** Three-year-old girl with endodermal sinus tumor, transaxial plane. (**a**) T1-weighted (800/20), and (**b**) T2-weighted (2000/70) images (1.5 T). The presacral tumor (En) contains areas of high signal intensity on the T1-weighted image corresponding to regions of low signal intensity on the T2-weighted image. These were found to be areas of hemorrhagic necrosis. b = bladder, r = rectum, s = sacrum

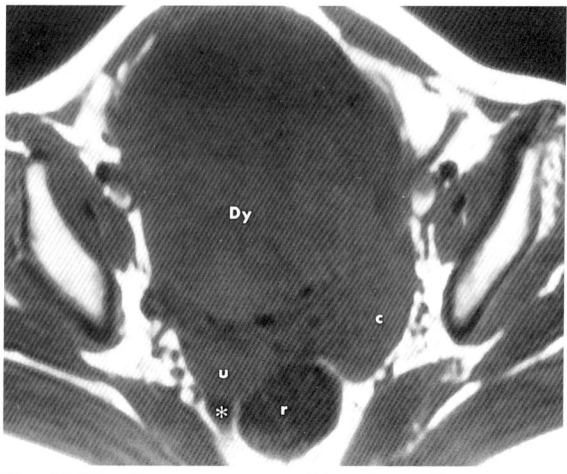

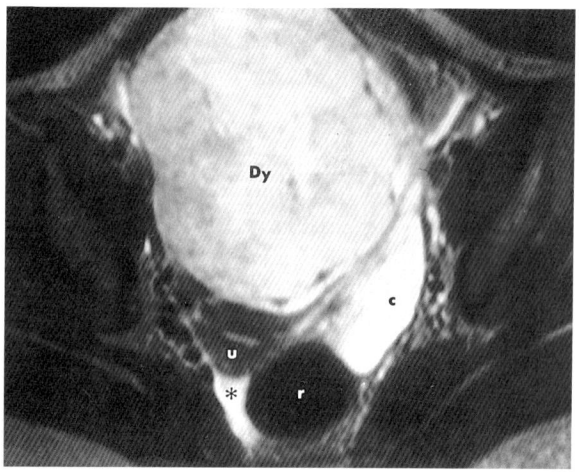

Fig. 10.**32** Seventeen-year old patient with positive pregnancy test and large pelvic mass, transaxial plane. (**a**) T1-weighted (400/15), and (**b**) T2-weighted (2500/70) images (1.5 T). The large, well-encapsulated, predominantly solid mass with extensive necrosis was found to be a dysgerminoma (Dy) at the time of surgery. No trophoblastic giant cells were identified. The other ovary contained a hemorrhagic corpus luteum cyst (c). u = uterus, r = rectum, * = cul-de-sac fluid

sence of tumor markers such as Ca-125, AFP, and HCG are crucial in making the correct diagnosis. MRI provides information regarding the intratumoral architecture and extent of disease, which are of paramount importance to the surgeon. Identification of a predominantly solid component within a suspected teratoma, for example, alerts the surgeon to the possibility that the lesion may represent an immature of malignant lesion rather than a benign cystic teratoma. Similarly, invasion of or adhesions to surrounding organs may suggest a teratoma's malignant nature. Because a number of the germ cell neoplasms are bilateral, evaluation of both ovaries is important. MRI allows improved evaluation of the contralateral ovary, which might be distorted or compressed by a large unilateral tumor (Fig. 10. **32**).

Sex cord–stromal tumors. Sex cord-stromal tumors comprise approximately 8% of all ovarian tumors. These tumors arise from either the sex cords of the embryonic gonad or from the ovarian stroma (53). Fibromas, which are almost never associated with endocrine manifestations, account for half of the sex cord-stromal tumors, and the remainder are composed of granulosa-theca cell tumors, Sertoli-Leydig cell tumors, and gynandroblastomas.

Granulosa-theca cell tumors. Approximately half of granulosa-theca cell tumors are thecomas, one-fourth consist of granulosa cells alone, and the remaining fourth are a mixture of both types of cells. Two-thirds of granulosa cell tumors occur in postmenopausal women and their importance lies in the ability of these tumors to elaborate large amounts of estrogen. They are the most common clinically estrogenic ovarian tumor. Whereas in prepubertal girls granulosa cell tumors may produce precocious sexual development, in adult women they may be associated with endometrial hyperplasia, cystic disease of the breast, and endometrial carcinoma (5–25%). Rarely, androgenic changes such as hirsutism or frank virilization may be seen (62). Ninety-five percent of granulosa cell tumors are unilateral with an average size of 12 cm. They may either be predominantly solid or predominantly cystic. After removal of a granulosa cell tumor, manifestations of hyperestrinism typically regress.

Five percent of granulosa cell tumors are diagnosed before puberty and differ histologically from their adult counterparts. These are termed juvenile granulosa cell tumors. Ninety-seven percent appear in the first three decades and 80% of these result in isosexual precocity. The gross appearance of the juvenile granulosa cell tumor is similar to that of the adult form (59).

Thecomas occur most commonly in postmenopausal women. They are usually unilateral and are almost never malignant. Most are 5 cm to 10 cm in diameter, solid and firm. Mixed granulosa-theca tumors are firm and solid due to the fibrotic thecal component. These tumors closely resemble fibromas (53).

Fibromas. Fibromas are usually seen in perimenopausal and postmenopausal women. Ninety percent are unilateral and 10% are multiple. Ascites is noted in approximately 50% of patients with fibromas greater than 5 cm in diameter. The constellation of findings seen in Meigs syndrome (ovarian tumor, hydrothorax, and ascites) occurs in 1–3% of patients with ovarian fibromas (62). Ascites and hydrothorax resolve following excision of the tumor. Fibromas are almost always benign. In patients with basal cell nevus syndrome, fibromas are typically bilateral, multinodular, and calcified (59).

Sertoli-Leydig cell tumors (arrhenoblastoma, androblastoma). Sertoli-Leydig cell tumors contain Sertoli cells, Leydig's cells, fibroblasts, or all of these in varying proportions and varying degrees of differentiation (62). These neoplasms constitute less than 1% of all ovarian tumors. The most common type contains mixtures of Sertoli and Leydig's cells as well as tissues similar to those of the fetal testis. Although Sertoli-Leydig cell tumors are usually virilizing ovarian neoplasms, they are occasionally associated with estrogenic or progestational manifestations. 15% demonstrate no hormonal activity (59). Average age at diagnosis is 25 years. Patients typically present with oligomenorrhea followed by amenorrhea, loss of female secondary sex characteristics, and progressive masculinization. Sertoli-Leydig cell tumors average 10 cm in size, and 3% are bilateral. They roughly resemble granulosa cell tumors in appearance. After removal of the tumor, normal menses characteristically resume, although clitoromegaly and deepening of the voice are less apt to regress.

Pure Sertoli cell tumors are rare. Average age at diagnosis is 27 years, and 65% of patients have signs of estrogen production. Tumors are usually unilateral, solid, and often lobulated. Malignant behavior is unusual.

Leydig's cell tumors, in contrast to Sertoli cell tumors, occur predominantly after the age of 50. These tumors produce testosterone, are unilateral, and almost invariably benign. Leydig's cell tumors must be distinguished from adrenal causes of androgen excess. High testosterone levels generally indicate an ovarian tumor whereas high dihydroepiandrostenedione levels suggest an adrenal origin (59).

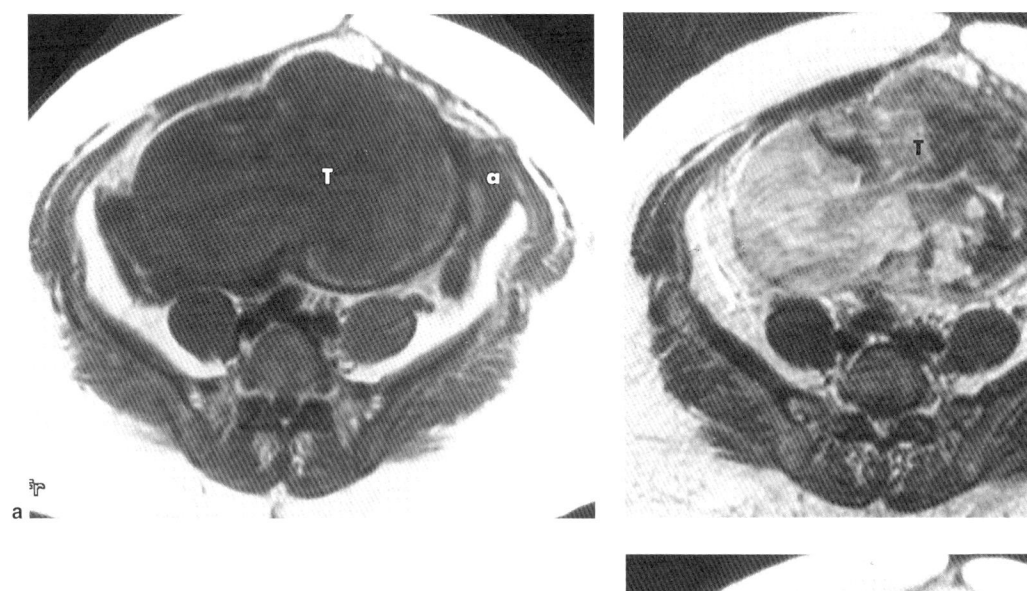

Fig. 10.**33** Forty-six-year old woman with ovarian granulosa cell tumor, transaxial plane. (**a**) T1-weighted (600/12), (**b**) fast spin-echo T2-weighted (3000/85 effective TE, 8 echo train length), and (**c**) gadolinium-DTPA-enhanced T1-weighted (600/20) images (1.5 T). On the T1- and T2-weighted images alone, regions of necrosis within solid portions of the tumor (T) cannot be appreciated. The intratumoral architecture is best appreciated on the gadolinium-enhanced image. At the time of surgery, focal rupture of the ovarian capsule was noted. a = ascites

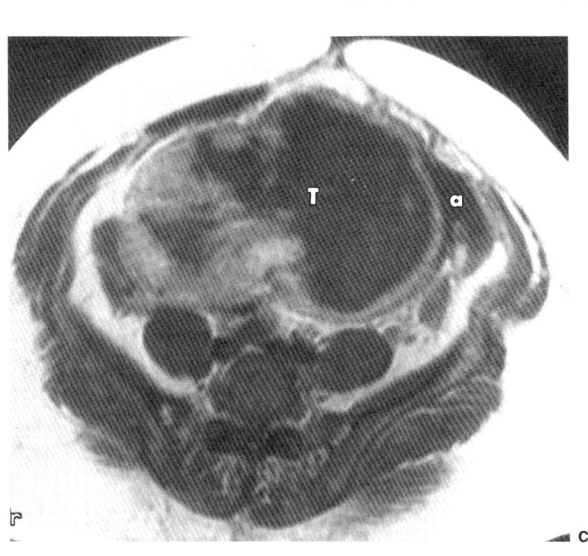

312   10 Ovary

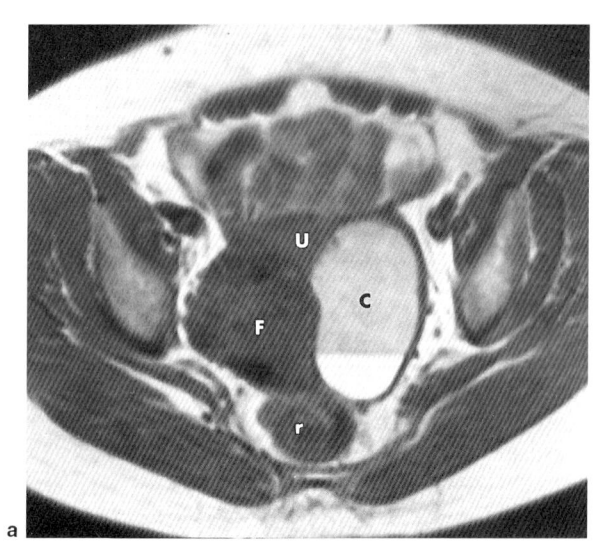

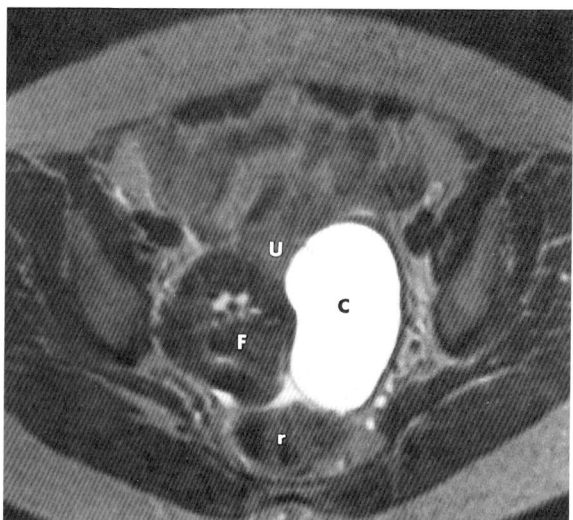

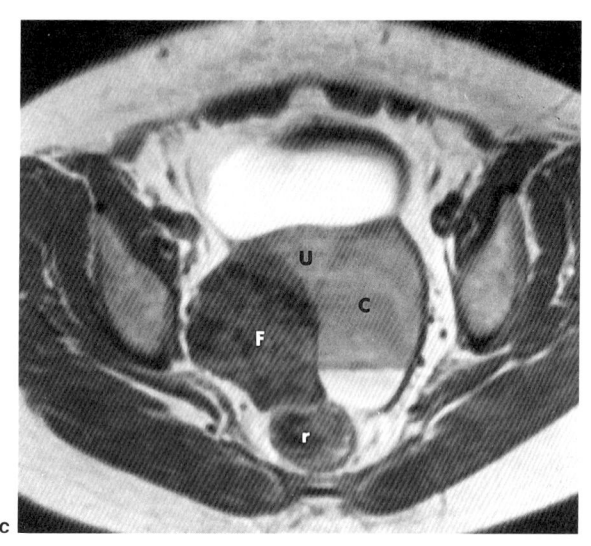

Fig. 10.**34** Right ovarian fibroma and left adnexal mucinous cystadenoma, transaxial plane. (**a**) T1-weighted (700/20), (**b**) T2-weighted (2500/70), and (**c**) gadolinium-DTPA-enhanced T1-weighted (700/20) images (1.5 T). The right ovarian fibroma (F) has intermediate to low signal intensity on both T1- and T2-weighted images. Irregular foci of bright signal intensity within the lesion noted on the T2-weighted image corresponded to regions of hyalinization and myxomatous change. There is little enhancement after gadolinium administration. The left ovarian mucinous cystadenoma (C) has a fluid-fluid level. U = uterus, r = rectum

Gynandroblastoma. Gynandroblastomas are extremely rare tumors that contain both granulosa-theca cell and Sertoli-Leydig cell patterns (50). They may be associated with either androgen or estrogen production.

MRI of sex cord–stromal tumors. The MRI appearance of sex cord stromal tumors may resemble that of either germ cell or epithelial tumors (Fig. 10.33). Notable exceptions include fibromas and thecomas, both of which are usually well-defined solid tumors that demonstrate low signal intensity on both T1- and T2-weighted images. They both may have irregular foci of bright signal on T2-weighted images, which correspond to regions of hyalinization and myxomatous change similar to that seen in degenerating leiomyomas (Fig. 10.**34**) 67, 63). Occasionally, differentiation of an ovarian fibroma from an exophytic subserosal leiomyoma may prove difficult (25).

For the remainder of the sex cord-stromal tumors, the role of MRI lies in detecting adnexal lesions in patients with endocrine abnormalities in whom non-tumor-related etiologies have been excluded, and in whom sonography or CT remain nondiagnostic (6). In patients with known tumors, the role of MRI lies in lesion characterization and staging.

References

1 Hamlin DJ, Fitzsimmons JR, Pettersson H, Riggall FC, Morgan L, Wilkinson EJ. Magnetic resonance imaging of the pelvis: Evaluation of ovarian masses et 0.15 T. AJR. 1985;145:585–590.
2 Dooms GC, Hricak H, Tscholakoff D. Adnexal structures: MR imaging. Radiology. 1986;158:639–646.
3 Mitchell DG, Mintz MC, Spritzer CE, et al. Adnexal masses: MR imaging observations at 1.5 T, with US and CT correlation. Radiology. 1987;162:319–324.
4 Mawhinney RR, Rowell MC, Worthington BS, Symonds EM. Magnetic resonance imaging of benign ovarian masses. Brit J Radiol. 1988;61:179–186.

5. Smith FW, Cherryman GR, Bayliss AP, et al. Comparative study of the accuracy of ultrasound imaging, x-ray computerized tomography and low field MRI diagnosis of ovarian malignancy. Magn. Reson Imaging. 1988;6:225–227.
6. Ayalon D, Graif M, Hetman-Peri M, et al. Diagnosis of a small ovarian tumor (androgen secreting) by magnetic resonance: A new noninvasive procedure. Am J Obstet Gynecol. 1988;159:903–905.
7. Stevens SK, Hricak H, Stern JL. Ovarian lesions: Detection and characterization with gadolinium-enhanced MR imaging at 1.5 T. Radiology. 1991;181:481–488.
8. Thurnher S, Hodler J, Baer S, Marincek B, von Schulthess GK. Gadolinium-DOTA enhanced MR imaging of adnexal tumors. JCAT. 1990;14(6):939–949.
9. Riccio TJ, Adams HG, Munzing DE, Mattrey RF. Magnetic resonance imaging as an adjunct to sonography in the evaluation of the female pelvis. Mag Reson Imaging. 1990;8:699–704.
10. Ghossain MA, Buy J-N, Lignères C, et al. Epithelial tumors of the ovary: Comparison of MR and CT findings. Radiology. 1991;181:863–870.
11. Andreotti RF, Zusmer NR, Sheldon JJ, Ames M. Ultrasound and magnetic resonance imaging of pelvic masses. Surg Gynecol Obstet. 1988;166:327–332.
12. Lewis E. Imaging techniques in gynecologic cancer. In: Rutledge FN, Freedman RS, Gershenson DM, eds. Volume 29: Gynecologic Cancer: Diagnosis and Treatment Strategies. Vol. 29. Austin: University of Texas Press; 1987:397–427.
13. Fukuda T, Ikeuchi M, Hashimoto H, et al. Computed tomography of ovarian masses. JCAT. 1986;10(6):990–996.
14. Amendola MA. The role of CT in the evaluation of ovarian malignancy. CRC Crit Rev Diagn Imaging. 1985;24(4):329–368.
15. Stevens SK. The adnexa. In: Higgins CB, Hricak H, Helms CA, eds. Magnetic Resonance Imaging of the Body. 2nd ed. New York: Raven Press; 1992:865–890.
16. Kier R, McCarthy SM, Scoutt LM, Viscarello RR, Schwartz PE. Pelvic masses in pregnancy: MR imaging. Radiology. 1990;176:709–713.
17. Weinreb JC, Brown CE, Lowe TW, Cohen JM, Erdman WA. Pelvic masses in pregnant patients: MR and US imaging. Radiology. 1986;159:717–724.
18. Nishimura K, Togashi K, Itoh K, et al. Endometrial cysts of the ovary: MR imaging. Radiology. 1987;162:315–318.
19. Arrivé L, Hricak H, Martin MC. Pelvic endometriosis: MR imaging. Radiology. 1989;171:687–692.
20. Zawin M, McCarthy S, Scoutt L, Comite F. Endometriosis: Appearance and detection at MR imaging. Radiology. 1989;171:693–696.
21. Togashi K, Nishimura K, Kimura I, et al. Endometrial cysts: Diagnosis with MR imaging. Radiology. 1991;180:73–78.
22. Togashi K, Nishimura K, Itoh K, et al. Ovarian cystic teratomas: MR imaging. Radiology. 1987;162:669–673.
23. Stevens SK, Hricak H, Campos Z. Differentiation of teratomas from cystic hemorrhagic adnexal lesions: Utility of proton selective fat saturation magnetic resonance imaging. Radiology. [In press].
24. Kier R, Smith RC, McCarthy SM. Value of lipid- and water-suppression MR images in distinguishing between blood and lipid within ovarian masses. AJR. 1992;158:321–325.
25. Weinreb JC, Barkoff ND, Megibow A, Demopoulos R. The value of MR imaging in distinguishing leiomyomas from other solid pelvic masses when sonography is indeterminate. AJR. 1990;154:295–299.
26. Carr BR. Disorders of the ovary and female reproductive tract. In: Wilson JD, Foster DW, eds. Williams Textbook of Endocrinology. 8th ed. New York: Saunders; 1992:733–798.
27. Peters H, Himelstein-Braw R, Faber M. The normal development of the ovary in childhood. Acta Endocrinol. 1976;82:617–630.
28. Nicosia SV. Morphologic changes of the human ovary throughout life. In: Serra GB, ed. The Ovary. New York: Raven Press; 1983:57–81.
29. Francis CC. Female genitalia. In: Francis CC. The Human Pelvis. St. Louis: CV Mosby; 1952:156–170.
30. Clement PB. Anatomy and histology of the ovary. In: Kurman RJ, ed. Blaustein's Pathology of the Female Genital Tract. 3rd ed. New York: Springer; 1987:438–470.
31. Zawin M, McCarthy S, Scoutt LM, Comite F. High-field MRI and US evaluation of the pelvis in women with leiomyomas. Mag Reson Imaging. 1990;8:371–376.
32. Robboy SJ, Lombardo JM, Welch WR. Disorders of abnormal sexual development. In: Kurman RJ, ed. Blaustein's Pathology of the Female Genital Tract. 3rd ed. New York: Springer; 1987:15–35.
33. Carrington BM, Hricak H. The uterus and vagina. In: Hricak H, Carrington BM, eds. MRI of the Pelvis: A Text Atlas. London: Martin Dunitz; 1991:93–184.
34. Hricak H, Chang YCF, Thurnher S. Vagina: Evaluation with MR imaging. Part I. Normal anatomy and congenital anomalies. Radiology. 1988;169:169–174.
35. Jaffe RB. Disorders of sexual development. In: Yen SSC, Jaffe RB, eds. Reproductive Endocrinology. 2nd ed. New York: WB Saunders; 1986:283–312.
36. Secaf E, Nuruddin R, Hricak H, et al. Evaluation of ambiguous genitalia with MR imaging. Radiology. 1989;173(P):371.
37. Gambino J, Caldwell B, Dietrich R, Walot I, Kangarloo H. Congenital disorders of sexual differentiation: MR findings. AJR. 1992;158:363–367.
38. Lierse W. Applied Anatomy of the Pelvis. Chapter XVII. Ovary. Berlin: Springer; 1987:272–276.
39. Murphy GF, Welch WR, Urcuyo R. Brenner tumor and mucinous cystadenoma of borderline malignancy in a patient with Turner's syndrome. Obstet Gynecol. 1979;54:660.
40. Rosenwaks Z, Wentz AC, Jones GS, et al. Endometrial pathology and estrogens. Obstet Gynecol. 1979;53:403.
41. Merrill JA. Endometriosis. In: Danforth DN, Scott JR, eds. Obstet Gynecol. 5th ed. Philadelphia: JB Lippincott; 1986;995–1007.
42. Friedman H, Vogelzang RL, Mendelson EB, Neiman HL, Cohen M. Endometriosis detection by US with laparoscopic correlation. Radiology 1985;157:217–220.
43. Binkovitz LA, King BF, Ehman RL. Sciatic endometrioisis: MR appearance. JACT. 1991;15(3):508–510.
44. Wolf GC, Kopecky KK. MR imaging of endometriosis arising in cesarean section scar. JCAT. 1989;13(1):150–152.
45. Clement PB. Endometriosis, lesions of the secondary müllerian system, and pelvic mesothelial proliferations. In: Kurman RJ, ed. Blaustein's Pathology of the Female Genital Tract. 3rd ed. New York: Springer; 1987:516–559.
46. Morrow CP, Townsend DE. Tumors of the ovary: Soft tissue and secondary (metastatic) tumors; tumor-like conditions. In: Morrow CP, Townsend DE, eds. Synopsis of Gynecologic Oncology. 3rd ed. New York: Churchill Livingston; 1987:335–343.
47. van Look PFA. Hypothalamic-pituitary-ovarian relationships in the polycystic ovary syndrome. In: Coutts JRT, ed. Functional Morphology of the Ovary. Baltimore: University Park Press; 1981:167–177.
48. Clement PB. Nonneoplastic lesions of the ovary. In: Kurman RJ, ed. Blaustein's Pathology of the Female Genital Tract. 3rd ed. New York: Springer; 1987:471–515.
49. Francis GL, Getts A, McPherson JC III. Preliminary results suggesting exaggerated ovarian androgen production early in the course of polycystic ovary syndrome. Adolesc Health Care. 1990;11:480–484.
50. Kraus FT. Female genitalia. In: Kissane JM, ed. Volume 2: Anderson's Pathology. 9th ed. St. Louis: CV Mosby; 1990:1620–1725.
51. Mitchell DG, Gefter WB, Spritzer CE, et al. Polycystic ovaries: MR imaging. Radiology. 1986;160:425–429.
52. Faure N, Prat X, Bastide A, Lemay A. Assessment of ovaries by magnetic resonance imaging in patients presenting with polycystic ovarian syndrome. Human Reprod. 1989;4(4):468–472.
53. Cotran RS, Kumar V, Robbins SL. Female genital tract. In: Cotran RS, Kumar V, Robbins SL, eds. Robbins Pathologic Basis of Disease. 4th ed. Philadelphia: WB Saunders; 1989;1127–1180.
54. Young RC, Fuks Z, Hoskins WJ. Cancer of the ovary. In: DeVita VT, Hellman S, Rosenberg SA, eds. Cancer Principles & Practice of Oncology. 3rd ed. Philadelphia: JB Lippincott; 1989:1162–1196.
55. Morrow CP, Townsend DE. Tumors of the ovary: General considerations; classification; the adnexal mass. In: Morrow PC, Townsend DE, eds. Synopsis of Gynecologic Oncology. 3rd ed. New York: Churchill Livingston; 1987:231–255.

56. Czernobilsky B. Common epithelial tumors of the ovary. In: Kurman RJ, ed. Blaustein's Pathology of the Female Genital Tract. 3rd ed. New York: Springer; 1987:560–606.
57. Dooms GC, Hricak H, Crooks LE, Higgins CB. Magnetic resonance imaging of the lymph nodes: Comparison with CT. Radiology. 1984;153:719–728.
58. Talerman A. Germ cell tumors of the ovary. In: Kurman RJ, ed. Blaustein's Pathology of the Female Genital Tract. 3rd ed. New York: Springer; 1987:660–721.
59. Morrow CP, Townsend DE. Tumors of the ovary: Sex cord stromal tumors and germ cell tumors. In: Morrow CP, Townsend DE, eds. Synopsis of Gynecologic Oncology. 3rd ed. New York: Churchill Livingston; 1987:305–333.
60. Dooms GC, Hricak H, Sollitto RA, Higgins CB. Lipomatous tumors and tumors with fatty component: MR imaging potential and comparison of MR and CT results. Radiology. 1985; 157:479–483.
61. Smith RC, Lange RC, McCarthy SM. Chemical shift artifact: Dependence on shape and orientation of the lipid-water interface. Radiology. 1991;181:225–229.
62. Young RH, Scully RE. Sex cord-stromal, steroid cell, and other ovarian tumors with endocrine, paraendocrine, and paraneoplastic manifestations. In: Kurman RJ, ed. Blaustein's Pathology of the Female Genital Tract. 3rd ed. New York: Springer; 1987:607–658.
63. Talerman A. Nonspecific tumors of the ovary, including mesenchymal tumors and malignant lymphoma. In: Kurman RJ, ed. Blaustein's Pathology of the Female Genital Tract. 3rd ed. New York: Springer; 1987:722–741.

Hyperandrogenism

R. Sörensen and L. Moltz

Anatomy

Among endocrinopathies in woman, hyperandrogenism is one of the most common. Its cause may be glandular or extraglandular. Extremely high peripheral plasma androgen can be a sign of an androgen-producing ovarian or adrenal tumor. The source of androgen excess is determined using selective catheterization and blood sampling from the veins of the ovaries and adrenal glands.

Knowledge of the anatomy of these veins and their variations is essential for correct placement of the catheter (Fig. 10.35). Anatomical studies of complete venographic examinations demonstrate the vascular collaterals and anastomoses (1, 2, 3).

The **left ovarian vein** empties into the left renal vein opposite the adrenal vein (Fig. 10.36). Catheterization of this vein may be difficult because venous valves sometimes present in its proximal portion. With the new guidewire (Terumo) and catheter systems (tracker), valves can be surpassed to collect samples. Multiple veins contribute blood to the ovarian venous effluent creating an admixture of blood in the ovarian sample. They are shown in Fig. 10.37 (1, 3). Ascending lumbar veins can have connections to renal veins in 9% of patients and may give incorrect samplings if catheterized by mistake (Fig. 10.38). Retroaortic venous rings have to be identified before sampling (Fig. 10.39). In these cases, the adrenal vein

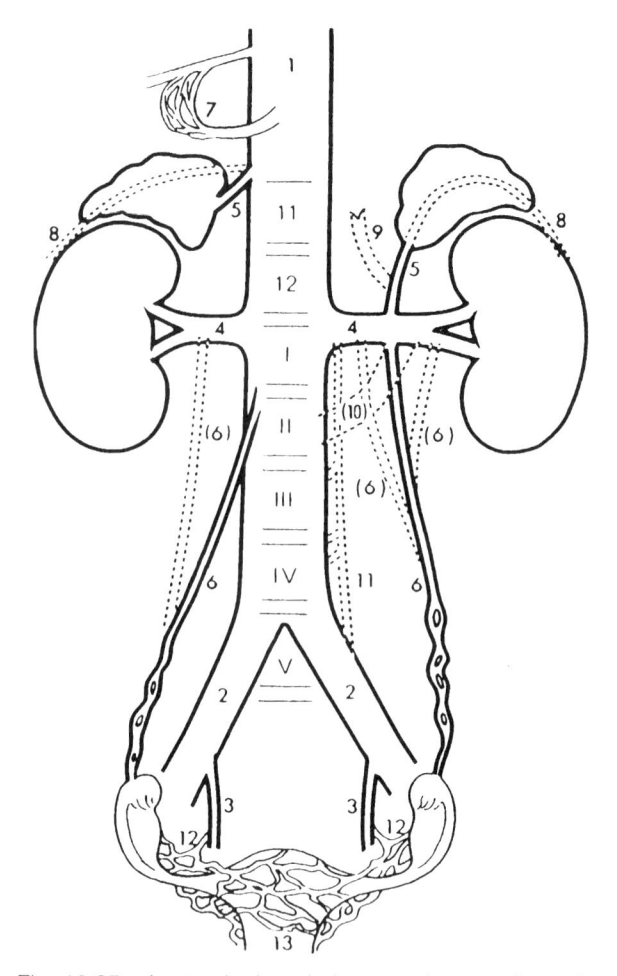

Fig. 10.**35** Anatomical variations and anomalies of adrenal and ovarian veins in women. 1. Inferior Vena caca, 2. Common iliac vein, 3. Internal iliac vein, 4. Renal vein, 5. Adrenal vein, 6. Ovarian vein, 8. Capsular vein, 9. Inferior phrenic vein, 10. Retroaortic renal vein, 11. Ascending lumbar vein, 12. Ovarian plexus, 13. Uterine plexus

drains into the upper portion and the ovarian vein drains into the preaortic or into the undivided renal vein. The renal vein can have a retroaortic portion only. The adrenal vein then drains either prehilar or directly into the inferior vena cava.

The inferior vena cava gets blood directly from the **right ovarian vein,** either at the mouth of the right renal vein or up to 5 cm below. The contributing veins are demonstrated in Fig. 10.40. The ovarian vein drains into the renal vein in about 3% to 11% (Fig. 10.**41**).

The **left adrenal vein** drains into the left renal vein (Fig. 10.42). The purity of the effluent hormone is influenced by multiple contributing veins indicated in Fig. 10.43. The adrenal vein may be duplicated. The inferior phrenic vein regularly joins the left adrenal vein and should not be selectively catheterized because hormone levels will be faulty (Fig. 10.44).

Hyperandrogenism

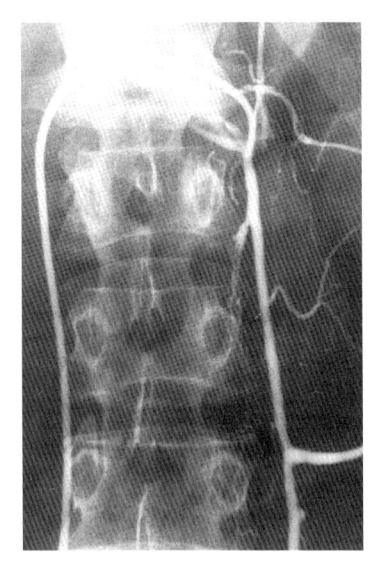

Fig. 10.36 Left ovarian vein. Single left ovarian vein emptying into the left renal vein

The **right adrenal vein** is smaller and thinner than the left adrenal vein. This vein drains into the inferior vena cava approximately 2 to 3 cm above and posterolateral to the right renal vein (Fig. 10.45). It is usually more difficult to be catheterized due to its proximity to the right hepatic vein. Small hepatic veins are very difficult to differentiate from right adrenal veins. Lecky (4) published a table that characterizes signs for differentiation (1, 2, 3; Fig. 10.46). Anastomoses are shown in Fig. 10.47 (1, 2, 3).

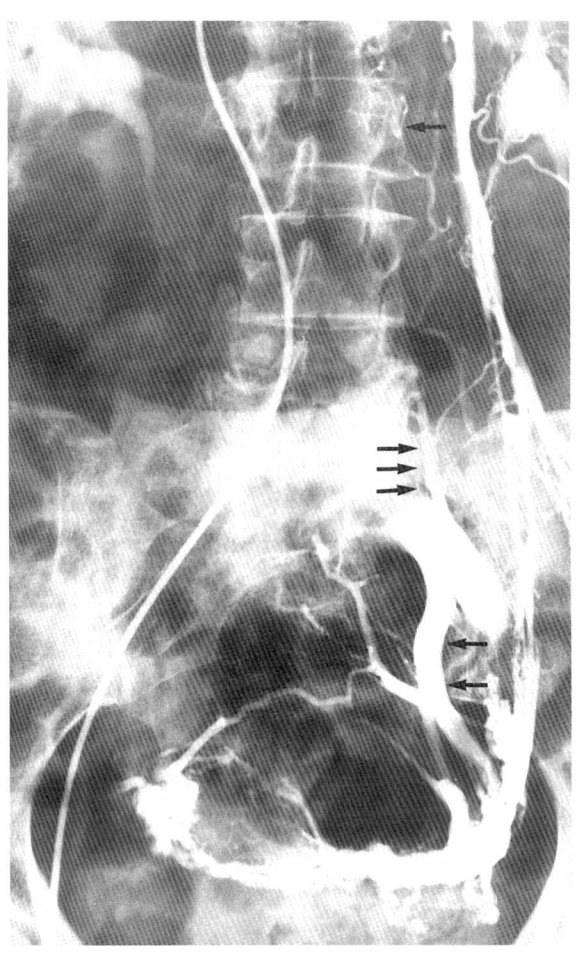

Fig. 10.37 Left ovarian vein. Venography of the most common contributary and connecting veins: peridural plexus (1 arrow), internal iliac vein (2 arrows), and multiple ovarian veins (concommitant veins); ascending lumbar vein (3 arrows)

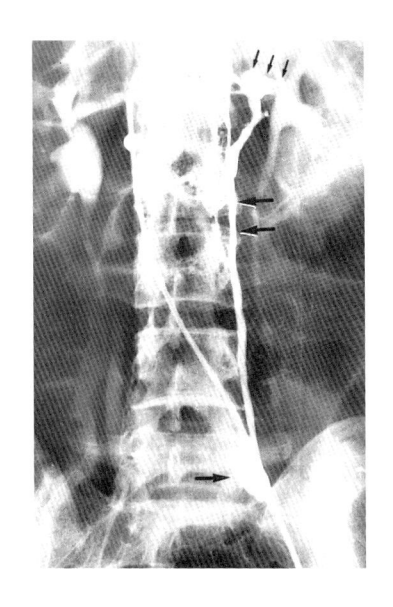

Endocrinology

Catheterizing ovarian and adrenal veins and determining of hormone levels differentiates nontumorous and tumorous hyperandrogenism and is essential for medical management. Except in rare cases of women with tumors, hyperandrogenism is due to increased hormone production by the ovaries and the adrenal glands or both. Many methods have been used to try to locate the source of excess hormone production, but most of these techniques proved unreliable. Catheterization procedures should be performed if the patient's peripheral plasma testosterone (T) levels are greater than 1.5 ng/mL, plasma DHEA-S levels are greater than 7,000 ng/mL, and if other imaging modalities have failed to locate the lesion (these values apply only if normal plasma levels of T-assay method are less than 0.5 ng/mL).

Fig. 10.38 Ascending lumbar vein (2 arrows), connecting vein between the renal vein (3 arrows) and the internal iliac vein (1 arrow). This is not an ovarian vein

316   10 Ovary

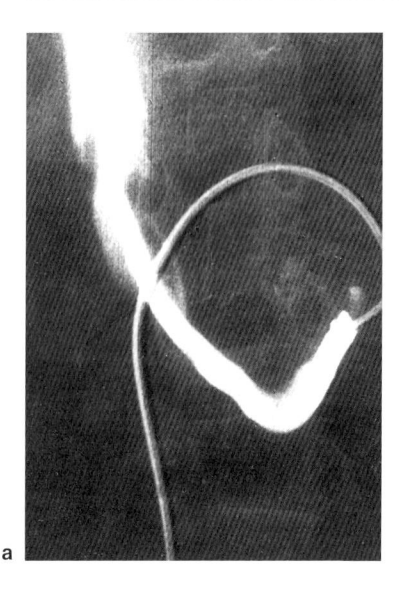

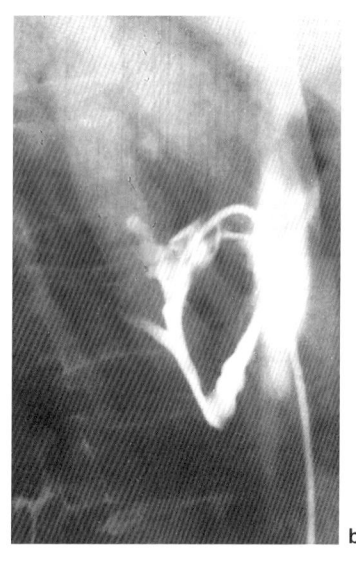

Fig. 10.**39** Circumaortic venous ring. (**a**) anterior-posterior projection. (**b**) lateral projection

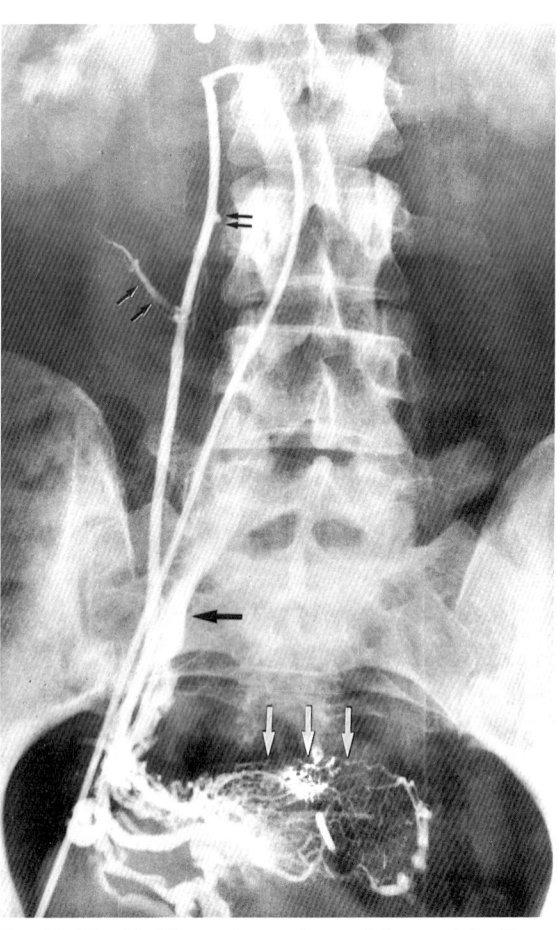

Fig. 10.**40** Right ovarian vein and its contributions: uterine plexus with veins to the contralateral side (3 arrows), parietal veins (2 arrows), internal iliac vein (1 arrow)

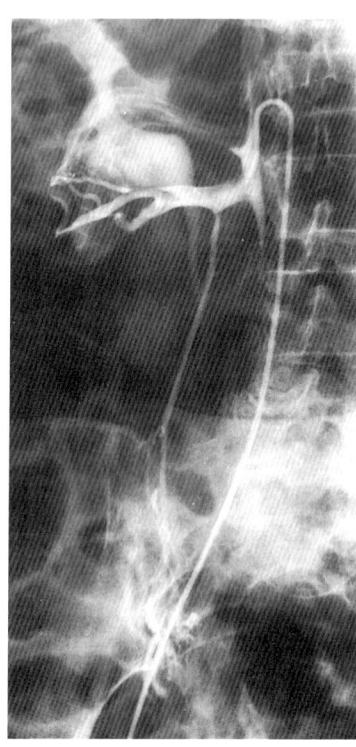

Fig. 10.**41** Right ovarian vein draining into the right renal vein

Hyperandrogenism 317

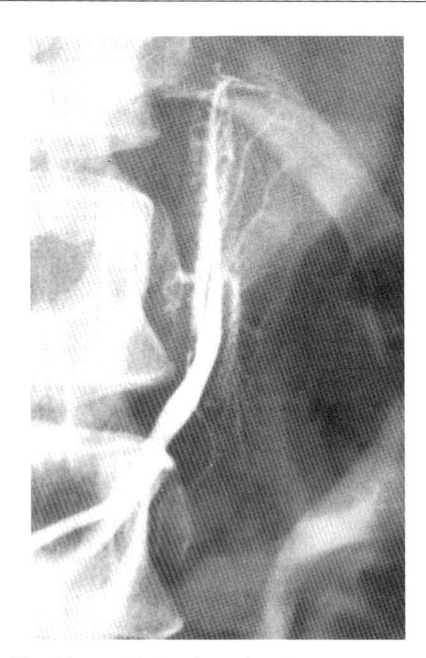

Fig. 10.**42** Normal left adrenal vein

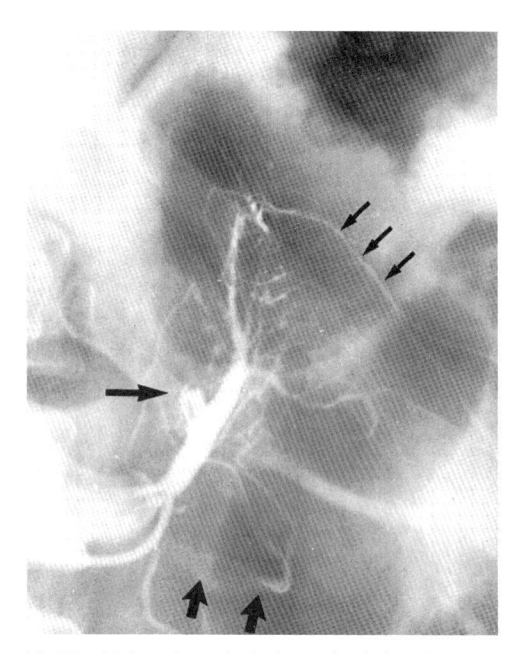

Fig. 10.**43** Veins that drain into the left adrenal vein. Inferior phrenic vein (arrow) with venous valve, renal vein (2 arrows), capsular veins (3 arrows)

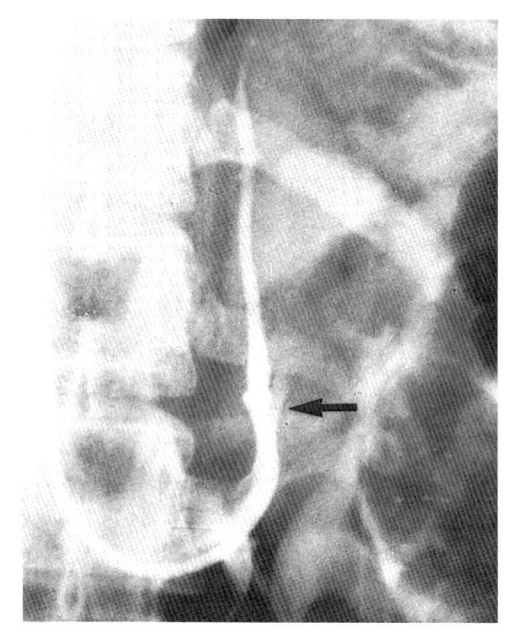

Fig. 10.**44** Selective catheterization of the inferior phrenic vein. The arrow demonstrates the origin of the left adrenal vein

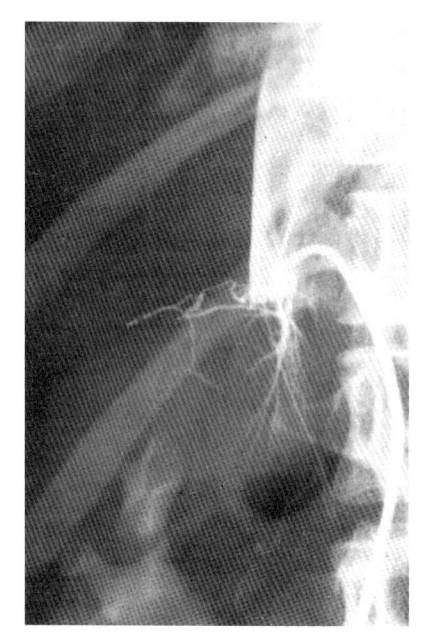

Fig. 10.**45** Normal right adrenal vein

318 10 Ovary

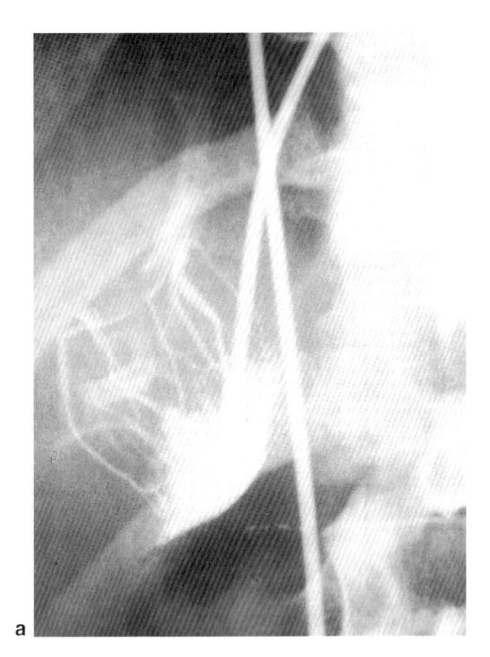

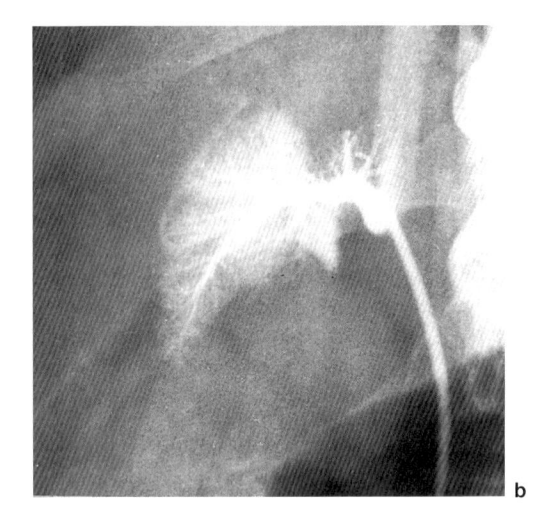

Fig. 10.46 Right hepatic veins mimicking right adrenal veins

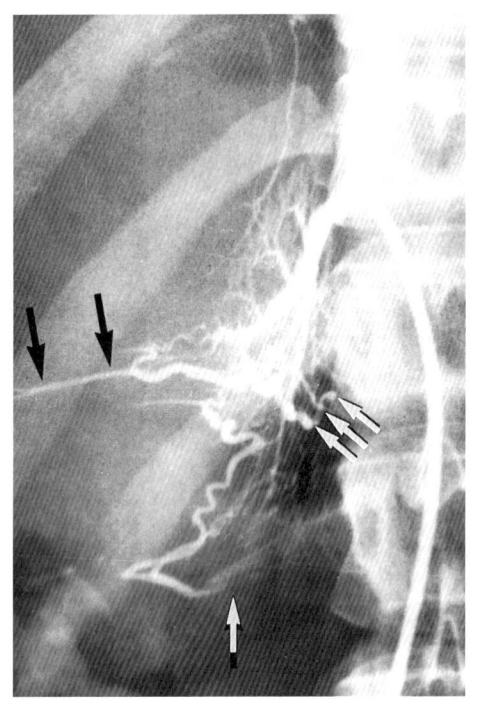

Fig. 10.47 Venous contributions to the right adrenal vein: connecting vein to the renal vein (1 arrow), renal capsular veins (2 arrows), epidural and paravertebral veins (3 arrows)

At present, selective catheterization is the most sensitive method for preoperative identification of an androgen-secreting neoplasm.

Clinical History

This clinical history is important for providing information on the following: start, duration, and progression of signs of hyperandrogenism; race, family history, growth, and weight; thelarche, pubarche, menarche, and menopause; partus, abortion, basal temperature, and previous surgery; methods and frequency of hair removal, and the amount of daily hairloss; irregularities of the menstrual cycle, amenorrhea, sterility, medication, and therapeutic trials; accompanying disease of thyroid, liver, kidneys, neurological disorders, and anorexia.

Nontumorous patients are divided into three subgroups. Nontumorous patients without clinical signs of polycystic ovaries (PCO), nontumorous patients with laparoscopically confirmed PCO, and nontumorous patients with histologically proven hyperthecosis (40). All patients have either elevated (T) and DHEA-S levels or both. They should have a laparoscopy prior to catheterization to rule out a visible neoplasm. Another group are the patients with histologically proven ovarian tumors. Patients should avoid taking any hormone drugs during the 6 months preceding catheterization.

Physical Examination

The physical examination provides information on the type, localization, distribution, and the grade of hyperandrogenism, the symptoms of virilism, and the various other stigmata, such as habitus, weight, height, striae, struma, preliminary pubes, and distribution of fat. A gynecological examination evaluates the external and internal genital parts (clitoris, ovaries, the quality of the cervical mucus, and the cytology of the vagina).

Laboratory Tests

Multiple laboratory tests have been used to determine the excess of androgen production because none of the circulating androgens has an exclusive gonadal or adrenal source. Plasma concentration reflects the sum of entry into the circulation from glandular secretions and extraglandular tissue production, as well as the hepatic and extrahepatic clearance. The estimation of secretion rates is complicated by the complexities of ovarian and adrenal steroidogenesis (episodic, diurnal, cyclic, and age-related variation. Dynamic function tests discriminate between steroids of ovarian and adrenal origin; they are however not reliable due to nonspecific pharmacodynamic effects. Estrogen-suppressible ovarian and glucocorticoid-suppressible adrenal neoplasms as well as ACTH-responsive ovarian and HCG-responsive adrenal tumors, have been described. CT and ultrasound do not detect ovarian and adrenal tumors if their sizes are smaller than the sizes of the organs itself (6, 7). The gradients of the steroids serve as semiquantitative estimates; they reflect hormone output more closely when compared with the absolute effluent levels (8, 9). This approach, however, is associated with significant errors: 1. the inability to calculate secretion rates without determination of actual glandular blood flow during the procedure; 2. the lack of knowledge of intraglandular androgen metabolism; 3. the influence of premedication stress, 4. the application of contrast media on the secretion of hormones, and 5. the uncertainty of problems related to correct identification of catheter placement during the sampling procedures. This could result in an admixture of peripheral blood with the effluent of the secreting organ (1). Nevertheless, the method of catheterization and venous sampling provides useful information on ovarian and adrenal nontumorous androgen secretion.

Plasma testosterone and DHEA-S are the most important hormones in the workup of patients with hyperandrogenism: T is the indicator of ovarian and adrenal androgen secretion; DHEA-S is almost exclusively the product of the zona reticularis of the adrenal gland. No androgen-producing tumors without elevation of plasma T and DHEA-S have been described so far (7). All tests for determination of plasma hormone content should be done according to a standardized protocol in order to reduce the influence of cyclic, circadian, and episodic variations of steroid secretion (Table 10.6).

Table 10.6 Standardized protocol for ovarian and adrenal vein sampling

- Discontinuation of hormone therapy 6 weeks prior to catherization
- No premedication or sedation
- Catheterization within the early follicular phase (day 3–7), except in oligo-and amenorrhoic patients
- Catheterization between 8 and 10 a.m.
- Three serial blood samples at 5 to 10 min. intervals of all four vessels in a randomized fashion

Dexamethasone is known to suppress adrenal androgen secretion and is used to differentiate adrenal and ovarian hyperandrogenism. If androgen levels are examined before and after dexamethasone suppression, the origin of androgen excess can be localized. Adrenals are adequately suppressed if hydrocortisone (compound F) is less than 40 ng/mL and DHEA-S is less than 400 ng/mL. The problem is that the dexamethasone long-term suppression test is not reliable, because it not only suppresses adrenal androgens but also ovarian androgen biosynthesis.

Stress

Stress has an effect on hormone release. Catheterization causes only little stress. Peripheral compound F during the procedure prior to venography is not significantly different ($p > 0.05$) from that of a normal women. Likewise, peripheral F does not differ significantly according to the literature (1, 11, Fig. 10.**48**). Other radiographic procedures such as retrograde venography fail to demonstrate ovarian tumors and cause a stress-induced, uncontrolled output of adrenal steroids. Moreover, gross morphology and functional pathology do not necessarily correlate (8, 12). Selective catheterization techniques are known to be reliable methods for studying direct glandular secretion (13, 14).

Normal Women

Normal women have a wide range of individual T and DHEA-S concentrations evaluated in peripheral veins as well as in the four glandular effluents (4, 11). Large interindividual variations of dihydrotestosterone (DHT), DHEA-S, 17α-hydroxyprogesterone (17-OHP), and F levels are observed in each vessel as well. These studies reveal that the gonads do not secrete significant amounts of T during the early follicular phase (11). There is also an ovarian contribution

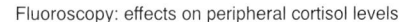

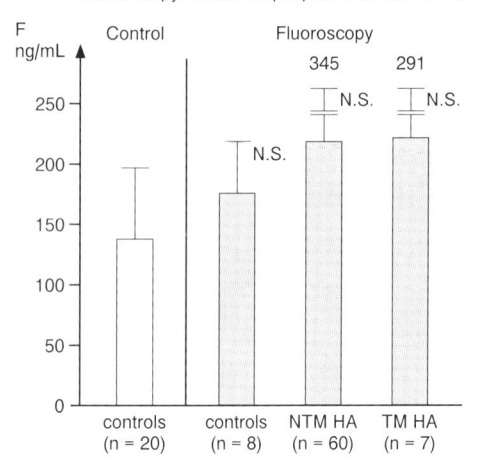

Fig. 10.**48** Peripheral hydrocortisone (F) levels during the catheterization procedure of 75 women in comparison with a control group of normal outpatients (N = 20)

of 33% to 66% to the circulating T, which changes after dexamethasone administration (15, 16). The discrepancy is understandable in view of the nonspecificity of glucocorticoid suppression tests (10). In contrast to the absence of gonadal T, DHT, and F secretion, the ovaries generate significant quantities of Delta-4-A, DHEA-S, and 17-OHP between day 3 and 7 of the cycle (17). The adrenals are considerably more active than the gonads. DHT is directly secreted by normal adrenals (18). The adrenal DHEA-S gradients are relatively small. They reflect the low metabolic clearance rate characteristic of this steroid (16). Random, nonsimultaneous catheterization of the four glandular veins reveal no significant differences between the respective effluent concentrations on the left and right sides. The ovaries have parallel androgen secretion during the early follicular phase; the same applies to the adrenal steroid output. The problems of data interpretation due to episodic, circadian, and cyclic variations of glandular steroidogenesis can be overcome by serial sampling and uniform timing of the procedure.

Nontumorous Hyperandrogenism

In cases of nontumorous hyperandrogenism the type, frequency, and extent of hormonal changes vary considerably between patients. The degree of deviation does not correlate to either the severity of symptoms or to the laparoscopic, angiographic, or histological findings.

There is a marked overlap of T and DHEA-S levels between healthy and hirsute women. This observation also applies to DHT, Delta-4-A, DHEA, and F levels. Compared to the normal cohort, the mean levels of all steroids, except F, in peripheral blood is significantly elevated in women with nonneoplastic disease as a group. Peripheral concentrations of T and DHEA-S during catheterization are above normal in about one-third of nontumorous androgenic women, whereas Delta-4-A, DHEA, and 17-OHP were increase in about half of the patients. Peripheral elevation of androgen levels is evident in only 65%, when hormone analysis is restricted to the measurement of peripheral T and DHEA-S; however, in 90% when all seven steroids are taken into consideration.

There is a direct ovarian and adrenal secretion of DHT in hirsute women according to Moltz that confirms the preliminary results presented by Maroulis (19, 20). In absolute terms, adrenal steroid release is significantly greater than gonadal steroid output during the early follicular phase; this applies to all seven hormone assays ($p < 0.001$). Compared to the group of healthy women, the mean ovarian peripheral gradients for T, Delta-4-A, and 17-OHP, and the APG for 17-OHP surpasses the normal upper limit, but these differences are significant only in regard to gonadal output of 17-OHP ($p < 0.05$).

The excess output of ovarian and adrenal androgen or both is assumed in a given individual, if one or more of the respective T, DHT, Delta-4-A, and DHEA-S gradients exceed the upper 95% confidence limit of normal secretions. Combined hypersecretion can be expected in 41% of patients. Purely ovarian (27%) or adrenal overproduction (12%) is identified less often; normal glandular androgen output is found in 20% of hirsute patients.

Polycystic Ovary Syndrome

It is still a matter of controversy whether PCO constitutes a nosological entity or a nonspecific morphologic substrate associated with hyperandrogenism. Hirsute women should undergo laparoscopy to rule out a macroscopically visible ovarian neoplasm. The changes suggestive of polycystic ovary syndrome are a thickened and whitish cortex, multiple subcapsular cysts, and gross gonadal enlargement. There is no correlation between morphological, clinical and endocrine changes; a PCO-specific hormonal pattern is not identifiable (21). Analysis of gradient data reveal that combined ovrian–adrenal androgen hypersecretion is present in 46% of PCO cases; purely ovarian (21%) or adrenal (12%) overproduction are not as frequent (21). Gradient evaluation in each individual case showed that glandular hypersecretion of at least one androgen is present in 80%. The percentage incidence of elevated OPG and adrenal peripheral gradients (APG) does not deviate substantially from those found in a whole group of 60 patients with nontumorous hyperandrogenism (22). From these data it is concluded that PCO is not a nosological entity, but rather a nonobligatory sign of hyperandrognism.

Ovarian Hyperthecosis

Ovarian hyperthecosis has repeatedly been described as a tumor-like disease separate from PCO and characterized by a pathognomonic histology as well as a distinct clinical and endocrine feature (23). This assertion remains a topic of debate.

A specific hormone profile can not be identified. There is overlap of testosterone levels in peripheral and glandular effluent blood between healthy women and patients with hyperthecosis as well as androgen-secreting ovarian neoplasms. In several individuals described in in the literature testosterone secretion fell within the tumorous range (12). Gradient analysis of all androgens indicate ovarian hypersecretion, but also significant adrenal involvement. The minor differences between hyperthecosis and PCO represent only variable manifestation of the same condition of a disturbed androgen metabolism. A tumor, however, should be ruled out in patients with hyperthecosis.

Androgen-secreting Ovarian Neoplasm

This tumor is rare. Neoplastic hyperandrogenism should be ruled out in women with severe, sudden or late onset, and with progressive hirsutism. Other signs of virilism are suggestive of tumorous hyperandrogenism. Selective catheterization has been used to study glandular secretion of several ovarian and adrenal androgen-secreting tumors (12). Representative secretion pattern or criteria differentiating nontumorous and tumorous hyperandrogenism can not be established because investigations constituted single case reports.

According to the literature, it appears that virilizing adrenal tumors secrete predominantly either T or DHEA-S, although simultaneous elevated output of Delta-4-A and DHEA was described.

Standarized bilateral ovarian–adrenal vein catheterization was found to be successful in preoperatively assessing glandular steroid release in seven occult virilizing gonadal neoplasms (12). The histology of the involved ovaries is demonstrated in a published series and reveals three lipid cell, two Leydig's cell and two Sertoli–Leydig cell tumors measuring between 0.6 and 2.2 cm in diameter. Endoscopy and radiography failed to locate the functional lesions. Prior to catheterization, peripheral T surpassed the upper 95% confidence limit of the nontumorous group (1.5 ng/mL in all instances). This may indicate unpredictable episodic T secretion by the ovarian lesion. Antecubital vein DHT exceeded the nontumorous range in two patients. The peripheral concentrations of the other steroids fell within the nonneoplastic range in all instances. Selective sampling displays a unilateral increase of T in the effluent draining in neoplastic gonade which exceeds the upper 95% confidence limit of the nontumorous group (2.7 ng/mL).

Catheterization Techniques

Catheterization is performed following a standardized protocol (Table 10.**6**). The patient receives no premedication to avoid iatrogenic secretion of adrenal steroids. The procedure takes place during the early follicular phase (days 3 to 7) except in postmenopausal or amenorrhoic individuals between 8 a.m. and 10 a.m. to reduce interference from cyclic and circadian variations of androgen seretion.

A femoro–visceral catheter (Fig. 10.**49**) is introduced percutaneously under local anesthesia using a femoral approach. This catheter can be turned into different shapes (1, 2, 3, 4, 24) to fit the different angled origins of both adrenal and ovarian veins. The high-flow, thin-wall catheters are used now, however, they have poorer torque control, especially if they are shaped within the venous system. The catheter is guided into the adrenal and ovarian veins in random sequence. Three serial samples (8 to 10 mL) are obtained at 5- to 15-minute intervals for all four vessels to compensate for episodic variations in steroid secretions. After each sampling, fluoroscopic control during the injection of up to 0.5 mL of a nonionic contrast medium is used to confirm the correct position of the catheter tip. This is routinely followed by flushing with saline solution after withdrawal of the catheter tip. Steroid levels determined in samples considered subselective by radiographic criteria are disregarded. In androgenized patients, samples are drawn both before, and 20 to 30 minutes after intravenous injection of 8 to 12 mg of dexamethasone. In addition, three peripheral blood samples are drawn. Retrograde venography is not carried out because of accompanying complications. Retrograde venography has a definite effect on adrenal steroid release; 0.5 mL is well

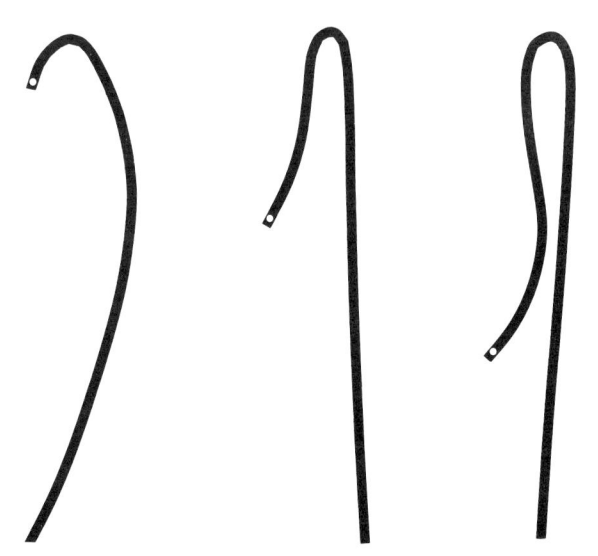

Fig. 10.**49** Angiographic catheters for sampling of adrenal and ovarian veins

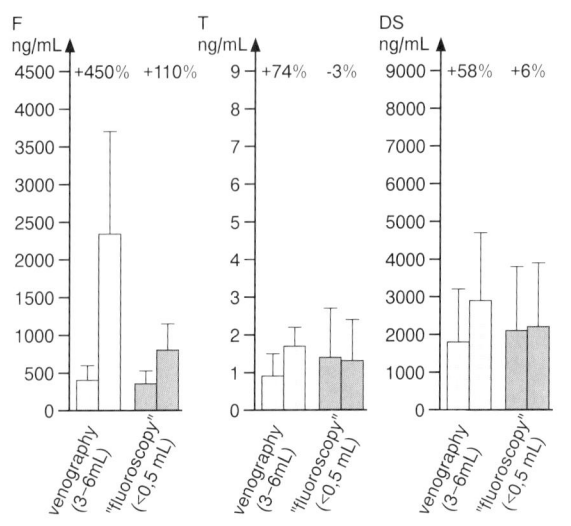

Fig. 10.**50** Effects of contrast media on adrenal steroid release in nine patients with hyperandrogenemia. F = cortisol; T = testosterone, DHEA-S (DS) = dehydroepiandrosterone sulfate. The percentage values denote the mean changes of adrenal vein steroid levels induced

tolerated and does not effect hormone effluence (Fig. 10.**50**). Accurate placement of the catheter (**selectivity**) at the orifices of adrenal and ovarian effluents can be expected for the left adrenal vein in 97.3%, the left ovarian vein in 66.7%, the right adrenal and ovarian veins in 82.7% and 79.7%, respectively. Accurate placement of all four glandular effluents can be achieved in 45%, in three of four, and in two of four veins in 81% and 100%, respectively (Table 10.**7**).

Retrograde injection of contrast media into adrenal veins induces changes in the adrenal secretory activity. These depends on the amount injected (Fig. 10.**50**). While venography (3 to 6 mL) causes extremely high elevation of adrenal vein hydrocortisone, less elevation is observed for testosterone and DHEA sulfate Injections of minute volumes of contrast medium (less than 0.5 mL: "fluoroscopic control") has no significant effect on adrenal androgen release (3).

Table 10.**7** Accuracy of catheterization

	NL (n = 8)	NTM (n = 60)	TM (n = 7)	Total (n = 75)
LOV	8	36	6	50 (66.7%)
ROV	7	47	5*	59 (78.7%)
LAV	8	58	7	73 (97.3%)
RAV	6	49	7	62 (82.7%)

NL: normal volunteers, NTM: nontumorous patients, TM: patients with tumors, LOV: left ovarian vein, ROV: right ovarian vein, LAV: left adrenal vein, RAV: right adrenal vein, * ovarectomy

Side Effects

These are usually related to contrast media injected into the gland. They are minor according to the literature (1, 2, 3, 24, 25) and include extravasation of contrast into the adrenal parenchyma, small hematomas at the puncture site, and allergic reactions. Serious complications are described (4, 25) to be rare. The procedure lasts approximately 45 minutes on the average and causes minor discomfort.

Radiation Exposure

Twenty minutes of fluroscopy results in a total radiation dose of 800 mrem at the level of the gonads (1, 3). Radiographs are not necessary.

Conclusion

Today, selective ovarian-adrenal sampling is the most sensitive method for semiquantitative estimation of glandular androgen secretion. It is the only technique that allows separate analysis of each ovary and each adrenal gland. The procedure is reliable and safe provided that it is performed at centers with adequately experienced staff under strict, standardized conditions to reduce the interference of episodic, circadian, and cyclic variations of steroidogenesis. The evolutionary pathophysiology of glandular androgen hypersecretion must be regarded as a continuous process without sharp borderlines from normal to nontumourous conditions, such as polycystic ovaries and hyperthecosis, to neoplastic disease. Hirsutism and related symptoms are caused by excess androgens of ovarian and of adrenal origin. Combined hypersecretion occurs more frequently than either purely gonadal or adrenal overproduction. Preoperative verification and localization of a virilizing neoplasm is important, because it reduces the number and the extent of the surgical procedure.

References

1 Sörensen R, Moltz L, Schwartz U. Technical difficulties of selective venous blood sampling in the differential diagnosis of female hyperandrogenism. Cardiovasc Intervent Radiol. 1986;9:75–82.
2 Sörensen R, Moltz L. Diagnostik bei progredientem Hirsitismuns. Kathetertechnik und Ergebnisse. Fortschr Röntgenstr. 1981;135:257–266.
3 Moltz L, Sörensen R. Selective venous sampling for the differential diagnosis of female hyperandrogenemia. In: Uflacker, eds. Percutaneous Venous Blood Sampling in Endocrine Disease. New York: Springer; 1992.
4 Lecky JW, Wolfman NT, Modic CW. Current concepts of adrenal angiography. Radiol Clin N Amer. 1976;14:309–352.
5 Schwartz U, Moltz L, Pickartz H, Sörensen R. Die Hyperthecose – eine tumorähnliche Ovarialveränderung bei androgenisierten Frauen. Geb Frauenhk. 1986;46:391–397.
6 Abrams HL, Siegelmann SS, Adams DF, et al. Computed tomography versus ultrasound of the adrenal gland: A prospective study. Radiology 1. 1982;143:121–128.

7. Mitty HA, Yeh HC. Radiology of the adrenals with sonography and CT. Philadelphia: Saunders; 1982:56–57.
8. Moltz L, Pickartz H, Sörensen R, Schwartz U, Hammerstein J: A Sertoli-Leydig cell tumor and pregnancy-clinical, endocrine, radiologic, and electron microscopic findings. Arch Gynecol 1983;233:295–308.
9. Soules MR, Abraham GE, Bossen EH: The steroid profile of a virilizing ovarian tumor. Obstet Gynecol 1978;52:73–78.
10. Moltz L. Rationeller Einsatz endokrinologischer und radiologischer Verfahren bei der Differentialdiagnose von Androgenisierungserscheinungen der Frau. Geburtsh u Frauenheilk. 1982;42:321–326.
11. Moltz L, Sörensen R, Schwartz U, Hammerstein J. Ovarian and adrenal vein steroids in healthy women with ovulatory cycles-selective catheterization findings. J Steroid Biochem. 1984;20:901–905.
12. Moltz L, Pickartz H, Sörensen R, Schwartz U, Hammerstein J. Ovarian and adrenal vein steroids in seven patients with androgen-secreting ovarian neoplasms: selective catheterization findings. Fertil Steril. 1184;42:585–593.
13. Kirschner MA, Jacobs JB. Combined ovarian and adrenal vein catheterization to determine the sites of androgen overproduction in hirsute women. J Clin Endocrinol Metab. 1971;33:199–209.
14. Moltz L. Differential-diagnostic clarification of androgen-producing tumors. In: Hammerstein J, Lachnit-Fixson U, Neumann F, Plewig G, eds. Adrogenization in women. Exc Med, Int Congr Ser No. 493, North Holland: Elsevier; 1979:114–124.
15. Genazzani AR, Magrini G, Facchinetti, F, et al. Behaviour and origin of plasma androgens throughout the menstrual cycle. In: Martini L, Motta M eds. Androgens and Antiandrogens. New York: Raven Press; 1977:247–261.
16. Vermeulen A, Rubens R. Adrenal virilism. In: James VHT, ed. The Adrenal Gland. New York: Raven Press; 1970:259–282.
17. Abraham GE, Chakmakjian ZH. Serum steroid levels during the menstrual cycle in a bilaterally adrenalectomized women. J Clin Endocrinol Metab. 1973;37:581–592.
18. Maroulis GB, Abraham GB. Concentration of adrogens and cortisol in the various zones of the human adrenal cortex. In: Genazzani A, Thijssen JHH, Siiteri P, eds. Adrenal Androgens. New York: Raven Press; 1980:49–53.
19. Maroulis GB. Evaluation of hirsutism and hyperandrogenemia. Fertil Steril. 1981;36:273–305.
20. Maroulis GB, Lindstrom R, Abraham GE, Marshall JR. Testosterone and dehydrotestosterone secretion by the adrenal and ovary in hirsute patients. Endocrine Society Meeting Abstract. 1975;471:286.
21. Moltz L, Sörensen R, Römmler A, Schwartz U, Hammerstein J. Polyzystische Ovarien: eigenständiges Krankheitsbild oder unspezifisches Symptom? Geb Frauenhk. 1985;45:107–114.
22. Moltz L, Schwartz U, Sörensen R, Pickartz H, Hammerstein J. Ovarian and adrenal vein steroids in patients with nonneoplastic hyperandrogenism: selective catheterization findings. Fertil Steril. 1984;42:69–75.
23. Karam K, Haji S. Hyperthecosis syndrome. Acta Obstet Gynecol Scand. 1979;58:73–78.
24. Sörensen R, Moltz L. Technical Aspects and anatomical difficulties of adrenal and gonadal phlebography and blood sampling. Exc Med, Amsterdam, International Congress, series No. 550. 1980;78–88.
25. Lamarque JL, Bruel LN, Lopez P, et al. Les complications del'angiographie surrenalienne. Ann Radiol. 1979;22:401–408.

11 Quantification of Osteoporosis

P. Lang, S. Grampp, M. Jergas, P. Steiger,
S. Majumdar, C. Glüer, and H. K. Genant

Table 11.1 Comparison of bone densitometry techniques

Technique	Site	Relative Sensitivity*	Precision* (%)	Accuracy* (%)	Duration of Examination (min)	Absorbed Dose (mrem [mSv])	Cost ($)
Standard technique							
SPA	proximal radius (cortical)	1×	2–3	5	15	10 (100)	75
DPA	spine, hip, total body mineral (integral)	2×	2–4	4–10	20–45	5 (50)	100–150
QCT	Spine (trabecular)	3–4×	2–5	5–20	10–20	100–1000 (1000–10000)	100–200
Newer developments							
SPA-R	Distal radius, calcaneus (integral)	2×	1–2	5	10–20	5–10 (50–100)	50″
AP-DXA pencil beam	Spine, hip, total bone mineral (integral), forearm	2×	0.5–2	3–5	2–5	1–3 (10–30)	75″
Lateral DXA pencil beam, decubitus	Spine (integral or predominantly (trabecular)	2×	2–5	3–8	4–15	10–15 (100–150)	150″
AP-DXA fan beam	Spine, hip, total bone mineral (integral), forearm	2×	0.5–2	3–5	5 sec–90 sec	3–12 (30–120)	75″
Lateral DXA fan beam, supine	Spine (integral or predominantly trabecular)	3×	1–2	3–8	2	27 (270)	100″
QCT-A	Spine, hip (trabecular and integral)	3–4×	1–2	5–10	10	100–300) (1000–3000)	150″

Note: SPA = single-energy photon absorptiometry, DPA = dual-energy absorptiometry, QCT = quantitative computed tomography, SPA-R = rectilinear SPA, AP-DXA = dual-energy x-ray absorptiometry in anteroposterior projection, lateral DXA = DXA in lateral projection, QCT-A = QCT with advanced software and hardware capabilities; * see text for definitions; ″ projected cost

Numerous methods have been used for quantitative assessment of the skeleton in osteoporosis with variable precision, accuracy, and sensitivity (Table 10.8). The first methods to be developed were radiogrammetry (26) and photon absorptiometry (9), which measure primarily cortical bone of the peripheral appendicular skeleton. In the past decade, techniques have become available that can quantify bone mineral content in the spine, which is the site of early osteoporosis. Quantitative computed tomography (QCT) (11–13, 29, 31, 32, 39, 61, 84, 91, 101, 113, 130) provides a measure of purely trabecular bone of the vertebral spongiosum, or other sites, whereas dualphoton absorptiometry (DPA) (56, 87, 95) and its offspring dual–X-ray absorptiometry (DXA) (5, 53, 71, 72, 86, 102, 106, 120, 122) measure an integral of compact and cancellous bone of the spine, hip, or entire skeleton. Newer techniques include ultrasound measurements and quantitative MRI. This chapter describes the capabilities of commonly available bone densitometry techniques, addresses the controversies regarding their clinical utility, delineates the criteria for their appropriate use, and provides a perspective on future techniques for assessing bone mineral density, fracture risk, and bone strength.

Single Photon Absorptiometry

Photon absorptiometry was first introduced by Cameron and Sorensen in 1963 (8, 9). Many single photon absorptiometry (SPA) devices have been developed in the past 20 years, but the most widely distributed is the Norland Cameron device. With this method, a quantitative assessment of the bone mineral content at a peripheral site of the skeleton (e.g., distal or ultradistal radius, calcaneus) is possible. A highly collimated photon beam from a radionuclide source (usually ^{125}I) is used to measure photon attenuation at the site of measurement. The measured attenuation is then converted to bone mineral content (BMC) or bone mineral density (BMD) using a known standard.

SPA works only when soft-tissue thickness is constant. Beam intensity in SPA is influenced by both bone mineral density as well as soft-tissue thickness. Variations in soft-tissue thickness may cause underestimation or overestimation of bone mineral density (Fig. 11.1a). However, if the forearm is embedded or immersed in a material with absorption properties for ^{125}I photons identical to soft-tissue, the absorption due to the soft-tissue alone becomes constant (Fig. 11.1b). Fortunately, such materials do exist and the most common is water. Separate measurements of trabecular and cortical bone are not possible with SPA. For example, a measurement of the distal third of the radius includes mainly cortical bone. The relatively uniform structure at this site with 95% cortical bone ensures good precision (107), yet the metabolically active trabecular bone is barely included. On the

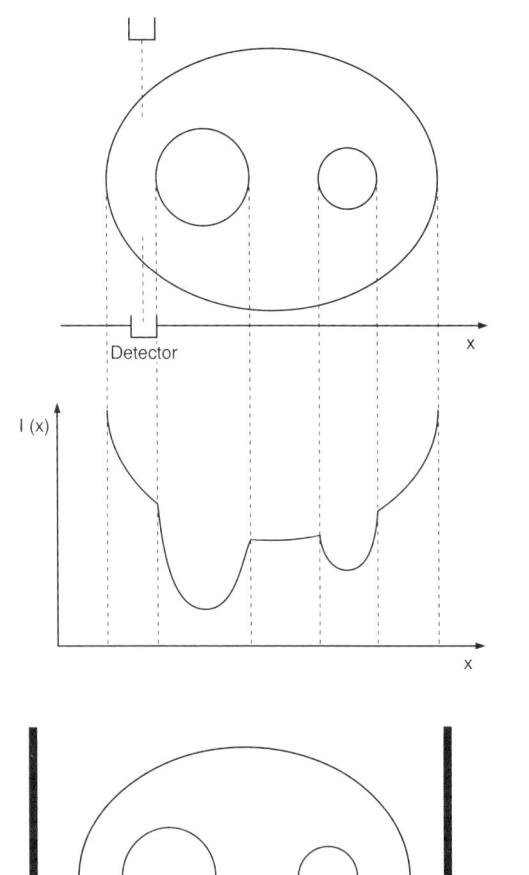

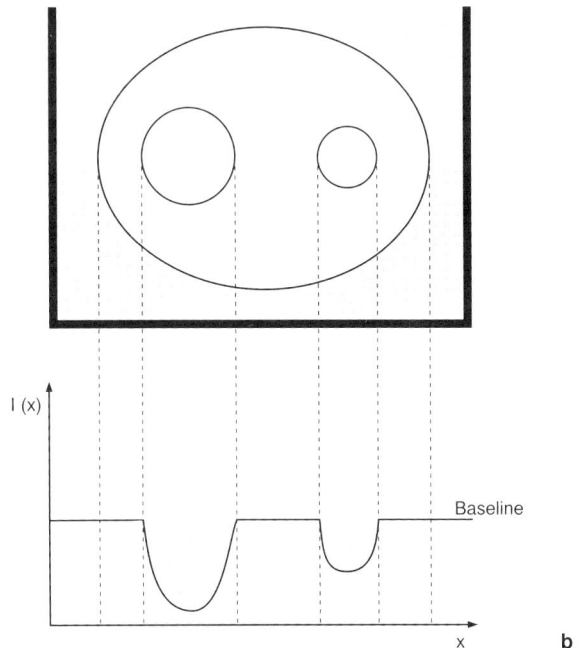

Fig. 11.1 Principle of single photon absorptiometry.
a The beam intensity I(x) is demonstrated as a function of position x of for a simulated forearm. Because the arm is surrounded by air, the soft-tissue absorption is not uniform
b The beam intensity I(x) with the use of a soft-tissue equivalent bolus (water). The absorption caused by soft tissue is constant, and any excess absorption is caused by bone tissue. The hatched area therefore is proportional to the amount of bone mineral present along the scan line (with permission from reference 28)

other hand, measurements of the ultradistal radius include more trabecular bone (up to 40%), but difficult localization and inhomogeneity of the trabecular bone content cause deterioration in precision at this site, at least with earlier devices (123). Newly developed rectilinear scanning devices show a significantly enhanced precision at this site. The value of bone mineral measurements at the calcaneus has been controversial because of the uncertain relationship between BMD and body weight or exercise at this site (118, 131). Nevertheless, recent studies show promising results documenting the value of calcaneus measurements in predicting osteoporotic fractures (121, 124, 133). SPA has proven to be a valuable tool in the diagnosis of osteoporosis, providing reasonable precision and low radiation exposure (Table 11.1). Therefore, it is still in use at many centers, with a distribution of about 1500 systems. In more recently developed devices, the radionuclide source is replaced by an X-ray tube (SXA), resulting in improved precision and cost effectiveness for these systems.

Dual Photon Absorptiometry

DPA has been studied extensively as a technique used to measure mineral content of the spine as well as of the hip and total body (56, 87, 95). DPA represents an extension of the principle of SPA. SPA requires a constant soft-tissue thickness. Furthermore, soft tissue is composed of more than just one material. For the peripheral skeleton, a limb can be assumed to be composed of bone, muscle, and other types of soft tissue that can be simulated by immersion of the extremity in water. For the axial skeleton, however, this assumption is not valid, and significant amounts of fat may also lie within the scan path. In addition, bolusing is not possible at these scan sites. This problem can, however, be solved by the use of two distinct photon energy sources. In the DPA technique, a high-purity, high-activity gadolinium source, which has photons of predominantly 44 keV and 100 keV, is used as the transmission source, and the scans are performed on a whole-body rectilinear scanner.

In both bone and soft tissue, the low-energy beam (44 keV) is attenuated more than the high-energy beam (100 keV), but to a much greater extent in bone (Fig. 11.2). In other words, bone yields a higher contrast at low energies than at high energies. DPA is based on this contrast difference. By multiplying the high-energy intensity curve by an appropriate factor, K, the soft-tissue portion of the intensity profile can be made to match exactly that of the low-energy curve. When this rescaled high-energy profile is subtracted from the low-energy profile, the soft-tissue contribution is eliminated, leaving only the bone contribution (Fig. 11.2).

The principal advantages of DPA are low radiation dose, clinically sufficient accuracy, and a large number of accessible measurement sites such as spine, hip, and total body. Shortcomings include a relatively long scanning time (20–45 minutes) and, more importantly, limitations in short-term precision. Short-term, in vivo precision errors range between 1.1% (117) and 2.3% (132), and long-term precision errors vary between 1.4% (109) and 3.7% (81). The precision of measurement by DPA in healthy, young patients is 2% to 3% (coefficient of variation). Specific problems, particularly those related to software and isotope source changes, may increase the precision error to 4–6% (17, 82, 100). Because DPA integrates compact and cancellous bone, the sensitivity of DPA is considered lower than that of QCT, which can selectively measure the metabolically more active trabecular bone. DPA bone density measurements may be incorrectly elevated by the presence of osteophytes, posterior element hypertrophy, or vascular calcifications at the scanned level.

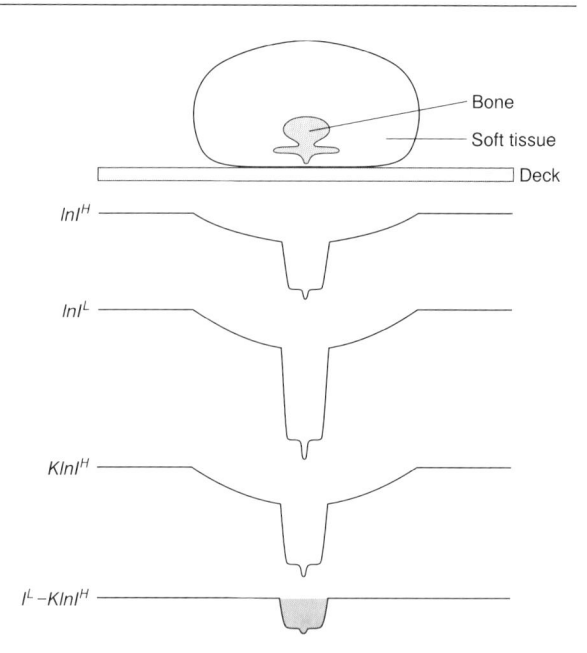

Fig. 11.2 Photon intensity profiles illustrating the theoretical background of dual photon absorptiometry. [Ln I^H] represents the high-energy profile (100 keV); [ln I^L] is the intensity profile at low energy (44 keV). Multiplication of [ln I^H] with an appropriate factor K results in [K ln I^H]; the soft-tissue portion of [K ln I^H] matches that of [ln I^L]. When [K ln I^H] is subtracted from the low-energy profile [ln I^L], the soft-tissue contribution is eliminated; the hatched area represents the bone contribution only (with permission from reference 28)

Dual X-Ray Absorptiometry

Although an x-ray–based technique for bone mineral densiometry had been developed already in the 1960s and 1970s (43, 48, 116), it did not gain widespread acceptance until recently. In 1987, the first commercially available x-ray–based dual-energy bone densitometers were introduced.

Because of the enhanced flux from an X-ray tube—as compared to an isotope source—the scan speed and the collimation of the X-ray beam could be enhanced, resulting in reduced scanning time and improved resolution. Numerous acronyms such as DER (dual-energy radiography), DRA (dual-energy radiographic absorptiometry), QDR (quantitative digital radiography), DEXA (dual-energy X-ray absorptiometry), and DXA (dual X-ray absorptiometry) have been suggested. We propose the use of DXA for this new family of bone densitometers (33).

At our institution, we have assessed the performance of the Hologic QDR-1000, QDR-1000/W, and QDR 2000 systems (Hologic Inc, Waltham Massachusetts), the Lunar DPX-L system (Lunar Radiation, Madison, Wisconsin), and the Norland XR26 MarkII system (Norland, Fort Atkinson, Wisconsin). The QDR-1000 (Hologic, Waltham, Massachusetts) (116) differs from the standard DPA scanners by a number of features, namely an X-ray tube instead of a Gd-isotope source, alternating X-ray generator voltage along with an integrating instead of a photon-counting detector, and an internal calibration wheel. The QDR-1000/W differs from the older QDR 1000 system in that it allows total body scans in addition to measuring sites in the peripheral and axial skeleton. Both systems use X-rays of two different energy levels (70 kVp and 140 kVp) to image and measure the bone mineral content of the designated area of the body. The soft tissues that are contained within the area of interest are subtracted and only the bones are imaged and measured. The Lunar DPX-L (Lunar Radiation, Madison, Wisconsin) (72) is an X-ray–based scanner that uses a heavily filtered constant beam along with an energy-discriminating photon-counting detector. The Norland XR26 (Norland, Fort Atkinson, Wisconsin) uses an X-ray tube along with two photon-counting detectors, one for each energy, and allows for variation of beam intensity to match patient thickness.

With the Hologic QDR 1000 and 1000W systems, the Lunar DPX-L, and the Norland XR 26 scanners, lateral DXA measurements of the spine can only be obtained by positioning the patient on the side; reproducibility of such measurements is consequently limited. However, the Hologic QDR 2000 system allows rotation of X-ray source and detectors from a vertical orientation into a horizontal orientation, so that the patient need not to relocated in a lateral position, but can remain in the initial supine position used for the AP scan. In addition, the Hologic QDR 2000 system employs a fan beam source and multiple detector array rather than a pencil beam and single or dual detectors like the other currently existing systems. Array detector systems offer increased scan speed and spatial resolution compared to pencil beam devices, but the source-detector geometry complicates the data acquisition. Since, at the present time, most studies have been performed using the Hologic QDR 1000 and 1000W, the Lunar DPX-L, and the Norland XR26, we will initially focus on the results obtained with these scanners using pencil beam technique. In the second half of this section, we will discuss newer results using the Hologic QDR 2000 with its fan beam, multi-detector array technique.

DXA systems can be used to determine bone material of the spine (Fig. 11.**3**), the hip (Fig. 11.**4**), the forearm, the total body (Fig. 11.**5**), and principally any body part. Most investigators have performed DXA bone mineral evaluations of the spine and hip in an anteroposterior (AP) projection. In the spine, these AP-measurements represent an integral of compact and cancellous bone. Measurements are typically performed from L1 or L2 to L4; each vertebral level is evaluated separately (Fig. 11.**3a**). In the hip, various regions of interest are evaluated; these include the femoral neck, the greater trochanter, the intertrochanteric region, Ward's triangle, as well as a region that incorporates the femoral head and neck, the greater and lesser trochanter, and portions of the femoral shaft (Fig. 11.**4**). Measurements in the intertrochanteric region and Ward's triangle reflect bone density in areas of principally trabecular bone with only small contributions from cortical bone at the anterior and posterior femoral surface; all other regions of interest assess an integral of cortical and trabecular bone analagous to AP measurements of the spine. DXA also allows for measuring bone mineral in the forearm, the calcaneus, and the total body (Fig. 11.**5**) (60, 83, 85).

Mazess et al. found a long-term in vitro precision error of 0.6% for DXA (72). Short-term in vivo precision ranged between 0.6% and 1.5% in the spine, and between 1.2% and 2.0% in the hip depending on the scanning speed (72). In a recent study, Mazess et al. (69) found a short-term in vivo precision between 0.48% and 0.55% for the spine and between 0.85% and 1.0% for the femoral neck depending on the scanning speed. When they immersed bone phantoms in different amounts of water simulating different soft-tissue thickness, there was no significant effect of tissue thickness on mass, area, or areal density (bone mineral density). Similarly, Pacifici et al. observed a short-term in vitro precision of 0.41%; short-term in vivo precision amounted to 1.00% (86).

Since DXA employs principles similar to those of DPA, DXA lends itself to comparison to DPA. Several studies independently found that bone mineral density values obtained with the Hologic DXA were consistently lower than those derived from DPA for both spine and hip measurements (5, 38). One of several explanations is a calibration offset difference caused by the use of different calibration phantoms (5).

In a study performed at University of California

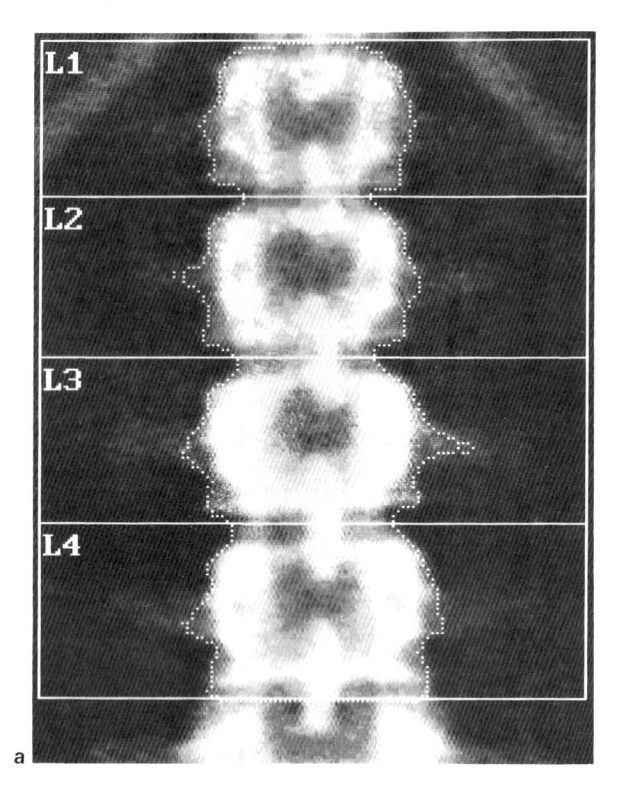

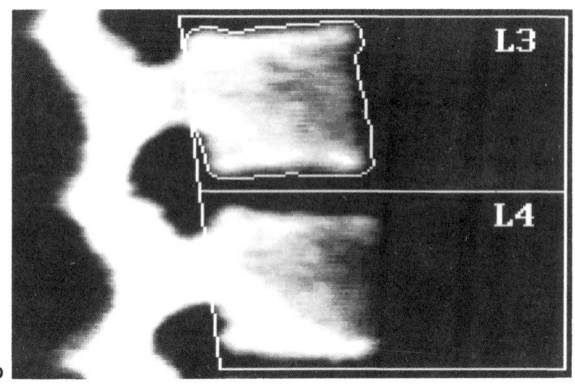

Fig. 11.3a Dual X-ray absorptiometry (DXA) of the lumbar spine in anteroposterior projection. The different vertebral levels L1 to L4 are evaluated separately; AP measurements include areas of purely trabecular bone located within the vertebral body as well as zones of predominantly compact bone located in the vertebral endplates and the posterior spinal elements
b DXA of the lumbar spine in lateral projection. The patient was placed on his side for this measurement. The posterior elements are not superimposed on the vertebral body thus permitting measurements of principally trabecular bone within the vertebral body with only small contributions from the cortical rim

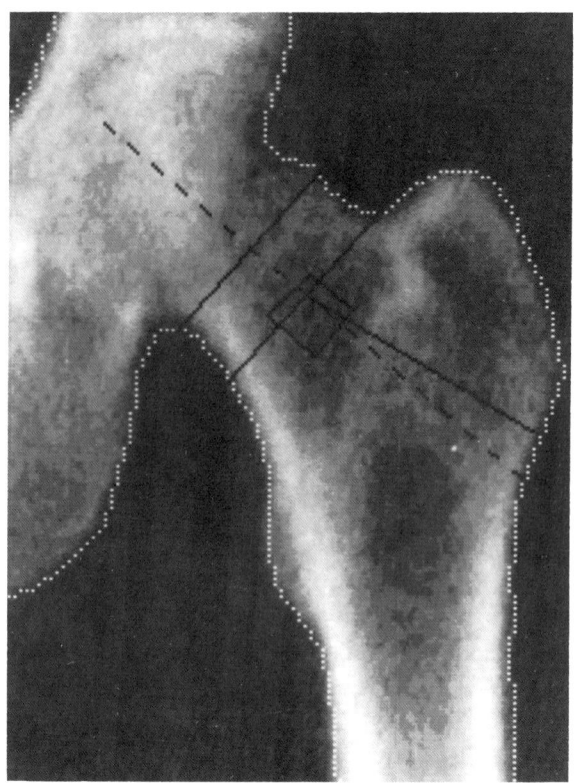

Fig. 11.4 Dual X-ray absorptiometry of the hip. Bone mineral density is assessed for various regions of interest such as the femoral neck, the greater trochanter, the intertrochanteric region, Ward's triangle, as well as an integral region representing the femoral head and neck, the trochanter, and portions of the femoral shaft

San Francisco (UCSF) (38), we found a long-term in vitro precision of 0.44% for the Hologic DXA compared to 1.33% for the Norland DPA (Fig. 11.6). Short-term in vivo presision ranged from 0.6% at the trochanter to 1.2% at the femoral neck for DXA. This represents a marked improvement over results obtained with DPA scanners, which at best achieve a short-term in vivo precision error of 2% to 3% (70).

Correlation of DXA and DPA at UCSF was found to be excellent in both the spine as well as the hip (Fig. 11.7) (38). In the spine, correlation coefficients varied from $r = 0.95$ to $r = 0.98$ (5, 38) (Fig. 11.7a); for the femoral neck, a correlation coefficient of $r = 0.95$ was described (38) (Fig. 11.7b). Since the correlation between DXA and DPA is so strong, normative data generated with DPA can be extrapolated to DXA with appropriate offsets. The bone mineral values for individual patients must then be corrected by the average differences between DXA and DPA for the spine and the femoral neck, respectively.

When AP-DXA was compared to QCT (38), correlation was only moderate ($r = 0.85$; coefficient of variation 11.9%). Although correlation between QCT

11 Quantification of Osteoporosis 329

and AP-DXA of the spine is statistically significant, the spread is relatively large and AP-DXA data can not be predicted for the individual patient on the basis of QCT and vice versa.

The moderate correlation between AP-DXA and QCT measurements of the spine can be explained by the different bone compartments that are assessed by both methods: QCT measures metabolically very active, purely trabecular bone; AP-DXA measurements, however, reflect an integral of trabecular and low-turnover compact bone. AP-DXA may, therefore, be less sensitive to bone loss related to primary or secondary osteoporosis. This limitation may, however, be overcome by acquisition of DXA measurements in a lateral projection (Fig. 11.3b). In the lateral view, the vertebral bodies are not superimposed on the posterior spinal elements which permits measurement of principally trabecular bone located in the vertebral body with only a small cortical rim contribution (Fig. 11.3b). However, only L4 projects free of ribs and/or pelvis (103).

In a study at UCSF that involved only 35 patients and that compared AP-DXA, lateral DXA obtained in decubitus position with a pencil beam technique, and QCT, the percentage decrement between normal premenopausal and normal postmenopausal women was for AP-DXA −8.4% (z-score = −0.75), for lateral DXA −39.9% (z-score = −1.36), and for QCT −25.6% (z-score = −1.46); the percentage decrement between normal premenopausal and osteoporotic postmenopausal women was for AP-DXA −15.9%,

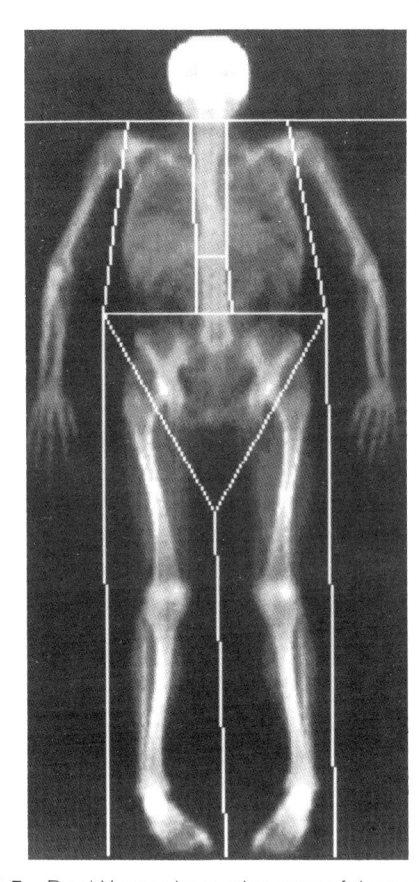

Fig. 11.5 Dual X-ray absorptiometry of the total body. Bone mineral density can be separately measured in the head, the left and right arms, the left and right rib cage, the T- and L-spine, the pelvis, and the left and right leg. In addition, total body bone mineral content (in grams) and bone mineral density (in grams/cm^2) can be calculated

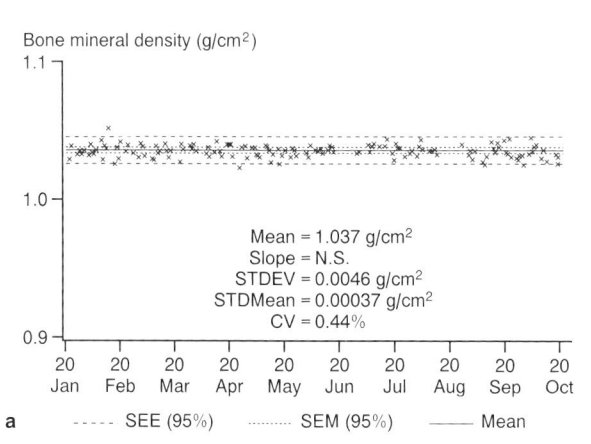

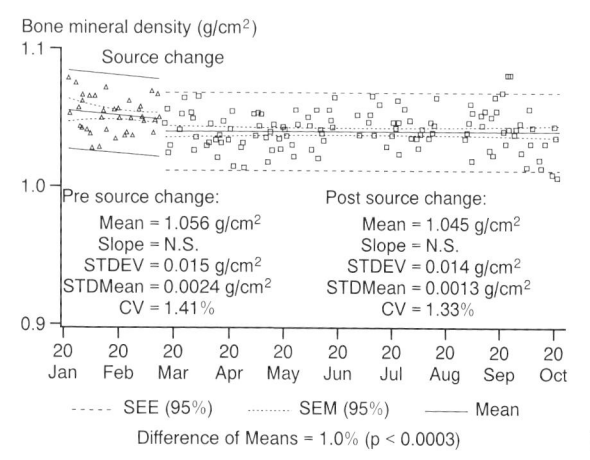

Fig. 11.6 Long-term in vitro precision data for DXA (in **a**) and DPA (in **b**) obtained from an anthropomorphic spine phantom. STDEV = standard deviation, STDMEAN = standard mean, CV = coefficient of variation, SEE = standard error of estimate, SEM = standard error of the mean. In **b**, measurements made before and after source change are indicated by a triangle and square, respectively. Precision of DPA is slightly improved after source change. CXA has approximately three fold better long-term in vitro precision than DPA (with permission from reference 38)

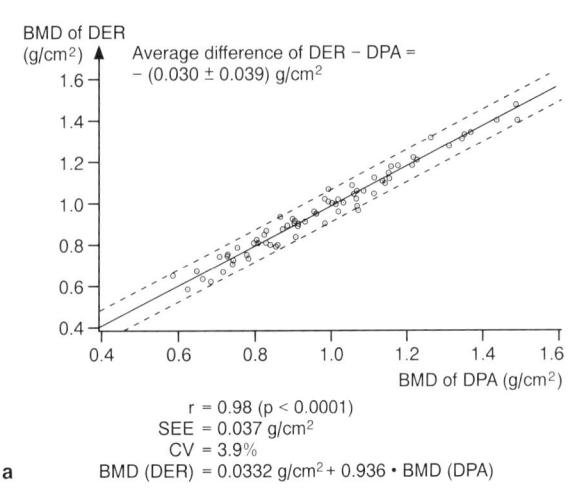

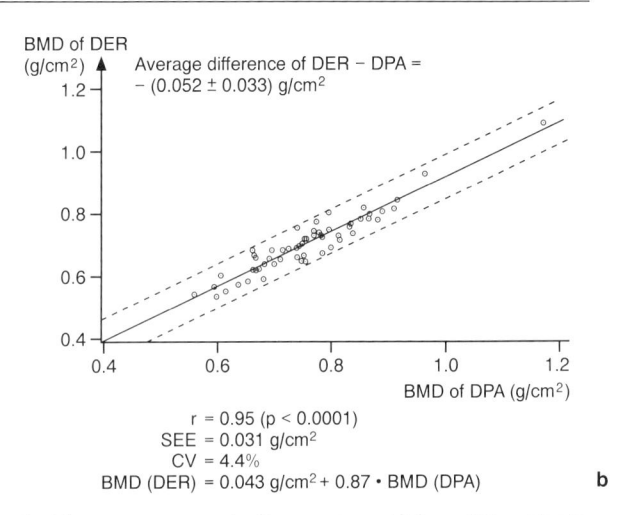

Fig. 11.7 Correlation of DXA and DPA results
a Spine measurements (L2–L4) from 72 patients
b Hip measurements (femoral neck) from 56 patients. SEE = standards error of the estimate.
DXA and DPA demonstrate excellent correlation in both the spine and the hip (with permission from reference 38)

(z-score = –1.41), for lateral DXA –58.7% (z-score = –1.99), and for QCT –50.4% (z-score = –2.9%) (58). These results indicate the improved sensitivity of lateral DXA over AP-DXA in assessing perimenopausal and postmenopausal bone loss. Similar results were reported by Slosman et al. (111). In the UCSF study, the correlation between lateral DXA and QCT was also better than that between AP-DXA and QCT (AP-DXA versus QCT: r = 0.75; lateral DXA versus QCT: r = 0.86) (58).

The precision and accuracy of lateral DXA obtained with the patient in a decubitus position is, however, affected by difficulties in placing the patient in a reproducible fashion in a decubitus lateral position. Slosman et al. found a coefficient of variation of BMD lateral decubitus spine measurements of 2.8% obtained in 20 healthy volunteers after repositioning (111). Similar results were reported by Mazess et al. (73).

This problem can be overcome with a device such as the Hologic QDR 2000 that affords rotation of the X-ray source and the detectors from a vertical orientation into a horizontal orientation, so that lateral spine measurements can be obtained with the patient in a supine position. Since the X-ray tube and the detectors are rotated, the patient does not need to be repositioned after the AP-scan and landmarks that have been established in the AP scan can be used for the lateral scan. Harper et al. (45) found comparable precision of 0.012 and 0.012 gms/cm² for AP and lateral supine measurements, respectively. Likewise, the measured biological variability, i.e., the average coefficient of variation, of the normal population in their study was similar (14.8% for AP and 15.4% for supine lateral measurements). The loss in bone mineral density observed in patients between the ages of 30 and 70 was significantly higher with lateral supine DXA (–34%) than with AP-DXA (–21%) (45). They concluded that supine lateral DXA is a precise technique that provides improved diagnostic sensitivity when compared to AP-DXA measurements (45). Improved sensitivity when compared to AP-DXA and higher precision when compared to decubitus lateral DXA was also reported by Slosman et al. (110).

With the pencil beam systems, both AP-spine and AP-hip measurements are generated with a radiation dose of approximately 2–3 mrem (38); the radiation dose for lateral scans of the spine obtained in decubitus position amounts to approximately 15 mrem. Examination time for an AP-spine measurement using a pencil-beam scanner ranges from 5 to 8 minutes; AP-hip pencil beam measurements take between 2 and 5 minutes. A total body measurement with pencil beam technique requires between 10 and 20 minutes.

With the fan beam technique currently available on the Hologic QDR 2000, AP-spine and AP-hip measurements have approximately 3–12 mrem radiation dose (Table 11.1); the examination time is, however, shortened by a factor of 4–5 or greater when compared to pencil beam systems. A total body examination in fan beam technique requires only approximately 5–6 minutes, which represents a marked improvement when compared to pencil beam scanners.

AP-DXA is readily available for braod clinical use (5, 38, 53, 71, 72, 86, 102, 106, 120, 122). The increased scan speed when compared to DPA represents a major advance. This is particularly important in osteoporotic patients who may complain about back pain when lying still for about 30 minutes. Moreover, errors resulting from patient motion are reduced and, finally, better utilization of the equipment is achieved, thereby reducing the overall costs of the examination. The improved precision of AP-DXA represents a major advantage over DPA and allows measurement of significant bone mineral changes over relatively short periods of time. AP-DXA is increasingly replacing DPA. The diagnostic sensitivity of lateral DXA surpasses that of AP-DXA and approaches that of QCT since it measures principally high-turnover trabecular bone. Lateral DXA obtained with the patient in a supine position has a precision that may come close to that of AP-DXA. The use of fan beam rather than pencil beam techniques helps to shorten scan times in measuring the spine, the hip, and the total body with DXA.

Quantitative Computed Tomography

For measuring the spine, quantitative computed tomography (QCT) (32, 91) affords capability for precise three-dimensional anatomic localization providing a direct density measurement, and allows the radiologist to spatially distinguish highly responsive cancellous bone from less responsive cortical bone. The lumbar vertebrae contain substantial amounts of compact bone and only part of the spinal bone mineral is high-turnover trabecular bone.

Technical Aspects of Vertebral QCT

QCT measurements developed at UCSF (11, 29) rely on commercially available CT scanners and use a mineral standard for simultaneous calibration (Fig. 11.8), a computed radiograph (scout view) for localization (Fig. 11.9a), and either single—or dual—energy techniques (12, 29, 61). Representative volumes (approximately 4 cm^3) of purely trabecular bone at the midplane of 2 to 4 lumbar vertebral bodies are quantified and averaged (Fig. 11.9b), and the results are expressed in mineral equivalents of solute dipotassium hydrogen phosphate (K$_2$HPO$_4$) in mg/ml a density measurement). The examination takes 5–10 minutes, and the radiation exposure is approximately 200 mrem, one-tenth the dose of a routine CT study. (The radiation dose is higher on some CT systems be

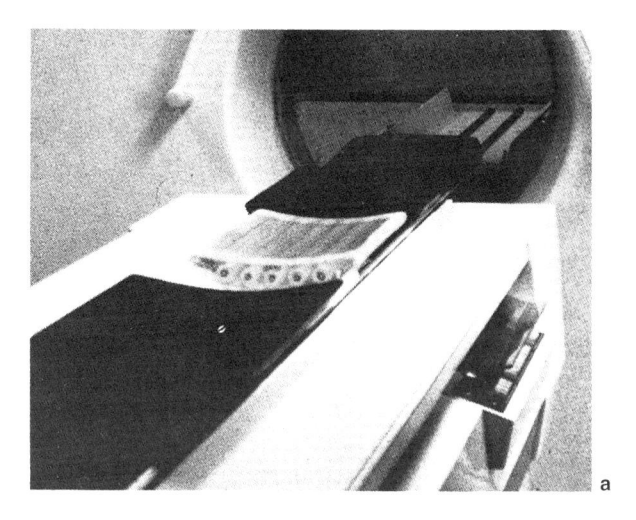

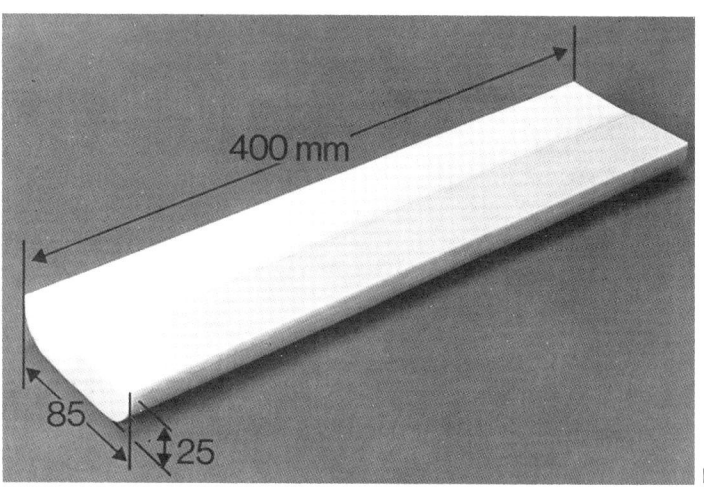

Fig. 11.8a Standardized version of Cann-Genant calibration phantom (11, 29) in use at over 500 centers worldwide
b Solid state phantom with small cross-sectional area. The phantom consists of two samples, a 200 mg/mL hydroxy-apatite and a water equivalent (with permission from reference 27)

332   11 Quantification of Osteoporosis

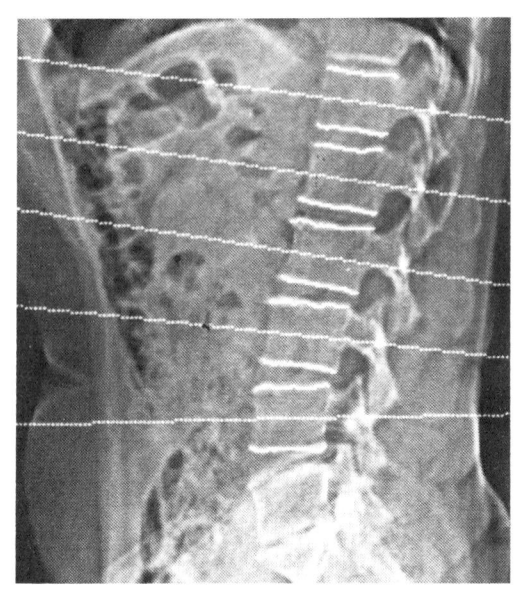

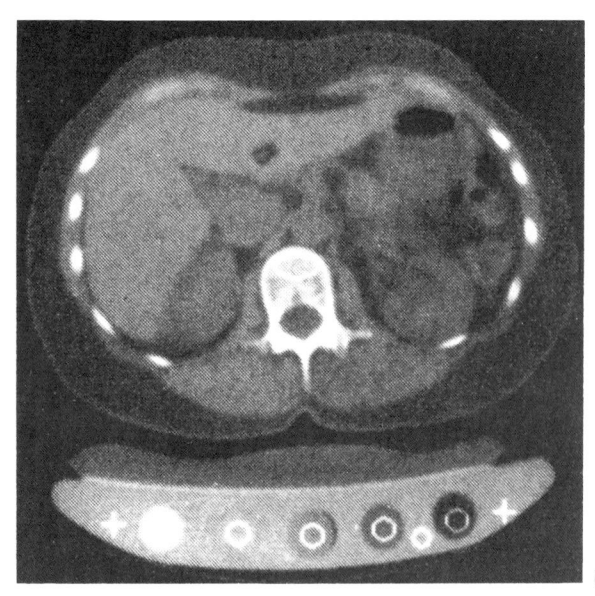

Fig. 11.**9a**   QCT spine technique using GE 9800 scanner. Lateral scout view provides a rapid and simple localization approach in which the midplane of four vertebral bodies are defined on the video monitor and a single 10-mm thick section is obtained at each level
b An oval region of interest, centered in the mid-vertebral body, is used to determine cancellous bone mineral content (mg/ml), while circular regions of interest are used to quantify the K_2HPO_4 solutions in the phantom (with permission from reference 27)

cause the manufacturers have restricted the ability to reduce kVp or mAs settings).

Simultaneous and nonsimultaneous calibration techniques are available. Simultaneous calibration (11) is used nowadays in most clinical applications (Fig. 11.**8**). For simultaneous calibration, the patient is placed on top of a calibration phantom that has inserts of known mineral density oriented perpendicular to the plane of the CT slices. The Cann-Genant phantom has cylindrical channels of solute dipotassium hydrogen phosphate (K_2HPO_4) of 50 mg/cc, 100 mg/mL, and 200mg/ml along with a water and a fat equivalent channel (Fig. 11.**8a**) (11). K_2HPO_4 has attenuation characteristics very similar to those of calcium hydroxyapatite ($Ca_{10}(PO_4)_6(OH)_2$), which closely represents the bulk of mineral found in bone. Since the K_2HPO_4 concentrations of the cylindrical inserts is known, they can serve as a calibration reference for determination of intravertebral bone mineral.

Aqueous solutions, as are used in this phantom, have the potential drawback of limited long-term stability due to the production of gas bubbles, precipitation of dissolved materials, and impurities (88). Because of these problems, solid-state phantoms have been developed. Solid-state phantoms are totally stable, i.e., their attenuating properties do not change with time, and they are sturdier and more resistant to damage (3, 51, 52).

Simultaneous calibration corrects to a large extent for short– and long-term scanner instability. Non-simultaneous calibration was used with limited success (10) in earlier studies (1); with the introduction of fourth generation CT scanners, there is increased interest in nonsimultaneous calibration. With nonsimultaneous calibration, a quasianthropomorphic tissue equivalent calibration phantom is scanned before the patient and after the patient or both (40). By mounting one or two additional attenuator rings, the phantom can be matched approximately to the patient's size. Obviously, nonsimultaneous reference phantoms can not correct for scanner instabilities between the calibration measurements, and the subjective choice of attenuator rings is only an approximation of patient size and composition. Moreover, it might lead to reproducibility errors if chosen differently.

Slices, 8–10 mm thick, are taken parallel to the vertebral endplates by tilting the gantry appropriately. The operator can address the coordinate system that is logged to the image and use trackballs to define the positions of the scans to be taken. Automated determination of the midvertebral CT slice, which has been presented recently (50), helps to further reduce precision errors (63).

Currently, in most centers, evaluation is performed by the operator by placing an elliptical ROI manually in the vertebral body (Fig. 11.**9b**); using this technique, reproducibility of bone mineral measurements is influenced by operator performance. Automated evaluation optimizes reproducibility and simplifies the operator's task. Recent image-evaluation software incorporating contour-tracking techniques allows for anatomically adapted and automatically placed ROIs (51, 105, 114, 115) (Fig. 11.**10**).

Steiger and Genant (114, 115) propose an automated image evaluation that automatically yields vertebral bone mineral density for an integral, a peeled, and an elliptical ROI. The integral ROI includes the cortex and the trabecular portions of the vertebral body and the spinous process; transverse processes are excluded from analysis (Fig. 11.**10 a**). The peeled ROI is defined at a constant disfance from the bone edge similar to the peeled ROI that had been initially described by Sandor (105). The peeled ROI is designed to exclude cortical bone (Fig. 11.**10c**). The elliptical ROI has been traditionally used in the determination of vertebral bone mineral content (Fig. 11.**10 d**). Calibration is also performed automatically, with the option of operator interference in case the calibration ROIs are misplaced. Similar automated image-evaluation packages are already being offered commercially (51, 52).

Steiger and Genant (114) tested the proposed ROIs in a series fo 214 women. ROIs were tested with both single and dual energy techniques. Decreasing bone mineral density with age was evident in all ROIs with both single and dual energy techniques (Fig. 11.**11 a**). The different ROIs were compared with use of percentage decrements and z-scores. Percentage decrements are helpful in observing group differences in cross-sectional studies, whereas z-scores have individual diagnostic value, because they account for the group variance. In terms of percentage decrements, the elliptical and peeled ROIs showed equivalent results; however, the elliptical ROI yielded larger z-scores in most comparisons and may, therefore, be slightly more useful in diagnosis than the peeled ROI. These recent data do not support the switch from the use of the elliptical ROI for clinical reasons (114). However, an automated placement of the elliptical ROI will reduce the precision error caused by the interactive and operator-dependent sizing and placement of the ROI (51, 52, 105).

The limitation of the integral ROI used by Steiger and Genant (114) is that it excludes the vertebral endplates and parts of the pedicles, laminae, and spinous processes; nonetheless, substantial portions of these structures are still included. Jones, (49) as well as Steiger and Genant (114), observed that patients with osteoporosis have a lower ratio of trabecular bone to integral bone than do normal control subjects. The integral ROI is necessary in order to determine this ratio and may thus add some new information about bone status in health and disease (114).

For single-energy QCT, a low-dose, low-energy setting should be selected resulting in an organ dose of typically 200 mrem and essentially no gonadal exposure. The low-voltage setting also provides a relatively high sensitivity to mineral variations and less to fat variations.

For dual-energy QCT, the lower energy setting should be as slow as possible, with an optimum effective energy of about 40 keV (119) or a peak voltage setting of 65 kVp (134); current scanners allow measurements to be taken at about 80 kVp, which corresponds to approximately 55 keV effective energy. This setting is almost as good as 40 keV (119). The upper energy should be as high as possible (typically 120 or 140 kVp), and the dose, theoretically, should be about equal at both energies (119), although it is generally greater at the higher energy level.

The precision of vertebral QCT in humans is 1% to 3% for single-energy (80 kVp) and 3% to 5% for dual-energy (80 kVp/120 kVp) techniques (32). The accuracy of single-energy QCT is 1% to 2% for K_2HPO_4 solutions and 5% to 15% for human vertebral specimens spanning a wide age range (30, 31, 91).

The density of yellow marrow is less than that of red marrow because of the presence of fat, which falsely reduces the measured spinal mineral value (by approximately 7 mg per 10% fat by volume at 80 kVp), and can result in inaccuracies of 20% to 30% in measurements in the elderly osteoporotic population. Dual-energy QCT (12, 29, 61), which is now offered by several manufacturers, can reduce the magnitude of this error due to fat in the marrow of the elderly to approximately 5%, but at the expense of reduced precision. Dual-energy QCT is considered unnecessary for most clinical applications; however, when highly accurate measurements are needed (for instance in special research applications), both single— and dual—energy QCT can be performed initially at baseline. Single-energy QCT can then be applied for longitudinal follow-up, thus maintaining high precision.

Steiger and Genant recommend a modified quantitative CT protocol for clinical applications in which bone mineral density of only L1 and L2 are measured at a fixed gantry tilt (114). They found that BMD decreases from T12 to L3 on an average of 9–13 mg/mL (Fig. 11.**12 a**). The correlation between average spinal BMD of T12 to L3 and average BMD of L1 and L2 was strong (r = 0.997) (Fig. 11.**12 b**). Thus, the average BMD of T12 to L3 can be accurately predicted by the average of BMD of L1 and L2 (114).

The gantry tilt necessary to align the CT slice parallel to the vertebral endplates in greatest between L2 and L3 and least evident between T12 and L1 (114). With the assumption that the average anterior vertebral body extends over 40 mm, to 50 mm and that the average tilt adjustement in a normal postmenopausal group is 3.6^0(114), the use of a fixed gantry tilt for measuring L1 and L2 would result in a shift of effective section position of 0.6 mm to 0.8 mm. The additional variation introduced by this technique is negligible in clinical settings in which the one-time assess-

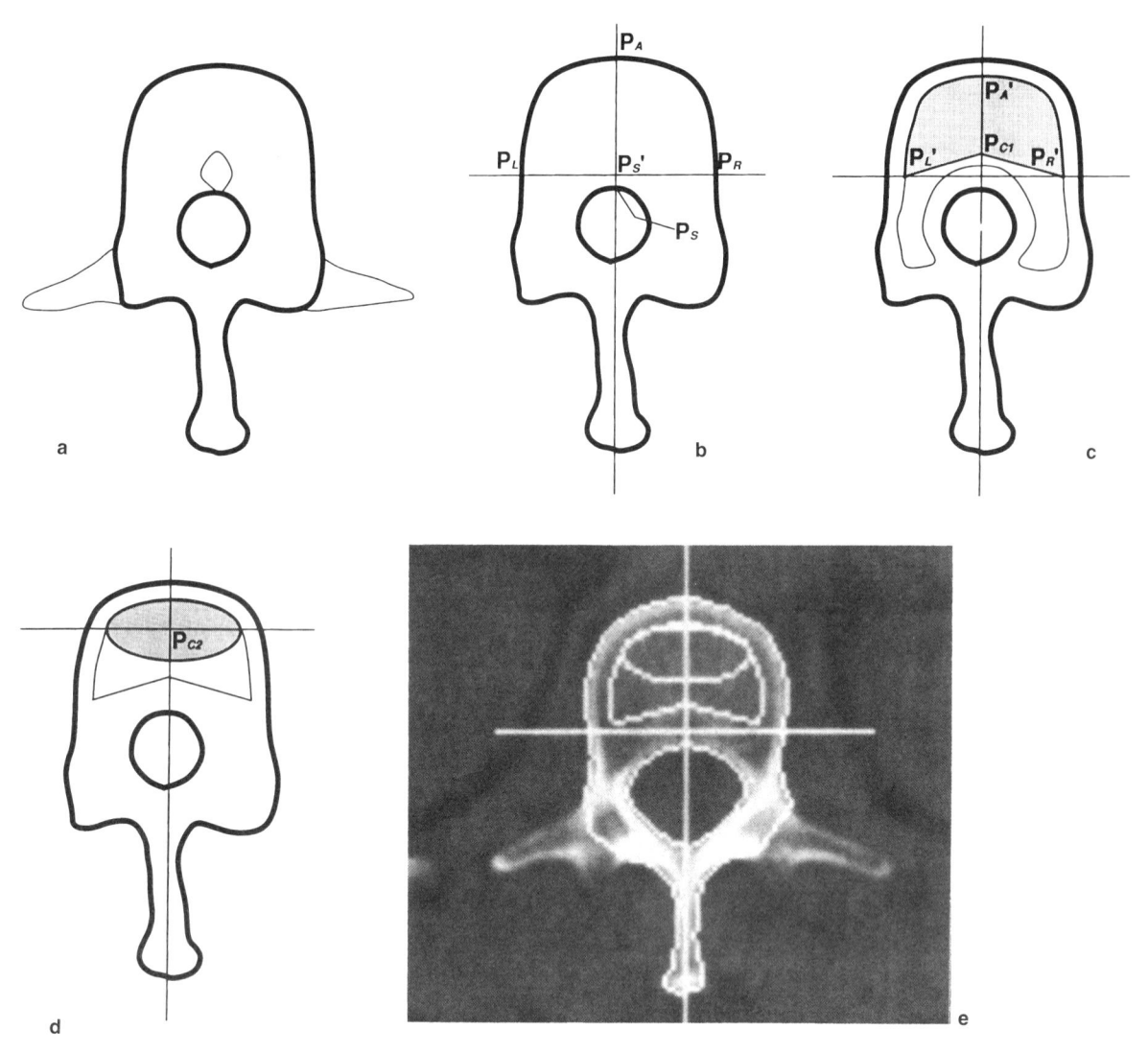

Fig. 11.10 Automated evaluation of a vertebral body with the Quantitative Image Evaluation Technique (QUIET) software system. The automatic execution as outlined below takes approximately 2–3 seconds on a VAX station 3250. The operator can intervene if the automatic ROI determination should fail or if manual corrections are needed for anatomic irregularities. The evaluation is fully automatic in most cases. Only approximately 3% of cases require complete manual placement of the elliptical ROI. The evaluation of the calibration phantom, measured simultaneously with the patient study by following the technique described by Cann and Genant (11, 29), is also localized and evaluated automatically

a Contour detection and integral ROI. The contours of the vertebral body and the spinal canal are automatically tracked. The spinal canal contour is automatically smoothed to avoid inclusion of the base venous complex. The transverse processes are clipped by eliminating convex contour segments that turn more than 135° over 9 mm. The posterior spinous process is not eliminated. The bold lines represent the resulting integral ROI

b Principal axis determination. The vertical principal axis of the vertebral body without the transverse processes is computed along with its intersections with the outer and spinal cord contours, PA and PS. The height of the anterior vertebral body h is computed as the distance PAPS. A line perpendicular to the principal axis (the baseline) is drawn through PS', located on the principal axis 0.1 h above PS. The intersection of the baseline with the outer contour yields PL and PR and the vertebral body width W as the distance PLPR

c Peeled ROI. A new contour is defined at a constant distance (0.12 w) from the bone edge (thin line). Its intersections with the principal axis and the baseline yield PA', PL', and PR'. PC1 is located on the principal axis at 0.275 h from PS. The anterior portion of the peeled contour along with the triangle PL'PC1PR' defines the peeled ROI (shaded area). This ROI closely resembles the one proposed by Sandor et al. (105)

d Elliptical ROI. The elliptical ROI has been traditionally used in the determination of vertebral body content. A line perpendicular to the principal axis is drawn through PC2, located at 0.63 h above PS. This line is one of the ellipse axes, and, along with its intersections with the peeled contour and PA', it defines the elliptical ROI

e The three different ROIs and the principal axis system for lumbar vertebral (L1) (with permission from reference 114)

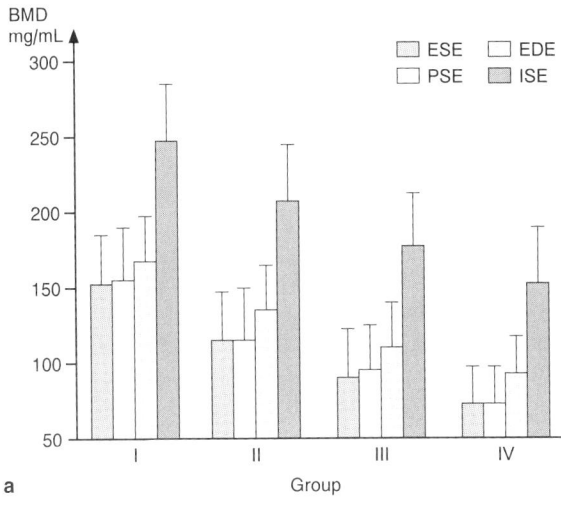

Fig. 11.**11a** Bone mineral density as a function of patient group and ROI. (214 women; group I: healthy premenopausal women; group II: healthy early postmenopausal women; group III: healthy late postmenopausal women; group IV: osteoporotic postmenopausal women). ESE = elliptical ROI, single energy; PSE = peeled ROI, single energy; EDE = elliptical ROI, dual energy; ISE = integral ROI, single energy

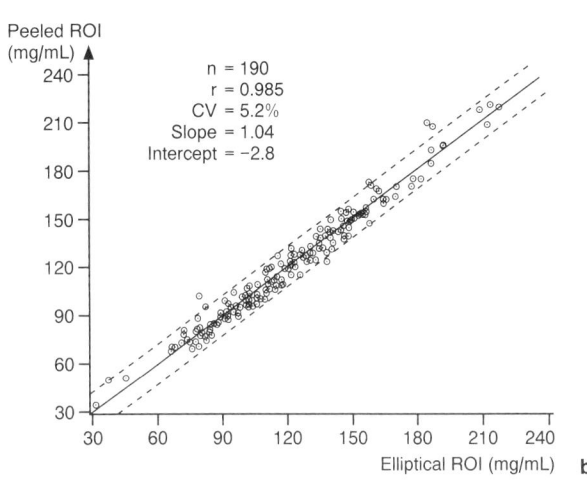

b Correlation of elliptical and peeled ROIs in healthy pre- and postmenopausal women (groups 1–3) (with permission from reference 114)

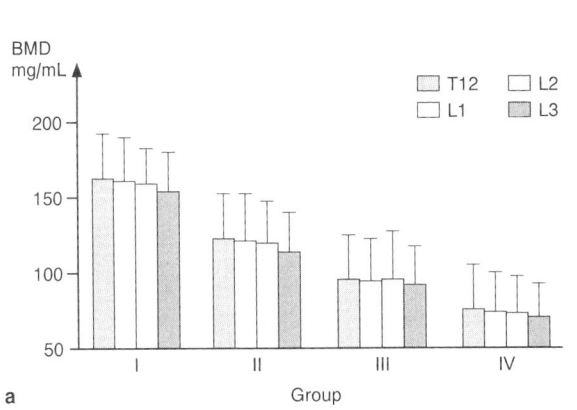

Fig. 11.**12a** Bone mineral density (BMD) as a function of vertebral level in 214 women. (Group I: healthy premenopausal women; group II: healthy early postmenopausal women; group III: healthy late postmenopausal women; group IV: osteoporotic postmenopausal women). BMD decreases from T12 to L3 on an average of 9 – 13 g/ml

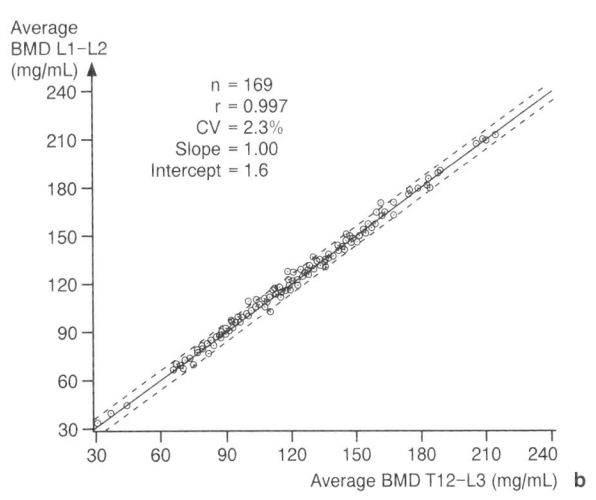

b Correlation of BMD expressed as average of T12 through L3 versus average of L1 and L2 in healthy pre- and postmenopausal women (with permission from reference 114)

ment of an individual's BMD is the primary goal. The use of a constant gantry tilt and the assessment of L1 and L2 only would reduce the time required to perform quantitative CT scanning of the spine to approximately 5 minutes and decrease radiation exposure. In research settings, however, where highly precise longitudinal measurements are needed, scanning of three vertebral levels may be preferable.

Finite Element Analysis

Finite element analysis (FEA) is frequently employed by engineers to provide structural information in evaluating the strength of a new design. Mechanical engineers use FEA in the design of buildings and other structures. In FEA, a complex structure with unknown mechanical properties is divided into a series of geometrically simplified elements. The behaviour of each individual element is determined from mathematical equations relating applied forces or stresses to the expected displacement or strain of the element. In order to describe the mechanical behaviour of a structure completely using finite element analysis, knowledge of 1. the geometry, 2. the material properties, and 3. the loads acting on the object are needed. Model geometry is usually obtained directly from the object itself. Loading conditions are estimated based on the intended use of the structure. The mechanical properties are determined in compression tests of the materials comprising the structure under appropriate loading conditions.

The first FEA-based investigations analyzing the mechanical behaviour of the skeleton were performed in 1972 (7, 104). Initial applications were focused on evaluating artificial joints and fracture-fixation devices. The models used in these studies were not representative for the individual patient, but rather designed to characterize the behavior of the prosthetic devices implanted into the bone. Mechanical tests of excised specimens served to define the material properties of cortical and trabecular bone. These early studies indicated the feasibility of FEA for evaluating the complex geometry and loading conditions of the human skeleton.

Finite element models that are specific for individual patients have recently been developed using three-dimensional contiguous slice QCT studies of the spine (22, 24) (Fig. 11.**13**) and of the hip (54, 62). The data obtained with patient-specific FEA were demonstrated to correlate with the measured mechanical in vitro behaviour of vertebral and femoral specimens. Faulkner et al. (22, 24) evaluated estimates of vertebral strength obtained with FEA for the ability to discriminate between normal, healthy, and osteoporotic patients (Fig. 11.**13**). They studied 28 normal patients and 15 patients with radiographically proved osteoporotic fracture. Three-dimensional QCT examinations were used to generate FEA models of L1 and L2 or both. A large variation in the FEA-estimated strength was found between models that were characterized by almost the same total bone content and trabecular mineral density (22, 24). Since these models contained the same amount of bone, the difference in FEA-estimated strength was thought to reflect the pattern with which the bone was distributed through the model. This pattern is not reflected in the bone density and bone mineral content measurements. Faulkner et al. (22, 24) concluded that FEA provides a reasonably valid model for estimating vertebral strength. Using receiver operating curve (ROC) analysis, they found that vertebral FEA strength measurements provide a slight, but statistically significant improvement over QCT measurements of trabecular density for differentiating between normal and osteoporotic patients (Fig. 11.**14**) (22, 24). The technique is, however, computationally very intensive and is therefore limited by long computing times. Improvements in computing time and precision may help to implement this technique into clinical routine for evaluating the osteoporotic patient and for identifying the patient who is at risk for osteoporotic fracture.

Ultrasound

Whereas bone mass has been established as a sensitive predictor for fracture risk in osteoporotic populations, other factors such as an accumulated burden of fatigue damage and ineffective trabecular architecture greatly influence bone fragility. Ultrasound has been proposed as a new, noninvasive technique for estimating bone mass that may also provide information on bone quality. In evaluating bone using ultrasound methods, two different technical approaches have become available. One technique measures the speed of sound (SOS) in bone, the other technique is based on broadband ultrasound attenuation (BUA) (Fig. 11.**15**) (2).

Initial SOS studies have focused on the in vivo measurement of the ultrasonic velocity in the cortical part of the femur or proximal radius, and in the patella (41, 46); more recently, SOS measurements have also been performed in the os calcis (59). SOS is a function of mass density and elastic modulus. The elastic modulus is influenced by the spatial configuration of the trabeculae, biomechanical properties of bone, and fatigue damage. Thus, bone mass and qualitative characteristics of bone contribute to SOS in bone. Greenfield et al. (41) suggested that SOS measurements may improve differentiation between normal and abnormal bone in osteoporosis and metabolic bone disease. Heaney et al. (46) reported that patellar SOS measurements can discriminate between normal and osteoporotic women as well as bone densitometry in the axial skeleton. In addition, low values of ultrasonic SOS have been reported to be predictive of future vertebral crush fracture. Brandenburger et al. (6)

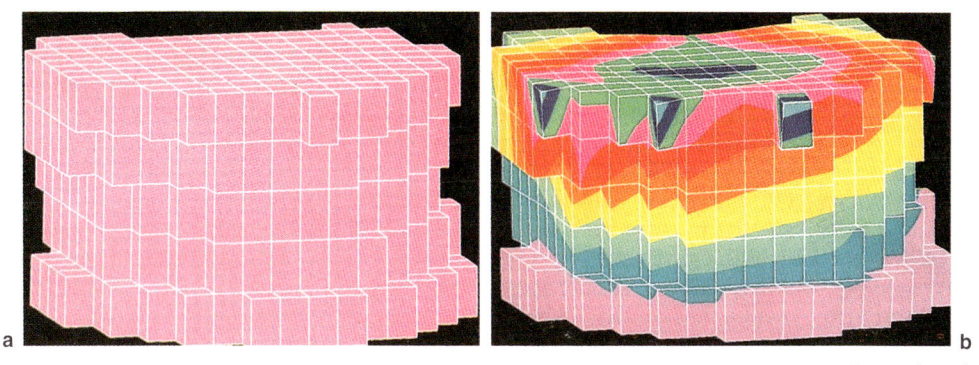

Fig. 11.**13a** Patient-specific finite element mesh of a vertebral body generated from three-dimensional quantitative CT data. In this case, the mesh is made of 575 rectangular solid elements
b Deformed mesh plot of (**a**) generated from analysis results. Banded displacement contours show regions of minimal displacement at inferior model surface (where model is contained not to move) up to large displacement regions at superior surface of model. These results can be used to estimate strength of vertebral body (with permission from 25)

demonstrated that subjects with SOS of one standard deviation or more below normal had three to five times higher risk of fracture in the next 2 years than those with normal readings. Short-term reproducibility data of SOS in the patella yielded an interoperator coefficient of variation of 1.85%; 6-month reproducibility data demonstrated a coefficient of variation of 2.3% (46).

Investigations have also concentrated on the use of BUA of the os calcis (4, 59, 89). The BUA value of the os calcis is measured as a function of frequency by using a receive and emit transducer on each side of the heel. The transducers and the heel are immersed in a water bath. Langton et al. (59) demonstrated that BUA is dependent on the bone mineral content of the os calcis and concluded that the technique can be used to determine bone loss and study the onset and progression of osteoporosis. Baran et al. (4) compared vertebral and femoral BMD measured by dual photon absorptiometry and BUA in women with vertebral osteoporosis, women with hip fractures, and age-matched controls. They demonstrated that BUA values were significantly decreased in women with osteoporosis and women with hip fractures; correlation between bone density measurements and BUA values was also significant. McKelvie et al. (77) found in vitro correlations between BUA and QCT of $r = 0.92$ and $r = 0.86$ for the os calcis and trabecular samples, respectively. Resch et al. (89) reported decreased BUA values in osteoporotic women; in vivo BUA values correlated significantly with QCT results ($t = 0.25$, $p < 0.005$). Short-term BUA reproducibility in the os calcis ranges between 1.35% (59) and 2.5% (77). Measuring BUA on excised human vertebrae, McKelvie et al. (76) described a correlation

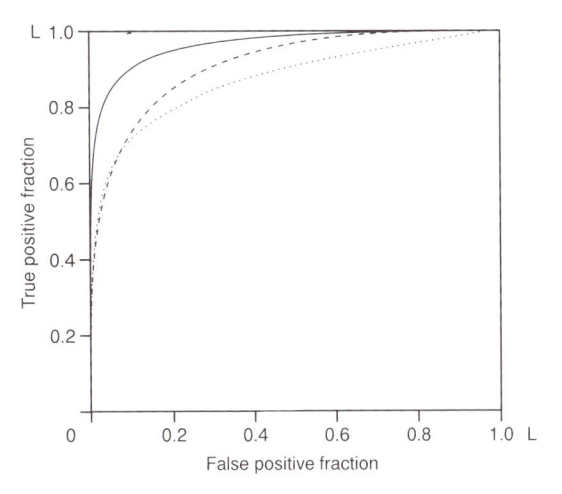

Fig. 11.**14** Receiver-operating-characteristic (ROC) curves for distinguishing control subjects from patients with osteoporosis on the basis of FEA estimated vertebral yield test (thick line), QCT-determined trabecular mineral density (dashed line), and total vertebral body bone content (thin line). Curves are based on results from 28 control subjects and 15 patients with osteoporosis. Area under the FEA ROC curve (0.964) is statistically larger ($p < 0.05$) than the areas under the density (0.907) and content (0.871) curves (with permission from 23)

between BUA and maximum compressive strength of $r = 0.46$. The correlation improved markedly to $r = 0.82$ when averaging 4 to 5 vertebrae obtained from the same cadaver, indicating the potential of BUA for direct assessment of bone strength.

Ultrasonic speed of sound and broadband ultrasound attenuation measurements represent new,

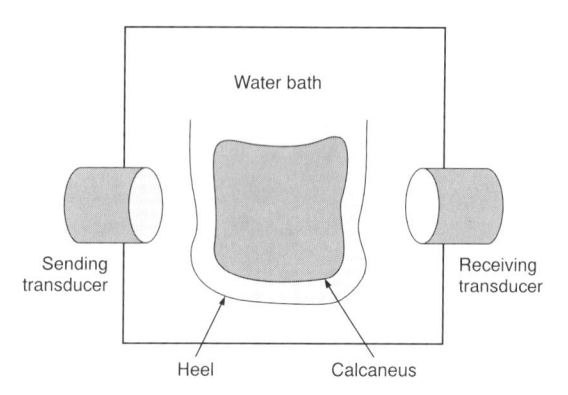

Fig. 11.**15** Schematic diagram shows method for measuring broadband ultrasound attenuation (BUA) and speed of sound (SOS) at the heel or both. For heel measurement, water immersion is necessary to eliminate air between transducers and facilitate transmission of sound wave to measurement site (with permission from 25)

simple, radiation-free methods to assess bone mass and quality that may become useful in the management of osteoporosis. The ultimate clinical value of ultrasound methods in evaluating osteoporosis remains to be established in larger prospective studies.

Magnetic Resonance Imaging

Recent reports indicate the potential use of MRI as a means of assessing bone mineral density and perhaps even bone structure without ionizing radiation (16, 18, 64, 66, 68, 108).

With increasing age, T1 and T2 relaxation times of the vertebral marrow have been demonstrated to decrease progressively (18, 90); histologically, there is loss in vertebral bone mineral, concomitant decrease in hematopoietic marrow, and increase in fatty marrow. Fatty marrow expands into the widened marrow spaces as trabecular rarefaction progresses. Consequently, the T1 relaxation times of vertebral marrow become similar to those of fat which is characterized by a relatively short T1 and T2 relaxation time. Since bone mineral density and the amount of intertrabecular fatty marrow are inversely related, it has been speculated that MR relaxation parameters may potentially be used in the future to assess bone mineral density (18). However, the amount of red and fatty marrow is also dependent on a large number of other factors such as hematopoietic demand, so that this approach does not appear promising at the present time.

More recent studies have focused on the influence of trabecular bone on marrow signal intensity. Davis et al. (16) performed experiments in which they immersed bone powder in water and cottonseed oil; as the bone surface to volume ratio increased, they observed a significant decrease in T2* relaxation for both water and oil (16). Similarly, Rosenthal et al. (97) have measured a reduction in the T2* of water present in the trabecular spaces compared to extratrabecular water using specimens of excised human vertebrae. These results suggest that the presence of trabecular bone in the marrow space will cause T2* shortening and thus signal loss.

The influence of trabecular density on MR signal intensity in gradient-echo images can be reproduced in vivo in imaging the knee joint (108). Fatty marrow demonstrates high signal intensity on gradient-echo MR images in the diaphysis with its relatively low trabecular density. In areas of high trabecular density such as the epiphysis, however, low signal intensity will be observed on gradient-echo MR images resulting from more pronounced T2*-shortening at the bone–marrow interface.

Bone density and T2* relaxation have been recently directly correlated in vitro and in vivo. Majumdar et al. (65, 68) found a strong correlation between vertebral bone density derterminded by QCT and the inverse of T2* relaxation (1/T2*) ($r = 0.92$; $p \leq 0.0001$) in an in vitro study (Fig. 11.**16**). In a second experiment, Majumdar et al. (67) also correlated elastic modulus of trabecular bone specimen with 1/T2*. In these preliminary studies, the correlation of 1/T2* with elastic modulus ($r = 0.98$) was greater than that between 1/T2* and bone density ($r = 0.82$) determined by quantitative computed tomography (67).

Wehrli et al. (128) obtained similar results using NMR interferometry. They found that T2* in healthy persons increases slightly with age (128). In patients with osteroporosis, however, T2* values are signifi-

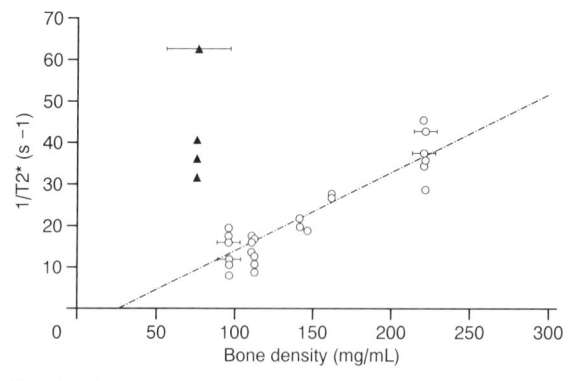

Fig. 11.**16** Variation of 1/T2* as a function of trabecular density (with permission from: 68). Bone mineral density was determined with quantitative computed tomography. 1/T2* was measured using a gradient-echo sequence with echo times varying from 10 to 50 ms. The correlation between 1/T2* and bone mineral density is high ($r = 0.92$, $p < 0.0001$). (Triangle: specimen which disintegrated during evacuation with a vacuum pump—excluded from statistical analysis)

cantly prolonged, which is likely to be caused by a enlargement of the intertrabecular space (128).

An additional new MR-based modality for evaluating trabecular microarchitecture is MR microscopy. Wehrli et al. (127, 129) were able to generate "microscopic" images with sufficient spatial resolution to demonstrate individual trabeculae. The in-plane resolution of these images ranged from 33×33 μm to 66×66 μm. The study had, however, been performed at a field strength of 9.4 T—significantly higher than what is currently available for in vivo studies in humans. In addition, the marrow had been removed from the specimen in order to avoid chemical shift artifact.

$T2^*$ decay may not only be influenced by trabecular density, but also by trabecular geometry as is suggested by the greater correlation of $1/T2^*$ with elastic modulus as compared with bone density (67). MR imaging may thereby provide unique information not only on trabecular density but also on trabecular structure and architecture. The information provided by quantitative MRI may be useful in the future in assessing bone strength and predicting fracture risk. However, both techniques require significant development before they can be used clinically.

Clinical Use of Bone Densitometry

Evaluation of Patients with Metabolic Disease Affecting the Skeleton

Many metabolic disorders including hyperparathyroidism, Cushing syndrome, and amenorrhea among premenopausal women, as well as chronic immobilization and chronic steroid and thyroid therapy have profound influence on calcium metabolism and may adversely affect the skeleton. In these secondary forms of osteoporosis, bone density measurements are important in the overall clinical evaluation, because they may prompt decisions such as reduction of corticosteroids in the case of steroid-induced osteoporosis (37, 93), subtotal parathyroidectomy in the case of hyperparathyroid bone disease (35, 55, 92), or initiation of estrogen replacement therapy in the case of amenorrhea or oligomenorrhea (14, 32, 94).

Evaluation of Perimenopausal Women for Initiation of Estrogen Therapy

The loss of bone due to accelerated resorption in women at menopause is a universally accepted phenomenon; loss of ovarian function profoundly influences the risk for development of osteoporosis. Most women who begin estrogen replacement therapy at the time of menopause or soon thereafter are spared the normal skeletal degradation that would otherwise occur at this point in the life cycle (21). Perhaps more important, long-term estrogen replacement therapy reduces the risk likelihood of fracture twofold (20).

Decisions about initiation of estrogen therapy may be contingent on a number of factors, including current level of bone density, severity of menopausal symptoms, patient or physician preferences, laboratory evidence of rapid bone loss, and possibly the long-term risk of cardiovascular disease (47). Many experts agree that compliance with estrogen therapy may be enhanced by quantitative information concerning fracture risk and efficacy of treatment.

The absolute level of bone density at menopause and the magnitude of subsequent bone loss are important considerations in assessing risk for fracture. Even considering menopausal and age-related decrements in bone mass, the subgroup of women who have high bone density at menopause will most likely have less risk of fracture due to their relatively dense skeletons and may not require estrogen or other interventions. Similarly, women with low to moderate levels of bone density appear to be at increased risk for fracture if therapy is not initiated early (80, 94, 124). The decision to begin prophylaxis against osteoporosis, therefore, can most appropriately be made with knowledge of the woman's bone density.

Detection of Osteoporosis and Assessment of its Severity

Recent reports suggest (15, 125) that historically based risk factors (e. g., low calcium intake, smoking, family history of osteoporosis, petite frame), taken either singularly or in combination, have limited predictive value for fracture risk or for bone density in the individual patient, but some characteristics such as female, postmenopausal, white, and elderly, may be helpful in targeting certain populations for study. Similarly, it is generally acknowledged that substantial bone loss may precede radiographically detectable osteoporosis or fracture. Furthermore, even the presence of osteoporotic fracture may confer uncertain and variable risk for future fracture.

For several reasons, bone density per se provides the primary standard of osteoporosis risk: First, most of the variance in bone strength is attributable to bone density (44, 75, 78). Second, recent studies suggest a gradient of increasing fracture risk corresponding to declining levels in bone density (79, 80, 98, 99, 126). Third, prophylactic agents such as estrogen that reduce occurence of hip and spine fractures undoubtedly do so by retarding bone loss.

It should be recommended, therefore, that bone densitometry of the skeleton be performed in individuals in whom osteoporosis is suggested or in whom a traumatic fracture is suggested based on radiographic findings. If fracture risk, assessed by means of bone densitometry, is low, conservative patient management, perhaps with calcium and exercise, should be employed. If fracture risk is high, more aggressive treatment, perhaps with estrogen and calcitonin, should be prescribed.

Monitoring of Treatment, Evaluation of Disease Course

In the past, bone density measurement techniques were associated with large precision errors relative to estimated rates of change and were therefore criticized, because they could not be used to monitor changes in bone density in individual patients. In response to this criticism, substantial improvements have been made in the recent years. At present, SPA with rectilinear scanning, DXA, and QCT with automatic image analysis have precision errors that approach 1% to 2% (Table 11.1). To achieve precision levels of this degree, however, adherence to strict quality assurance measures and careful technical monitoring are necessary.

Numerous studies have shown that large annual losses of 5% to 20% from sites rich in trabecular bone can be observed in women undergoing surgical or natural menopause (21, 32, 96), in patients beginning high-dose corticosteroid treatment (91), and in individuals who are completely immobilized (57, 74). Similarly, large annual gains of 5% to 15% have been observed in some osteoporotic patients receiving calcitonin treatment (36, 42) or investigational agents such as sodium fluoride (19), bisphosphonates (34), or parathyroid hormone (112).

Given the marked effect of some interventions, continued improvements in measurement precision and the speed at which bone density measurements can now be performed and their reduced cost, it is difficult to pose convincing arguments against monitoring individual patients when important therapeutic decisions are to be made.

References

1. Abols Y, Genant HK, Rosenfled D, Boyd DP, Ettinger B, Gordon GS. Spinal bone mineral determination using computerized tomography in patients, controls, and phantoms. In: Mazess RB, eds. Proceedings of the 4th International Conference on Bone Measurement. US Government Printing Office. Washington, D.C.; 1979:80–1928.
2. Antich PP, Andereson JA, Ashman RB, Dowdey JE, Gonzalez J, Murry RC, et al. Measurement of mechanical properties of bone material in vitro by ultrasound reflection: methodology and comparison with ultrasound techniques. J Bone Min Res. 1991;6:417–426.
3. Arnold B. Solid phantom for QCT bone mineral analysis. In: eds. Proceedings of the 7th International Workshop on Bone Densitometry. Palm Springs: 7th International Workshop on Bone Densitometry; 1989.
4. Baran DT, Kelly AM, Karellas A, et al. Ultrasound attenuation of the os calcis in women with osteoporosis and hip fractures. Calcif Tiss Int. 1988;43:138–142.
5. Borders J, Kerr E, Sartoris DJ, Stein JA, Ramos E, Moscona AA, et al. Quantitative dual energy radiographic absorptiometry of the lumbar spine: in vivo comparison with dual-photon absorptiometry. Radiology. 1989;170:129–131.
6. Brandenburger GH, Kwon S, S.W. M, et al. Preliminary results from a longitudinal clinical study of ultrasound velocity. Atlanta: American Society for Bone Mineral Research; 1990.
7. Brekelmans WAM, Poort HW, Sloof TJJH. A new method to analyse the mechanical behavious of skeletal parts. Acta Orthop Scand. 1972;43:301–317.
8. Cameron EC, Boyd RM, Luk D, et al. Cortical thickness measurements and photon absorptiometry for determination of bone quantity. J Can Med Assoc. 1977;116:145–7.
9. Cameron JR, Mazess RB, Sorenson MS. Precision and accuracy of bone mineral determination by direct photon absorptiometry. Inves Radiol. 1968;3:141–50.
10. Cann CE. Quantitative computed tomography for bone mineral analysis: technical considerations. In: Genant HK, eds. Osteoporosis Update 1987. San Francisco: University of California Printing Services; 1987:131–145.
11. Cann CE, Genant HK. Precise measurement of vertebral mineral content using computed tomography. J Comp Assist Tomogr. 1980;4:493.
12. Cann CE, Genant HK. Single versus dual-energy CT for vertebral mineral quantification. J Comp Assist Tomogr. 1983;7(3):551.
13. Cann CE, Genant HK, Kolb FO, et al. Quantitative computed tomography for prediction of vertebral fracture risk. Metab Bone Dis Relat Res. 1984;5:1–7.
14. Cann CE, Martin MC, Genant HK, et al. Decreased spinal mineral content in amenorrheic women. JAMA. 1984;251:626–9.
15. Citron JT, Ettinger B, Genant HK. Prediction of peak premenopausal bone mass using a scale of weighted clinical variables. In: Christiansen C, Johansen JS, Riis BJ, eds. Osteoporosis 1987: proceedings of the International Symposium on Osteoporosis. Copenhagen: Osteopress; 1987:146–152.
16. Davis CA, Genant HK, Dunham JS. The effects of bone on proton NMR relaxation times of surrounding liquids. Invest Radiol. 1986;21:472–477.
17. Dawson-Hughes B, Deehr MS, Berger PS, Dallal GE, Sadowski LJ. Correction of the effects of source, source strength, and soft-tissue thickness on spine dual-photon absorptiometry measurements. Calcif Tiss Int. 1989;44:251–257.
18. Dooms GC, Fisher MR, Hricak H, Richardson M, Crooks LE, Genant HK. Bone marrow imaging: magnetic resonance studies related to age and sex. Radiology. 1985;155:429–432.
19. Duursma SA, Glerum JH, Van Dijk Aea. Responders and nonresponders after fluoride therapy in osteoporosis. Bone. 1987;8:131–136.
20. Ettinger B, Genant HK, Cann CE. Long-term estrogen replacement therapy prevents bone loss and fractures. Ann Intern Med. 1985;102:319–324.
21. Ettinger B, Genant HK, Cann CE. Postmenopausal bone loss ins prevented by low dosage estrogen with calcium. Ann Intern Med. 1986;106:40–45.
22. Faulkner K. Quantitative computed tomography and finite element modelling to predict vertebral fractures. [Doctoral Dissertation] University of California San Francisco; 1990.
23. Faulkner KG, Cann CE. ROC analysis of vertebral finite element models for fracture prediction: comparison with QCT. In: Christiansen C, Overgaard K, eds. Osteoporosis 1990. Copenhagen: Osteopress; 1990:1029–1031.
24. Faulkner KG, Cann CE, Hasegawa BH. Effect of bone distribution on vertebral strength: assessment with patient-specific nonlinear finite element analysis. Radiology. 1991;179:669–674.
25. Faulkner KG, Gluer CC, Majumdar S, Lang P, Engelke K, Genant HK. Noninvasive measurements of bone mass, structure, and strength: current methods and experimental techniques. AJR. 1991;157:1229–37.
26. Garn SM. The earlier gain and later loss of cortical bone. In: Thomas CC, eds. Nutritional Perspective. Springfield: 1970:146.
27. Genant HK, Block JE, Ettinger B, Glüer CC, Steiger PW. Quantitative computed tomography. Primer on Osteoporosis. San Francisco: University of California Press. 1988;15–38.
28. Genant HK, Block JE, Ettinger B, Glüer CC, Steiger PW. Single and dual photon absorptiometry. Primer on Osteoporosis. San Francisco: University of California Press. 1988;39–51.
29. Genant HK, Boyd DP. Quantitative bone mineral analysis using dual-energy computed tomography. Invest Radiol. 1977;12:545.

30. Genant HK, Cann CE, Boyd DP, et al. Quantitative computed tomography for vertebral mineral determination. In: Frame B, Potts JT, eds. Clinical disorders of bone and mineral metabolism. Amsterdam: Excerpta Medica; 1983:40–47.

31. Genant HK, Cann CE, Ettinger B, et al. Quantitative computed tomography for spinal assessment: current status. J Comp Assist Tomogr. 1985;9(3):602.

32. Genant HK, Cann CE, Ettinger B, Gordan GS. Quantitative computed tomography of vertebral spongiosa: A sensitive method for detecting early bone loss after oophorectomy. Ann Int Med. 1982;97:699–705.

33. Genant HK, Gluer CC, Faulkner KG, Majumdar S, Harris ST, Engelke K, et al. Acronyms in bone densitometry. Radiology. 1992;184:878.

34. Genant HK, Harris ST, Steiger P, Davey PF, Block JE. The effect of etidronate therapy in postmenopausal women: preliminary results. In: Christiansen C, Johansen JS, Riis BJ, eds. Osteoporosis 1987: proceedings of the International Symposium on Osteoporosis. Copenhagen: Osteopress; 1987: 1177–1181.

35. Genant HK, Heck LL, Lanzl LH, Rossmann K, Vander Horst J, Paloyan E. Primary hyperparathyroidism. Radiology. 1973;109:513–519.

36. Gennari C, Chierichetti SM, Bigazzi S, et al. Comparative effects on bone mineral content of calcium and calcium plus salmon calcitonin given in two different regimens in postmenopausal osteoporosis. Curr Ther Res. 1985;38:455–464.

37. Gennari C, Imbimbo B. Effects of prednisone and deflazacort on vertebral bone mass. Calc Tiss Int. 1985;37:592–593.

38. Glüer CC, Steiger P, Selvidge R, Elliesen-Kliefoth K, Hayashi C, Genant HK. Comparative assessment of dual-photon-absorptiometry and dual-energy-radiography. Radiology. 1990;174:223–228.

39. Glüer G-C, Reiser U, Davis CA, Rutt BK, Genant HK. Vertebral mineral determination by quantitative computed tomography (QCT): Accuracy of single and dual energy measurements. J Compt Asst Tomogr. 1988;12:242–58.

40. Goodsitt M, Rosenthal DI. Quantitative computed tomography scanning for measurement of bone and bone marrow fat content: a comparison of single and dual energy techniques using a solid synthetic phantom. Invest Radiol. 1987;22:799–810.

41. Greenfield MA, Craven JD, Huddleston A, Kehrer ML, Wishko D, Stern R. Measurement of the velocity of ultrasound in human cortical bone in vivo. Radiology. 1981;138:701–710.

42. Gruber HE, Ivey JL, Baylink DJ, et al. Long-term calcitonin therapy in postmenopausal osteoporosis. Metabolism. 1984;33:295–303.

43. Gustavson L, Jacobson B, Kusoffsky L. X-ray spectrophotometry for bone mineral determinations. Med Biol Eng Comput. 1974;12:113–118.

44. Hansson T, Roos B, Nachemson A. The bone mineral content and ultimate compressive strength of lumbar vertebrae. Spine. 1981;5:46–55.

45. Harper KD, Wilkinson WE, Lobaugh B, King ST, Drezner MK. Supine lateral dual energy x-ray apsorptiometry of the spine provides improved diagnostic sensitivity. 14th Annual Meeting of the American Society for Bone Mineral Research. Minneapolis: Mary Ann Liebert; 1992:S139.

46. Heaney RP, Avioli LV, Chesnut CH, Lappe J, Recker RR, Brandenburger GH. Osteoporotic bone fragility: detection by ultrasound transmission velocity. JAMA. 1989;261:2986–2990.

47. Hillner BE, Hollenberg JP, Pauker SG. Postmenopausal estrogens in the prevention of osteoporosis: a benefit that is virtually without risk if cardiovascular effects are considered. Am J Med. 1986;80:1115–1127.

48. Jacobson B. X-ray spectrophotometry in vivo. AJR. 1964;91:202–210.

49. Jones CD, Laval-Jeanet AM, Laval-Jeanet MH, Genant HK. Importance of measurement of spongious vertebral bone mineral density in the assessment of osteoporosis. Bone. 1987;8:201–6.

50. Kalender WA, Brestowsky H, Felsenberg D. Bone mineral measurements: automated determination of the midvertebral CT section. Radiology. 1988;168:219–221.

51. Kalender WA, Klotz E, Süss C. Vertebral bone mineral analysis: an integrated approach. Radiology. 1987;164:419–423.

52. Kalender WA, Süss C. A new calibration phantom for quantitative computed tomography. Med Phys. 1987;9:816–819.

53. Kelly TL, Slovik DM, Neer RM. Calibration and standardization of bone mineral densitometers. J Bone Min Res. 1989;4(5):663–669.

54. Keyak JH, Meagher JM, Skinner HB, Mote CD. Automated three-dimensional finite element modelling of bone: a new method. J Biomed Eng 1990;12:389–397.

55. Kochersberger G, Buckley NJ, Leight GS, Martinez S, et al. What is the clinical significance of bone loss in primary hyperparathyroidism. Arch Intern Med. 1987;147.

56. Krølner B, Pors Nielsen S. Measurement of bone mineral content (BMC) of the lumbar spine, Part I. Theory and application of a new two-dimensional dual photon attenuation method. Scand J Clin Lab Invest. 1980;40:485.

57. Krølner B, Toft B. Vertebral bone loss: an unheeded side effect of therapeutic bed rest. Clin Sci. 1983;64:537–549.

58. Lang P, Schmitz S, Steiger P, Genant HK. Lateral dual x-ray absorptiometry of the spine: a comparison with AP dual x-ray absorptiometry and quantitative computed tomography. In: Christiansen C, Overgaard K, eds. Osteoporosis 1990. Copenhagen: Osteopress; 1990:859–862.

59. Langton CM, Palmer SB, Porter RW. The measurement of broadband ultrasonic attenuation in cancellous bone. Eng Med. 1984;13:89–91.

60. Larcos G, Wahner HW. An evaluation of forearm bone mineral measurement with dual-energy X-ray absorptiometry. J Nucl Med. 1991;32:2101–2106.

61. Laval-Jeanet AM, Cann CE, Roger BM, et al. A postprocessing dual-energy technique for vertebral CT densitometry. J Comp Assist Tomogr. 1984;9:1164.

62. Lotz JC. Hip fracture risk predictions by x-ray computed tomography. [Doctoral Dissertation] Boston: Massachusetts Institute of Technology; 1988.

63. Louis O, Luypaert R, Kalender W, Osteaux M. Reproducibility of CT bone densitometry: operator versus automated ROI definition. Eur J Radiol. 1988;8:82–84.

64. Majumdar S. Quantitative study of the susceptibility difference between trabecular bone and bone marrow: computer simulations. Magn Reson Med. 1991;22:101–110.

65. Majumdar S, Genant HK. Quantitation of susceptibility effects in trabecular bone and their correlation with bone density. Society for Magnetic Resonance Imaging, 8th Annual Meeting, Printed Program Supplement: Society for Magnetic Resonance Imaging; 1990:22.

66. Majumdar S, Genant HK. Quantitation of susceptibility effects in trabecular bone and their correlation with bone density. Society for Magnetic Resonance Imaging, 8th Annual Meeting, Printed Program Supplement: Society for Magnetic Resonance Imaging; 1990:22.

67. Majumdar S, Keyak J, Lee I, Genant HK, Skinner H. Relationship between the mechanical properties of trabecular bone and intratrabecular marrow relaxation time T2*. Society for Magnetic Resonance in Medicine, Book of Abstracts. Berlin: Society for Magnetic Resonance in Medicine; 1992:1301.

68. Majumdar S, Thomasson D, Shimakawa A, Genant HK. Quantitation of the susceptibility difference between trabecular bone and bone marrow: experimental studies. Magn Reson Med. 1991;22:111–127.

69. Mazess R, Chesnut CH, McClung M, Genant HK. Enhanced precision with dual-energy x-ray absorptiometry. Calc Tiss Int. 1992;51:14–17.

70. Mazess RB, Barden H, Ettinger M, Schulz E. Bone density of the radius, spine, and proximal femur in osteoporosis. J Bone Min Res. 1988;3:13–18.

71. Mazess RB, Barden HS. Measurement of bone by dual-photon absorptiometry (DPA) and dual-energy x-ray absorptiometry (DEXA). Ann Chir Gyn. 1988;77:197–203.

72. Mazess RB, Collick B, Trempe J, Barden H, Hanson J. Performance evaluation of a dual energy x-ray bone densitometer. Calcif Tissue Int. 1989;44:228–232.

73. Mazess RB, Gifford CA, Bisek JP, Barden HS, Hanson JA. DEXA measurement of spine density in the lateral projection. I: Methodology. Calc Tiss Int. 1991;49:235–239.

74. Mazess RB, Whedon GD. Immobilization and bone. Calcif Tissue Int. 1983;35:265–7.

75. McBroom RJ, Hayes WC, Edwards WT, Goldberg RP, White AA. Prediction of vertebral body compressive fracture using quantitative computed tomography. J Bone Joint Surg (Am). 1985;67:1206–1214.
76. McKelvie M, Palmer S. The interaction of ultrasound with cancellous bone. Meeting of the Physical Acoustics Group of the Institute of Physics and the Institute of Acoustics. Hull: Institute of Physics; 1987.
77. McKelvie ML, Fordham J, Clifford C, Palmer SB. In vitro comparison of quantitative computed tomography and broadband ultrasound attenuation of trabecular bone. Bone. 1989;10:101–104.
78. Melton LJI, Riggs BL. Risk factors for injury after a fall. Clin Geriatr Med. 1985;1:525–39.
79. Melton LJI, Wahner HW, Riggs BL. Bone density measurement (editorial). J Bone Min Res. 1988;3:ix.
80. Melton W, Wahner HW, Richelson LS, O'Fallon WM, Riggs BL. Osteoporosis and the risk of hip fracture. Am J Epidemiol. 1986;124:254–261.
81. Nilas L, Hassager C, Christiansen C. Long-term precision of dual-photon absorptiometry in the lumbar spine in clinical settings. Bone Miner. 1988;3:305–315.
82. Nilas L, Pødenphant J, Riis BJ, Gotfredsen A. Usefulness of regional bone measurements in patients with osteoporotic fractures of the spine and distal forearm. J Nucl Med. 1987;28:960–965.
83. Nuti R, Martini G. Measurements of bone mineral density by DXA total body absorptiometry in different skeletal sites in postmenopausal osteoporosis. Bone. 1992;13:173–178.
84. Orphanoudakis SC, Jensen PS, Rauschkolb EN, et al. Bone mineral analysis using single energy computed tomography. Invest Radiol. 1979;14:122.
85. Overgaard K, Hansen MA, Riis BJ, Christiansen C. Discriminatory ability of bone mass measurements (SPA and DEXA) for fractures in elderly postmenopausal women. Calcif Tissue Int. 1992;50:30–35.
86. Pacifici R, Rupich R, Vered I, Fischer KC, Griffin M, Susman N, et al. Dual energy radiography (DER): a preliminary comparative study. Calcif Tissue Int. 1988;43:189–91.
87. Peppler WW, Mazess RB. Total body bone mineral and lean body mass by dual photon absorptiometry. Calcif Tiss Int. 1981;33:353.
88. Reiser U, Heuck F, Faust U, Genant HK. Quantitative Computertertomografie zur Bestimmung des Mineralgehaltes in Lendenwirbeln mit Hilfe eines Festkörper-Referenzsystems. Biomed Techn. 1985;30:187–188.
89. Resch H, Pietschmann P, Bernecker P, Krexner E, Willvonseder R. Broadband ultrasound attenuation: a new diagnostic method in osteoporosis. AJR. 1990;155:825–828.
90. Richards MA, Webb JA, Jewell SE, Gregory WM, Reznek RH. In-vivo measurement of spin lattice relaxation time (T1) of bone marrow in healthy volunteers: the effects of age and sex. Br J Radiol. 1988;61:30–33.
91. Richardson M, Genant H, Cann C. Assessment of metabolic bone diseases by quantitative computed tomography. Clin Orthop. 1985;185:224–238.
92. Richardson ML, Pozzi-Mucelli RS, Kanter AS, Kolb FO, Ettinger B, Genant HK. Bone mineral changes in primary hyperparathyroidism. Skeletal Radiology. 1986;15:85–95.
93. Rickers H, Deding AA, Christiansen CC. Mineral loss in cortical and trabecular bone during high-dose prednisone treatment. Calcif Tiss Int. 1984;36:269–273.
94. Riggs BL, Wahner HW. Bone densitometry and clinical decision-making in osteoporosis. Ann Int Med. 1988;107:293–5.
95. Riggs BL, Wahner HW, Dunn WL, et al. Differential changes in bone mineral density of the appendicular and axial skeleton with aging. J Clin Invest. 1981;67:328–35.
96. Riis B, Thomsen K, Christiansen C. Does calcium supplementation prevent postmenopausal bone loss? New Engl J Med. 1987;316:173–7.
97. Rosenthal H, Thulborn KR, Rosenthal DI, Kim SH, Rosen BR. Magnetic susceptibility effects of trabecular bone on magnetic resonance imaging of bone marrow. Invest Radiol 1990;25:173–178.
98. Ross PD, Wasnich RD, Heilbrun LK, Vogel JM. Definition of a spine fracture threshold based upon prospective fracture risk. Bone. 1987;8:271–278.
99. Ross PD, Wasnich RD, Vogel JM. Detection of prefracture spinal osteoporosis using bone mineral absorptiometry. J Bone Min Res. 1988;3:1–11.
100. Ross PD, Wasnich RD, Vogel JM. Precision errors in dual-photon absorptiometry related to source age. Radiology. 1988;166:523–527.
101. Ruegsegger P, Elsasser U, Anliker M, et al. Quantification of bone. Radiology. 1976;121:93.
102. Rupich R, Pacifici R, Delabar C, Susman N, Avioli LV. Lateral dual energy radiography: new technique for the measurement of L3 bone mineral density. J Bone Mineral Res. 1989;4:S194.
103. Rupich RC, Griffin MG, Pacifici R, Avioli LV, Susman N. Lateral dual-energy radiography: artifact error from rib and pelvic bone. J Bone Miner Res. 1992;7:97–101.
104. Rybicki EF. On the mathematical analysis of stress in the human femur. J Biomechanics. 1972;5:203–215.
105. Sandor T, Kalender WA, Hanlon WB, Weissman BN, Rumbaugh C. Spinal bone mineral determination using automated contour detection: application to single and dual-energy CT. SPIE Med Imaging Instrum. 1985;555:188–194.
106. Sartoris DJ, Resnick D. Dual energy radiographic absorptiometry for bone densitometry: current status and perspective. AJR. 1989;152:241–246.
107. Schlenker RA, Von Seggen WW. The distribution of cortical and trabecular bone mass along the lengths of the radius and ulna and the implications for in vivo bone mass measurements. Calcif Tiss Res. 1970;20:41.
108. Sebag GH, Moore SG. Effect of trabecular bone on the appearance of marrow in gradient-echo imaging of the appendicular skeleton. Radiology. 1990;174:855–859.
109. Slemenda CW, Johnston CC. Bone mass measurement: which site to measure? Am J Med. 1988;84:643–5.
110. Slosman DO, Rizzoli R, Donath A, Bonjour J-P. Bone mineral density of lumbar vertebral body determined in supine and lateral decubitus. Study of precision and sensitivity. 14th Annual Meeting of the American Society for Bone Mineral Research. Mary Ann Liebert; Minneapolis: 1992:S192.
111. Slosman DO, Rizzoli R, Donath A, Bonjour JP. Vertebral bone mineral density measured laterally by dual-energy X-ray absorptiometry. Osteoporos Int. 1990;1:23–29.
112. Slovik DM, Rosenthal DI, Doppelt SH, et al. Restoration of spinal bone in osteoporotic men by treatment with human parathyroid hormone (1-34) and 1,25-dihydroxyvitamin D. J Bone Miner Res. 1986;1:377–381.
113. Stebler B, Ruegsegger P. Special purpose CT system for quantitative bone evaluation in the appendicular skeleton. Biomed Tech. 1983;28:196.
114. Steiger P, Block JE, Steiger S, Heuck A, Friedlander A, Ettinger B, et al. Spinal bone mineral density by quantitative computed tomography: effect of region of interest, vertebral level, and technique. Radiology. 1990;175:537–543.
115. Steiger P, Steiger S, Ruesegger P, Genant HK. Two- and three-dimensional quantitative image evaluation techniques for densitometry and volumetrics in longitudinal studies. In: Genant HK, eds. Osteoporosis Update 1987. San Francisco: University of California Printing Services; 1987:171–180.
116. Stein J, Hochberg AM, Lazetawsky L. Quantitative digital radiography for bone mineral analysis. In: Dequeker JV, Geusens P, Wahner HW, eds. Bone mineral measurements by photon absorptiometry: methodological problems. Louvain: Leuven University Press; 1987:411–414.
117. Stevenson JC, Lees B, Devenport M, Cust MP, Ganger KF. Determinants of bone density in normal women: risk factors for future osteoporosis? BMJ. 1989;298:924–928.
118. Suominen H, Heikkinen E, Vaino P, Lahtinen T. Mineral density of calcaneus in men at different ages: a population study with special reference to life-style factors. Age Ageing. 1984;13:273.
119. Talbert AJ, Brooks RA, Morgenthaler DG. Optimum energies for dual-energy computed tomography. Phys Med Biol. 1980;25(2):261–269.
120. Uebelhart D, Braillon P, Meunier PJ, Delmas PD. Lateral dual photon absorptiometry of the spine in vertebral osteoporosis and osteoarthritis. Comparison with quantitative computed tomography (abstract). J Bone Mineral Res 1989;4(suppl):S328.

121 Vogel JM, Wasnich RD, Ross PD. The clinical relevance of calcaneus bone mineral measurements: a review. Bone Miner. 1988;5:35–58.
122 Wahner HW, Dunn WL, Brown ML, Morin RL, Riggs BL. Comparison of dual-energy x-ray absorptiometry and dual photon absorptiometry for bone mineral measurements of the lumbar spine. 1988;63:1075–1084.
123 Wahner HW, Eastell R, Riggs BL. Bone mineral density of the radius: Where do we stand? J Nucl Med. 1985;26:1339–41.
124 Wasnich R. Fracture prediction with bone mass measurements. In: Genant H, eds. Osteoporosis Update 1987. Berkeley: University of California Press; 1987:95–101.
125 Wasnich RD. Screening for osteoporosis: pro. In: Genant HK, eds. Osteoporosis Update 1987. San Francisco: Radiology Research and Education Foundation; 1987:123–27.
126 Wasnich RD, Ross PD, Heilbrun LK, Vogel JM. Prediction of postmenopausal fracture risk with use of bone mineral measurements. Am J Obstet Gynecol. 1985;153:745–51.
127 Wehrli FW, Chung J, Kugelmass SD, Williams J, Wehrli SL. Relationship between Young's modulus and morphometric parameters in human trabecular bone studied by NMR microscopy. Society for Magnetic Resonance in Medicine, Book of Abstracts. Berlin: Society for Magnetic Resonance in Medicine; 1992:973.
128 Wehrli FW, Ford JC, Attie M, Kressel HY, Kaplan FS. Trabecular structure: preliminary application of MR interferometry. Radiology. 1991;179:615–621.
129 Wehrli FW, Wehrli SL, Williams J, Attie M. Anisotropy of trabecular microstructure studied by high-field NMR microscopy and linewidth measurements. Society for Magnetic Resonance in Medicine, Book of Abstracts, New York, NY: Society for Magnetic Resonance in Medicine; 1990:127.
130 Weissberger MA, Zamenhof RG, Aronow S, et al. Computed tomography for the measurement of bone mineral in the human spine. J Comp Assist Tomogr. 1978;2:253.
131 Williams JA, Wagner J, Wasnich R, Heilbrun L. The effect of long-distance running upon appendicular bone mineral content. Med Sci Sport Exercise. 1984;16:223.
132 Wilson CR. Bone mineral content of the femoral neck and spine versus the radius or ulna. J Bone Joint Surg (Am). 1977;59A:665–669.
133 Yano K, Wasnich RD, Bogel JM, Heilbrun LK. Bone mineral measurements among middle-aged and elderly Japanese Residents in Hawaii. Am J Epidemiol. 1984;119:751–764.
134 Zamenhof RGA. Optimization of spinal bone density measurement using computerized tomography. In: Genant HK, eds. Osteoporosis Update 1987. San Francisco: University of California Printing Services; 1987:145–169.

12 Positron Emission Tomography in Endocrine Disease

C. Muhr

Positron emission tomography (PET) has been established as an important research tool for several years and has, in recent years, also become a valuable clinical instrument. PET offers unique opportunities for performing in vivo biochemical observations, with examples such as observations and measurements of glucose metabolism, amino acid transport and metabolism, receptor characterization, enzyme activity, blood flow, and oxygen consumption measurement (6, 12, 17, 25, 27).

For the past ten years, our group, working within the field of endocrinology, has been working with pituitary adenomas, focusing on metabolic mapping, dopamine receptor determinations, the enzyme MAO-B, and pharmacokinetics.

The new technology of the PET camera, with its advanced computer technique, has led both to increased sensitivity in registering radioactive uptake and to considerably improved images. Cameras for both brain studies and whole-body studies are now available at several PET centers. The most commonly used radionucleides are ^{11}C (with a half-life of 20 minutes), ^{18}F (with a half-life of 110 minutes), ^{15}O (with a half-life of 2 minutes) and ^{13}N (with a half-life of 10 minutes). These radionucleides are newly produced for each individual examination in a cyclotron, which in ideal circumstances is located at the PET center. The chemistry involved in labeling and synthezizing the substances demands special skills. A large number of different substances have been labeled with positron emitting radionucleides and are now available for use in a variety of PET studies (17).

The labeled substance is usually administered intravenously or inhaled, as in oxygen uptake studies, and then distributes throughout the body. During the study, the dynamics of the accumulation and elimination of the substance within the specific organ or area of interest will be registered. The duration of the examination depends on the half-life of radionucleide, for ^{11}C with a half-life of 20 minutes, registration continues for about 30 minutes and for ^{15}O with a 2-minute half-life, only a few minutes of registration are necessary.

PET technique is a tracer technique that has the two big advantages that only minimal amounts of tracer are used and that low concentrations of the target substance can be registered.

The emitted positrons from the radionucleides collide with electrons in the tissue and annihilate, and the particle mass transforms into energy in the form of 2 photons directed 180° to each other. These photons are registered by detectors in a system of rings (Fig. 12.**1**). These data are then transformed into images via computers (28). Registrations are usually continued during the entire span of the examination and a sequence of images are taken. All the data is saved and can also be analyzed at a later stage, according to different principles, to obtain desired information. Different types of models have been proposed for analyzing this data (10, 26, 29).

Slice thickness in most modern cameras is around 4 mm and their spatial resolution is 5–7 mm. Detectable volume depends much on contrast to the surrounding structures. If there is a specific uptake, i.e., a high ratio between uptake within a given area and uptake in the surroundings, volumes on the order of a few cubic millimeters can be visualized. For registration of quantitatively true values, a somewhat larger volume is necessary to compensate for partial volume effects.

Metabolic Mapping

The first and most commonly used tracer for metabolic studies is 18-fluorodeoxyglucose (^{18}FDG). This substance enables an estimation of glucose utilization in the tissue under examination (6, 7, 30). Glucose has also been labeled with ^{11}C and this substance has some advantages over ^{18}FDG (17).

PET with ^{11}C-labeled L-methionine provides information related to amino acid metabolism. Uptake of ^{11}C-L-methionine mainly demonstrates the transport of this particular amino acid, because of the A and L systems of transport within the brain (2, 4, 5, 13, 14, 16, 20, 21).

The pituitary gland is, however, located outside the blood–brain barrier and the availability of the labeled substance will therefore not be affected to the same degree by transport limitations.

We have demonstrated that ^{11}C-L-methionine uptake is high in all pituitary adenomas.

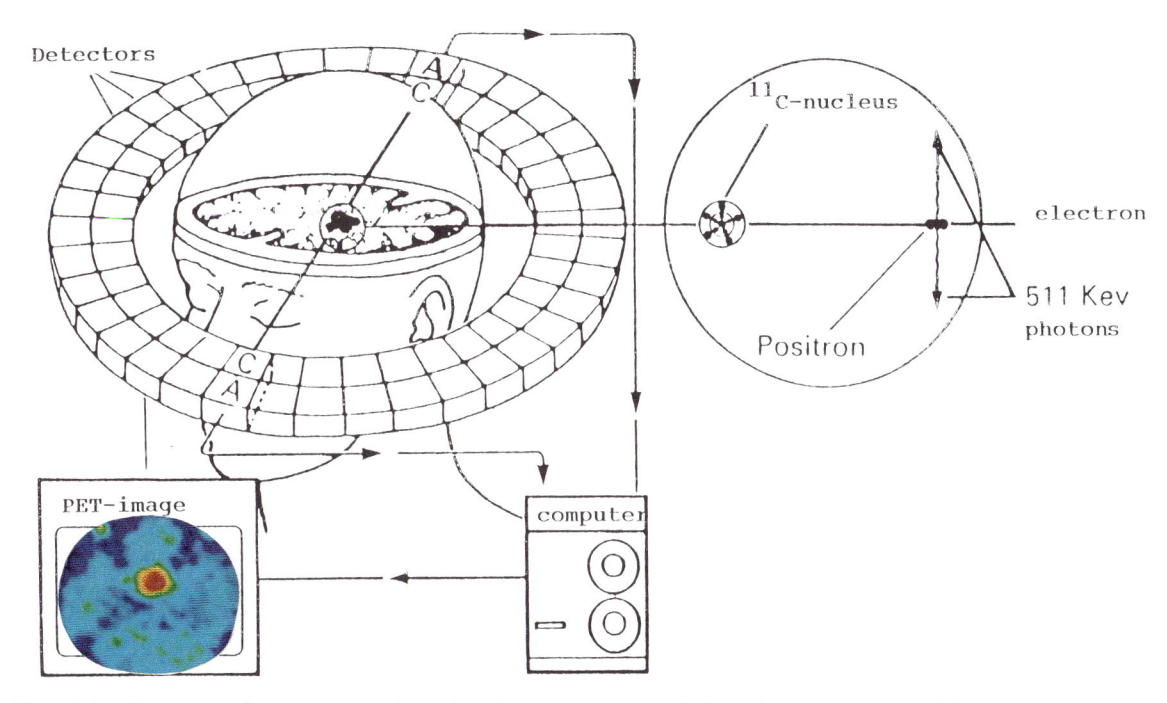

Fig. 12.1 The rings of detectors register the photons generated when the positrons annihilate. All data is taken up by the computer and can be transformed into an image demonstrating the uptake of the labeled substance

^{11}C-L-methionine is only taken up in viable tissue and is therefore very useful for diagnosing and outlining viable tumor tissue (Fig. 12.2). In this respect, PET with ^{11}C-L-methionine is superior to both MRI and CT and is valuable for differentiating between active tumor tissue on the one hand and postoperative fibrosis and cystic necrotic areas on the other.

Hormonally active adenomas, especially prolactinomas, have the highest ^{11}C-L-methionine uptake of all the adenomas we have studied. Metabolic mapping using more than one metabolic tracer opens up possibilities for further differential diagnostic aspects. In a comparison between ^{11}C-L-methionine and ^{18}FDG tumor uptake, a relatively high ^{11}C-L-methionine uptake was obtained in all adenomas whereas glucose use was notably high in some adenomas but considerably lower in others (Fig. 12.3). The different PET patterns correspond in all probability to adenoma subgroups (25). PET with tracer combinations offers in vivo biochemical characterization that may provide even more information than a biopsy. Furthermore, a biopsy can of course only furnish information concerning the very small biopsied portion.

An in vivo technique is of special value in endocrinology, where there are so many biofeedback mechanisms. These normal control mechanisms are absent in all in vitro systems, which are thus quite artificial.

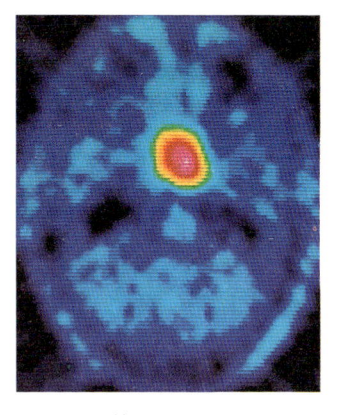

Fig. 12.2 PET with ^{11}C-L-methionine, which will only be taken up in, and thus reveal, viable tumor tissue such as in this prolactinoma, in axial projection

Receptor Studies

Dopamine-D$_2$-receptors are considered prerequisite for treatment effect with dopamine agonists, and have been of special interest. They can be studied with the help of the specific D$_2$-antagonist raclopride, labeled with ^{11}C. D$_2$-binding is measured by combined experiments with both the s-form of raclopride, which actively binds to receptors and reveals total binding, and with the r-form, which reveals nonspecific binding. A quantitative value for specific binding is then ob-

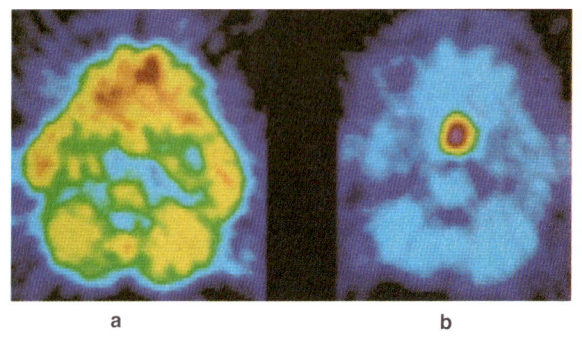

Fig. 12.**3** PET images, in axial projections, demonstrating high accumulation of ^{11}C-L-methionine and relatively lower accumulation of ^{18}FDG within the same pituitary adenoma.

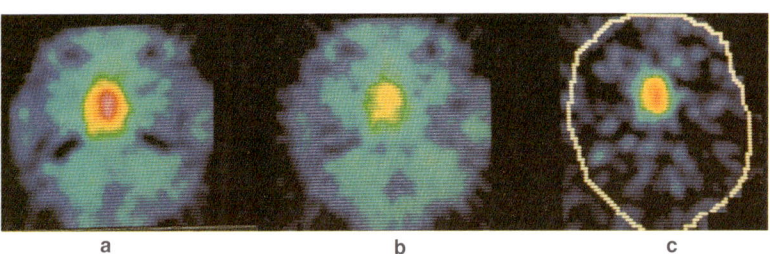

Fig. 12.**4** PET images, in axial projections, using the specific D$_2$-antagonist ^{11}Craclopride, demonstrating in a prolactinoma (**a**) total binding, (**b**) nonspecific binding and (**c**) high specific D$_2$binding

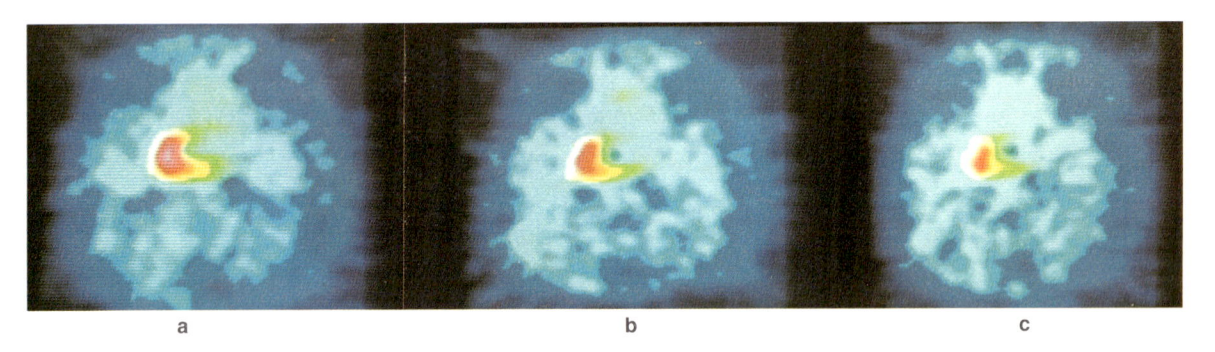

Fig. 12.**5** PET images demonstrating, in axial projections, (**a**) high D$_2$-binding before start on medication with the dopamine agonist bromocriptine (**b**) 20% decrease in free D$_2$-receptors 3 $^1/_2$ hours after administration of medication, and (**c**) 13 hours after administration of medication a further decrease in the number of free dopamine receptors

tained by subtracting nonspecific binding from total binding (8, 9, 15, 19, 23, 25, 32, 33) (Fig. 12.**4**).

By performing repeated PET during a period of medication, it is possible to determine the number of receptors that are occupied by the drug (Fig. 12.**5**). This can then be correlated to drug effect and thus facilitates determination of optimal dosage.

We have also studied somatostatin receptors with an ^{11}C-labeled somatostatin analog.

Other groups have also used PET with ^{18}F-labeled receptor ligands to demonstrate estrogen and progesterone receptors in tumors (15).

Evaluation of Medical Treatment

PET using ^{11}C-L-methionine has proven to be a useful and sensitive tool for evaluating the medical treatment of pituitary adenomas (3, 22, 24, 25). The uptake of ^{11}C-L-methionine appears to correspond closely to the hormonal activity of pituitary adenomas; prolactinomas with high levels of hormone production and secretion demonstrate the highest L-methionine uptake of all adenoma types.

Within a few hours after initiation of bromocriptine treatment methionine uptake in a prolactinoma is considerably decreased (Fig. 12.**6**). The occurrence of this finding indicates that the medical treatment is effective. Methionine can also be used to ascertain optimal dosage and to evaluate the duration of medication effect (Fig. 12. **7**).

Hyperprolactinemia—Prolactin-secreting Pituitary Adenoma

Prolactin-secreting adenomas originate from lactotroph cells in the anterior pituitary. The earliest symptoms of these tumors are due to elevated prolactin levels in serum and lead to infertility, with anovula-

Fig. 12.6 PET images, in axial projections, demonstrating the high sensitivity of this technique. Using ^{11}C-L methionine (**a**) high amino acid metabolism is seen in the prolactinoma, (**b**) a considerable decrease is seen already 2 hours after bromocriptine i.m. injection, and (**c**) 7 days later a dramatic further decrease is observed

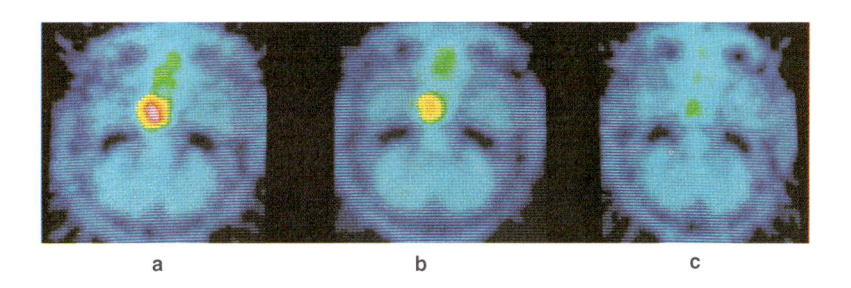

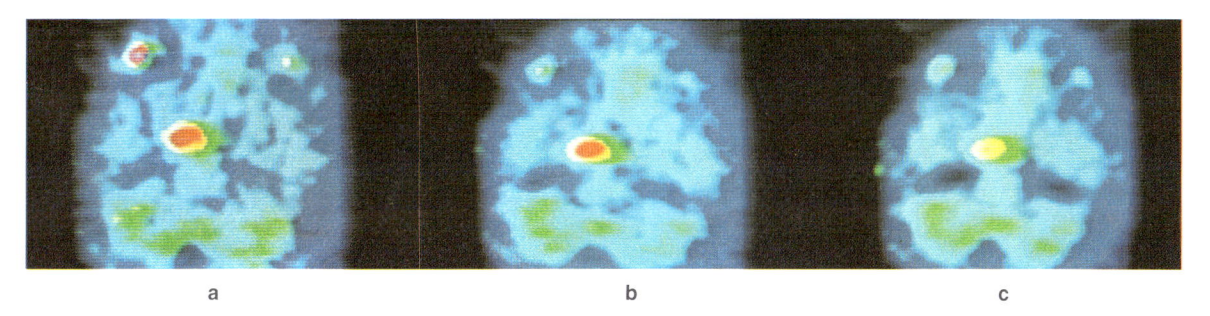

Fig. 12.7 PET images, in axial projections, showing the value of this technique in establishing dosage level in this GH-secreting adenoma treated with a somatostatinanalogue. (**a**) high ^{11}C-L methionine uptake in the adenoma, (**b**) no significant change in the amino acid metabolismon the dosis 250 µg/day and (**c**) considerable decrease in amino acid metabolism on the dosis 1200 µg/day

tion and amenorrhea in women and decreased libido in both sexes. The lactotroph cells of the normal pituitary gland are controlled by an inhibitory mechanism. The inhibitory substance is dopamine, which is secreted in the hypothalamus and transported to the pituitary by way of the portal vessels of the pituitary stalk. This means that anything which diminishes this inhibition will lead to an elevation in serum prolactin. It is therefore of great importance to differentiate prolactin-secreting adenomas from other type of lesions in this area. Serum prolactin levels higher than 200 µg/L (normal < 20 µg/L) speak strongly in favur of a prolactinoma as the lactotrophs in the normal pituitary gland rarely secrete enough prolactin to exceed this value. On the other hand, tumors with lower prolactin values cannot be properly diagnosed on this basis. The treatment of choice for prolactinomas is medication with a dopamine agonist. The most commonly used is bromocriptine, administered either in a long-acting form for i.m. injection (4 weeks duration) or perorally (1, 20). Treatment with a dopamine agonist will result at least in a decrease and most probably a normalization of serum prolactin levels, whether the hyperprolactinemia is caused by a disturbance of inhibition or by a prolactinoma.

Demonstration of high levels of D_2 dopamine receptors in an adenoma indicate that it is a prolactinoma (Fig. 12.4).

When PET indicates a considerably decreased methionine uptake, i.e., a considerable decrease in metabolism, after initiation of dopamine agonist treatment, the adenoma has thus been proved to be a prolactinoma (Fig. 12.6).

Other forms of hypersecreting pituitary adenomas are diagnosed by elevated serum values of their specific hormones. Microadenomas (less than 10 mm in size) are best localized with MRI, but PET, using labeled substances specific for each adenoma type, may in the future provide further help in identifying these small tumors. There are still a number of microadenomas, especially ACTH adenomas, that are not properly visualized with MRI.

Differential Diagnosis of Hormonally Inactive Pituitary Adenomas versus Suprasellar Meningiomas

Clinically nonsecreting pituitary adenomas usually attain considerable size before they are diagnosed. The symptoms that lead to diagnosis are either impaired vision, in the classical form of bitemporal hemianopsia caused by compression of the optic chiasma, or symptoms of pituitary insufficiency caused by pressure on the normal pituitary gland. One frequent location of meningiomas is the suprasellar space, and in many cases it is difficult with CT and MRI to distinguish between a meningioma and a nonsecreting pituitary adenoma. However, PET using ^{11}C-L-deprenyl makes

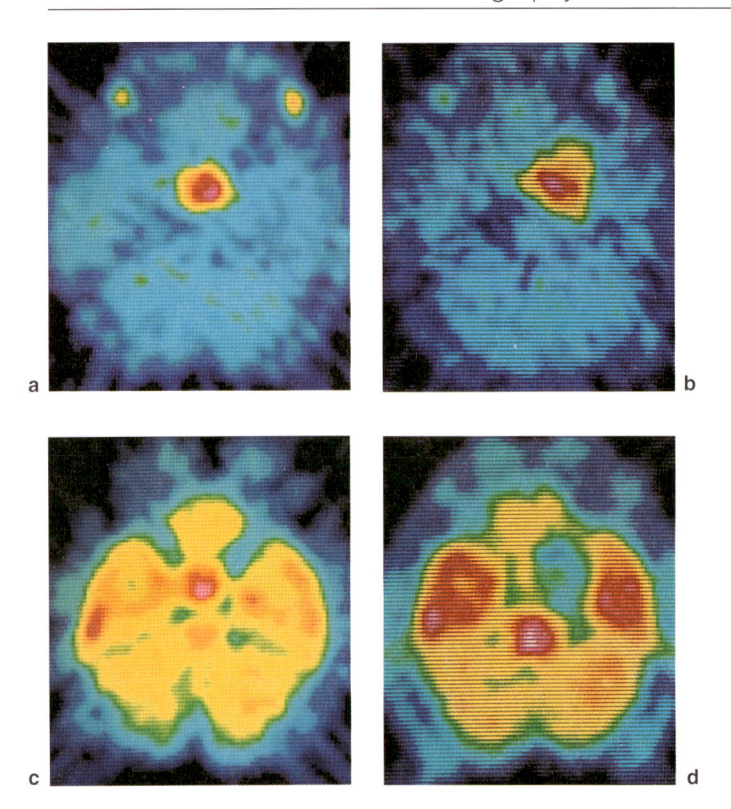

Fig. 12.**8** PET images, in axial projections, demonstrating high accumulation of ^{11}C-L-methionine in both (**a**) the clinically nonsecreting pituitary adenoma and (**b**) the meningioma and (**c**) high ^{11}C-L-deprenyl accumulation in the pituitary adenoma but (**d**) very low uptake in the meningioma enabling differential diagnosis to be made between these two tumors

possible this differential diagnosis. Deprenyl binds irreversibly to the enzyme MAO-B, the levels of which are considerably higher in pituitary adenomas in comparison to the very low levels found in meningiomas. No overlapping has been seen so far in the 40 patients studied (Fig. 12.**8**).

Pharmacokinetics and Pharmaceutical Distribution

The distribution of a particular medication can be followed by labeling the different medications used (11, 21, 18, 25). By interfering with the modulating system

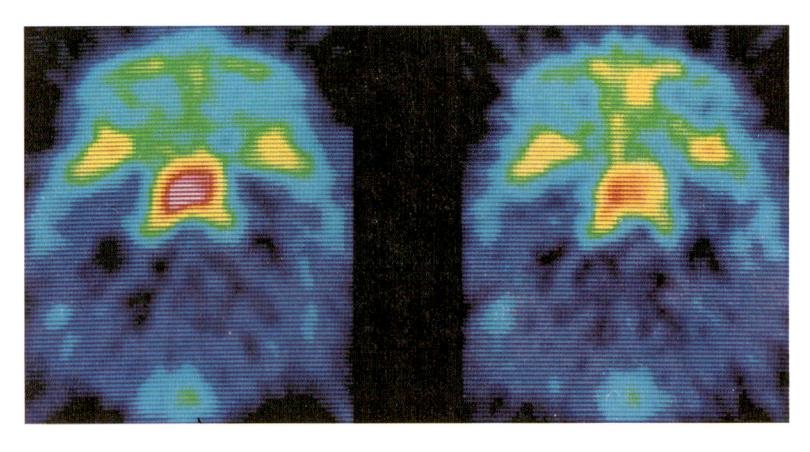

Fig. 12.**9** PET image, in axial projections, demonstrating (**a**) high accumulation of dopamine agonist medication ^{11}C-labeled bromocriptine in a prolactinoma and (**b**) decreased accumulation of ^{11}C-bromocriptine after protection of the receptors with Haloperidol, as a sign of bromocriptine interference with D_2-receptors

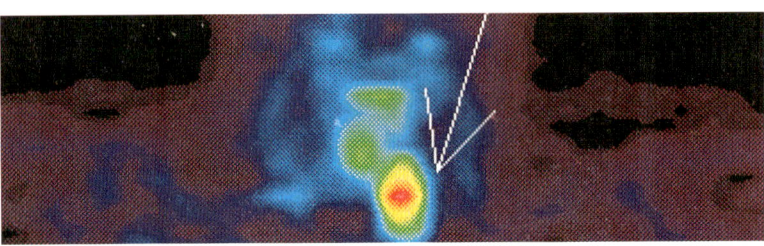

Fig. 12.**10** PET image, in a frontal reconstruction, demonstrating high uptake of ^{11}C-L-methionine in a parathyroid adenoma. (Courtesy of Dr J Rastad)

it is also possible to evaluate in part the mode of action of the medication. The dopamine agonist bromocriptine has been labeled with ^{11}C and shown, with PET, to accumulate in all pituitary tumors. ^{11}C-bromocriptine has been shown to interact with dopamine D$_2$-receptors in prolactinomas, where decreased accumulation was found when the receptors had been protected by premedication with haloperidol (Fig. 12.**9**).

Parathyroid Adenomas

Parathyroid adenomas may be difficult to localize, and a wide range of possible locations have been described, so that extensive surgery is sometimes needed before these adenomas can be removed. Rastad et al., Department of Surgery, Uppsala Akademiska Hospital, Sweden (to be published) have demonstrated that PET with ^{11}C-methionine is very valuable for revealing even small parathyroid adenomas (Fig. 12.**10**).

Acknowledgement: The work referred to has been carried out in collaboration with Professor PO Lundberg at the Department of Neurology, and the group at Uppsala University PET-center, Uppsala, led by Professor Bengt Långström, to whom I want to express my deep gratitude and to Dr Rastad. The work was supported by funds from the Swedish Medical Research Council and the Swedish Society for Cancer Research.

References

1. Benker G, Gieshoff B, Freundlieb O, Windeck R, Schulte HM, Lancranjan I, Reinwein D. Parenteral bromocriptine in the treatment of hormonally active pituitary tumors. Clin Endocrinol. 1986;24:505–513.
2. Bergström M, Muhr C, Lundberg PO, Bergström K, Lundqvist H, Antoni G, Fasth K-G, Långström B. In vivo study of amino acid distribution and metabolism in pituitary adenomas using positron emission tomography with ^{11}C-D-methionine and ^{11}C-L-methionine. J Comput Assist Tomogr. 1987;1;11:384–389.
3. Bergström M, Muhr C, Lundberg PO, Bergström K, Gee AD, Fasth K-G, Långström B. Rapid decrease in amino acid metabolism in prolactin-secreting pituitary adenomas after bromocriptine treatment–a PET study. J Comput Assist Tomogr. 1987;2(11):815–819.
4. Bergström M, Muhr C, Ericson K, Lundqvist H, Lilja A, Långström B, Johnström P. The normal pituitary examined with positron emission tomography and (C-11-methyl)-L-methionine and (C-11-methyl)-D-methionine. Neuroradiology. 1987;4(29):221–225.
5. Bustany P, Chatel M, Derlon JM, Darcel F, Sgourpoulus P, Soussaline F, Syrota A. Brain tumor protein synthesis and histological grades: a study by positron emission tomography (PET) with ^{11}C-L-methionine. J Neuro-Oncol. 1986;3:379–404.
6. Di Chiro G. Positron emission tomography using (^{18}F)fluorodeoxyglucose in brain tumors. A powerful diagnostic and prognostic tool. Investigative Radiology. 1987;22:360–371.
7. Di Chiro G, Books RA, Patronas NJ, et al. Issues in the in vivo measurement of glucose metabolism of human central nervous system tumors. Ann Neurol. 1984;15:138–146.
8. Eckernäs S-Å, Aquilonius SM, Hartvig P, Hägglund J, Lundqvist H, Någren K, Långström B: Positron emission tomography (PET) in the study of dopamine receptors in the primate brain: evaluation of a kinetic model using ^{11}C-N-methyl-spiperone. Acta Neurol Scand. 1987;75:168–178.
9. Farde L, Ehrin E, Eriksson L, Greitz T, Hall H, Hedström C-G, Litton J-E, Sedvall G. Substituted benzamides as ligands for visualization of dopamine receptor binding in the human brain by positron emission tomography. Proc Natl Acad Sci. 1985;82:3863–3867.
10. Gjedde A. High- and low-affinity transport of D-glucose from blood to brain. J Neurochem. 1981;36,1463–1471.
11. Hartvig P, Någren K, Lundberg PO, Muhr C. Terenius L, Lundqvist H, Lärkfors L, Långström B: Kinetics of four ^{11}C-labelled enkephalin peptides in the brain, pituitary and plasma of rhesus monkeys. Regulatory Peptides. 1986;16:1–13.
12. Heiss W-D, Pawlik G, Herholz K, Wienhard K, eds. Clinical efficacy of positron emission tomography. Proceedings of a workshop held in Cologne, FRG. Dordrecht: Martinus Nijhoff; 1987.
13. Ishiwata K, Vaalburg W, Elsinga PH, Paans AMJ, Woldring MG. Comparison of L-(^{11}C)methionine and L-methyl-(^{11}C)methionine for measuring in vivo protein synthesis rates with PET. J Nucl Med. 29:1419–1427, 1988.
14. Lilja A. Radiological aspects of the diagnosis of glioma. [Doctorial thesis]. Uppsala: Uppsala University; 1985.
15. Logan J, Wolf AP, Shiue C-Y, Fowler JS. Kinetic modeling of receptor-ligand binding applied to positron emission tomographic studies with neuroleptic tracers. J Neurochem. 1987;48(1):73–83.
16. Lundqvist H, Stålnacke CG, Långström B, Jones B. Labeled metabolites in plasma after i.v. administration of ^{11}C-methyl-L-methionine. In: Greitz T, et al., eds. The metabolism of the human brain studied by positron emission tomography. New York: Raven Press; 1985:223–240.
17. Långström B, Hartvig P. Positron emitting tracers in studies of neurotransmission and receptor binding. In: Nunn AD, ed. Radiopharmaceuticals Chemestry and Pharmacology. New York: Marcel Dekker; 1992:221–265.
18. Mintun MA, Raichle ME, Kilbourn MR, Wooten GF, Welch MJ. A quantitative model for the in vivo assessment of drug binding sites with positron emission tomography. Ann Neurol. 1984;15:217–227.
19. Muhr C, Bergström M, Lundberg P-O, et al. Dopamine receptors in pituitary adenomas: PET visualization with ^{11}C-N-methyl-spiperone. J Comput Assist Tomogr. 1986;(110):175–180.
20. Muhr C, Bergström M, Lundberg PO, et al. Malignant prolactinoma with multiple intracranial metastases studied with positron emission tomography. Neurosurgery. 1988;1(22):374–379.
21. Muhr C, Lundberg PO, Antoni G, Bergström K, Hartvig P, Lundqvist H, Långström B, Ståhlnacke C-G. The uptake of ^{11}C-labelled bromocriptine and methionine in pituitary tumors studied by positron emission tomography (PET). In: Lamberts, Tilders, van der Veen, Assies, eds. Trends in diagnosis and treatment of pituitary adenomas. Amsterdam: Free University Press. 151–155, 1984.
22. Muhr C, Bergström M, Lundberg PO, Bergström K, Långström B. Positron emission tomography for the in vivo characterization and follow up of treatment in pituitary adenomas. Adv Biosci. 1988;2(69):163–170.
23. Muhr C, Bergström M, Lundberg PO, Bergström K, Långström B. In vivo measurement of dopamine receptors in pituitary adenomas using positron emission tomography. Acta Radiol. Proceedings: Symposium Neuroradiologicum; 1986:3.
24. Muhr C, Bergström M, Lundberg PO, Långström B. PET in neuroendocrinology. Recent advances in basic and clinical neuroendocrinology. Casanueva FF, Dieguez C, eds. Amsterdam: Elsevier Science Publishers BV; 1989:313–319.
25. Muhr C, Bergström M. Positron emission tomography applied in the study of pituitary adenomas. J Endocrinol Invest. 1991;14:509–528.
26. Patlak CS, Blasberg RG, Fenstermacher JD. Graphical evaluation of blood-to-brain transfer constants from multiple-time uptake data. J Cereb Blood Flow Metab. 1983;3:1–7.
27. Patronas NJ, Di Chiro G, Kufta C, et al. Prediction of survival in glioma patients by means of positiron emission tomography. J Neurosurg. 1985;62:816–822.
28. Phelps ME, Hoffman EJ, Mullani NA, Ter-Pogossian MM. Application of annihilation coincidence detection to transaxial reconstruction tomography. J Nucl Med. 1975;16:210–224.

29 Phelps ME, Barrio JR, Huang SC, Keen RE, Chugani H, Mazziotta JC. Criteria for the tracer kinetic measurement of cerebral protein synthesis in humans with positron emission tomography. Ann Neurol. 1984;15:192–202.
30 Phelps ME, Huang SC, Hoffman EJ, Selin C, Sokoloff L, Kuhl DE. Tomographic measurement of local cerebral glucose metabolic rate in humans with (F-18)2-fluoro-2-deoxy-D-glucose: validation of method. Ann Neurol. 1979;6:371–388.
31 Reubi JC, Heitz PU, Landolt AM. Visualization of somatostatin receptors and correlation with immunoreactive growth hormone and prolactin in human pituitary adenomas: evidence for different tumor subclasses. J Clin Endocrinol Metab. 1987;65:65–73.
32 Wong DF, Gjedde A, Wagner HN. Quantification of neuroreceptors in the living human brain. I. Irreversible binding of ligands. J Cerebr Blood Flow Metab. 1986;1(6):137–146.
33 Wong DF, Gjedde A, Wagner HN, Dannals RF, Douglass KH, Links JM, Kuhar MJ. Quantification of receptors in the living human brain. II. Inhibition studies of receptor density and affinity. J Cerebr Blood Flow Metab. 1986:2(6):147–163.

Index

Bold numbers refer to figure legends.

A

abscess, epididymis, 259
absorptiometry
   dual photon (DPA), 326, **326**, **329**
   dual X-ray (DXA), 326–31, **328**, **329**
   single photon (SPA), **325**, 325–6
acromegaly, 12–13
   change in facial appearance, **12**
   typical clinical findings, 13
ACTH (adrenocorticotropic hormone), 161, 162, 163
adenocarcinoma
   adrenal gland, **139**
   ovary, peritoneal and hepatic metastases, **306**
   rete testis, 272
adenohypophysis, 28
adenolipoma, adrenal gland, **136**
adenoma
   adrenal gland, 136, **138**, **143**, 148, **162**, 177
   anaplastic, MR appearance, 65
   autonomous, **53**, 53–4, **72**, 72, 82
   follicular, hyperfunctioning, **62–3**
   gonadotropin-secreting, 16
   hypophyseal, 38
      chromophobic, **37**
   MRI, 61–2
   nonfunctioning, adrenal gland, **154**
   parathyroid, **57**, **64**, **87**, **88**, **89**, **91**, **93**, **94**, **96**, **101**, 101–2, **103**, **107**, **108**, 124, **124**
      CT contrast enhancement, **100**, **102**
      ectopic, **102**, 125–6
      Gd-DTPA enhancement, **107**
      and PET imaging, 348–9
      preoperative localization, 99, 111–12, 126, 127
      shoulder-streak artifacts, **99**
      transcatheter ablation, 122
      vs. thyroid nodule, **110**
   pituitary, 11–16, **21**, **22**, 30–3
      and adrenal enlargement, **145**
      calcified, **26**
      classification, 12
      CT classification, 23
      cystic, **23**, **24**, **25**
      PET imaging, **346**, 346–7
      radiologist's view, 40–1
      vs. suprasellar meningioma, 347–8
   thyrotropin-producing, 15–16
adenopathy, retroperitoneal, with ovarian carcinoma, **306**
ADH secretion, inappropriate, *see* SIADH
adnexa uteri
   endometrioma, **308**
   mucinous cystadenoma, **312**
   teratoma, cystic, **308**
Adosterol scintigraphy, 169, **170**, 171
adrenal cortex, and radiopharmaceuticals, 5
adrenal cortical carcinoma, 149, **150**

adrenal gland, **129**, 129–79, **142**
   adenocarcinoma, **139**
   adenolipoma, **136**
   adenoma, **138**, **143**, **149**, **162**, 177
   anatomy, 129–30
      CT, 142
      MRI, 147, **148**
   angiography, 159–68
   angioma, **138**
   atrophy, 135
   bronchial carcinoma metastasis, **141**, **145**
   calcification, 178
   carcinoma, **141**, **144**, 178
      liver metastasis, **140**
      transhepatic biopsy, **141**
   congenital adrenal hyperplasia, 133
   CT, 142–6
   cyst, 178
   embryology, 130
   endocrinology, 131–5
   fetal tumor, **140**
   hemorrhage, **137**, 177
   hyperplasia, 136, **137**, 143, **164**, 177
   malignancy, 138–9
   mass, **156**, **157**
   metastasis, 178
   MRI, 146–58
   myelolipoma, 178
   nononcologic mass, 154
   normal, **136**
   oncologic mass, 154–6
   pathology, ultrasound, 135–6
   pheochromocytoma, 138, **138**, **139**, 164–8, **165**, **166**, **167**, 178
   physiology, 131
   radiologist's view, 177–8
   scintigraphy, 169–76
   steroid biosynthesis, **133**
   surgeon's view, 178–9
   tumors, 142–3, 144–5
      hyperfunctioning, 148–56
      localization and diagnosis, 178–9
   ultrasound, 135–41
   vascular anatomy, 159
   venous sampling, 160, 163
adrenaline, 130
adrenal medulla, pheochromocytoma, 134–5
adrenocortical tumors, 134
adrenocorticotropic hormone (ACTH), 161, 162, 163
adrenogenital syndrome, **137**, 287
AFP (alpha-fetoprotein), 271, 309
aldosteronism, **164**
   primary, 162–3
aldosteronoma, 149–50, **151**
   episodic hormone secretion, 161
   venous sampling results, 163

Index

alpha-fetoprotein (AFP), 271, 309
amenorrhea, 286
anaplastic carcinoma, thyroid gland, **56**
anatomy
   adrenal gland, 129–30
      CT, 142
      MRI, 147
      vascular, 159
   carcinoid, 211
   carcinoid syndrome, 222
   eye, and Graves ophthalmopathy, **77**
   hyperandrogenism, 314–15
   ovary, 282–3
   pancreas, 180
      MRI, **191**
   parathyroid gland, 85
      CT, 100
      MRI, 104–5
      variations, **85**
   pituitary gland, 7–9
      MRI, 28–30, **29**
   sella turcica
      CT, **19**, **20**
      MRI, 28–30
   testis, 246–7
      MRI, 268–9
   thyroid gland, 43–6
      CT, 55, **55**
      MRI, 58–9
   vascular, 221
   veins
      distorted after thyroidectomy, **117**
      parathyroid, 114
androgen
   biosynthesis, 247, 250
   effects, 248
androgens, insensitivity, 252
androsterone, 247
aneurysm
   carotid artery, **40**
   pituitary gland, radiologist's view, 41
   vs. pituitary adenoma, 35
angiography
   adrenal gland, 159–68
      technique, 159–61
   carcinoid syndrome, 221–32, 222–4, **226**, **228**
   catheters for adrenal and ovarian sampling, **321**
   pancreas
      contrast medium, 197
      technique, 194–5
   parathyroid gland, 113–22
   pituitary gland, 35–40
      normal findings, 36
      pathological findings, 36–40
      technique, 35–6
angioma, adrenal gland, **138**
anorchism, congenital, 251
appendiceal carcinoid, 211
apudoma, 197, 243
   pancreatic head, **187**
   pancreatic tail, **188**
   vs. pancreatic lobule, **184**
APUD system, 45, 175, 181
arteriography, pancreas, radiologist's view, 206
arteriovenous malformation
   scrotum, **276**
   testis, 275–6
artery
   adrenal, 130, **130**
   carotid, 57, **96**
      aneurysm, **40**

      encasement, **32**
      in thyroid carcinoma, **56**
   carotid–cavernous sinus fistula, 79, **80**
   gastroduodenal (GDA), 195, 202, **203**, 205
   hepatic, 205
      embolization (HAE), 228–9, 233
   hypophyseal, **38**
   inferior thyroid, **105**
   intra-arterial stimulation test, 202–5, 205
   ovarian, 283
   parathyroid, 120–1
      DSA complications, 121–2
   renal, stenosis, 168
   splenic, 205
      vs. insulinoma, **185**
   subclavian, DSA, **120**
   superior mesenteric (SMA), 195, 202, **203**, 205, 221
      carcinoid syndrome, **222**, **225**, **228**, **230**
   thyrocervical trunk, 121
   thyroid, **45**, 85
   thyroid ima, 121
   see also blood; catheterization; vascular
artifacts
   CT, 1
   DSA, 3
ascites
   with fibroma, 310
   with ovarian carcinoma, **305**
aspermia, 250
aspiration cytology device, **93**
asthenozoospermia, 250
atrophy
   adrenal, 135
   testicular, 263
autonomous adenoma, **53**, 53–4, 82
autonomy
   disseminated, thyroid, 73
   multifocal, 82
      thyroid, 72–3, **73**
   multinodular, thyroid, 82
azoospermia, 250

B

benign prostatic hyperplasia (BPH), 253
biosynthesis
   androgen, 247, 250
   progesterone, **284**
   serotonin, **213**
   sex hormones, **249**
   steroid, adrenal gland, **133**
bladder implant, ovarian carcinoma, **303**
blastoma, adrenal gland, 143
blindness, cortical, and parathyroid arteriography, 122
blood
   circulation, testis, **247**
   supply
      ovary, **283**
      thyroid gland, 45
   vessels, hypothalamic–pituitary axis, **8**
BMD (bone mineral density), **334**, **335**
bone, mineral density (BMD), **334**, **335**
bone densitometry
   clinical use, 339–40
   comparison of techniques, 324
BPH (benign prostatic hyperplasia), 253
breast, estrogen and progesterone effects, 285
[11]C-bromocriptine, **348**
bronchus carcinoid, 211

C

CAH (congenital adrenal hyperplasia), 133
calcification
    adrenal gland, 178
    testicular, 264, **265**
calibration phantom, Cann–Genant, **331**
camera, scintillation, 69
cAMP, and hypoparathyroidism, 85
Cann–Genant calibration phantom, **331**
capillary blush, 197
carcinoembryonic antigen, 75
carcinoid syndrome, 211–34, **222, 223, 226, 227, 228, 230, 231**
    anatomy, 211, 222
    angiographic findings, 222–4
    angiography, 221–32
    CT, 214–21
    diagnosis, 212–13
    differential diagnosis, 225–7
    liver metastases, 216
    nuclear medicine, 232–3
    pathophysiology, 212
    radiologist's view, 233
    retroperitoneal metastases, 216
    serotonin metabolic pathway, **213**
carcinoid tumor, midgut, **224**
carcinoid tumors, 211–13, 213, 221–2
carcinoma
    adrenal cortical, 149, **150**, 163–4
    adrenal gland, **141, 143, 144**, 178
        liver metastasis, **140**
        transhepatic biopsy, **141**
    anaplastic, thyroid gland, **56**
    C cell, 83
    cervical, 289
    embryonal, 309
    embryonal cell, **274**
    endometrial, 289
    endometrioid, ovarian, **302**
    medullary, 66
        thyroid gland, 75, 83, 238
    MRI, 63–8
    ovarian, 298–312
        bladder implant, **303**
    ovary, ascites, **305**
    papillary, thyroid gland, 54, **54**
    parathyroid gland, 103
    prostatic, 252–3
    thyroid, 49, **65–6**
    vagina, 289
    vulva, 289
carotid–cavernous sinus fistula, 79, **80**
catheterization, 114
    adrenal vein, 321–2
    adrenal veins, accuracy, **322**
    inferior phrenic vein, **317**
    inferior vena cava, 168
    ovarian vein, 321–2
    ovarian veins, accuracy, **322**
    pancreatic angiography, 195
    and peripheral hydrocortisone levels, 319, **320**
    thyroid veins, 128
catheters
    jugular vein, **119**
    for parathyroid venous sampling, **118**
cavernous sinus, **8**, 30
C cell carcinoma, 83
cervical carcinoma, 289
cervical ganglia, vs. ectopic parathyroid gland, 109, **110**
cervix, estrogen and progesterone effects, 285
chest imaging, ECG-gated, with thyroid disease, 58
choriocarcinoma, 309
chromaffin cells, adrenal gland, 131
classification
    ovarian carcinomas (FIGO), 288
    pituitary adenomas, 12, 23
    testicular tumors, histologic, 260
    thyroid gland inflammations, 47
    thyroid tumors, 50
    thyroid tumors (TNM), 50
    thyroid tumors (WHO), 50
clear cell tumors, ovary, 300, **304**
clitoromegaly, **293**
Coca-Cola sign, 78
cold nodules, thyroid, scintigraphic appearance, 47, **53**, **71**, 71–2, 73
collimator, gamma camera, 4
colorectal carcinoid, 211
common epithelial tumors, ovary, 300
computed tomography, *see* CT
congenital adrenal hyperplasia (CAH), 133
congenital cystic dysplasia, testis, 263–4
Conn syndrome, 149–50, 179
contrast media
    and adrenal steroid release, **322**
    CT, 1
    DSA, parathyroid glands, 121
    MRI, 2
        parathyroid glands, 111
    for pancreatic angiography, 197
corpus luteum cyst, 297
craniopharyngioma, **34**
    pituitary gland, radiologist's view, 41
    vs. pituitary adenoma, 33
cryptorchidism, 251
CT (computed tomography)
    adrenal gland, 142–6
    carcinoid syndrome, 214–21
    and Graves ophthalmopathy, 77, **78**
    and multiple endocrine neoplasia, 240–4
    pancreas, 182–9
        normal findings, 183–4
        pathology, 184–8
        radiologist's view, 206
        technique, 182–3
    parathyroid gland, 98–103
        shoulder-streak artifacts, **99**, 100
        technique, 99–100
    pituitary gland, 18–27
    quantitative, 328, 329, 331–6
    sensitivity for hyperparathyroid diagnosis, 112
    technique, 1
    thyroid gland, 55–6
Cushing syndrome, 14–15, 132, 148, **162**, 179, 287
    adenoma, **143**, 149
    adrenal gland scintigraphy, 170
    typical clinical findings, 14
cyst
    adrenal gland, 144, 147, 178
    epidermoid, testis, **275**
    intrasellar, vs. pituitary adenoma, 33
    ovary, nonneoplastic, 297–8
    parathyroid gland, 89, **90**
    testicular, 263–4, **264**
    thyroid, MRI, 63
    thyroid gland, **53**
cystadenoma
    mucinous, adnexal, **312**
    serous, ovary, **300**
cystic degeneration, 63
    thyroid adenoma, **64**

D

dehydroepiandrosterone sulfate (DHEA-S), 318–21
densitometry, bone
   clinical use, 339–40
   comparison of techniques, 324
[11]C-L-deprenyl, 347, **348**
DHEA-S (dehydroepiandrosterone sulfate), 318–21
diabetes insipidus, 16
diazoxide (DZX), 191
dicarboxypropandiphosphonate (DPD), 75
differential diagnosis
   carcinoid syndrome, 225–7
   Graves ophthalmopathy, 78–81
   pituitary adenomas vs. other sellar diseases, 31–5
digital subtraction angiography, *see* DSA
5-α-dihydrotestosterone, 247
dimercaptosuccinic acid (DMSA), 75
DMSA (dimercaptosuccinic acid), 75
Doppler sonography, 280
DPA, *see* dual photon absorptiometry
DPD (dicarboxypropandiphosphonate), 75
DSA (digital subtraction angiography), 97
   pancreas, 197
   parathyroid glands, 121–2
   subclavian arteries, **120**
   technique, 3–4
dual photon absorptiometry (DPA), 326, **326**, 329
dual X-ray absorptiometry (DXA), 326–31, **328**, **329**
duplex sonography, and Graves disease, 51
DXA, *see* dual X-ray absorptiometry
dysgenesis, gonadal, 293–5
dysgerminoma, 306, **310**
DZX (diazoxide), 191

E

ECG gating
   ectopic parathyroid gland, **110**
   substernal goiter, 60
   thyroid disease chest imaging, 58
ectopic thyroid, 74
embolization, 96
   materials, 229, 233
   technique, 231
embryology, adrenal gland, 130
embryonal carcinoma, 309
embryonal cell carcinoma, **274**
empty sella, **34**
   vs. pituitary adenoma, 33
endocrine orbitopathy, 48
endocrinology
   carcinoid syndrome, 211–13
   hyperandrogenism, 315
   multiple endocrine neoplasia, 235–40
   ovary, 283–9
   pancreas, 180–2
   parathyroid gland, 85–6
   pituitary gland, 9–16
   testis, 247–53
   thyroid gland, 46–50
endodermal sinus tumor, 309, **309**
endometrial carcinoma, 289
endometrioid carcinoma, ovarian, 300, **302**
endometrioma
   adnexal, **308**
   ovarian, **296**
endometriosis, 288–9, **295**, 295–6
endosonography, 210
   see also sonography; ultrasound
endocrinology, adrenal gland, 131–5
epididymis
   abscess, **259**
   aplasia, 257
   tumors, 253, 261
epididymitis
   acute, **271**
   chronic, **259**
epididymo-orchitis, 259, 270
epinephrine, 130
epiorchium, 246
epithelial tumors, ovary, MRI, 300–2
esophagus, **57**
estradiol, and ovarian cycle, 284
estrogen
   biosynthesis, ovary, **284**
   metabolic effects, 286
   sex-specific effects, 285
estrone, and ovarian cycle, 284
etiocholanolone, 247
examination technique
   hyperandrogenism, 319
   testis, 254–5
   thyroid gland, 46
exophthalmos, Graves disease, **79**, **80**
exsiccosis, 86
eye, anatomy, and Graves ophthalmopathy, **77**
eye muscles, 79

F

fallopian tubes, estrogen and progesterone effects, 285
family screening, thyroid carcinoma, 83
[18]FDG (18-fluorodeoxyglucose), 344
femoral neck, absorptiometry, **330**
fertility disorders, 250–2
fetal tumor, adrenal gland, **140**
fibroma, ovary, 310–11, **312**
FIGO classification, ovarian carcinoma, 288, 299
finite element analysis, osteoporosis, 336, **337**
fistula, carotid–cavernous sinus, **79**, **80**
18-fluorodeoxyglucose ([18]FDG), 344
follicle-stimulating hormone (FSH), 286
follicular adenoma, hyperfunctioning, **62–3**
follicular cyst, 297, **297**
FSH (follicle-stimulating hormone), 286
functioning nodules, scintigraphy, thyroid, 72

G

galactorrhea-amenorrhea syndrome, 287
gamma camera, **4**, 4, 170
gastric blush, insulinoma, **195**
gastric carcinoid, 211
gastrinoma, 181, 184, 185
   anatomic triangle, **187**
   CT pattern, 187
   diagnostic accuracy, 188, 201
   localization, 202–5
   pancreatic head, **197**
   peripancreatic nodules, **200**
   radiologist's view, 207–8
gastroenteropancreatic system, 209
GDA, *see* artery, gastroduodenal
Gd-DTPA
   adenoma vs. nonadenoma, 152
   distinguishing benign and malignant thyroid tumor, 65
   dosage, 58
   and ovarian malignancy, 290

Index

and parathyroid glands, 111
   regions not enhancing with goiter, 60
Gd-DTPA enhancement, parathyroid adenoma, **107**, 108
germ cell tumors, 302–3
   MRI, 309–10
glandular cystic endometrial hyperplasia, 288
glioma, optic nerve, vs. pituitary adenoma, 35
GnRH (gonadotropin-releasing hormone), 248, 286
goiter, 46–7
   benign nodular, **54**
     ultrasound findings, 51–2
   diffuse, **71**
     ultrasound findings, 51
   indications for preoperative imaging, 82
   MRI findings, 59–60
   multinodular, **58–9**, **71**, **72**, 81
   retrosternal, **56**
   scintigraphy, 70
gonadal dysgenesis, 293–5
gonadoblastoma, 309
gonadotropin-secreting adenoma, 16
gonadotropin-releasing hormone (GnRH), 248, 286
granulosa–theca cell tumor, 310
Graves disease, 48, **60–1**, 60–1, 73, **73**, **74**, 81, 82
   inferno effect, sonographic appearance, 88
   ophthalmopathy, diagnostic imaging, 76–81
   ultrasound findings, **52**
     51
   vs. other hyperthyroidism, MRI limitations, 61
Graves ophthalmopathy
   differential diagnosis, 78–81
   MR appearance, **79**
gynandroblastoma, 312

H

HAE (hepatic artery embolization), 228–9, 233
hairless woman syndrome, 252
halo appearance, thyroid gland sonography, 52, **53**
haloperidol, **348**
Hashimoto disease, 47, 49, 90
   ultrasound findings, 51
HCG, *see* human chorionic gonadotropin
Helmholtz coil, 57
hematocele, chronic testicular, **277**
hematoma, adrenal gland, 147–8
hemorrhage, adrenal gland, 177
hemosiderin rim, MRI, and cystic degeneration, 63
Henoch–Schönlein purpura, 258, 262
hepatic artery embolization (HAE), 228–9, 233
hepatic capsular metastases, ovarian adenocarcinoma, **306**
hermaphroditism, true, 292, **292**
hernia
   meconium, 277–8, **278**
   scrotum, 277, **277**
5-HIAA (5-hydroxyindoleacetic acid), 212, **219**
hip, absorptiometry, **330**
Hippel–Lindau syndrome, 261
hirsutism, 134
   idiopathic, 287
histopathology, thyroid gland, 50
hormones
   hypothalamic hypophysiotropic, 10
   menstrual cycle, **285**
   pituitary, major physiological actions, 10
   sex, biosynthesis, **249**
hot nodules, 82
hot spots, adrenal gland scintigraphy, 175, 177
Hounsfield unit, 1

HPT, *see* hyperparathyroidism
human chorionic gonadotropin (HCG), 271, **285**, 309
hydrocele, testis, **262**, 262–3
hydrocortisone, peripheral, during catheterization, 319, **320**
hydrothorax, 310
5-hydroxyindoleacetic acid (5-HIAA), 212
   and inteferon treatment, **219–21**
5-hydroxytryptophan, 213
hyperaldosteronism, 131–2, 149–50
   symptomatology, 131
hyperandrogenemia, 134, **322**
hyperandrogenism, 314–23
   anatomy, 314–15
   endocrinology, 315
   nontumorous, 320–1
hypercalcemia, 86, 98
hypercalcemic crisis, 86
hypercorticism, 161–2
hypercortisolism, 132
hyperparathyroidism (HPT), 85–6, 105–12, 235
   comparison of diagnostic techniques, 112
   effect of surgical treatment, **113**
   familial, 91
   persistent, 102–3, **103**, 125
   recurrent, 102–3, 125, 128
   reoperation, 128
   risk factors, 92
   scintigraphic findings, 124–5
   secondary, 91
   treatment, 95–6, 122
hyperplasia, adrenal gland, 136, **137**
hyperprolactinemia, 287
   effects, 13
   and PET imaging, 346–7
hyperthecosis
   ovarian, 298, **299**, 321
   ovary, 287
hyperthyroid, indications for preoperative imaging, 82
hyperthyroidism, 47–9, 81–2
   clinical symptoms, 48
   Graves type, 48
   iatrogenic, 73
   iodine-131 uptake, 70
   prevalence, 98
   primary, 103
   treatment, 99
hypertrichosis, 134
hypoadrenocorticism, 132–3
   symptoms, 132
hypoaldosteronism, 132
hypocalcemia, 86
hypocorticoidism, 132–3
   symptoms, 132
hypogonadism, 250–1
hypoparathyroidism, 85
   with hypercalcemia, symptoms, 86
   with hypocalcemia, symptoms, 86
hypophyseal adenoma, **38**
   chromophobic, **37**
hypophysis, **8**
hypopituarism, causes, 11
hypothalamic–pituitary axis, blood vessels, **8**
hypothalamo-pituitary regulatory system, **9**
hypothyroidism, 49–50
   causes, 49
   clinical symptoms, 49
   iodine-131 uptake, 70

I

IAS, see intra-arterial stimulation test
idiopathic testicular infarction, 259–60
imaging
    parathyroid gland, 96–7
        sensitivity, 97
        three-dimensional
            sella turcica, 26, **27**
            with thyroid mass, 60
Imperato–McGinley syndrome, 252
incidentaloma, 154
    adrenal gland, 142
infarction, testicular, 259
inferno effect, sonographic appearance, Graves disease, 87
infertility, endocrine syndromes, 251–2
infundibulum, pituitary gland, 28
inguinal testis, **256**
insulinoma, 181, **183**, 184, **186**
    diagnostic accuracy, 188, 201
    gastric blush, **195**
    localization, 202–5
    multiple, **204**
    pancreatic distribution, **185**
    pancreatic head, **193**, **198**
        cystic, **200**
    pancreatic isthmus, **193**
    pancreatic tail, **192**, **196**, **198**, **199**
    radiologist's view, 207
    vs. splenic artery loop, **185**
inteferon treatment, 219–21
interventional radiology, carcinoid syndrome, 227–31
    contraindications, 229
intra-arterial stimulation (IAS) test, 202–5, **203**, **204**
iodine-123, 5
iodine-131, 69
    thyroid uptake, 70
iodine-131, see also MIBG
islet cell tumor, 181
    arteriographic localization, 194, 195
    characteristics, 182
    factors affecting arteriography, 201
    MRI appearance, 192
    step-by-step imaging tests, **208**

K

Kallmann syndrome, 251–2
    in women, 288
Klinefelter syndrome, 251, 263

L

lamina parietalis, 246
lamina visceralis, 246
Langerhans islet, **181**
larynx, carcinoid tumor, 211
Laurence–Moon–Biedl syndrome, 252
Leydig's cells, testis, 247
Leydig's cell tumor, **261**, 280, 311, 321
    testis, 279
LH (luteinizing hormone), 286
LHRH (luteinizing hormone–releasing hormone), 248
liver, carcinoid metastases, 216, **217**, **218**, **219**, 225–7
localization
    arteriographic, islet cell tumor, 194, 195
    gastrinoma, 202–5
    insulinoma, 202–5
    pancreatic tumor, 188–9

    intraoperative ultrasound, 209
    preoperative
        abnormal parathyroid, 106, 128
        adrenal gland tumors, 178–9
        pancreatic tumors, 210
        parathyroid adenoma, 99, 111–12, 126, 127
luteinizing hormone (LH), 286
luteinizing hormone–releasing hormone (LHRH), 248
lymph nodes
    cervical, inflammatory changes, 68
    retroperitoneal, carcinoid syndrome, **217**
lymphoma
    adrenal gland, **155**
    orbital, 79, **80**
    thyroid, **67**
        MR appearance, 65

M

macroadenoma, pituitary gland, **31**, **32**
macro-orchia, 256–7, **257**
macroprolactinoma, **14**
magnetic resonance imaging, see MRI
male genitalia, **246–7**
malignancy, adrenal gland, 138–9
Meckel's diverticula, carcinoid, 211
meconium hernia, 277–8, **278**
mediastinum testis, 246
medullary carcinoma, 66, 75
    thyroid gland, 75, 83, 238
Meigs syndrome, 310
MEN, see multiple endocrine neoplasia
meningioma
    pituitary gland, **39**
        radiologist's view, 41
    suprasellar, vs. pituitary adenoma, 347–8
    vs. pituitary adenoma, 35
menstrual cycle, hormonal situation, **285**
Merseburg triad, 48
mesentery
    carcinoid metastases, 214–16, **226**
    mass, **215**, **216**, **217**
mesothelioma, juxtatesticular, 272
metaiodobenzylguanidine, see MIBG
metastasis, adrenal gland, 178
^{11}C-L-methionine, 344, 345, **348**
methylglucamine diatrizoate, 100
MIBG (metaiodobenzylguanidine) scanning, 164, **165**, 169, 179, 232–3
    carcinoid syndrome, **231**
microadenoma, pituitary gland, **31**
microlithiasis, testicular, 264
monorchism, congenital, 251
moon face, **15**
MRI (magnetic resonance imaging)
    adrenal gland, 146–58
        techniques, 146–7
    applied sequences, pituitary gland, 28
    contrast media, parathyroid glands, 111
    epithelial tumors, ovary, 300–2
    and Graves ophthalmopathy, 77
    hyperparathyroid diagnosis, 112
    osteoporosis, **338**, 338–9
    ovary, 289–312
        indications, 289
        techniques, 290–1
    pancreas, 190–4
        method, 190–1
        normal findings, 191
        pathology, 191–4

radiologist's view, 206
parathyroid gland, 104–12
  pitfalls, 109–10
  technique, 104
pituitary gland, 27–35
  technique, 27–8
sex cord–stromal tumors, 312
spectroscopy, 156
technique, 1–2
testis, 267–78
  indications, 267
  technique, 267–8
thyroid gland, 57–68
  technique, 57–8
mucinous tumors, ovary, 300
multiple endocrine neoplasia (MEN), 83, 91–2, 181, 235–45
  endocrinology, 235–40
  imaging, 240–4
  with pheochromocytoma, **175**
  type I, 235–8
    biochemical diagnosis, 238
    biochemical screening program, 236
    prognosis, 238
  type II, 238–40
    biochemical screening program, 239
mumps, and orchitis, 258
muscle, MRI, 66
myelolipoma, adrenal gland, 144, 147, 178
myoma, uterine, 288–9

N

nerve, recurrent laryngeal, **105**, 122
neuroblastoma, 152–3, **153**
  adrenal gland, 143–4, **176**
neurohypophysis, 28
Noonan syndrome, 252
Norland Cameron device, single photon absorptiometry, **325**
normozoospermia, 250
nuclear imaging, techniques, 4–5
nuclear medicine
  adrenal gland, 169–76
  carcinoid syndrome, 232–3
  parathyroid gland, 123–5
    imaging technique, 123
  thyroid gland, 69–76

O

octreotide, 175, 243
oligozoospermia, 250
omental cake, **305**
ophthalmopathy, Graves disease
  diagnostic imaging, 76–81
  differential diagnosis, 76–81
  MR appearance, **79**
optic nerve glioma, vs. pituitary adenoma, 35
orbitomeatal line, **18**
orbitopathy, endocrine, 48
orchiectomy, 279, 280
orchitis, 260, **271**
  acute, **258**
  primary, 258–9
  secondary, 259
osteoporosis
  finite element analysis, 336, **337**
  MRI, **338**, 338–9
  quantification, 324–43
  regions of interest (ROIs), 333, **334**, **335**

ultrasound, 336–8, **338**
ovary, **282**, 282–323
  adenocarcinoma, peritoneal and hepatic metastases, **306**
  agenesis and dysgenesis, 283
  anatomy, 282–3
  androgen-secreting neoplasm, 321
  blood supply, **283**
  carcinoma, 288, 298–312
    bladder implant, **303**
    FIGO staging, 299
    peritoneal implant, **305**
  endocrinology, 283–9
  endometrioma, **296**
  fibroma, 310–11, **312**
  granulosa cell tumor, **311**
  hyperthecosis, 287, 298, **299**, 321
  MRI, 289–312
  nonneoplastic cysts, 297–8
  normal MRI appearance, **290**, 290–2, **291**
  pathology, MRI, 292–312
  physiology, 283
  polycystic ovarian disease, 298, **298**, **307**
  primary carcinoid tumor, 304
  serous cystadenoma, **300**
  stromal hyperplasia, 298
  teratoma, 303–5

P

pampiniform plexus, 246
pancreas, 180–210
  anatomy, 180
    MRI, **191**
  angiography, 194–205
  CT, 182–9
  development, **180**
  and duodenum, **181**
  endocrinology, 180–2
  lesion, in multiple endocrine neoplasia, 235–6
  lobule, **181**
  MRI, 190–4
  in multiple endocrine neoplasia type I, **237**
  multiple tumors, imaging, **241–4**
  pathology, CT, 184–8
  radiologist's view, 206–8
  surgeon's view, 209–10
  tumor, 187
    localization, 188–9
    tumor marker sensitivity, 238
pancreatic polypeptide (PP), 236
papillary carcinoma
  metastatic, thyroid, **75**
  thyroid gland, 54, **54**
parathyroid adenoma, **57**, **64**, **88**, **89**, **91**, **93**, **94**, **96**, **101**, 101–2, **103**, **107**, **108**, 124, **124**
  CT contrast enhancement, **100**, **102**
  ectopic, **102**, 125–6
  Gd-DTPA enhancement, **107**
  and PET imaging, 349
  preoperative localization, 99, 111–12, 126, 127
  shoulder-streak artifacts, **99**
  transcatheter ablation, 122
  vs. thyroid nodule, **110**
parathyroid gland, 85–128, **105**
  abnormal, **106**
    preoperative MRI localization, 106
  anatomy, 85
    CT, 100
    MRI, 104–5
    variations, **85**

parathyroid glands, angiography, 113–22
  arteries, 120–1
  autotransplanted tissue, 117
  biopsy, 92
  cancer, 94–5
  carcinoma, **95**, 103
  CT, 98–103
  cysts, 89, **90**
  disease, in MEN type II, 239
  disorders, MRI characteristics, 106–7
  DSA, 121–2
  ectopic, **109**, 109, **110**, **114**, 121
    vs. cervical ganglia, 109, **110**
  endocrinology, 85–6
  hyperplastic, **92**, 94, **95**, **101**
  lesion, in multiple endocrine neoplasia, 235
  MRI, 104–12
  nuclear medicine, 123–5
  pathology, 100–3
  physiology, 85
  radiologist's view, 125–6
  and radiopharmaceuticals, 5
  surgeon's view, 127–8
  surgical procedures and preoperative localization, 128
  ultrasound, 86–97
  variants, 93
  venous sampling, 113–22
    technique, 117–18
parathyroid hormone (PTH), 85, 105–6, 118
parathyroid hyperplasia, 100–1
pathology
  adrenal gland
    CT, 142–6
    ultrasound, 135–6
  adrenal medulla, scintigraphic findings, 174
  pancreas
    angiography, 195–201
    CT, 184–8
    MRI, 191–4
  parathyroid gland, 100–3
  pituitary gland, computed tomography, 22–6
  testis, MRI, 269–78
pathophysiology, Graves ophthalmopathy, 76–7
PCO, *see* polycystic ovary syndrome
PCOD, *see* polycystic ovarian disease
penis tumors, 253
perchlorate discharge test, scintigraphy, 70
percutaneous transhepatic portography (PTP), 241
  see also portal venous sampling
perineuritis, orbit, 79
periorchium, 246
periscleritis, 79
peritoneum, ovarian adenocarcinoma metastases, **306**
PET, *see* positron emission tomography
pharmacokinetics, and PET imaging, 348
phenoxybenzamine hydrochloride, 166
phentolamine, 166
pheochromocytoma, 83, 151–2, **152**, **176**
  adrenal gland, **138**, **139**, 143, 164–8, **165**, **166**, **167**, 178
  adrenal medulla, 134–5
  extra-adrenal, scintigraphy, **174**
  in multiple endocrine neoplasia type II, 239
Philadelphia collar, 57
photomultipliers, 4
physiology
  adrenal gland, 131
  ovary, 283
  pituitary gland, 9–10
  testis, 247–8
  thyroid gland, 46
pitfalls, parathyroid gland
  MRI, 109–10
  sonography, 89–90
pituitary adenoma, 11–16, **21**, **22**, 30–3
  and adrenal enlargement, **145**
  calcified, **26**
  classification, 12
  CT classification, 23
  cystic, **23**, **24**, **25**
  PET imaging, **346**, 346–7
  radiologist's view, 40–1
  vs. suprasellar meningioma, PET imaging, 347–8
pituitary gland, 7–42, **18**
  anatomy, 7–9
    MRI, 28–30, **29**
  aneurysm, radiologist's view, 41
  angiography, 35–40
  craniopharyngioma, radiologist's view, 41
  CT, 18–27
    normal findings, 20–2
  endocrinology, 9–16
  lesion, in multiple endocrine neoplasia, 236
  meningioma, **39**
    radiologist's view, 41
  MRI, 27–35
  pathology, computed tomography, 22–6
  and PET imaging, 344
  physiology, 9–10
  posterior, diseases, 16
  radiography, 16–18
  radiologist's view, 40–1
  rare disturbances, 35
  surgeon's view, 41–2
pituitary hormones, major physiological actions, 10
plexus thyroideus impar, 45
Plummer disease, 82
polycystic ovarian disease (PCOD), 298, **298**, **307**
polycystic ovary syndrome (PCO), 286–7, **287**
  and hyperandrogenism, 318, 320
polyorchia, 256
portal venous sampling (PVS), 202, 205
  transhepatic percutaneous
    radiologist's view, 206–7
    surgeon's view, 209
  see also percutaneous transhepatic portography
positron emission tomography (PET), 344–50, **345**
  metabolic mapping, 344–5
  and pharmacokinetics, 348
  receptor studies, 345–6
  slice thickness, 344–50
  and treatment evaluation, 346
potassium perchlorate, and scintigraphy, 69
PP (pancreatic polypeptide), 236
Prader–Labhart–Willi syndrome, 252
Prader syndrome, **137**
preoperative localization
  abnormal parathyroid, and surgical procedures, 128
  pancreatic tumors, 210
  parathyroid adenoma, 127
    prospective accuracy, 126
  parathyroid gland
    abnormal, 106
    adenoma, 99, 111–12
primary hypothyroidism, 49
progesterone
  biosynthesis, ovary, **284**
  metabolic effects, 286
  and ovarian cycle, 284
  sex-specific effects, 285
prolactinoma, 13–14, **14**, **21**, **22**, **23**, **24**, **25**
  PET imaging, **345**, **346**, **348**
propanolol hydrochloride, 166

proptosis, Graves ophthalmopathy, 78
prostatic carcinoma, 252–3
prosthesis, testicular, 274, **275**
pseudohermaphroditism, 293
    and dysgerminoma occurrence, 306
    female, **293**
pseudohypoparathyroidism, 85
pseudomyxoma peritonei, **301**
PTH, *see* parathyroid hormone
PTP, *see* percutaneous transhepatic portography
pubertal disorders, 248
pubertas praecox, 248
pubertas tarda, 248
PVS, *see* portal venous sampling
pyocele, testis, 277
pyramidal lobe, **43**, 44

Q

quantitative computed tomography (QCT), 328, 329, 331–6
quantitative image evaluation technique (QUIET), **334**

R

radio frequency (RF) pulses, 1
radiography
    interventional, 96
    parathyroid venous sampling, 118–19
    pituitary gland, 16–18
radioisotopes, 5
radiologist, and pancreatic tumor research, 189
radiologist's view
    adrenal gland, 177–8
    carcinoid syndrome, 233
    pancreas, 206–8
    parathyroid gland, 125–6
    pituitary gland, 40–1
radiology, interventional
    carcinoid syndrome, 227–31
    contraindications, 229
radiopharmaceuticals, 5
    thyroid, 69
Recklinghausen disease, 211
recurrent nerve, and thyroid gland, 46
5-α-reductase deficiency, 252
regions of interest (ROIs), in osteoporosis, 333, **334**, **335**
Reifenstein syndrome, 252
RF (radio frequency) pulses, 1
Riedel disease, 47
road-mapping, parathyroid venous sampling, 118–19
ROI (region of interest), in osteoporosis, 333, **334**, **335**
Rokitansky–Küster–Hauser syndrome, 286, 288
Rokitansky nodules, 305

S

scar tissue, MRI, 66, **67**
Schwartz–Bartter syndrome, 16
scintigraphy
    adrenal cortex, principles, 169
    adrenal gland, 169–76
        dosimetry, 169
        principles, 173–7
        technique, 169–70
    adrenal medulla
        principles, 171–5
        technique, 172
    cold nodules
        goiter, 47
        thyroid, **53**, **71**, 71–2, 73
    dual tracer, 97
    normal thyroid, 70
    parathyroid gland, 123–5
    perchlorate discharge test, 70
    and small pancreatic tumors, 243
    static, 5
    suppression test, 70
    thyroid, 69, 82
    whole body, 5
        thyroid carcinoma, 74–5
scrotal disease, acute, 257–60
scrotum, 255–6, 280
    arteriovenous malformation, **276**
    benign masses, 276–8
    fluid collections, 276–8
    hernia, 277, **277**
secondary hypothyroidism, 49
selenium-75, 5
sellar diaphragm, 29–30
sella turcica, 27
    anatomy
        CT, **19**, **20**
        MRI, 28–30
    computed tomography, 19–27
    measurement, **17**
    pathological findings, 17–18
    radiography, **17**, 17–18
    three-dimensional imaging, 26, **27**
    see also empty sella
semen, normal values, 250
seminal vesicle tumors, 253
seminoma, **261**, **273**, **274**
serotonin
    biosynthesis and degradation, **213**
    metabolic pathway in carcinoid syndrome, **213**
serous tumors, ovary, 300
Sertoli cell only syndrome, 250
Sertoli–Leydig cell tumor, 288, 311, 321
Sestimibi scanning, 128
sex cord–stromal tumor, 310
    MRI, 312
sex hormones, biosynthesis, **249**
sexual differentiation, disorders, 292–5
shoulder-streak artifacts, parathyroid gland CT, **99**, 100
SIADH (syndrome of inappropriate ADH secretion), 16
single photon absorptiometry (SPA), **325**, 325–6
SMA, *see* artery, superior mesenteric
small bowel
    and mesenteric masses, **215**, **216**
    multifocal carcinoid, **231**
solenoid coil, 57
solid state phantom, **331**
somatostatin, 175, 191
somatostatinoma, 181
somatostatin receptor scintigraphy, 209
sonography
    color-coded, 51, **88**
        and autonomous adenoma, 53
    see also endosonography; ultrasound
Soranus of Ephesus, 286
SPA, *see* single photon absorptiometry
spermatic cord
    torsion, 270–1
    tumor, 261
spermatocele, **257**, 277
spermatocytes, 246
spermatogenesis, **247**
    disturbed, 250
SPGR, *see* spoiled gradient recalled imaging

spine
    absorptiometry, **330**
    quantitative computed tomography (QCT), 331–6, **332**
spin-echo imaging, MRI, 2
spoiled gradient recalled imaging (SPGR), 156
steroid biosynthesis, adrenal gland, **133**
strap muscle, **89**, **92**, **95**, **96**
struma ovarii, 74, **307**
suppression test, scintigraphy, 70
suprasellar cistern, 30
surgeon's view
    adrenal gland, 178–9
    parathyroid gland, 127–8
    pituitary gland, 41–2
    testis, 279–80
    thyroid gland, 81–3
surgery
    parathyroid gland, 128
    and primary hyperthyroidism, 95–6
Swyer syndrome, 287
syndrome of inappropriate ADH secretion (SIADH), 16

T

tachykinin, 221
TBG (thyroxine-binding globulin), 46
technetium-99m, 5
technetium-99m-pertechnetate, 69, 123
technetium–thallium subtraction, **124**
techniques, of endocrine imaging, 1–6
teratoma, 211
    cystic
        adnexal, **308**
        ovary, **307**
    immature, **308**
    ovary, 303–5
teratozoospermia, 250
test
    intra-arterial stimulation (IAS), 202–5
    laboratory, hyperandrogenism, 319
    perchlorate discharge, scintigraphy, 70
    step-by-step imaging, islet cell tumors, **208**
    suppression, scintigraphy, 70
testicular capsule tumors, 253
testicular feminization, 252
testicular infarction, 259
testicular tumors, diagnosis, 262
testis, 246–81
    anatomy, 246–7
        MRI, 268–9
    arrested descent, 255–6
    arteriovenous malformation, 275–6
    atrophy, 263
    blood circulation, **247**
    calcification, 264, **265**
    congenital abnormalities, 269
    congenital anomalies, 255–6
    congenital cystic dysplasia, 263–4
    cyst, 263–4, **264**
    endocrinology, 247–53
    epidermoid cyst, **275**
    examination technique, 254–5
    hematocele, **277**
    hydrocele, 262–3
    idiopathic infarction, 259–60
    infarct, **275**
    inflammatory processes, 269–70
    inguinal, **256**
    leukemic infiltration, **261**
    maldescended, 256, 260
    microlithiasis, 264
    MRI, 267–78
    neoplasm, 271–4
    normal, **255**
    pathology, MRI, 269–78
    physiology, 247–8
    prosthesis, 274, **275**
    pyocele, 277
    spermatocele, 277
    surgeon's view, 279–80
    torsion, **272**, 280
    tumor, 252, 260–2, 271–4, 279–80
        histologic classification, 260
    tunica albuginea, fibrosis and calcification, 264
    ultrasound, 253–65
    undescended, **270**
    varicocele, 263, **263**, 277
testosterone, 248
TG (thyroglobulin), 46, 50
thallium-201, 5, 123
thallium scintigraphy, 74
theca–lutein cysts, 297–8
thecoma, 310
three-dimensional imaging
    sella turcica, 26, **27**
    with thyroid mass, 60
thymic carcinoid, 211
thyroglobulin (TG), 46, 50
thyroid autonomy, 48
thyroid bed, inflammatory changes, **68**
thyroidectomy, 50, 83, 85
thyroid gland, **43**, 43–84, **105**, **124**
    adenoma, cystic degeneration, **64**
    anatomy, 43–6
        MRI, 58–9
    anterior view, **44**
    blood supply, 45
    carcinoma, 63–8, **65–6**, 82–3
        whole body scintigraphy, 74–5
    CT, 55–6
    cyst, **53**
    diseases, 46–50
    echo-free nodules, 53
    ectopic, 74
    endocrinology, 46–50
    examination methods, 46
    halo appearance, 52, **53**
    histology, 44
    histopathology, 50
    hyperechoic nodules, 52, **53**
    hypoechoic nodules, 53
    imaging, and radiopharmaceuticals, 5
    indications for preoperative imaging, 82
    inflammation, 47
        classification, 47
    isoechoic nodules, 52
    isthmus, 44
    lymphoma, **67**
        MR appearance, 65
    medullary carcinoma, 75, 83
        in MEN type II, 83, 238
    mixed echoic nodules, 53
    MRI, 57–68
    nodule, vs. parathyroid adenoma, **110**
    normal location, **114**
    nuclear medicine, 69–76
    pathological changes, MRI, 55–6
    pathological findings, 59–68
    physiology, 46
    posterior view, **45**
    radiopharmaceutical uptake, 69–70

nodular vs. single lobe, 72
and recurrent nerve, 46
relationships, **44**
scintigraphy, 69
  normal scan, 70
sonogram, **51**
surgeon's view, 81–3
tumor, 49–50
  MR appearance, 65
  TNM classification, 50
  WHO classification, 50
ultrasound, 50–4, **52**
  normal findings, 51
  pathological findings, 51–4
veins, **115**
vs. muscle, MRI, **61**
thyroiditis, 47, 61, 73, **74**
  autoimmune, ultrasound findings, 51
thyroid lobe, and ectopic parathyroid gland, 109
thyroid-stimulating hormone (TSH), 46, 47
thyroid storm, 48–9
thyrotropin-producing adenoma, 15–16
thyrotropin-releasing hormone (TRH), 46, 47, 286
thyroxine, and scintigraphy, 69
thyroxine-binding globulin (TBG), 46
TNM classification, thyroid tumors, 50
torsion
  spermatic cord, 270–1
  testicular, **272**, 280
trachea, 57
  and thyroid carcinoma, **56**
TRH (thyrotropin-releasing hormone), 46, 47, 286
tricuspid insufficiency, **230**
tryptophan, 212
TSH (thyroid-stimulating hormone), 46, 47
T1 (spin-lattice relaxation), MRI, 2
T2 (spin-spin relaxation), MRI, 2
tubuli seminiferi, 246
tumor markers, sensitivity, 238
tumors
  adrenal gland, 144–5
    hyperfunctioning, 148–56
  adrenocortical, 134
  androgen-secreting ovarian neoplasm, 321
  carcinoid, 211–13, 221–2
  clear cell, ovary, **304**
  common epithelial, ovary, 300
  endodermal sinus, 309, **309**
  endometrioid, ovarian, 300, **302**
  epididymis, 261
  germ cell, 302–3
    MRI, 309–10
  granulosa cell, ovarian, **311**
  granulosa–theca cell, 310
  intrasellar, **38**
  mucinous, ovary, 300
  ovary, 298–312
    classification, 288
  prolactinoma, PET imaging, **345**, **346**
  serous, ovary, 300
  Sertoli–Leydig cell, 311
  sex cord–stromal, 310
    MRI, 312
  spermatic cord, 261
  surface epithelium, ovary, 300
  testicular, 252, 260–2, 271–4, 279–80
    diagnosis, 262
    histologic classification, 260
  thyroid, malignant, 49–50
tunica albuginea, 246
  cysts, 263

testis, fibrosis and calcification, 264, **264**
Turner syndrome, **294**, 294

U

Ullrich–Turner syndrome, 248, 252, 287
ultrasound
  adrenal gland, 135–41
    normal findings, 135
    pathology, 135–6
    technique, 135
  Doppler sonography, 280
  intraoperative
    pancreatic tumor localization, 209
    parathyroid gland, 95–6
  osteoporosis, 336–8, **338**
  pancreas, intraoperative, 207
  parathyroid gland, 86–97
    clinical setting, 90–1
    normal findings, 87
    pathologic findings, 87–96
    pitfalls, 89–90
    technique, 86–7
  sensitivity for hyperparathyroid diagnosis, 112
  testis, 253–65
    indications, 253–4
    mandatory cases, 280
  thyroid gland, 50–4
  see also endosonography; sonography
undescended testis, **270**
uterine myoma, 288–9
uterus, estrogen and progesterone effects, 285
uterus myomatosus, 288–9

V

vagina
  carcinoma, 289
  estrogen and progesterone effects, 285
varicocele, 251
  testis, 263, 277
vascular anatomy, 221
vascular rim, parathyroid sonogram, **88**
vasculitis, testicular, 275, **275**
vas deferens tumors, 253
vasoactive intestinal polypeptide (VIP), 236
vein
  adrenal, 130, **130**, **317**, **318**
    in women, 314, **314**
  anatomy distorted after thyroidectomy, **117**
  azygos, 114
  circumaortic ring, **316**
  hepatic, vs. adrenal, **318**
  inferior thyroid, **105**
  inferior thyroid trunk, **115**
  inferior vena cava, catheterization, 168
  internal jugular, **114**
  jugular, **57**, 118
    catheter, **119**
    compression on MRI, **68**
    and parathyroid sonography, 87
  lumbar, ascending, **315**
  mediastinal, **116**
  ovarian, 314, **314**, **315**, **316**
    vs. ascending lumbar vein, **315**
  parathyroid, 113–17, **114**
  phrenic, inferior, **317**
  portal, 202
  renal, **317**

vein, renal, and ovarian, **316**
  superior ophthalmic, and carotid–cavernous sinus fistula, **80**
  thoracic, **116**
  thyroid, 114, **114**
    catheterization, 128
  uterine plexus, **316**
  vertebral, 114
  see also blood; catheterization; vascular; venogram; venous
venogram
  adrenal, **162**
  adrenal gland, normal, **160**
  hepatic, **161**
venography, adrenal, 168
venous catheterization, 210
venous sampling
  adrenal gland, 160, 163
  adrenal vein, standardized protocol, 319
  ovarian vein, standardized protocol, 319
  parathyroid gland, 113–22
    results, 119–20
    road-mapping, 118–19
    technique, 117–18
results
  adrenal hyperplasia, 164
  aldosteronoma, 163
  thyroid, **114**
  transhepatic portal, 202
vertebra, quantitative computed tomography (QCT), **332**, **334**
vipoma, 181
virilization, 134
vulvar carcinoma, 289

W

warm nodules, 82
Wermer syndrome, 181
WHO classification, thyroid tumors, 50
Wilms tumor, vs. neuroblastoma, 152
window adjustment, CT, 1

Z

Zollinger–Ellison syndrome, 92, 189, 198, 201, **241**